FRCEM Final

Clinical Short Answer Question

Volume 1

Moussa Issa

Disclaimer

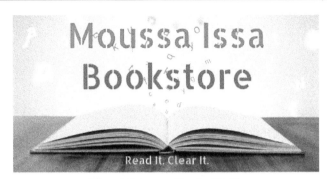

Your Ultimate Study Guide

First Edition 2019 by Moussa Issa Bookstore Limited.
Distributed by Moussa Issa Bookstore
Reprinted with Revisions 2020

ISBN-13: **978-1916029620**

8.5" x 11" (21.59 x 27.94 cm)
BISAC: Medical / Emergency Medicine
Authored by Moussa Issa
Published by: Moussa Issa Bookstore Ltd

TERMS OF USE

Copyright © 2020 Moussa Issa Bookstore Limited.
Distributed by Moussa Issa Bookstore Ltd
Website: www.moussaissabooks.com
Email: info@moussaissabooks.com
eBook subscription: www.moussaissabooks.com/ebook

Preface

FRCEM FINAL Clinical SAQ book, is designed to present concise, easy-to-read, practical information on the diagnosis and treatment of a wide spectrum of conditions that present to the emergency department.

The chapters emphasize the immediate management of life-threatening problems & then present the evaluation and treatment of specific disorders.
In keeping with the curriculum spanning ST 1- ST 6 I have strived to provide the reader with a broad-based text written in a clear and point form manner.

My goal was to not only provide practicing emergency physicians quick access to accurate and useful information that will aid in their everyday practice of emergency medicine but also mainly to help trainees throughout their 6 year training in Emergency Medicine.

Because this text focuses on the practical aspects of emergency care, there is little discussion of the basic science or pathophysiology of disease processes.
This is the only book of its kind available which covers the entire curriculum and helps prepare for the FINAL Clinical SAQ. The book will be useful to all practitioners of Emergency Medicine, including Physicians, Residents, Medical Students as well as Physician Extenders.

This edition of the FINAL Clinical SAQ contains the curriculum in totality. You need not go through any other material for the preparation of the Final SAQ Exam. I have in clear and concise format covered the most asked topics as well as the probable topics that could be questioned for the exams. In addition with helping one prepare for the exam, this book is valuable to learn from in all years of training. The guidelines followed are according to NICE & Royal College of Emergency Medicine.

Relevant pictures are added where needed to provide better understanding of the topic as well as cover probable images that could be questioned on.

I would like to thank my wife and children for the never ending support throughout this journey.

Dr Moussa Issa

Acknowledgments

To my wife and children: Marlene, Tatiana, Kevin, Ryan and Brandon. I thank you for your love and support. You've always been by my side and never complained watching me working on my books when you needed me the most.

To my co-Editors: Tina Cardoza, Muhammad Amjad, Faizan Alam and Nasir Mahmood. Thank you for taking the time to lay this out and providing me the inspiration to do this. **Muhammad Amjad** you are an amazing colleague, a kind brother and a great friend; thank you and I appreciate you more than you'll ever know.

To some other important people: Sayed Ramadan, Zain Ul Abadin, Russel Hall, Robyn Pretorius, Rana Tanweer, Moez Ibrahim, Mohanad Ibrahim, Yasser Mohamad, Awwad El Mahdi, Luke Joseph Chirayil, Donna Edano, Abubakar Bin Omer Badam, Pintu Syed, and all the others who took the time to help me find some needed corrections to my books that only made this workbook and latest printing even better. I would like to thank you for your interest in my work and I encourage you to continue to send me your invaluable feedback and ideas for further improvement of the FRCEM Exam book series. I am grateful to you.

To all my clients and Colleagues: Your continued patronage has helped me keep this book running. For this, I never mind the arthritis on my writing hand. We have ventured many roads together, some new and some well-travelled, but we have continued to sharpen each other with patience, perception and perseverance. The pain cannot overcome the happiness that I am feeling right now, thanks to you.

To you: The only thing that can stop you from showing the best results is you being so extremely nervous. There's no need to be scared, buddy. You are ready to show everyone that you are the smartest fella in the world! Good luck!

I feel blessed that social media have given me the chance to reconnect or stay connected with many colleagues all over the world. I am grateful to you all and wish you success throughout your exams. Remember, few years ago, I was also at the beginning like you, with little effort and perseverance, I managed to clear all FRCEM Exams.

An exam is not a game. It's a background for your future.
Wish you to pass all exams.

Dr Moussa Issa
MBChB MRCEM FRCEM

My sources:

Many guidelines presented in this book originated from:
- ⤮ Royal College of Emergency Medicine (www.rcem.ac.uk),
- ⤮ National Institute for Health and Care Excellence (www.nice.org.uk),
- ⤮ British Thoracic Society (www.brit-thoracic.org.uk),
- ⤮ Resuscitation Council UK (www.resus.org.uk),
- ⤮ American Heart Association (www.heart.org),
- ⤮ Advanced cardiovascular Life Support (ACLS),
- ⤮ Advanced Trauma Life Support (ATLS),
- ⤮ Advanced Paediatric Life Support (APLS),
- ⤮ Toxbase (www.toxbase.org),
- ⤮ Life in the fast lane (www.lifeinthefastlane.com)

I owe my dedicated work to the above organizations.

Disclaimer:
Information and images included in these notes originate from multiples sources such as academic journals, textbooks, published articles, Emergency Medicine websites and Blogs etc.
The Editor and the Publisher have gone to every effort to seek permission from and acknowledge the sources of clinical guidelines and images which appear in this compilation that is public on the internet. Nevertheless, should there be any cases where Copyright holders have not been identified or suitably acknowledged, the author welcome advice from such Copyright holders and will endeavor to amend the text accordingly on future prints.

Table of Contents

Ebook for only £3/month!

Get our Reading App for your Android smartphone or tablet to start enjoying the Moussa Issa eBookstore discovery and digital reading experience.

Download our APP on your Smart device Now.

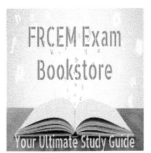

FRCEM Exam eBookstore

FRCEM Exam Bookstore   Books & Reference

PEGI 3

Offers in-app purchases
ⓘ This app is compatible with all of your devices.

Installed

A static eBook with little interactivity cannot draw your attention any more. Thus it is essential to engage readers with interactive reading experience.
Moussa Issa eBookstore proves to be on top of the interactive eBook game, enabling readers to watch integrated videos related to the subject directly on the page.
The additional flipping effect makes the eBook fully interactive and dynamic.

Customize your experience with multiple font and page styles and social sharing tools.

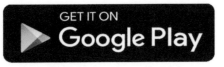
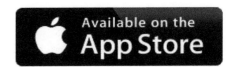

Distributed by Moussa Issa Bookstore Ltd
Website: www.moussaissabooks.com
Email: info@moussaissabooks.com
eBook subscription: www.moussaissabooks.com/read-ebook-online

Section I: Major and Acute Presentations

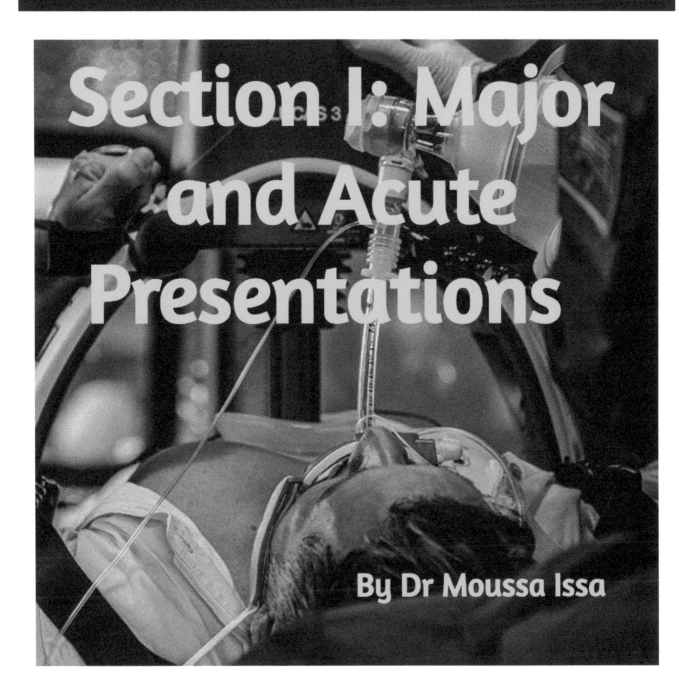

Section I: Major and Acute Presentations

By Dr Moussa Issa

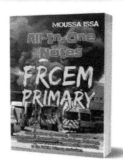
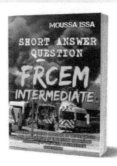
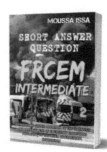
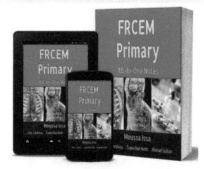
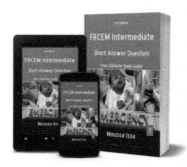
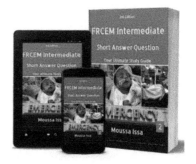
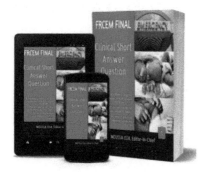
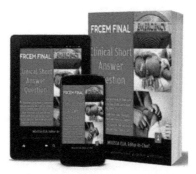
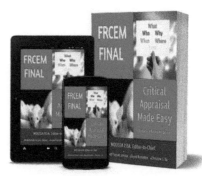
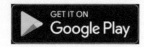
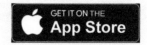

1. Abdominal Pain
I. ED APPROACH TO ABDOMINAL PAIN

INTRODUCTION

- Large numbers of patients with abdominal pain present to their general practitioners and emergency departments every year. Most require no specific medical intervention but some will require urgent hospital admission. The elderly and paediatric patient present particular challenges. The very young often give a poor history or can very quickly deteriorate.
- The elderly may have a very complicated medical history and misleading signs. A longitudinal study found that 50% of elderly patients (65 or over) with abdominal pain required admission.[1]
- Because of the difficulty of assessment in these groups of patients EP should have a lower threshold for referral.

AETIOLOGY OF ABDOMINAL PAIN

Gastrointestinal		Gynaecological
• Oesophagitis	• Diverticular Disease	• Ectopic Pregnancy
• Gastritis	• IBS	• PID
• PUD	• Ischaemic bowel	• Ruptured Ovarian cyst
• Gallstones	• Incarcerated hernia	
• Pancreatitis	• Gastroenteritis	
• Acute liver failure	• Constipation	
• Bowel obstruction		

Urological	Medical	Vascular
• Renal colic	• AMI	• AAA
• Pyelonephritis	• DKA	• Mesenteric Ischaemia
• UTI	• Pneumonia	
• Testicular Torsion	• Mesenteric Adenitis	
• Epididymorchitis	• Hypercalcaemia	

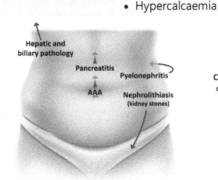

Common patterns of pain radiation

Courtesy-Strong Medicine

[1] Dang C, Aguilera P, Dang A, et al. Acute abdominal pain: four classifications can guide assessment and management. Geriatrics2002;57:30–2

Differential diagnosis based on age group

AGE	DIFFERENTIAL DIAGNOSIS
Infants	• Meconium ileus • Hypertrophic pyloric stenosis • Intussusception • Appendicitis • Hernia • Volvulus • Testicular torsion
Adolescents	• Appendicitis • Testicular torsion • Epididymorchitis • Ectopic pregnancy
Elderly	• Aortic aneurysm • Urinary retention • Mesenteric infarction • Acute cholecystitis

PATHOPHYSIOLOGY OF PAIN[2]

- **Visceral pain** comes from the abdominal viscera, which are innervated by autonomic nerve fibers and respond mainly to the sensations of distention and muscular contraction—not to cutting, tearing, or local irritation. Visceral pain is typically vague, dull, and nauseating. It is poorly localized and tends to be referred to areas corresponding to the embryonic origin of the affected structure. Foregut structures (stomach, duodenum, liver, and pancreas) cause upper abdominal pain. Midgut structures (small bowel, proximal colon, and appendix) cause periumbilical pain. Hindgut structures (distal colon and GU tract) cause lower abdominal pain.
- **Somatic pain** comes from the parietal peritoneum, which is innervated by somatic nerves, which respond to irritation from infectious, chemical, or other inflammatory processes. Somatic pain is sharp and well localized.
- **Referred pain** is pain perceived distant from its source and results from convergence of nerve fibers at the spinal cord. Common examples of referred pain are scapular pain due to biliary colic, groin pain due to renal colic, and shoulder pain due to blood or infection irritating the diaphragm.

[2] Parswa Ansari, Acute Abdominal Pain [MSD Manual]

CLINICAL ASSESSMENT
HISTORY

- When possible, the history should be obtained from a nonsedated patient. The initial differential diagnosis can be determined by a delineation of the pain's location, radiation, and movement (e.g., appendicitis-associated pain usually moves from the periumbilical area to the right lower quadrant of the abdomen). After the location is identified, the physician should obtain general information about onset, duration, severity, and quality of pain and about exacerbating and remitting factors.
- Associated symptoms often allow the physician to further focus the differential diagnosis.
- **For bowel obstruction**, constipation is the symptom with the highest positive predictive value.
- **For appendicitis**, right lower quadrant pain has the highest positive predictive value, although migration from periumbilical to right lower quadrant pain and fever also suggest appendicitis. Some conditions that were historically considered useful in diagnosing abdominal pain (e.g., anorexia in patients with appendicitis) have been found to have little predictive value.
- **Colic** (i.e., sharp, localized abdominal pain that increases, peaks, and subsides) is associated with numerous diseases of hollow viscera. The mechanism of pain is thought to be smooth muscle contraction proximal to a partial or complete obstruction (e.g., gallstone, kidney stone, small bowel obstruction). Although colic is associated with several diseases, the location of colic may help diagnose the cause. The absence of colic is useful for ruling out diseases such as acute cholecystitis; less than 25 percent of patients with acute cholecystitis present without right upper quadrant pain or colic.
- Peptic ulcer disease is often associated with Helicobacter pylori infection (75 to 95 percent of duodenal ulcers and 65 to 95 percent of gastric ulcers),[3] although most patients do not know their H. pylori status. In addition, many patients with ulcer disease and serology findings negative for H. pylori report recent use of nonsteroidal anti-inflammatory drugs.
- Other symptoms of peptic ulcer disease include concurrent, episodic gnawing or burning pain; pain relieved by food; and nighttime awakening with pain.
- Symptoms in patients with abdominal pain that are suggestive of surgical or emergent conditions include fever, protracted vomiting, syncope or presyncope, and evidence of gastrointestinal blood loss.

---

[3] Srinivasan R, Greenbaum DS. Chronic abdominal wall pain: a frequently overlooked problem. Practical approach to diagnosis and management. Am J Gastroenterol. 2002;97(4):824–830.

CLINICAL FEATURES SUGGESTING PARTICULAR CAUSES OF ABDOMINAL PAINCLINICAL

FEATURES	DIFFERENTIAL DIAGNOSIS
Abdominal pain in patients with AF or Atherosclerotic disease.	• Aortic aneurysm • Mesenteric infarction (embolic or thrombotic)
Abdominal pain out of proportion to clinical findings.	• Aortic aneurysm • Mesenteric infarction • Renal colic
Flank pain radiating to the groin.	• Renal colic • Pyelonephritis • Testicular torsion • Aortic aneurysm
Severe abdominal pain radiating through to back.	• Aortic aneurysm • Acute cholecystitis • Ascending cholangitis • Acute pancreatitis • Peptic ulcer disease
Abdominal pain associated with shoulder tip pain (due to diaphragmatic irritation).	• Ectopic pregnancy • Acute pancreatitis • Acute cholecystitis • Ascending cholangitis • Aortic aneurysm • Bowel perforation
Abdominal pain with collapse or signs of shock.	• Aortic aneurysm • Ectopic pregnancy • Massive GI bleed • Myocardial infarction
Abdominal distension	• Bowel obstruction • Pregnancy • Ascites • Cancer
Evidence of GI bleeding (haematemesis or melena).	• Peptic ulcer • Diverticular disease • Malignancy • Varices • Angiodysplasia
Abdominal bruising	• Trauma • Aortic aneurysm • Acute pancreatitis Haemorrhagic fluid collecting in the paracolic gutters **(Grey Turner's sign)** or around umbilicus **(Cullen's sign)**
Constipation	• Bowel obstruction • Bowel ischaemia • Diverticular disease

PHYSICAL EXAMINATION
- The patient's general appearance and vital signs can help narrow the differential diagnosis.
- Patients with peritonitis tend to lie very still, whereas those with renal colic seem unable to stay still.
- Fever suggests infection; however, its absence does not rule it out, especially in patients who are older or immunocompromised. Tachycardia and orthostatic hypotension suggest hypovolemia.

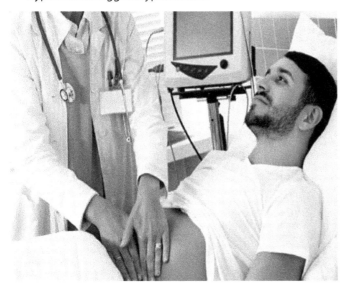

- The location of pain guides the remainder of the physical examination. Physicians should pay close attention to the cardiac and lung examinations in patients with upper abdominal pain because they could suggest pneumonia or cardiac ischemia.
- There are several specialized maneuvers that evaluate for signs associated with causes of abdominal pain. When present, some signs are highly predictive of certain diseases. These include:
  o **Carnett's sign** (i.e., increased pain when a supine patient tenses the abdominal wall by lifting the head and shoulders off the examination table) in patients with abdominal wall pain[4];
  o **Murphy's sign** in patients with cholecystitis (although it is only present in 65 percent of adults with cholecystitis and is particularly unreliable in older patients);
  o **Psoas sign** in patients with appendicitis.
- Other signs such as rigidity and rebound tenderness are nonspecific.
- Rectal and pelvic examinations are recommended in patients with lower abdominal and pelvic pain.

- **A rectal examination** may reveal fecal impaction, a palpable mass, or occult blood in the stool. Tenderness and fullness on the right side of the rectum suggest a retrocecal appendix.
- **A pelvic examination** may reveal vaginal discharge, which can indicate vaginitis. The presence of cervical motion tenderness and peritoneal signs increase the likelihood of ectopic pregnancy[5] or other gynecologic complications, such as salpingitis or a tuboovarian abscess.

Diagnostic Testing
Lab testing
- According to the SAEM Academy article published by Dr Luz Silverio[6], the diagnostic testing should be guided by the patient's history and physical examination findings which can be used to initially narrow the differential diagnosis.
- Standard "abdominal labs" must be tailored to the patient's presentation:
  o Urine analysis
  o Beta- HCG (females only)
  o Full Blood Count
  o Electrolytes
  o Liver function tests
  o Lipase
- Further labs that can be helpful in particular presentations of abdominal pain include: troponin, coagulation studies including prothrombin time and partial thromboplastin time, lactate, CRP, and gonococcal/chlamydia testing.

Imaging
- Portable x-ray and ultrasound can serve as immediate diagnostic tools that can be performed at the bedside when there is concern for pneumoperitoneum or hemoperitoneum, respectively.
- An upright chest x-ray or lateral decubitus abdominal film has been demonstrated to reveal free air in 80% of cases with perforated viscus.
- Ultrasound is an excellent tool for the evaluation of many urgent causes of abdominal pain.
- Bedside ultrasound can be used to search for abdominal free fluid suggestive of hemoperitoneum along with possible etiologies such as a ruptured abdominal aortic aneurysm (AAA) or ruptured ectopic pregnancy.

[4] Srinivasan R, Greenbaum DS. Chronic abdominal wall pain: a frequently overlooked problem. Practical approach to diagnosis and management. Am J Gastroenterol. 2002;97(4):824–830.

[5] Buckley RG, King KJ, Disney JD, Gorman JD, Klausen JH. History and physical examination to estimate the risk of ectopic pregnancy: validation of a clinical prediction model. Ann Emerg Med. 1999;34(5):589–594.
[6] Luz Silverio, MD, Santa Clara Valley Medical Center. Approach to abdominal pain [online]

- Bedside and radiology-performed ultrasound can also be diagnostic of nephrolithiasis, abdominal aneurysms, and in slender patients, appendicitis.
- An ultrasound verifying intrauterine pregnancy can help to rule out ectopic pregnancy in the case of the pregnant female. It may not entirely rule out ectopic or heterotopic pregnancy. Ultrasound is the diagnostic modality of choice for patients with suspected biliary pathology and ovarian and testicular torsion[7].
- For patients presenting with concerning findings in whom ultrasound is unlikely to be diagnostic, CT should be considered.
- The use of CT scans can improve diagnosis and treatment of acute abdominal pain and decrease return visits by up to 30%. On the other hand, computed tomography carries significant radiation exposure and cost, can lead to false positives, and does not completely rule out all serious life-threatening illnesses causing abdominal pain.

Treatment

- **Antibiotics:** The abdomen is a frequent site of infection in the development of sepsis. Patients with abdominal pain who are found to be septic should receive early administration of antibiotics as part of their initial resuscitation. Antibiotics should also be given promptly to patients with peritonitis or a perforated viscus.
- **Antiemetics:** Abdominal pain is frequently associated with nausea and vomiting. Two commonly used drugs for nausea and vomiting in the emergency department are ondansetron and metoclopramide and they have been demonstrated to be roughly equivalent in efficacy. Ondansetron is given 4-8 milligrams orally or intravenously every 4 hours; metoclopramide is given 10 milligrams intravenously, sometimes with the addition of diphenhydramine to prevent extrapyramidal side effects.
- **Analgesia:** Patients presenting in significant abdominal discomfort and a history and physical suggesting a concerning diagnosis should be provided with immediate pain relief. Narcotic medication should not be withheld out of concern that the abdominal exam may become unreliable and the diagnosis therefore obscured. Fentanyl provides a nice option if a shorter acting agent is desired or if the blood pressure is tenuous.

- **Specialty Consultation:** Immediate surgical consultation should be obtained in patients whose presentation of abdominal pain involves hemodynamic instability and/or a rigid abdomen. It is important to consider which specialty to consult based on the likely diagnosis. For instance, a ruptured AAA will be managed by vascular surgery, a perforated viscus by general surgery, testicular torsion by urology, and a ruptured ectopic pregnancy by OB/GYN. Nonsurgical consultation such as gastroenterology for a GI bleed or the medical ICU for DKA may also be necessary.
- **Outpatient Follow-up:** Approximately 25% of patients presenting to the emergency department with abdominal pain ultimately receive the diagnosis of "nonspecific abdominal pain," and follow-up is an essential part of their disposition plan. Of these patients, 30-hour follow-up can yield a difference in diagnosis or treatment in up to 20%. In addition to expedited outpatient follow-up, many patients presenting with nonspecific abdominal pain may benefit from outpatient specialty follow-up for further, non-emergent

Pearls and Pitfalls[8]

- Monitor vital signs for impending hemodynamic collapse. Patients with a peritoneal examination warrant early surgical consult.
- Elderly patients may present with very atypical symptoms but have high morbidity and mortality associated with the complaint of abdominal pain.
- CT is diagnostic of an urgent intra-abdominal condition in 50% of these patients.
- Every female of childbearing age with abdominal pain must receive a pregnancy test.
- Diffuse or upper abdominal pain should warrant thorough cardiac and pulmonary evaluation; diaphragmatic irritation can present as abdominal discomfort.
- The most frequent causes of emergency department missed CT diagnoses are right upper quadrant pathology (only 15-20% of gallstones are radiopaque) and urinary tract infections.
- Patients with significant intra-abdominal conditions tend to have exams that evolve over time. Frequent re-examinations will help with both diagnosis and early treatment.
- Manage and treat pain when appropriate.
- When in doubt, arrange close follow-up.

---

[7] *Luz Silverio, MD, Santa Clara Valley Medical Center. Approach to abdominal pain* [online]

[8] *Luz Silverio, MD, Santa Clara Valley Medical Center. Approach to abdominal pain* [online]

II. APPENDICITIS

1. INTRODUCTION

- Appendicitis, an inflammation of the vestigial vermiform appendix, is one of the most common causes of the acute abdomen and one of the most frequent indications for an emergent abdominal surgical procedure worldwide.[9]

2. CLINICAL ASSESSMENT:

History

- Abdominal pain is the most common symptom and is reported in nearly all confirmed cases of appendicitis.
- The clinical presentation of acute appendicitis is described as a constellation of the following classic symptoms:
  - Right lower quadrant (right anterior iliac fossa) abdominal pain
  - Anorexia
  - Nausea and vomiting
- In the classic presentation, the patient describes the onset of abdominal pain as the first symptom. The pain is typically periumbilical in nature with subsequent migration to the right lower quadrant as the inflammation progresses.
- Although considered a classic symptom, migratory pain occurs only in 50 to 60 percent of patients with appendicitis.
- Nausea and vomiting, if they occur, usually follow the onset of pain. Fever-related symptoms generally occur later in the course of illness.
- In many patients, initial features are atypical or nonspecific and can include:
  - Indigestion
  - Flatulence
  - Bowel irregularity
  - Diarrhea
  - Generalized malaise
- Because the early symptoms of appendicitis are often subtle, patients and clinicians may minimize their importance. The symptoms of appendicitis vary depending upon the location of the tip of the appendix.
- For example, an inflamed anterior appendix produces marked, localized pain in the right lower quadrant, while a retrocecal appendix may cause a dull abdominal ache.
- The location of the pain may also be atypical in patients who have the tip of the appendix located in the pelvis, which can cause tenderness below **McBurney's point.**

Physical examination

- The early signs of appendicitis are often subtle. Low-grade fever reaching 38.3°C may be present. The physical examination may be unrevealing in the very early stages of appendicitis since the visceral organs are not innervated with somatic pain fibers.
- However, as the inflammation progresses, involvement of the overlying parietal peritoneum causes localized tenderness in the right lower quadrant and can be detected on the abdominal examination.
- Rectal examination, although often advocated, has not been shown to provide additional diagnostic information in cases of appendicitis. In women, right adnexal area tenderness may be present on pelvic examination, and differentiating between tenderness of pelvic origin versus that of appendicitis may be challenging.
- High-grade fever 38.3°C occurs as inflammation progresses.
- Patients with a retrocecal appendix may not exhibit marked localized tenderness in the right lower quadrant since the appendix does not come into contact with the anterior parietal peritoneum[10].
- The rectal and/or pelvic examination is more likely to elicit positive signs than the abdominal examination. Tenderness may be more prominent on pelvic examination and may be mistaken for adnexal tenderness.
- Several findings on physical examination have been described to facilitate diagnosis, but these findings predated definitive imaging for appendicitis, and the wide variation in their sensitivity and specificity suggests that they be used with caution to broaden, or narrow, a differential diagnosis.
- There are no physical findings, taken alone or in concert, that definitively confirm a diagnosis of appendicitis.

Commonly described physical signs include:

- **McBurney's point tenderness** is described as maximal tenderness at 1.5 to 2 inches from the anterior superior iliac spine (ASIS) on a straight line from the ASIS to the umbilicus.
- **Rovsing's sign** refers to pain in the right lower quadrant with palpation of the left lower quadrant. This sign is also called indirect tenderness and is indicative of right-sided local peritoneal irritation.

---

[9] Williams GR. Presidential Address: a history of appendicitis. With anecdotes illustrating its importance. Ann Surg 1983; 197:495.

[10] Guidry SP, Poole GV. The anatomy of appendicitis. Am Surg 1994; 60:68.

- **The psoas sign** is associated with a retrocecal appendix. This is manifested by right lower quadrant pain with passive right hip extension. The inflamed appendix may lie against the right psoas muscle, causing the patient to shorten the muscle by drawing up the right knee. Passive extension of the iliopsoas muscle with hip extension causes right lower quadrant pain.
- **The obturator sign** is associated with a pelvic appendix. This test is based on the principle that the inflamed appendix may lie against the right obturator internus muscle. When the clinician flexes the patient's right hip and knee, followed by internal rotation of the right hip, this elicits right lower quadrant pain. The sensitivity is low enough that experienced clinicians no longer perform this assessment.

3. DIFFERENTIAL DIAGNOSIS:

Gastro-intestinal	Gynaecological	Urological
• Terminal ileitis • Acute cholecystitis • Mesenteric Adenitis • Gastroenteritis • Meckels Diverticulitis • Bowel obstruction • Diverticulitis • Non-specific abdominal pain	• Ectopic pregnancy • PID • Ruptured ovarian cyst • Ovarian torsion	• Renal colic • Urinary Tract Infection • Pyelonephritis

4. INVESTIGATION STRATEGIES

- o Urinalysis/ Urinary beta hCG
- o FBC, C-reactive protein
- o Plain abdominal x-ray: there is no role for plain films in patients with RIF pain, unless to look for another diagnosis (such as obstruction).
- ⎼ *Migration of pain, RIF rigidity* and *guarding* with *raised inflammatory markers* in combination strongly suggest appendicitis.

ALVARADO SCORE

ALVARADO score = MANTRELS (TL=2)		
M	Migration of pain to RIF	1
A	Anorexia	1
N	Nausea and vomiting	1
T	Tenderness in RIF	2
R	Rebound pain	1
E	Elevated temperature	1
L	Leukocytosis	2
S	Shift of WBC to left	1
Total		10

- *As the Alvarado Score is numerical, it has been evaluated for ruling in and ruling out appendicitis.*
  - o *Alvarado < 3-4*: *Studies ruling out appendicitis (sensitivity of 96%);*
  - o *Alvarado > 6-7*: *Studies ruling in appendicitis (sensitivity of 58-88%, depending on the study and score cut-offs used).*
- *The 2007 McKay study recommends:*
  - o *Alvarado ≥ 7*: *Surgical consultation,*
  - o *Alvarado 4-6:* *CT scan,*
  - o *Alvarado ≤ 3:* *no CT for diagnosing appendicitis, as appendicitis is unlikely.*

5. INVESTIGATIONS

- No single lab test specific for the diagnosis
- Both an elevated CRP and WBC have a combined sensitivity of 98%, and if both labs are within normal limits the diagnosis is less likely.
- Urine studies should be obtained. Useful for determining pregnancy, and evaluating for infection and hematuria.
- Ultrasound, the preferred imaging modality in children and pregnant patients with suspected appendicitis due to the absence of radiation. One multicenter cohort study found ultrasound to be 72.5-86% sensitive and 96% specific for appendicitis in children.
- CT is currently the preferred imaging study for evaluating acute appendicitis in adult males and nonpregnant females. CT of the abdomen/pelvis is also more useful for evaluating alternative diagnoses, and diagnosing complications of appendicitis (perforation, abscess, etc.). The overall sensitivity for IV contrast enhanced CT ranges from 95-100%, which is considerably better than ultrasound.
- Similarly, specificity is around 96%. Non-contrast CT scans are also quicker to obtain.
- MRI is typically reserved for pregnant patients after a non-diagnostic ultrasound. MRI has a similar diagnostic accuracy compared to CT, however emergent MRI often has limited availability, is expensive, and is more time consuming.

6. Treatment

- Acute appendicitis is traditionally treated surgically.
- Once the diagnosis is confirmed the patient should be made NPO and IV antibiotics should be started in the emergency department.
- Prompt resuscitation if sepsis
- IV fluid resuscitation,
- Pain control and antiemetics.
- Analgesia with reasonable doses of opioids has not been shown to alter the abdomen al exam.
- Surgical Referral

III. ACUTE PANCREATITIS

1. INTRODUCTION

- Acute pancreatitis is a relatively common and serious cause of acute abdominal pain. It is acute inflammation of the pancreas that results in the release of enzymes that cause autodigestion of the organ.
- The commonest causes of acute pancreatitis are **Gallstones and Alcohol**.
- Many cases are also idiopathic. The mnemonic 'I GET SMASHED'[11] is a useful memory aid for remembering the various causes:
  - *I*: Idiopathic
  - *G*: Gallstones
  - *E*: Ethanol
  - *T*: Trauma
  - *S*: Steroids
  - *M*: Mumps
  - *A*: Autoimmune
  - *S*: Scorpion stings
  - *H*: Hyperlipidaemia/hypercalcaemia
  - *E*: ERCP
  - *D*: Drugs

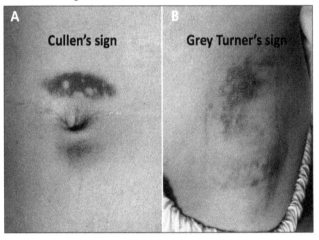

- **Clinical features of acute pancreatitis include:**
  - Epigastric pain (can be severe)
  - Nausea and vomiting
  - Referral **to T6-T10 dermatomes** (or shoulder tip via phrenic nerve if diaphragmatic irritation)
  - Pyrexia/sepsis
  - Epigastric tenderness
  - Jaundice
  - **Gray-Turner sign** (ecchymosis of the flank)
  - **Cullen sign** (ecchymosis of peri-umbilical area)

---

[11] *Medical Mnemonics: Causes of Pancreatitis – "I GET SMASHED"* [Online]

- **Signs of tetany,** such as fasciculations, twitching and a **positive Trousseaus or Chvostek's test**, should also be looked for since hypocalcaemia can develop secondary to intra-abdominal fat necrosis.

2. INVESTIGATIONS IN THE ED:

- **Serum amylase**: raised (> 1000 U/mL or ~3x upper limit of normal). Level not related to disease severity. May be normal even if severe disease as levels start to fall within 24-48h. (Cholecystitis, mesenteric infarction & GI perforation can cause small rises in amylase. Excreted renally, so renal failure raises levels.)
- **Serum lipase**: raised. More sensitive & specific test than amylase, but more expensive, so no prize for guessing which one is used in hospital
- **FBC:** raised WCC
- **U&Es, Glucose:** high, **Calcium** high
- **CRP:** elevated inflammatory marker. > 150 mg/L at 36h after admission is a predictor of severe pancreatitis.
- **LFTs:** may be deranged if gallstone or alcoholic pancreatitis
- **ABG:** monitor oxygenation and acid base status, for hypoxia and metabolic acidosis
- **Abdominal X-ray:** *absence of **psoas** (muscle) **shadow*** suggesting retroperitoneal fluid, ***sentinel loop*** of proximal jejenum.

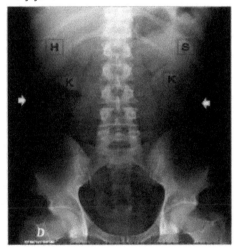

K = normal psoas shadow (slideshare.net)

- A **sentinel loop** is a dilation of an isolated segment of small intestine near the site of an inflamed organ, indicating localised ileus due to the inflammation leading to local muscle paralysis, distention and gas accumulation. In acute pancreatitis the sentinel loop is usually seen in left hypochondrium. (Acute cholecystitis = right hypochondrium. Acute appendicitis = right iliac fossa).

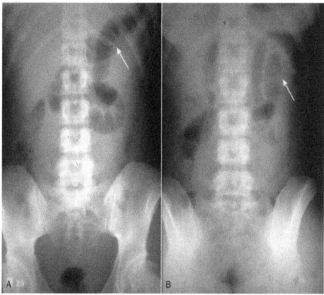

Sentinel loops in pancreatitis (Radiologykey.com)

- **Erect chest X-ray:** exclude other causes e.g. perforation (would show air under diaphragm). There may also be pleural effusion.
- **CT:** standard choice of imaging if diagnosis uncertain or to assess severity and complications- e.g. necrosis, deterioration
- **MRI:** may be better than CT, but more expensive, less available. See where this is going...
- **U/S:** look for gallstones or biliary dilation
- **ERCP**: if liver function tests worsen (but ERCP is also a cause of pancreatitis so take care)

3. RISK ASSESSMENT
1. RANSON CRITERIA

Criteria at time of patient admission to hospital:
Age > 55 (1 point)
Glucose > 10 (1 point)
WBC > 16 (1 point)
AST > 250 (1 point)
LDH > 350 (1 point)
Criteria that may develop over the first 2 hospital days:
BUN rises more than 5 mg/dL (1 point)
Base deficit > 4 (1 point)
Hct drops 10% or greater (1 point)
PO2 < 60 (1 point)
Calcium < 8 (1 point)
Fluid sequestration > 6L (1 point)

0-2 points:	Mortality is 1%
3-4 points:	Mortality is 16%
5-6 points:	Mortality is 40%
7-11 points:	Mortality almost 100%

2. GLASGOW PROGNOSTIC CRITERIA
- **Mnemonic "PANCREAS"**[12]
  - **P**aO2 < 8kPa
  - **A**ge >55yrs
  - **N**eutrophilia: WCC >15×109/L
  - **C**alcium: <2mmol/L (normal: 2.12mmol-2.65mmol/L)
  - **R**enal function: Urea>16mmol/L
    (normal: 2.5- 6.7mmol/L)
  - **E**nzymes : LDH > 600iU/L (normal : 70-250iU/L) ; AST > 200iU/L (normal : 5-35iU/L)
  - **A**lbumin: < 32g/L (serum)
  - **S**ugar: Blood Glucose >10mmol/L

- **A score ≥ 3** indicates Acute Severe Pancreatitis
- **A score = 2** indicates Acute Moderate Pancreatitis
- **A score < 2** indicates Acute Mild Pancreatitis

4. COMPLICATIONS
Early complications include:
- Severe sepsis and circulatory shock
- Acute renal failure
- Disseminated Intravascular Coagulation
- Hypocalcaemia
- Acute Respiratory Distress Syndrome
- Pancreatic encephalopathy
- Multi-organ failure

Late complications include:
- Insulin dependent diabetes mellitus (IDDM)
- Pancreatic pseudo-cyst
- Pancreatic abscess
- Chronic pancreatitis

5. MANAGEMENT OF ACUTE PANCREATITIS
- **Aim for SaO2% >95% and a urine output of >0.5 ml/Kg.**
- **Resuscitate** if dehydrated or signs of sepsis
- **Oxygen-** high flow through variable delivery mask
- **Intravenous access x2**
- **IV Normal Saline 1-2L** then reassess (may require several litres of fluid resuscitation)
- **Analgesia opiate** titrated to effect (**Tramadol**); **avoid Morphine**
- **Anti-Emetic**
- **Keep nil by mouth**
- **NG tube** only if there is evidence of an ileus
- **Urinary catheter** and hourly urine volumes
- **IV broad spectrum antibiotics** only if signs of sepsis
  Surgical referral: Involve surgical team and admit **ALL** patients with suspected pancreatitis.

---

[12] Ambonsall, Acute Pancreatitis [*PDF available*]

IV. BOWEL OBSTRUCTION

1. INTRODUCTION
- Intestinal obstruction can be classified in several different ways, most traditionally into small and large bowel obstruction.
- Bowel obstruction carries a high morbidity and mortality if managed incorrectly.

2. CAUSES OF INTESTINAL OBSTRUCTION

COLON
- **Tumours** (usually in left colon),
- **Volvulus of sigmoid or cecum,**
- Diverticulitis (usually in sigmoid),
- Faecal impaction,
- Hirschsprung disease,
- Crohn disease

DUODENUM

Adults
- Cancer of The Duodenum,
- Cancer of Head of Pancreas,
- Ulcer disease

Neonates
- Atresia,
- Volvulus,
- Bands,
- Annular pancreas

JEJUNUM AND ILEUM

Adults
- **Adhesions (common),**
- **Hernias,**
- Tumours,
- Foreign body,
- Meckel diverticulum,
- Crohn disease (uncommon),
- Ascaris infestation,
- Midgut volvulus,
- Intussusception by tumour (rare)

Neonates
- **Intussusception**
- Meconium ileus,
- Volvulus of a malrotated gut,
- Atresia,

- The most common causes of bowel obstruction are:
  o **Small bowel: Adhesions** (60% in UK), **Hernias, Intussusception** (Paediatric group)
  o **Large bowel: Malignancy** (developed countries), **Volvulus** (developing countries)
  o **Functional** (also referred to as paralytic) obstruction is relatively rare as a presentation to the emergency department.
- Functional obstruction results from atony of the intestine and loss of normal peristalsis.

- Atony of the bowel can be localised to a particular segment or generalised throughout the entire bowel.
- Localised atony is thought to result from an abnormality in the myenteric plexus of the bowel wall, whereas more generalised atony probably results from an imbalance in autonomic nerve supply, although there is little direct evidence for this.
- Different terms are often used to describe functional obstruction of the small or large bowel: **paralytic ileus** and **pseudo-obstruction** respectively.

HERNIAS

HERNIA	ANATOMY	INCIDENCE
Indirect inguinal hernia	Bowel passes through inguinal canal via a congenital weakness of the internal inguinal ring	most common
Direct inguinal hernia	Hernia exits abdominal cavity directly through the deep layers of the abdominal wall	uncommon
Femoral hernia	Abdominal contents pass through femoral canal just below inguinal ligament	rare

- **Inguinal hernias** are the most common type of hernia in both men and women, the indirect type accounting for 2/3 of cases.
- Almost all femoral hernias occur in women because of the wider bone structure of the female pelvis; however inguinal hernias are still more common in women than femoral hernias.

3. CLINICAL ASSESSMENT
The **cardinal features** of bowel obstruction are[13]:
- **Abdominal pain** - colicky or cramping in nature (secondary to the bowel peristalsis)
- **Vomiting** - occurring early in proximal obstructions and late in distal obstructions
- **Abdominal distension**
- **Absolute constipation** - occurring early in distal obstruction and late in proximal obstruction
Initially of gastric contents, before becoming bilious and then eventually faeculent

---

[13] *Bowel Obstruction-Teach me Surgery [online]*

- On examination, patients may show evidence of the **underlying cause** (e.g. surgical scars, cachexia from malignancy, or obvious hernia) or **abdominal distension**. Ensure to assess the patient's **fluid status**, as third-spacing can occur in bowel obstruction.
- Palpate for **focal tenderness*** (including guarding and rebound tenderness on palpation). Percussion may reveal a **tympanic sound** and auscultation may reveal 'tinkling' bowel sounds, both signs characteristic of bowel obstruction[14].
- *Patients with bowel obstruction may have abdominal tenderness, however should not have features of guarding or rebound tenderness, unless ischaemia is developing*

> ✦ **Closed Loop Obstruction**
> ✦ *If there is a second obstruction proximally (such as in a volvulus or in large bowel obstruction with a competent ileocaecal valve) this is termed a closed-loop obstruction.*
> ✦ *This is a surgical emergency as the bowel will continue to distend, stretching the bowel wall until it becomes ischaemic or perforates.*

4. INVESTIGATION STRATEGIES

GENERAL / BASIC

- **ABG** if signs of sepsis or strangulated bowel,
- **Urinalysis, ECG**
- Blood tests: **FBC, U&E, LFT, GLUCOSE, AMYLASE, GROUP&SAVE.**
- **Clotting screen** if septic or on anticoagulants.
- **Plain film X-ray erect** and **supine abdominal x-ray/ Chest x-ray**

SPECIFIC IMAGING

- CT
- Small bowel follow-through
- Water-soluble contrast enema

RADIOLOGICAL SIGNS OF BOWEL OBSTRUCTION

- If a patient presents with clinical features of obstruction then radiological assessment can be very helpful in determining the level of obstruction, and occasionally the cause.
- There are features visible on a plain abdominal X-ray that may help locate the level of obstruction.
- These are partly determined by a knowledge of small and large bowel anatomy.

---

[14] *Bowel Obstruction-Teach me Surgery [online]*

1. SMALL BOWEL OBSTRUCTION

- **KEY FEATURES OF SBO:**
  - *Dilated small bowel loop >2.5cm in diameter*
  - *The relatively central position of the small bowel and restriction in dilatation to 5cm also helps to distinguish small from large bowel on plain films.*
  - *Presence of valvulae conniventes,* which completely cross the bowel wall.
  - *The taeniae coli of the large bowel are incomplete across the bowel wall.*

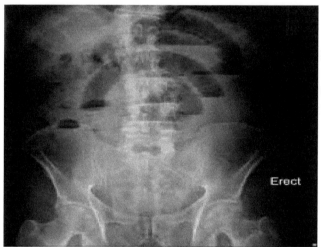

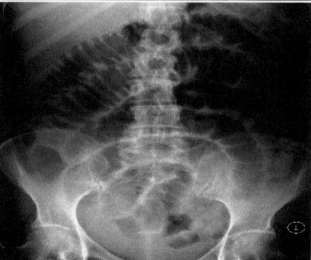

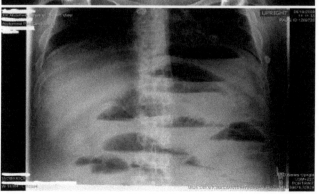

Small Bowel obstruction (Source-Medscape)

PARALYTIC ILEUS

- Paralytic ileus, also called **pseudo-obstruction**, is one of the major causes of intestinal obstruction in infants and children.
- **Causes of paralytic ileus may include:**
  - Bacteria or viruses that cause intestinal infections (gastroenteritis)
  - Chemical, Electrolyte, or Mineral imbalances (such as decreased potassium level)
  - Abdominal surgery
  - Decreased blood supply to the intestines
  - Infections inside the abdomen, such as appendicitis
  - Kidney or lung disease
  - Use of certain medicines, especially narcotics

SENTINEL LOOP

  - Intra-abdominal inflammation, such as with pancreatitis, can lead to a localized ileus.
  - This may appear as a single loop of dilated bowel known as a **'sentinel loop.'**

2. LARGE BOWEL OBSTRUCTION

- *The most common causes of large bowel obstruction are **colo-rectal carcinoma and diverticular strictures**.*
- *Less common causes are **hernias or volvulus** (twisting of the bowel on its mesentery). **Adhesions** do not commonly cause large bowel obstruction.*
- Radiological appearances of large bowel obstruction differ from those of small bowel obstruction, however, with large bowel obstruction there is often co-existing small bowel dilatation proximally.
- Abdominal X-ray cannot reliably differentiate mechanical obstruction from pseudo-obstruction.

- **KEY FEATURES OF LBO:**
  - *Dilatation of the caecum **>9cm** is abnormal*
  - *Dilatation of any other part of the colon **>6cm** is abnormal*
  - *Abdominal X-ray may demonstrate the level of obstruction.*

- **CT Scan**
  - It is the most useful in differentiating the specific cause and location of mechanical obstruction.
  - A **CT scan with IV contrast** of the abdomen and pelvis is the imaging modality of choice in **suspected bowel obstruction** and a shift in modern practice is moving towards **CT scanning as the initial imaging** used where possible[15].

---

15 Bowel Obstruction-Teach me Surgery [online]

  - CT imaging is more useful than AXRs as they are:
    - (1) more sensitive for bowel obstruction;
    - (2) can differentiate between mechanical obstruction and pseudo-obstruction;
    - (3) can demonstrate the site and cause of obstruction (hence useful for operative planning); and
    - (4) may demonstrate the presence of metastases if caused by a malignancy (which is likewise useful in operative planning).

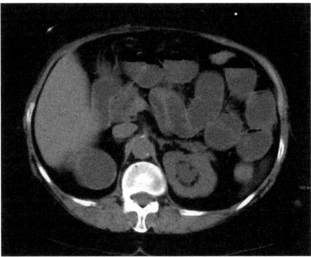

CT scan demonstrating features of small bowel obstruction-by James Heilman, MD [CC BY-SA 3.0 (https://creativecommons.org/licenses/by-sa/3.0)], from Wikimedia Commons

ED MANAGEMENT OF BOWEL OBSTRUCTION
A. GENERAL ED MANAGEMENT
  - **O2 and fluid resuscitation** if the patient is haemodynamically unstable
  - **Insert an IV cannula** (taking and sending blood as mentioned above)
  - **Move the patient to an appropriate area of the department and involve an ED senior in their management.**
  - **Start an IVI of 0.9% Saline**
  - **Titrate IV analgesia** (morphine) **with an antiemetic**
  - **Insert a nasogastric tube** and declare the patient **Nil by Mouth** (NBM)
  - **Insert a urinary catheter**
  - **Consider more invasive monitoring if required for accurate fluid resuscitation** (CVP and/or arterial line)
  - **Broad spectrum antibiotics** are commonly administered because of concerns that bacterial translocation may occur in the setting of small bowel obstruction; however, there are no controlled data to support or refute this approach.
  - **Refer to the surgical team**

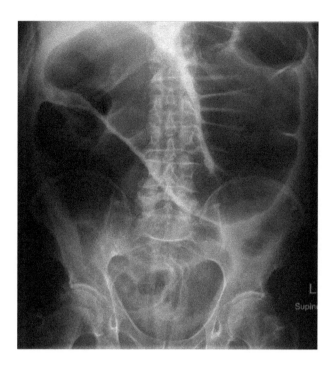

3. SIGMOID VOLVULUS

- Rotation (clockwise = anticlockwise) of section of intestine on its mesentery.
- Sigmoid volvulus occurs when a redundant portion of sigmoid colon twists around its mesentery.
- The sigmoid is the commonest site of volvulus but it can occur at other sites, especially the caecum (caecal volvulus).
- It often occurs in elderly or institutionalised patients with a history of chronic constipation.

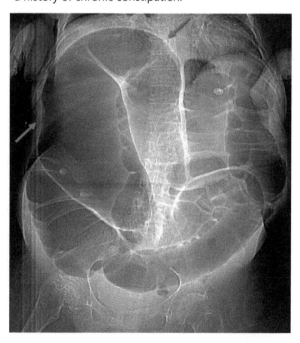

- Volvulus usually presents with **pain, abdominal distension, vomiting and absolute constipation**, but in elderly or confused patients' pain may be surprisingly limited.
- The blood supply is compromised and venous congestion occurs.
- There is progressive accumulation of gas and bowel fluid proximal to the obstruction and perforation will occur without prompt diagnosis and definitive management.
- Plain abdominal x-ray will demonstrate a **grossly distended sigmoid colon** with the a "**coffee bean sign**" created by the stretched haustrae.

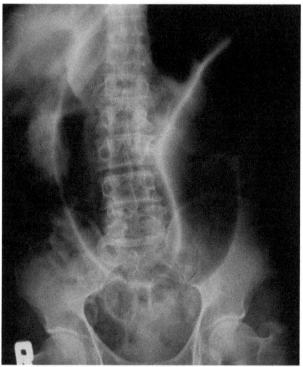

Coffee bean appearance with three dense lines converging towards the site of obstruction (**Frimann-Dahl sign**), which supports the diagnosis of sigmoid volvulus.

- Once a diagnosis of volvulus has been made, **prompt surgical referral is crucial**.
- The patient may require resuscitation and there can be significant fluid shifts and signs of sepsis due to bowel necrosis.

- *A **sigmoidoscope** will successfully decompress the majority of uncomplicated sigmoid volvulus, but definitive surgery may be required if there is evidence of necrosis or perforation.*

V. BOWEL PERFORATION

1. INTRODUCTION

- Bowel perforation results from insult or injury to the mucosa of the bowel wall resulting from a violation of the closed system. This exposes the structures within the peritoneal cavity to gastrointestinal contents. Bowel perforation can be secondary to many factors, most commonly inflammation, infection, obstruction, trauma, or invasive procedure.
- Patients presenting with abdominal pain and distension, especially in the appropriate historical setting, must be evaluated for this entity as delayed diagnosis can be life-threatening due to the risk of developing infections such as peritonitis. Management includes stabilizing the patient while making the surgical consultation. Even appropriately managed, bowel perforation can lead to increased morbidity and mortality from post repair complications such as adhesions and fistula formation.[16]

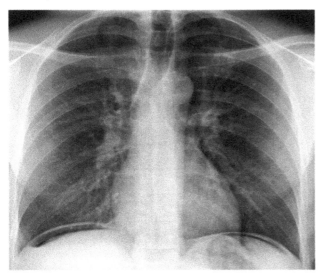

2. CAUSES OF BOWEL PERFORATION

Bowel perforations can be separated based on their anatomic locations, but many causes are overlapping:

- **Small bowel:** Erosion from duodenal ulcerations, tumor, infection or abscess, Meckel's diverticulum, hernia with strangulation, IBD/colitis, mesenteric ischemia, foreign body, obstruction, medication/radiation related, iatrogenic, blunt or penetrating abdominal trauma
- **Large bowel:** Tumor, diverticulitis, infection or abscess, colitis, foreign body, obstruction, volvulus, iatrogenic, blunt or penetrating abdominal trauma.

---

[16] Long B, Robertson J, Koyfman A. Emergency Medicine Evaluation and Management of Small Bowel Obstruction: Evidence-Based Recommendations. J Emerg Med. 2019 Feb;56(2):166-176.

3. SPECIFIC INVESTIGATIONS FOR BOWEL PERFORATION

- **Erect CXR**—aims to identify **free intra-peritoneal gas under the diaphragm** due to hollow viscus perforation. Patients should be sat upright for at least 10 minutes before the CXR.
- **Figures vary but an erect CXR identifies 70–80% of pneumoperitoniums**, so can be used as a rule-in but a not rule-out test.
- **A lateral CXR (left lateral decubitus shoot through)**
  - Has better sensitivity than an anteroposterior film for free air.
  - Patient is allowed to lie down in left lateral decubitus for around 10 minutes, so that **intraperitoneal air** in the lesser sac can pass through foramen of Winslow into the greater sac and **accumulate between lateral margin of liver and lateral abdominal wall.**

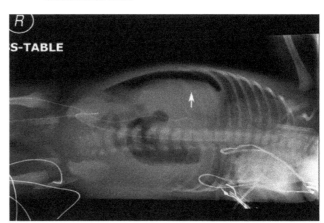

Left Lateral Decubitus: This is the preferred decubitus position. The free intraperitoneal gas is seen easily because it is contrasted against the liver. Although it is described as a "left lateral decubitus" it is marked with a right marker (Source- Radiography

- **Ultrasound**—in trained hands has a greater sensitivity for free intra-peritoneal air than CXR and has the advantage that it can be performed in the resuscitation room.
- **CT abdomen with contrast**—is the most sensitive investigation and is very useful in patients where there is diagnostic uncertainty.

4. ED MANAGEMENT OF BOWEL PERFORATION

- Fluid resuscitation.
- Intravenous analgesia and anti-emetic.
- Intravenous broad-spectrum antibiotics.
- Nil by mouth.
- Urgent surgical referral.

VI. ACUTE MESENTERIC ISCHAEMIA

INTRODUCTION

- Acute mesenteric ischaemia (AMI) is a condition due to a sudden decline in blood flow through the mesenteric vessels. Without appropriate and timely treatment, necrosis of the small and large intestine results, leading to sepsis and potentially death.
- Mortality rates for AMI range between 60% and 80%.
- AMI is classified as either **occlusive or nonocclusive mesenteric ischemia (NOMI)**.
- **Occlusive mesenteric arterial ischemia (OMI)** is subdivided into acute thromboembolism and acute thrombosis. A mesenteric venous thrombosis is a form of AMI that is covered in a different chapter.[17]

ETIOLOGY

- **The Embolic patients**
  - Commonly have a positive medical history of cardiovascular diseases including recent myocardial infarction, congestive heart failure, and atrial fibrillation.
  - Causes include peripheral arterial emboli, cardiac emboli, and an atheromatous plaque that ruptured or dislodged after surgery.
- **The typical thrombotic patient**
  - Experiences a history of postprandial abdominal pain, leading to food avoidance and weight loss.
  - Causes include atheromatous vascular disease (e.g., atherosclerosis, aortic aneurysm, aortic dissection) and decreased cardiac output due to a secondary cause (e.g., dehydration, myocardial infarction, congestive heart failure).
- **The NOMI patient**
  - The patient is typically critically ill, presents with several severe comorbidities, and is hemodynamically unstable.
  - Causes include drugs that reduce blood flow (e.g., vasopressors and ergotamines), hypotension from severe medical conditions (e.g., myocardial infarction, sepsis, CHF, and renal disease), and patients that recently received major surgery (e.g., cardiac and abdominal surgery).

HISTORY AND PHYSICAL EXAMINATION

- AMI patients typically present with abdominal pain that does not correlate with physical exam findings.

- Tenderness to palpation occurs when the entire bowel wall is involved, which is a later presentation when necrosis begins to occur.
- Patients with an embolic disease typically have a history of the bowel emptying violently, followed by severe pain. The syndrome rapidly advances to ischemia and necrosis because collateral blood flow is limited.
- Thrombosis may take days or weeks to progress, with abdominal pain gradually worsening. Patients also may have a combination of diarrhea, distention, bloody stool, and most importantly, a history of postprandial pain, suggesting chronic mesenteric ischemia.
- NOMI progresses slowly, and the associated abdominal pain is not localized and varies in severity and consistency. These patients are critically ill (e.g., septic shock, cardiac disease, and respiratory failure), hypotensive, and usually on vasopressor agents.

EVALUATION

- Laboratory values and biomarkers for AMI are nonspecific and do not have diagnostic power:
  - **An ECG** can be a useful investigation to identify AF and indicate the source of a possible embolus.
  - **Elevated D(-)-lactate and lactate dehydrogenase** are seen in late-stage AMI.
  - **CT angiography** is the preferred method for AMI.
  - **Catheter-directed angiography** has fallen out of favor during the initial stages of AMI diagnosis.
  - **Plain abdominal radiography,**
  - **Duplex ultrasonography,**
  - **Magnetic resonance angiography I.**

TREATMENT / MANAGEMENT

- **Fluid resuscitation** and correcting electrolyte imbalances.
- **Avoid vasopressors and alpha-adrenergic agents**, which may cause vasospasm.
- **Broad-spectrum antibiotics** should be given before surgery to avoid abdominal sepsis if the necrotic bowel is resected.
- **Early surgical exploration** is required to assess the level of ischemia and spread of necrosis.
- As NOMI is secondary to vasospasm rather than occlusion, treatment is medically focused and relies upon reversing the underlying cause of the low-flow state.
- **Catheter-directed papaverine** (phosphodiesterase inhibitor) delivered by a side-hole catheter or thrombolysis catheter is an interventional option.

---

[17] Khan SM, Emile SH, Wang Z, Agha MA. *Diagnostic accuracy of hematological parameters in Acute mesenteric ischemia-A systematic review. Int J Surg. 2019 Apr 16;66:18-27.*

VII. ABDOMINAL AORTIC ANEURYSM

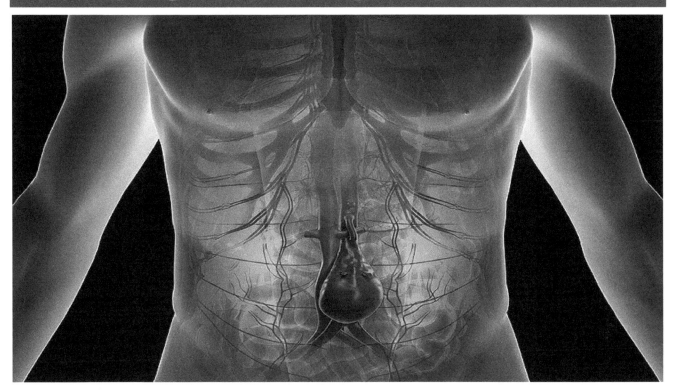

1. INTRODUCTION

- An Abdominal Aortic Aneurysm (AAA) is a permanent localised or diffuse dilatation of the abdominal aorta to 1.5 times its normal diameter that involving all three layers of the vessel wall. Normal infrarenal aortic diameters in patients >50y are 1.5 cm in women and 1.7 cm in men. An infrarenal aorta 3 cm in diameter or more is considered aneurysmal.
- True aneurysms of the Abdominal aorta involve all 3 layers of the vessel wall, and are defined as being >3cm in diameter or having increase >50% from baseline
- **False aneurysms (or pseudoaneurysms)** are deficient in at least one layer
- **Fusiform aneurysms** have a "bulbous" shape and are usually true aneurysms
- **Saccular aneurysms** have a lateral out-pouching like a Berry aneurysm and are often false aneurysms
- Most abdominal aortic aneurysms occur in the infra-renal segment (90-95%). AAAs to extension above the renal arteries is rare but extension into the iliac arteries is common.

2. CAUSES OF AAA

- **Strongly associated risk factors:**
  - Male gender
  - Age
  - Smoking
  - Hypertension
  - Genetic/familial disposition (e.g. inherited connective tissue disorders such as Marfans and Ehlers-Danlos)

- **Identified and postulated causes include:**
  - Atherosclerotic injury and associated degeneration
  - Primary connective tissue degeneration
  - Inflammatory arteritis with associated aneurysmal degeneration
  - Traumatic injury and pseudoaneurysm
  - Mycotic injury and pseudoaneurysm
  - Aortic dissection-related aneurysmal degeneration

3. CLINICAL FEATURES OF AAA

- The classic presentation is **central abdominal and back pain** in a patient with a known aneurysm.
- However, presentation may vary from a PEA arrest to painless, sudden collapse.
- Patients may be mistaken as having renal colic due to the presence of **haematuria** caused by **irritation of the ureter or rupture into the renal artery**.
- Examination may reveal a **tender pulsatile mass.**
- One or both **femoral pulses may be absent.**
- In the obese or elderly, the diagnosis can be particularly challenging and a high index of suspicion should be maintained.

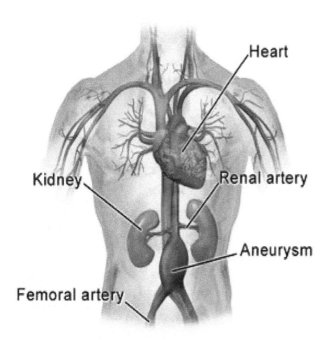

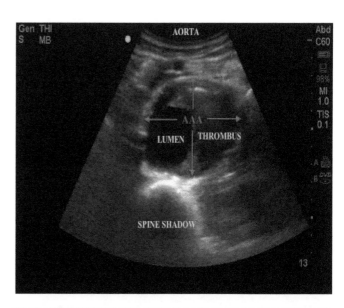

- There may be variations in measurement of the aneurysm size depending on technique.
- **The aneurysmal sac should be measured from outer wall to outer wall with a longitudinal image.**

4. INVESTIGATIONS FOR AAA

- Diagnosis is largely clinical supplemented by the use of **Emergency Ultrasound.** Ultrasound is now considered a core skill of Emergency Medicine trainees and one of the main indications is the diagnosis of AAA.
- Emergency ultrasound is a useful rule-in test for identifying an aneurysm but poor for detecting a leak.
- Ultrasound is user dependent and if there is ongoing clinical suspicion of a AAA further imaging is required.
- **CT** is rarely used in the unstable patient with a suspected AAA but maybe used if diagnostic uncertainty persists and the patient is stable.

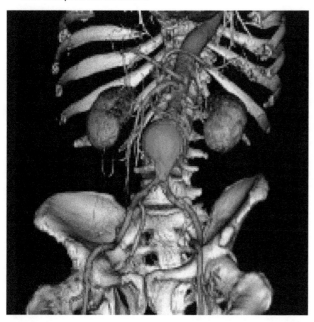

5. ED MANAGEMENT OF AAA

- **ABC** approach.
- **Cautious fluid resuscitation**:
  - Should be instituted, aiming for a **SBP >90 mmHg.**
  - Aggressive fluid resuscitation has been shown to worsen outcome in patients with leaking AAA.
  - Therefore, if the patient is conscious and passing urine, minimal fluid should be given until the aorta is cross-clamped in theatre.
  - The blood bank should be informed and **10 units of blood and 2 units of platelets** should be cross-matched.
  - **Refer to vascular surgeon** if surgical candidate,
  - Urgency depends on AAA size and presence/ absence of symptoms
    - <2cm diameter is normal
    - 2-5.5 cm diameter and asymptomatic requires follow up with regular ultrasound
    - > 5.5 cm diameter requires operative intervention regardless of symptoms in patients suitable for surgery

6. COMPLICATIONS

  - Death
  - Major haemorrhage
  - Aortic branch involvement resulting in ischaemia (e.g. Renal, spinal, pancreatitis)
  - Distal embolisation (e.g. Trash foot)
  - Rhabdomyolysis

MANAGEMENT AND TRANSFER OF PATIENTS WITH A DIAGNOSIS OF RUPTURED ABDOMINAL AORTIC ANEURYSM TO A SPECIALIST VASCULAR CENTRE.

RCEM[18] SUMMARY OF RECOMMENDATIONS

1. A clinical diagnosis of ruptured abdominal aortic aneurysm (rAAA) should be considered:

- In patients over the age of 50 years presenting with abdominal/back pain AND hypotension;
- In patients with a known AAA and symptoms of either abdominal/back pain OR hypotension/collapse;
- In patients where an alternative diagnosis is considered more likely on clinical grounds, rAAA still must be excluded, with radiological confirmation made prior to referral. Level 3, strong recommendation

2. All decisions concerning treatment and transfer should, where possible, be made in conjunction with the patient and/or their family.

3. Avoid hypertension in patients with a clinical diagnosis of rAAA to maintain an alert patient and systolic blood pressure 90-120mmHg is acceptable.

4. If a specialist vascular service cannot be provided on-site, the patient will require transfer to a centre with appropriate facilities and expertise. Transfer agreements with the local ambulance service should be in place. Level 4, strong recommendation

5. Rapid and co-ordinated transfer can reduce delays in the patient journey and improve outcome. Level 3, strong recommendation

To expedite transfer, the most senior doctor available should lead and be actively involved in the care of any patient with suspected rAAA. Outgoing referrals should go to a senior vascular trainee or consultant.

Items 6-18, below, are all Level 5, strong recommendation

6. All patients with a clinical or radiological diagnosis of rAAA should be assessed as to their current clinical state AND premorbid level of function to determine suitability for transfer.

7. Patients aged ≤85 years with no/mild/moderate systemic disease should be referred to the receiving hospital's on-call vascular service without delay.

8. Patients age >85 years or with severe systemic disease will benefit from a consultant*- consultant discussion prior to transfer to a vascular unit.

9. Impaired mental capacity is not a contraindication to assessment and transfer.

10. Patients who have been previously turned down for elective surgery should still be discussed via a consultant*-consultant referral.

11. Contraindications to transfer are restricted to those with:

- Cardiac arrest in the current admission;
- Patients requiring intubation due to acute deterioration;
- Patients requiring inotropic support (vasoactive drugs), except in certain rare situations.

Such patients are unlikely to survive transfer and surgery and should only be transferred after consultant*-consultant discussion.

12. There are no ESSENTIAL investigations required prior to transfer. However, a blood gas and an Emergency Department (ED) ultrasound are considered useful, if these incur no delay.

13. Investigations, including FBC, U&E, amylase, X-match, CT scans, MUST not delay transfer to a centre that can provide definitive care. If an alternative diagnosis is more likely, or the investigation can be performed without causing delay, it is reasonable to perform these investigations before transfer.

14. Patients should be treated, if necessary, with both analgesia (according to the Royal College of Emergency Medicine (RCEM) guidelines) and if required, fluids before and during transfer.

15. A time-critical transfer in a 999 ambulance, preferably with a paramedic crew is required, although this is not essential.

16. The facility to transfer CT images electronically must be in place to ensure all images are transferred to the receiving hospital. If electronic transfer is not possible, a copy of the DICOM files (CD or DVD or USB memory stick) must accompany the patient.

17. Patients should not usually travel with blood products, unless transfusion already commenced.

18. Patients who remain haemodynamically stable should be transferred to either an ED resuscitation area or local equivalent. Patients who are unstable may need rapid transfer to theatres.

19. Transfer to a specialist vascular centre should occur within 30 minutes of diagnosis.

---

[18] RCEM. *Management and Transfer of Patients with a Diagnosis of Ruptured Abdominal Aortic Aneurysm to a Specialist Vascular Centre. Jan 2019 [Online]*

VIII. BILIARY TRACT DISORDERS

INTRODUCTION

- The commonest biliary tract disorder presenting to the ED is **Gallstones.**
- Gallstones are precipitants of bile that form in the gallbladder. Bile contains cholesterol, bile pigments (from haemoglobin breakdown), and phospholipids.
- The varying concentrations of these components results in 3 main types of stone:
  - **Cholesterol**: large, often solitary stones that account for the majority of UK gallstone disease. Risk factors include increasing age, female sex, obesity, family history, hyperlipidaemia, diabetes, and cystic fibrosis.
  - **Pigmented**: small, dark stones composed of bilirubin and calcium salts. Risk factors for pigmented stones include haemolytic anaemias and cirrhosis.
  - **Mixed**: contain varying amounts of cholesterol, calcium salts, and bilirubin. The calcium salts allow the stones to be seen radiographically. Approximately 10% of gallstones are radio-opaque.

- An **ultrasound scan** is indicated to confirm the presence of gallstones. Blood tests are usually normal.
- If symptoms settle, then outpatient management is appropriate, pending a cholecystectomy.

2. ACUTE CHOLECYSTITIS

- In 95% of acute cholecystitis, a gallstone or biliary sludge becomes impacted at the neck of the gallbladder.
- Only 5% of patients have no stone; these are usually patients that have been admitted for trauma, burns, or have diabetes. **Acalculous acute cholecystitis** has a worse prognosis than those with gallstones.
- The obstructed gallbladder becomes distended, inflamed, and ischaemic. Bacteria are able to penetrate the gallbladder wall causing infection. Prolonged obstruction may result in a **gallbladder empyema.**

Gallstones

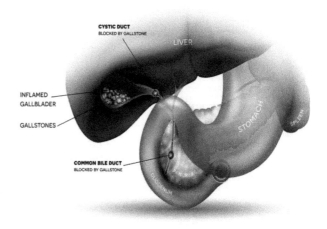

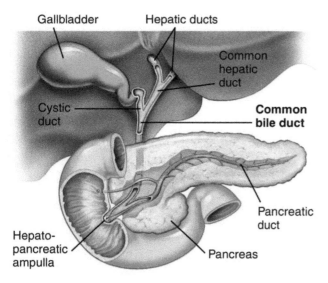

1. BILIARY COLIC

- Biliary colic occurs when a gallstone lodges in the neck of the gallbladder, the cystic duct, or common bile duct.
- The blockage causes increased intraluminal pressure and distension of the gallbladder. The gallstone then dislodges and passes out of the biliary tract.
- The patient experiences abdominal pain, often located in the right upper quadrant, associated with nausea and vomiting. The symptoms resolve when the stone passes.
- Patients may suffer recurrent episodes of biliary colic when further stones pass and therefore are diagnosed with chronic cholecystitis.

- **CLINICAL FEATURES OF ACUTE CHOLECYSTITIS**
  - **Abdominal pain**—typically located in the right-upper quadrant.
    - Pain is often dull and poorly localized initially due to distension of the gallbladder and stimulation of the visceral peritoneum.
    - As the inflammatory process progresses, inflammatory fluid leaks out stimulating the local parietal peritoneum, which is innervated by intercostal nerves and felt as a sharp, well-localized pain.
  - **Murphy's sign**—this is an indication of local peritonism.

- Deep palpation in the right-upper quadrant, during inspiration, causes pain as the inflamed gallbladder impinges on the palpating hand.
  - This causes a sudden inspiratory arrest.
  - The test is only positive if repetition in the left-upper quadrant doesn't cause pain.
- **Jaundice**—may occur if the stone moves and obstructs the common bile duct or if the gallbladder causes compression of the common hepatic duct (**Mirizzi's syndrome**).

SPECIFIC INVESTIGATIONS

- **Ultrasound scan**—is the most useful investigation for confirming the diagnosis. It may show gallbladder wall thickening, pericholecystic fluid, and an impacted gallstone.
- **Amylase or lipase** should be sent to exclude pancreatitis.
- **Urinary pregnancy test.**
- **ECG**—to exclude a MI or ACS
- **CXR**—to exclude pneumonia and look for evidence of air under the diaphragm in a suspected perforation.

- **ED MANAGEMENT OF ACUTE CHOLECYSTITIS**
  - **Fluid resuscitation**—if the patient has signs of sepsis or dehydration
  - **Analgesia**—intravenous morphine titrated to effect
  - **Antibiotics**—usually a 3rd generation cephalosporin but local antibiotic policy should be followed
  - **Nil by mouth**
  - **Urgent surgical review**—surgical options depend on the severity of illness ranging from medical therapy, to endoscopic retrograde cholangiopancreatography (ERCP), to cholecystectomy (open or laparoscopic).

3. CHOLEDOCHOLITHIASIS

- Choledocholithiasis is when a gallstone becomes stuck in the common bile duct resulting in jaundice and hepatic damage. Investigations are the same as acute cholecystitis. Treatment is removal of the stone via **ERCP.**

4. OBSTRUCTIVE JAUNDICE

- A gallstone in the common bile duct is a cause of post-hepatic jaundice. The patient will have dark urine and pale stools. **Cholangio-/pancreatic carcinomas** may present in a similar manner but are usually not painful.
- If the gallbladder is palpable a pancreatic carcinoma is the more likely diagnosis (**Courvoisier's law**: 'In the presence of jaundice, if the gallbladder is palpable, the cause is unlikely to be a stone').

5. GALLSTONE ILEUS

- Prolonged obstruction and inflammation of the gallbladder may result in a fistula developing between the gallbladder and the duodenum.
- The gallstone can then enter the GI tract and obstruct the terminal ileum.
- An abdominal X-ray may show air in the biliary tree and evidence of small bowel obstruction. Patients should be resuscitated and referred urgently for surgical review.

6. ASCENDING CHOLANGITIS

- Occurs when the common bile duct becomes infected, often secondary to a stone in the common bile duct (choledocholithiasis) that has caused chronic bile stasis.
- The classic presentation of ascending cholangitis is with **Charcot's triad:**
  - *Jaundice*
  - *Fever (usually with rigors)*
  - *Right upper quadrant pain*
- Ascending cholangitis is a potentially life-threatening medical emergency and patients are frequently septic.
- 10-20% of patients present with the additional features of **altered mental status and hypotension** secondary to septic shock. When the two additional features are present in addition to Charcot's triad the patient is said to have the **Reynold's Pentad.** *The treatment of ascending cholangitis is **urgent biliary drainage.***

➕ *Generally speaking Murphy's sign is usually positive in acute cholecystitis but negative in biliary colic and ascending cholangitis.*

- The **white cell count** and **CRP** are usually elevated in ascending cholangitis. **Jaundice** is often present and **ALP** and **bilirubin** levels can be markedly elevated.
- There is a significant amount of overlap between the presentation of biliary colic, acute cholecystitis and ascending cholangitis and the following table helps to differentiate between these diagnoses:

	Biliary colic	Acute cholecystitis	Ascending cholangitis
Pain duration	< 12 hrs	> 12 hrs	Variable
Fever	Absent	Present	Present
Murphy's sign	Negative	Positive	Negative
WCC & CRP	Normal	Elevated	Elevated
AST, ALT & ALP	Normal	Normal or mildly elevated	Elevated
Bilirubin	Normal	Normal or mildly elevated	Elevated

IX. RENAL COLIC

INTRODUCTION

- Nephrolithiasis, also known as kidney stones, is a common condition affecting 5% to 15% of the population at some point, with a yearly incidence of 0.5% in North America and Europe, and is caused by a crystal or crystalline aggregate traveling from the kidney through the genitourinary system.[19]
- Renal colic is caused by renal calculi (stones) as they pass through the ureter to the bladder. Renal stones may develop and may travel spontaneously through the ureter and into the bladder where they are passed out.
- The pain caused by the passage of stones through the ureter is often compared to the **contractions of childbirth**.

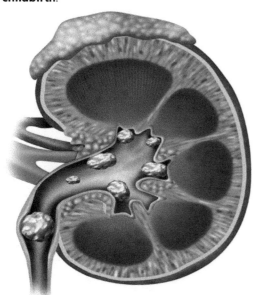

STONE COMPOSITION[20]

- *Calcium oxalate* and / or *phosphate: 60-80%*
- *Struvite 10-15%*
- *Cystine 1%*
- *Uric acid 1%.*
- *Occasionally: Xanthine, Indinavir and Triamterene.*

AETIOLOGY

The following are the most common:

1. **Inadequate urinary volume** -usually less than 1 L per day: increase the concentration of solutes and promote urinary stasis, which can cause supersaturation of solutes and lead to stone formation.

2. **Hypercalciuria:** It can be secondary to increased intestinal absorption of calcium, increased circulating calcium, hypervitaminosis D, hyperparathyroidism, high protein load, or systemic acidosis.

3. **Elevated urine levels of uric acid, oxalate, sodium urate, or cystine:** Often these can be secondary to a high protein diet, high oxalate diet, or a genetic defect causing increased excretion.

4. **Infection stones:** These are caused by urea-splitting organisms (*Proteus* or *Klebsiella* spp but not E. coli), that break down urea in the urine, increasing concentrations of ammonia and pH which promote stone formation and growth. Also called struvite or triple phosphate (Magnesium, Ammonium, Calcium) stones.

5. **Inadequate urinary citrate levels:** Citrate is the urinary equivalent of serum bicarbonate. It increases urinary pH, but it also acts as a specific inhibitor of crystal aggregation and stone formation. Optimal levels are approximately 250 mg/L to 300 mg/L of urine.

CLINICAL ASSESSMENT[21]

- **Patient History**
  - Patients with renal colic usually present with characteristic loin pain +/- radiation to the groin +/- vomiting and may have fever.
  - They usually but not always have haematuria (macroscopic or microscopic). However, 15% of patients with proven stone on imaging will not have haematuria.
  - They may have a previous history of renal calculus.

- **Physical Examination**
  - Abdominal examination is usually unremarkable. AAA may present with a similar presentation and should be considered in the appropriate patient age group- especially in males older than 50 years with a first presentation of suspected renal colic.

Differential Diagnosis	
• Pancreatitis	• Cholecystitis
• Appendicitis	• Renal carcinoma,
• Ovarian pathology and torsion	• Pyelonephritis
• PID	• Incarcerated hernia, e.g. abdominal and lumbar
• Pregnancy	• Diverticular disease
• Renal infarct	• Pneumonia
• Aortic aneurysm	

[19] Nadav G, Eyal K, Noam T, Yeruham K. Evaluation of the clinical significance of sonographic perinephric fluid in patients with renal colic. Am J Emerg Med. 2018 Dec 20; [PubMed]

[20] Frederic Coe. Kidney stone types [Online]

[21] Emergency Department Management of Renal Colic and Suspected Renal Calculus. IAEM Clinical Guideline p4. May 2014 [online]

EVALUATION

- Diagnosis is made through a combination of history and physical exam, laboratory and imaging studies.
- Urinalysis shows some degree of microscopic or gross hematuria in 85% of stone patients, but should also be evaluated for signs of infection (e.g., white blood cells, bacteria).
- Urinary pH greater than 7.5 may be suggestive of a urease producing bacterial infection, while pH less than 5.5 may indicate the presence of uric acid calculi.
- **Blood tests: FBC, U&E, Amylase, Phosphate, Urate, Bicarbonate and Calcium**
- Consider obtaining a **parathyroid hormone (PTH) level** if primary hyperparathyroidism is suspected as a cause of any hypercalcemia.

- **PLAIN KUB AND ABDOMINAL RADIOGRAPHY**
  - o An abdominal x-ray (KUB) can identify many stones, but 10% to 20% of renal stones are radiolucent and provide little information regarding hydronephrosis, obstruction or the kidneys.
  - o Additionally, bowel gas, the bony pelvis and abdominal organs may obstruct visualization of a stone. The KUB is recommended in kidney stone cases when the CT can is positive and the exact location of the stone is known.

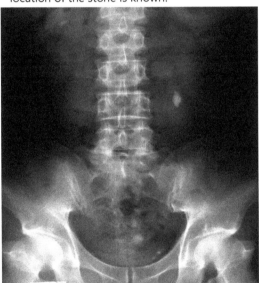

Abdominal Xray (KUB)

- **INTRAVENOUS UROGRAPHY (IVU)**
  - o Intravenous urography (IVU) is a traditional radiographic study of the renal parenchyma, pelvicalyceal system, ureters, and the urinary bladder.
  - o It involves the administration of intravenous contrast and require some degree of expertise the image.
  - o The delay in obtaining relevant information about the possible site of obstruction

  - o This exam has been largely replaced by non-contrast CT[22].
  - o Contraindications of IVU:
    - ↓ *Patients with renal failure,*
    - ↓ *Contrast allergy,*
    - ↓ *Pregnant women*
    - ↓ *Diabetics taking metformin.*

- **CT-KUB:**
  - o Non Contrast CT (NCCT)[23] has become the standard method for diagnosing acute flank pain.
  - o NCCT should be used to confirm a diagnosis in patients presenting with acute flank pain because it is superior to IVU. CT can demonstrate uric acid and xanthine stones which are radiolucent on plain films. CT also provides a better estimate of stone volume.
  - o A further advantage is the ability of CT to detect alternative diagnoses. Indinavir stones cannot be detected on NCCT.
  - o Immediate imaging is recommended with fever, a solitary kidney or when diagnosis is in doubt.
  - o Timing of imaging should be within 24 hours of ED presentation in order to confirm the diagnosis.

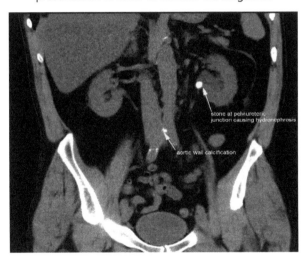

stone at pelviureteric junction causing hydronephrosis

aortic wall calcification

- **ULTRASOUND SCANNING**
  - o According to Radiopaedia[22], Ultrasound is frequently the first investigation of the urinary tract, and although by no means as sensitive as CT, it is often able to identify calculi. Small stones and those close to the corticomedullary junction can be difficult to reliably identify.
  - o Ultrasound compared to CT KUB reference showed a sensitivity of only 24% in identifying calculi. Nearly 75% of calculi not visualised were <3 mm.

---

[22] *Dr Adam Eid Ramsey and Dr Jeremy Jones et al. Urolithiasis. Radiopaedia [online]*

[23] *Emergency Department Management of Renal Colic and Suspected Renal Calculus. IAEM Clinical Guideline. May 2014 [online]*

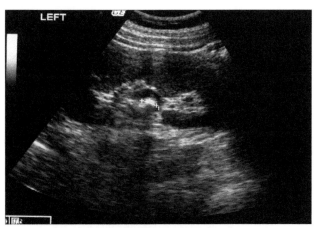
Ultrasound of the left Renal Stone

- **IMAGING IN PREGNANCY**
  o Incidence same as non-pregnant population
  o Like the non-pregnant person, 70-80% of the symptomatic stones pass spontaneously.
  o Ultrasound is the initial investigation of choice
  o Further investigations after discussion with radiologists

ED MANAGEMENT OF RENAL COLIC

- **Pain control:** either NSAIDs or opioids or combination of both.
  o NSAIDs: decrease spasm of ureter and decrease kidney capsule pressure by decreasing GFR.[24]
  o **Use caution** in those with underlying renal disease or problems with GI bleeding.
  o Opiates: fast onset.
  o Combination therapy with NSAID and opiate may decrease length of stay in ED.
- **Antiemetics:** Ondansetron (Zofran) and metoclopramide (Reglan) are commonly used. Reglan is the only antiemetic that has been studied in patients with renal colic. Reglan **not only has antiemetic properties, but enhances the effects of analgesia**. Two studies revealed that reglan provided equivalent pain relief compared to opioids.[25]
- **IV hydration:** routinely done, but **no studies show that fluids enhance stone passage or affect outcome**.
- **Medical expulsive therapy (MET):** Alpha-1 antagonists are frequently used to relax ureteral smooth muscle cells and improve stone passage. A recent systematic review concluded that Tamsulosin (Flomax) improved stone passage when compared to placebo.[26]

- While a few trials suggested that tamsulosin is an effective way to clear ureteral stones,[27] other studies suggest that there is no benefit.
- So, the bottom line is that it is **unclear if this is actually beneficial for the passage of renal stones**, and therefore is not employed as primary management of renal colic in the Emergency Department.
- **If septic:**
  o The presence of pyrexia mandates urgent full blood count, blood and urine cultures, creatinine and lactate levels should also be obtained.
  o Resuscitation using surviving sepsis guidelines in a High Dependency Unit environment is advised. A
  o ntibiotic options include **Gentamicin and Ceftazidime intravenously.**
- **If hydronephrosis**
  o **Urgent nephrostomy**- performed by a radiologist.
- **Stones causing significant ureteric obstruction and pain:** Stenting pending definitive treatment.

INDICATIONS FOR HOSPITAL ADMISSION

- Hospital admission is required if[28]:
  o The patient is in shock, has fever or signs of systemic infection.
  o There is pre-existing renal impairment or increased risk of loss of renal function.
  o There are bilateral obstructing stones.
  o There is no response to appropriate analgesia or abrupt recurrence of severe pain despite appropriate analgesia.
  o The patient is dehydrated and cannot take oral fluids due to vomiting.

LOW RISK PATIENTS

- Consider discharge for next day follow-up imaging in patients where[28]:
  o Urolithiasis is the likely diagnosis.
  o There is no suspicion of AAA.
  o There are no signs of sepsis.
  o Pain is controlled adequately.
  o The patient is able to pass urine.
  o Appropriate imaging is available the next day.
  o Social circumstances allow for discharge and return the next day

[24] Baun K, Easter J. Marx: Rosen's Emergency Medicine-Concepts And Clinical Practice. 8th ed. Elsevier Health Sciences; 2013:1336-1342.

[25] Pearle M, Goldfarb D, Assimos D et al. Medical Management of Kidney Stones: AUA Guideline. The Journal of Urology. 2014;192(2):316-324. doi:10.1016/j.juro.2014.05.006.

[26] Lu Z, Dong Z, Ding H, Wang H, Ma B, Wang Z. Tamsulosin for Ureteral Stones: A Systematic Review and Meta-Analysis of a Randomized Controlled Trial. Urologia Internationalis. 2012;89(1):107-115. doi:10.1159/000338909.

[27] Singh A, Alter H, Littlepage A. A systematic review of medical therapy to facilitate passage of ureteral calculi. Annals of emergency medicine. 2007;50(5):552–563.

[28] Emergency Department Management of Renal Colic and Suspected Renal Calculus. IAEM Clinical Guideline. May 2014 [online]

2. Acute Back Pain

INTRODUCTION

- For many individuals, episodes of back pain are self-limited. Patients who continue to have back pain beyond the acute period (four weeks) have subacute back pain (lasting between 4 and 12 weeks) and may go on to develop chronic back pain (persists for ≥12 weeks).
- Rarely, back pain is a harbinger of serious medical illness.

RED FLAG SYMPTOMS

- *Thoracic pain.*
- *Age of onset less than 20 or more than 55 years.*
- *Loss of control of the bowel or bladder.*
- *Weakness or numbness in a leg or arm.*
- *Foot drop, disturbed gait.*
- *High fever.*
- *Saddle anaesthesia (numbness of the anus, perineum or genitals).*
- *History of carcinoma.*
- *Structural deformity.*

ETIOLOGIES

1. Nonspecific back pain

- The vast majority of patients seen in primary care (>85 percent) will have nonspecific low back pain, meaning that the patient has back pain in the absence of a specific underlying condition that can be reliably identified.
- Many of these patients may have musculoskeletal pain.
- Most patients with nonspecific back pain improve within a few weeks.

2. Serious systemic etiologies

- Among patients who present with back pain to primary care settings, less than 1 percent will have a serious systemic etiology (cauda equina syndrome, metastatic cancer, and spinal infection).
- Almost all patients with these conditions will have risk factors or other symptoms.

a. Spinal cord or cauda equina compression

- There are many causes of cauda equina syndrome, the most common being herniation of the intervertebral disc.
- While the incidence of cord compression in patients known to have cancer varies depending on the cancer, among patients who are diagnosed with cord compression, it is the initial manifestation of malignancy in 20 percent[29].

- Metastatic disease from any primary cancer can cause cord compression.
- Pain is usually the first symptom of cord compression, but motor (usually weakness) and sensory findings are present in the majority of patients at diagnosis.
- Bowel and/or bladder dysfunction are generally late findings. Early diagnosis and treatment improves outcomes.

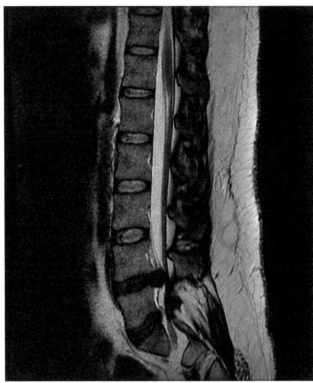

L4/5 disc extrusion causing cauda equina syndrome
Courtesy: radiopaedia

b. Metastatic cancer

- The bone is one of the most common sites of metastasis.
- A history of cancer (excluding nonmelanoma skin cancers) is the strongest risk factor for back pain from bone metastasis.
- Among solid cancers, metastatic disease from breast, prostate, lung, thyroid, and kidney cancers account for 80 percent of skeletal metastases.
- Approximately 60 percent of patients with multiple myeloma have skeletal lytic lesions present at diagnosis.
- Pain is the most common symptom.
- In patients with a history of cancer, sudden, severe pain raises concern for pathologic fracture.
- Patients may also have neurologic symptoms from either spinal cord compression or spinal instability.

---

[29] *Schiff D, O'Neill BP, Suman VJ. Spinal epidural metastasis as the initial manifestation of malignancy: clinical features and diagnostic approach. Neurology 1997; 49:452.*

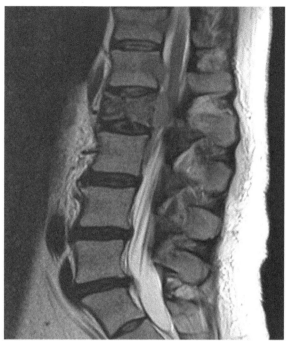

Metastatic Tumor to the Spine: Compression and Instability

c. Spinal epidural abscess

- Spinal epidural abscess is a rare but serious cause of back pain.
- Initial symptoms (eg, fever and malaise) are often nonspecific; over time, localized back pain may be followed by radicular pain and, left untreated, neurologic deficits.
- **Risk factors** include recent spinal injection or epidural catheter placement, injection drug use, and other infections (eg, contiguous bony or soft tissue infection or bacteremia).
- Immunocompromised patients may also be at higher risk. Treatment of spinal epidural abscess is reviewed in detail elsewhere.

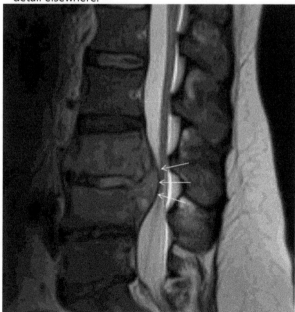

Spinal epidural abscess in brucellosis | BMJ Case Reports

d. Vertebral Osteomyelitis

- The majority of patients with vertebral osteomyelitis will present with back pain, which gradually increases over weeks to months; fever may or may not be present.

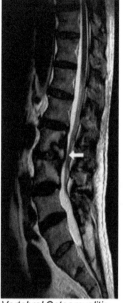

- The intervertebral disc may also be become infected (discitis), and the clinical presentation (positional discomfort, pain to palpation, neurologic signs/symptoms) may vary depending upon the extent of the infection.
- The incidence of vertebral osteomyelitis generally increases with age, and men are more commonly affected than women. Many cases are thought to be health care-related or postprocedural from hematogenous spread of bacteremia. Less specific risk factors include an immunocompromised state and injection drug use.

Vertebral Osteomyelitis

3. Less serious, specific etiologies
a. Vertebral compression fracture

- Approximately 4 percent of patients presenting in the primary care setting with low back pain will have a vertebral compression fracture[30]. While some produce no symptoms, other patients present with acute onset of localized back pain which may be incapacitating.
- There may be no history of preceding trauma.
- **Risk factors** for osteoporotic fracture include advanced age and chronic glucocorticoid use. A history of an osteoporotic fracture is a risk factor for subsequent fractures, which can be mitigated by pharmacologic therapy. Approximately 3 to 4 percent of patients who present in primary care settings with low back pain have a symptomatic disc herniation or spinal stenosis.

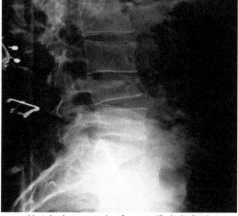

Vertebral compression fracture (Orthobullets)

[30] Jarvik JG, Deyo RA. Diagnostic evaluation of low back pain with emphasis on imaging. Ann Intern Med 2002; 137:586.

b. Radiculopathy

- Radiculopathy refers to symptoms or impairments related to a spinal nerve root.
- Damage to a spinal nerve root may result from degenerative changes in the vertebrae, disc protrusion, and other causes.
- The clinical presentations of lumbosacral radiculopathy vary according the level of nerve root or roots involved.
- Over 90 percent are L5 and S1 radiculopathies[31].
- Patients present with pain, sensory loss, weakness, and/or reflex changes consistent with the nerve root involved.
- Many patients with symptoms of acute lumbosacral radiculopathy improve gradually with supportive care.
- Sciatica is a nonspecific term used to describe a variety of leg or back symptoms.
- Usually, sciatica refers to a sharp or burning pain radiating down from the buttock along the course of the sciatic nerve (the posterior or lateral aspect of the leg, usually to the foot or ankle). Most sciatica is attributable to radiculopathy at the L5 or S1 level from a disc disorder.

c. Spinal stenosis

- Lumbar spinal stenosis is most often multifactorial. Spondylosis (degenerative arthritis affecting the spine) spondylolistheses, and thickening of the ligamentum flavum are the most common causes, typically affecting patients >60 years.
- Ambulation-induced pain localized to the calf and distal lower extremity resolving with sitting or leaning forward ("pseudoclaudication" or "neurogenic claudication") is a hallmark of lumbar spinal stenosis.
- Other symptoms of lumbar spinal stenosis can include back pain and sensory loss and weakness in the legs, though many patients may present with a normal neurologic exam.

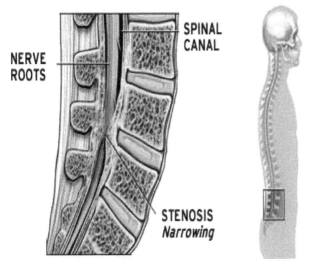

Spinal stenosis

- Symptoms of neurogenic claudication can usually be distinguished from vascular claudication. Rare patients develop a cauda equina syndrome.
- Patients often have symptoms only when active. Most patients with spinal stenosis related to osteoarthritis will have stable symptoms over time.

4. Other Etiologies
- Ankylosing spondylitis
- Osteoarthritis
- Scoliosis and hyperkyphosis
- Psychologic distress

5. Etiologies outside the spine
- Piriformis syndrome
- Sacroiliac joint dysfunction
- Bertolotti's syndrome

CLINICAL EVALUATION
HISTORY
- While it may not be possible to define a precise cause of low back symptoms for most patients, it is important to evaluate for evidence of specific etiologies of back pain.
- The history should include location, duration, and severity of the pain, details of any prior back pain, and how current symptoms compare with any previous back pain.
- We also ask about constitutional symptoms (eg, unintentional weight loss, fever, or night sweats), history of malignancy, precipitants or precipitating events, therapies attempted, neurologic symptoms (eg, weakness, falls or gait instability, numbness or other sensory changes, or bowel/bladder symptoms), stability or progression of symptoms, history of recent bacterial infections (particularly bacteremia), recent history or current use of injection drugs, history or current use of corticosteroid medications, and recent history of epidural or spinal procedures. Patients should also be evaluated for social or psychologic distress that may be contributing. Potentially useful items are a history of failed previous treatments, substance use disorder, and disability compensation. Screening for depression may be helpful. Features that may suggest underlying systemic disease include history of cancer, age >50 years, unexplained weight loss, duration of pain >1 month, nighttime pain, and unresponsiveness to previous therapies. Documented fevers, injection drug use, recent bacterial infection (particularly bacteremia), or recent epidural or spinal instrumentation increase the suspicion of spinal infection.

PHYSICAL EXAMINATION
- **Inspection of back and posture** – can reveal anatomic abnormalities such as scoliosis or hyperkyphosis.
- **Palpation/percussion of the spine** – usually performed to assess vertebral or soft tissue tenderness. Vertebral tenderness is a sensitive, but not specific, finding for spinal infection, and may also be seen in patients with vertebral metastases and osteoporotic compression fracture.

---

[31] *Acute low back problems in adults: assessment and treatment. Agency for Health Care Policy and Research. Clin Pract Guidel Quick Ref Guide Clin 1994; :iii.*

- **Neurologic examination** – Patients should have a neurologic examination including evaluation of the reflexes, strength, sensation, and gait. For patients suspected of having a radiculopathy, neurologic testing should focus on the L5 and S1 nerve roots, since most clinically significant radiculopathies occur at these levels.
- **Straight leg raising** – can be helpful in identifying whether symptoms are radicular in nature.
- **Nonorganic signs (Waddell's signs)** - Patients with psychologic distress that is contributing to back pain symptoms may have associated inappropriate physical signs, also known as "Waddell's signs". These include patient overreaction during physical examination, superficial tenderness, straight leg raise that improves when the patient is distracted, unexplainable neurological deficits (eg, nondermatomal distribution of sensory loss, sudden giving way or jerky movements with motor exam, inconsistency in observed spontaneous activity [dressing, getting off table]), and pain elicited by axial loading (pressing down on top of head, or rotating the body at hips or shoulders).

LABORATORY STUDIES

- Most patients with acute low back pain do not require any laboratory testing. In some patients with suspected infection or malignancy, we use the **ESR** and/or **CRP** in addition to plain radiographs to determine the need for advanced imaging.
- Because of its higher sensitivity, CRP may have similar or greater value than the ESR; however, CRP has not been similarly evaluated in the evaluation of low back pain.
- The ESR and CRP are also used in the diagnosis of ankylosing spondylitis.

IMAGING

- **Neurologic deficits** — Indications for imaging in the presence of neurologic symptoms depends upon the nature of the symptoms and the patient's risk factors for cancer and/or an infectious etiology of back pain.
  - Any patient with symptoms of spinal cord or cauda equina compression or progressive and/or severe neurologic deficits should have **immediate MRI** for further evaluation and urgent specialist referral. Such symptoms and signs include new urinary retention, urinary incontinence from bladder overflow, new fecal incontinence, saddle anesthesia, and significant motor deficits not localized to a single nerve root.

- **Infection** — For patients in whom there is a suspicion for spinal infection (including vertebral osteomyelitis or spinal epidural abscess), the evaluation should be guided by the degree of suspicion.

Moderate to high clinical suspicion for infection

- Immediate MRI without and with contrast is indicated.
- Sign and symptoms of infection may include objective fever, tenderness to palpation (vertebral osteomyelitis), and neurologic symptoms (spinal epidural abscess).

  - **Risk factors for infection include:**
    - Current immunosuppression
    - Current hemodialysis
    - Current or recent injection drug use
    - Current or recent invasive epidural/spinal procedure
    - Current or recent endocarditis or bacteremia

- MRI is the most sensitive imaging modality for detecting spinal infection with sensitivity of 0.96 and specificity of 0.92[32].
- For patients who are unable to obtain an MRI, a CT scan is a useful alternative to evaluate for epidural abscess, while radionuclide scans are an option to evaluate for osteomyelitis.
- The evaluation and diagnosis of these conditions are discussed in detail separately.

Lower concern for infection

- When there is a lower level of concern for the possibility of an infectious cause of back pain, it is reasonable to first evaluate patients with ESR and/or CRP. Patients with an elevated ESR and/or CRP should be evaluated with MRI.

- **Cancer** — Patients with cancer or risk factors for cancer and neurologic deficits should have immediate imaging as noted above. In patients without neurologic deficits, the decision to image is based on risk.

- **Compression fracture** — Patients with suspected vertebral compression fracture should have plain radiographs for evaluation. Features in the history that indicate an increased risk for vertebral fractures include prolonged glucocorticoid use, advanced age, significant trauma or presence of contusion or abrasion, or recent mild trauma in a patient with a known diagnosis of or risk factors for osteoporosis. Patients can have osteoporotic vertebral compression fractures in the absence of trauma.

- **Radiculopathy or lumbar spinal stenosis** — Patients with persistent symptoms due to a lumbosacral radiculopathy or spinal stenosis who have not responded to conservative treatment and who are candidates for and interested in invasive therapies (eg, surgery or epidural injection for radiculopathy) should have an MRI for further evaluation and be referred for consideration for these therapie.

- **Cancer risk** — In patients with low back pain who did not meet criteria for immediate imaging but who have risk factors for cancer and do not improve with conservative therapy after four to six weeks, we evaluate with plain radiographs and ESR (or CRP). Patients with a positive radiograph should have appropriate further evaluation for malignancy (eg, evaluation for primary site, other metastatic disease). Patients with a positive ESR (or CRP) but negative plain radiograph should be further evaluated with MRI.

---

[32] Jarvik JG, Deyo RA. Diagnostic evaluation of low back pain with emphasis on imaging. Ann Intern Med 2002; 137:586.

DIFFERENTIAL DIAGNOSIS

Possible diagnosis	Red flags
Spinal infection	• Fever. • Systemically unwell. • Recent bacterial infection. • Non-mechanical pain. • Pain worse at night. • IV Drug Users. • Immunosuppression. • HIV.
Tumour	• Age <20 or >50. • History of malignancy. • Non-mechanical pain. • Thoracic pain. • Systemically unwell. • Weight loss.
Vertebral fracture	• History of trauma (this may be minimal in the elderly or those with osteoporosis). • Prolonged steroid use.
Cauda equina syndrome	• Saddle anaesthesia. • Bladder or bowel dysfunction. • Gait disturbance. • Motor weakness (widespread or progressive) • Bilateral sciatica.
AAA	• Systemically unwell. • Cardiovascular compromise. • Pulsatile abdominal mass.
Inflammatory Rheumatic Disease (e.g. Ankylosing Spondylitis)	• Age <20. • Structural deformity of the spine. • Systemically unwell.

ED MANAGEMENT OF BACK PAIN

- **Symptomatic treatment of acute musculoskeletal lower back pain**
  - o Analgesia.
  - o Muscle relaxants.
  - o Patients should be advised to stay active.
  - o Physiotherapy.
  - o **Other treatments that have been investigated for low back pain are**:
    - ▪ Traction,
    - ▪ Massage,
    - ▪ Antidepressants.
    - ▪ Local heat,
    - ▪ Acupuncture,
    - ▪ Individual patient education for low back pain,
    - ▪ Spinal manipulative therapy,
    - ▪ Exercise therapy,
    - ▪ Lumbar supports,
    - ▪ Strong opiates (e.g. oramorph).
  - o Note that the above evidence largely relates to acute back pain.
  - o The results for chronic and subacute back pain may be different.
- **Treatment of Cauda Equina Syndrome**
  - o Urgent referral is required once the diagnosis has been made on MRI scanning.
- **Treatment of sciatica**
  - o Epidural
  - o Surgical discectomy
  - o Microdiscectomy
- **Treatment of vertebral compression fractures**
  - o **Osteoporosis** will also need to be investigated and managed.
  - o Postmenopausal women with an initial fracture are at much greater risk of subsequent fractures so this is very important and may help to prevent a future attendance with a hip fracture.
- **Treatment of metastatic disease**
  - o Patients with bone metastases and patients at high risk of developing bone metastases should be given information explaining what to do and who to contact if they develop symptoms of spinal metastases or spinal cord compression or if their symptoms progress while waiting for investigation.
  - o **Spinal cord compression** is an oncological emergency and treatment should be started within 24 hours. Most patients will be given **steroids** and will need **radiotherapy or surgery** *(See Chapter 27: Oncological emergencies)*.
  - o Patients with a risk of spinal instability should be nursed flat in neutral alignment.

3. Aggressive & Disturbed Behaviour in the ED

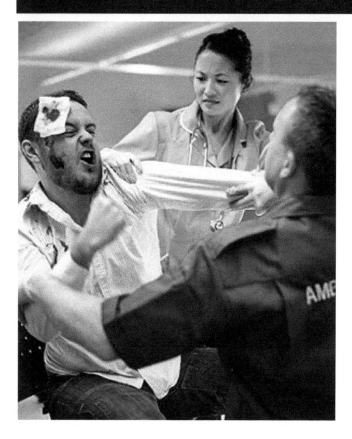

1. MEDICAL CAUSES OF VIOLENCE AND AGGRESSION IN PATIENTS
o   Head injury
o   Substance abuse and intoxication
o   Underlying Mental Illness
o   Hypoxia
o   Metabolic disturbances
o   Hypoglycaemia
o   Infection: Meningitis, Encephalitis, Sepsis
o   Hyperthermia or Hypothermia
o   Seizures: Post Ictal or Status Epilepticus
o   Vascular: Stroke or Subarachnoid Haemorrhage

2. RISK FACTORS FOR SUDDEN RELATED VIOLENCE
o   Younger age
o   Male gender
o   History of physical abuse by parent or guardian
o   History of violence
o   Past juvenile detention
o   Victimization in past year
o   Lower income
o   Unemployed and looking for work in the past
o   Substance dependence only
o   Comorbid mental health and substance disorder

3. INVESTIGATING THE VIOLENT AND AGGRESSIVE PATIENT
o   Blood sugar level
o   Full blood count
o   Urea, Electrolytes, Creatinine
o   Paracetamol,
o   Ethanol level
o   Urinalysis
o   Urine drug screen if available
o   +/- Head CT/MRI
o   +/- Lumbar Puncture

4. ED MANAGEMENT FOR VIOLENCE & AGGRESSION
A. DE-ESCALATION STRATEGIES
o   Consider personal safety at all times
o   Consider the safety of other patients and their visitors at all times
o   Place the person in a quiet and secure area and let staff know what is happening and why
o   Never turn your back on the individual
o   Don't walk ahead of the individual and ensure adequate personal space
o   Provide continuous observation and record behaviour changes in patient notes
o   Wear personal duress alarm if available
o   Let the person talk (everyone has a story to tell, let them tell it)
o   Never block off exits and ensure you have a safe escape route

B. INDICATIONS FOR RESTRAINING AND SEDATING A VIOLENT PATIENT
o   Preventing harm to the patient
o   Preventing harm to other patients
o   Preventing harm to caregivers and other staff

o Preventing serious disruption or damage to the environment
o To assist in assessing and management off the patient
o Restraints should never be use for ease of convenience

C. PHYSICAL/MECHANICAL RESTRAINTS

o Clinicians should beware of local policies, laws and acts before restraining patients.
o Applying physical restraint's is a team sport, **1 for each limb** and **1 to lead the restraint and manage the airway (Minimum of 5 persons).**
o Physical restraint should always be followed up with chemical and mechanical restraints.
o Physical restraints need to be secure enough to restrain the patient, but able to be easily removed if the patient begins to vomit, seizure, or loose's control of their airway.

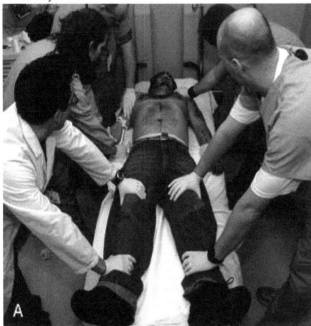

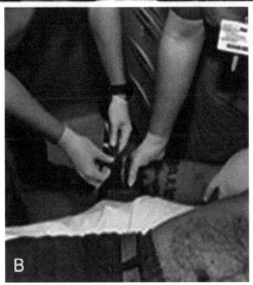

o Restraints must be applied in the least restrictive manner and for the shortest period of time.
o **Padding** should be applied between restraints and the patients to prevent neurovascular injury, and regular neurovascular observations should be performed every **15-30mins** whilst patient is physically restrained.
o The clinician ordering the restraints should **document the reason for restraints**, what limbs are restrained, how frequent neurovascular observations are needed, and when the restraints need reviewed, generally **every 2 hours'** restraints should be reviewed by treating clinician.

D. CHEMICAL RESTRAINTS/SEDATION

1. Benzodiazepines:
o **Lorazepam** 1-2mg PO
o **Midazolam** 2.5-5mg IV or IM increments and work upwards
o **Diazepam** 5-10 PO or IV increments and work upward

2. Antipsychotics:
o **Haloperidol** 2.5-10mg IV or IM
o **Olanzapine** 5-10mg PO or SL, or 10mg IM
o **Triperidol** 2.5-10MG IV or IM
o **Quetiapine** 25-200MG PO
o **Risperidone** 0.25-2mg PO/SL
o **Chlorpromazine** 100-200mg IV infusion over 24 hours

3. Barbiturates:
o **Thiopentone** 25mg IV increments until sedation has been achieved

Procyclidine is an anticholinergic drug principally used for the treatment of drug-induced Parkinsonism, Akathisia and Acute Dystonia; Parkinson disease; and idiopathic or secondary Dystonia.

5. COMPLICATIONS OF SEDATION AND RESTRAINING PATIENTS
o Respiratory Depression
o Pulmonary Aspiration
o Sudden cardiac death
o Excited delirium
o Hypotension,
o DVT & PE
o Rhabdomyolysis
o Dystonic reactions
o Neuroleptic Malignant Syndrome,
o Anticholinergic effects
o Delirium
o Lactic acidosis
o Lowered seizure threshold

4. Alcohol & Substance Abuse

ALCOHOL AND DRUG ABUSE IN ED

I. ALCOHOL USE DISORDER

- Alcohol Use Disorders (AUDs) carry considerable global morbidity and mortality, being identified by the World Health Organisation as directly responsible for 3.3 million deaths per year worldwide and contributing causally to more than 200 medical conditions including cardiovascular, gastrointestinal, neurological, and psychiatric disorders[33].
- Problematic alcohol consumption is classically associated with the younger population[34]; however, the 2014 National Psychiatric Morbidity Survey found that more than 1 in 6 adults aged 65-74 in England drink at hazardous levels or above, defined as a level of alcohol intake associated with risks of physical or psychological harm to the consumer .
- The ED may be the initial or only point of contact with the health care system for these patients.

1. UK RECOMMENDED ALCOHOL SAFE LIMITS

- According to the new guidelines, men should not drink more than **14 units of alcohol each week** – around 6 pints of beer.
- This is the same level as for women. Previous guidelines were 21 units for men and 14 units for women per week[35].
- The new guidelines move away from daily unit limits towards weekly limits, in order to demonstrate that it is not safe to drink every day.
- **No drinking during pregnancy:** The new guidelines state that pregnant women should not drink any alcohol at all. Previously they were advised to drink no more than 1 to 2 units of alcohol once or twice a week.

---

[33] World Health Organization Management of Substance Abuse Unit. Global status report on alcohol and health. World Health Organization (WHO). 2014.

[34] Griffin C, Bengry-Howell A, Hackley C, Mistral W, Szmigin I. 'Every time I do it I absolutely annihilate myself': Loss of (self-) consciousness and loss of memory in young people's drinking narratives. Sociology. 2009. 43(3):457-76.

[35] UK Chief Medical Officers' Low Risk Drinking Guidelines, published August 2016 [Online]

2. TERMINOLOGY
HARMFUL DRINKING
- It is defined as a pattern of alcohol consumption causing health problems directly related to alcohol.

HAZARDOUS DRINKING
- This is defined as drinking more than twice the recommended daily limit. This group can benefit from a brief intervention involving advice and information about reducing alcohol intake.

RISKY USE
- Risky alcohol use refers to consumption of an amount of alcohol that puts an individual at risk for health consequences. By definition, the condition of people with risky alcohol use is not so severe as to meet diagnostic criteria for an alcohol use disorder.
- Individuals with risky alcohol use may go on to develop an alcohol use disorder.

DEPENDENT DRINKING
- This is defined as drinking more than twice the recommended daily limit every day, **or demonstration of other signs of dependence.** This group do not benefit from brief intervention and need more complex management form specialist alcohol workers.

ALCOHOL DEPENDENCE
- It is characterised by craving, tolerance, a preoccupation with alcohol, and continued drinking in spite of harmful consequences. Someone who is alcohol-dependent may persist in drinking, despite harmful consequences.
- They will also give alcohol a higher priority than other activities and obligations.

BINGE DRINKING
- Binge drinking has been defined by as "drinking so much within about two hours that **blood alcohol concentration (BAC) levels reach 0.08g/dL".** Binge drinking is associated with acute injuries due to intoxication and may be associated with an increased cardiovascular risk.

2. ACUTE ALCOHOL WITHDRAWAL

- The physical and psychological symptoms that people can experience when they suddenly reduce the amount of alcohol they drink if they have previously been drinking excessively for prolonged periods of time.
- Alcohol use disorder (AUD) is defined by the World Health Organisation as consuming more than **40mg/day of alcohol for males and 30mg/day of alcohol for females**.

Definition

- Alcohol Withdrawal Syndrome (AWS) occurs as a spectrum of disease defined by DSM-5 as two or more of:
  - Insomnia
  - Autonomic dysfunction (tachycardia and sweating)
  - Tremor
  - Nausea and vomiting
  - Agitation
  - Anxiety
  - Seizures (generalised)
  - Hallucinations

- Symptoms can develop after anything from several hours to a few days following cessation of alcohol intake.
- Symptoms can range to mild tremor and anxiety through to Delirium Tremens (DT).
- DT represents the most severe form of AWS where patients develop a severe agitated delirium with hallucination.

- All patients who have Delirium tremens have Alcohol Withdrawal Syndrome but not all patients with Alcohol Withdrawal Syndrome have Delirium Tremens.

Clinical assessment and risk stratification
Screening for AUD

- Consider a comprehensive assessment for all adults referred to specialist services who score more than 15 on the Alcohol Use Disorders Identification Test (AUDIT).
- A comprehensive assessment should assess multiple areas of need, be structured in a clinical interview, use relevant and validated clinical tools, and cover the following areas[36]:
  - alcohol use, including:
    - consumption: historical and recent patterns of drinking (using, for example, a retrospective drinking diary), and if possible, additional information (for example, from a family member or carer)
    - dependence (using, for example, SADQ or Leeds Dependence Questionnaire [LDQ])
    - alcohol-related problems (using, for example, Alcohol Problems Questionnaire [APQ])
  - other drug misuse, including over-the-counter medication
  - physical health problems
  - psychological and social problems
  - cognitive function (using, for example, the Mini-Mental State Examination [MMSE])
  - readiness and belief in ability to change.

Requirement for Admission

NICE's guidance on alcohol use disorder states that patients:

- Presenting with or at risk of DT
- Presenting with or at risk of seizure
- Are frail, vulnerable or have multiple co morbidities
- Should be admitted for medically assisted withdrawal.
- Obviously, some patients will require admission as they have presented with another issue/condition.

Investigations

- Basic blood tests,
- ECG
- Basic imaging
- **CT Brain** might be mandated to rule out any occult head injury in patients presenting with confusion and agitation labelled as AWS.
- Patients with traumatic brain injury (TBI) may present with decreased cognition, confusion, somnolence, or unresponsiveness; all clinical pictures which are all easily mistakable for alcohol intoxication. The two also often occur in tandem, with alcohol use being a factor in at least 60% of TBIs[37].

Management (general and specific)
Management 1- symptom triggered scoring systems

- According to the IAEM guideline[38] , a **'Symptom-triggered treatment' (STT)** involves more frequent monitoring of withdrawal symptoms and involves earlier prescribing of benzodiazepines in most cases.
- Because of this, STT detoxification has a more favorable outcome than FDR . This has been shown to reduce hospital length of stay the number of readmissions, the overall dose of **benzodiazepine** required, and the severity of withdrawal symptom sequelae (i.e. seizures, agitation, hallucinations).

---

[36]Alcohol-use disorders: diagnosis, assessment and management of harmful drinking (high-risk drinking) and alcohol dependence . NICE CG115 [online]

[37] *Joe Bennett.* lcohol Intoxication Mimics: ED DDx + Approach to Management. [EMDocs online}

[38] IAEM CG: Management of acute Alcohol Withdrawal Syndrome in the Emergency Department Version 1, October 2019

- Furthermore, STT reduces the likelihood of under or over-treating a patient in AWS when compared to FDR.
- In general, **'Fixed-dose regimen' (FDR)** is more suitable for outpatient treatment where monitoring is not available. Benzodiazepines are proven to reduce withdrawal severity and incidence of both seizures and DTs. While any benzodiazepine can be used (chlordiazepoxide, lorazepam), diazepam is preferred in this guideline. Diazepam has the shortest time to peak effect, which facilitates rapid control of symptoms. It's long elimination half-life mediates a smoother withdrawal with a reduction in rebound and breakthrough symptoms[38].

MANAGEMENT OF PATIENTS ADMITTED TO WITH ALCOHOL WITHDRAWAL SYNDROME[38]

- Regular vital signs and neurological observation every 90 minutes.
- Routine blood investigations including FBC, U&E, Liver profile, Glucose and Coagulation test (if liver disease is suspected)
- Prophylaxis against Wernicke-Korsakoff syndrome should be given to all alcohol-dependent patients in ED/CDU as follows
  - ♣ **Pabrinex (1&2) once a day IV for 3 days** (or for the duration of their stay)
- In patients with signs of Wernicke-Korsakoff syndrome (delirium, ataxia, gaze palsy)
  - ♣ **Give IV thiamine** prior to glucose if possible
  - ♣ Give therapeutic dose of Pabrinex 2 pairs (1&2) TDS IV
- Regular CIWA-Ar scoring performed at 90 minutes intervals.
- Treat alcohol withdrawal with Diazepam based on CIWA-Ar score.
  - ♣ Absent to minimal withdrawal (score of 0-9): No treatment indicated, repeat CIWA-Ar in 90 min
  - ♣ Mild to moderate withdrawal (score of 10-19): **Diazepam 20mg stat PO**, repeat CIWAAr in 90 min
  - ♣ Severe withdrawal (score > 20): Diazepam 20mg stat PO, repeat CIWA-Ar in 90 min. CIWA-Ar can be repeated every 30-60 minutes in severe withdrawal.
- Look for deranged LFTs and for stigmata of chronic liver disease; consider Gastroenterology/Hepatology referral.
- Perform CT brain in FIRST seizure in patient with AWS. Recurrent withdrawal seizures can be treated with lorazepam/ phenytoin IV.
- If CIWA-Ar>10 after 24 hours, then:
  - ♣ Reassess and consider other diagnoses such as benzodiazepine dependency, drug seeking behavior, organic agitation as part of delirium or other cause.
  - ♣ Consider other drug treatment strategies and, if necessary, investigate further.

- ♣ SST can be extended after 24 hours after review by senior clinician.

Diazepam 10 mg = chlordiazepoxide 25mg = lorazepam 1mg

- SST aims at more frequent monitoring and scoring of withdrawal symptoms. By identifying moderate/severe symptoms earlier than would be indicated in a 'Fixed dose' treatment plan, patients benefit from a smoother and shorter withdrawal period.
- Patients in severe withdrawal may require PRN doses of Diazepam well before the next review/scoring period of 90 minutes. After patients have completed three successive assessments with a CIWA-Ar score of

Other complications of alcohol use disorder
1. Wernicke- Korsakoffs syndrome[39]

- Wernicke's encephalopathy is a degenerative brain disorder caused by the lack of thiamine (vitamin B1).
- It may result from alcohol abuse, dietary deficiencies, prolonged vomiting, eating disorders, or the effects of chemotherapy. B1 deficiency causes damage to the brain's thalamus and hypothalamus.
- Symptoms include mental confusion, vision problems, coma, hypothermia, low blood pressure, and lack of muscle coordination (ataxia).
- Korsakoff syndrome (also called Korsakoff's amnesic syndrome) is a memory disorder that results from vitamin B1 deficiency and is associated with alcoholism.
- Korsakoff's syndrome damages nerve cells and supporting cells in the brain and spinal cord, as well as the part of the brain involved with memory.
- Symptoms include amnesia, tremor, coma, disorientation, and vision problems, The disorder's main features are problems in acquiring new information or establishing new memories, and in retrieving previous memories. Although Wernicke's and Korsakoff's are related disorders, some scientists believe them to be different stages of the same disorder, which is called Wernicke-Korsakoff syndrome.
- **Wernicke's encephalopathy** represents the "acute" phase of the disorder and Korsakoff's amnesic syndrome represents the disorder progressing to a "chronic" or long-lasting stage. Most symptoms of Wernicke's encephalopathy can be reversed if detected and treated promptly and completely.
- Stopping alcohol use may prevent further nerve and brain damage. However, improvement in memory function is slow and, usually, incomplete. Without treatment, these disorders can be disabling and life-threatening.

---

[39] *Wernicke-Korsakoff Syndrome Information Page. The National Institute of Neurological Disorders and Stroke [Online]*

- **Treatment** involves replacement of thiamine and providing proper nutrition and hydration. In some cases, drug therapy is also recommended.
- Stopping alcohol use may prevent further nerve and brain damage.
- In individuals with Wernicke's encephalopathy, it is very important to start thiamine replacement before beginning nutritional replenishment.

2. Refeeding syndrome[40]

- Refeeding syndrome can be defined as the potentially fatal shifts in fluids and electrolytes that may occur in malnourished patients receiving artificial refeeding (whether enterally or parenterally).
- These shifts result from hormonal and metabolic changes and may cause serious clinical complications.
- The hallmark biochemical feature of refeeding syndrome is hypophosphataemia. However, the syndrome is complex and may also feature abnormal sodium and fluid balance; changes in glucose, protein, and fat metabolism; thiamine deficiency; hypokalaemia; and hypomagnesaemia.
- Electrolyte levels such as Urea&Electrolytes, Magnesium and Bone profile need to be checked regularly with dietician review.
- Correct any electrolyte abnormalitiesy if identified.

3. Hepatic Encephalopathy[41]

- Hepatic encephalopathy is a syndrome usually observed in patients with cirrhosis.
- Hepatic encephalopathy (HE) or portosystemic encephalopathy (PSE) is a reversible syndrome of impaired brain function occurring in patients with advanced liver failure. However, HE is not a single clinical entity. It may reflect either a reversible metabolic encephalopathy, brain atrophy, brain edema or any combination of these conditions.
- The mechanisms causing brain dysfunction in liver failure are still unknown. These factors are directly related to liver failure (e.g. decreased metabolism of ammonia).
- Unless the underlying liver disease is successfully treated, HE is associated with poor survival and a high risk of recurrence. Even in its mildest form, HE reduces health-related quality of life and is a risk factor for bouts of severe HE.
- The diagnosis of overt HE is based on a clinical examination and a clinical decision.
- Clinical scales are used to analyse its severity.

---

40 *Refeeding syndrome: what it is, and how to prevent and treat it. Hisham M Mehanna, Jamil Moledina, and Jane Travis. [Online]*

41 *Hepatic encephalopathy. Peter Ferenci. [Online]*

2. OPIATES

- Heroin is by far the most commonly abused opiate.
- Other drugs of abuse in this category include methadone, morphine, codeine, oxycodone, fentanyl (China white), and black tar (a potent form of heroin).
- Signs of intoxication are **decreased respiratory rate and pinpoint pupils.** Acute complications include **noncardiogenic pulmonary edema and respiratory failure.**

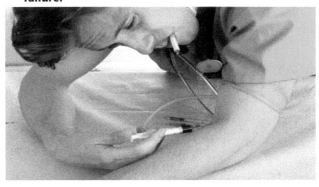

- Complications of chronic use are primarily infectious and include skin abscess at an injection site, cellulitis, mycotic aneurysms, endocarditis, talcosis, HIV, and hepatitis.
- Snorting of heroin is a recent trend that has expanded its user base in many areas.

3. COCAINE

- Cocaine may be smoked, inhaled, used topically, or injected. Acute cocaine intoxication may present with agitation, paranoia, tachycardia, tachypnea, hypertension, and diaphoresis.
- Complications of acute and chronic use can include myocardial ischemia or infarction, stroke, pulmonary edema, and rhabdomyolysis.

4. AMPHETAMINES

- Acute intoxication with amphetamines presents with signs of sympathetic nervous system stimulation, tachycardia, hypertension, anorexia, insomnia, and occasionally seizures.

5. HALLUCINOGENS

- Different hallucinogens present with a variety of organ system effects.
  - **Phencyclidine (PCP)** has been known to cause muscle rigidity, seizures, rhabdomyolysis, and coma.
  - **Anticholinergics** have been associated with delirium, supraventricular tachycardia, hypertension, and seizures.
  - **Other hallucinogens** (e.g., lysergic acid diethylamide [LSD], peyote, marijuana, nutmeg) rarely cause significant physical complications.

5. Anorectal Emergencies

I. ANAL PAIN

INTRODUCTION

- Anorectal disorders include a diverse group of pathologic disorders that generate significant patient discomfort and disability.
- Although these are frequently encountered in general medical practice, they often receive only casual attention and temporary relief. Diseases of the rectum and anus are common phenomena.
- Their prevalence in the general population is probably much higher than that seen in clinical practice, since most patients with symptoms referable to the anorectum do not seek medical attention.

Symptomatology of anorectal pathologies:

- Anal pain
- Bleeding per rectum
- Pus discharge from and around anus
- Prolapse
- Anal pruritus
- Presence of swelling or lumps in or around anus
- Passage of mucus per rectum
- Constipation or fecal obstruction
- Frequency of stool
- Difficulty in passing stool
- Incontinence to flatus or feces.

ETIOLOGIES[42]

- **The most common** anorectal lesions encountered in family practice are- (in the order of frequency):
  - Hemorrhoids [Internal or external]
  - Anal fissures [Acute or chronic]
  - Anal fistula [Low or high]
  - Abscesses [Perianal, ischio-rectal, submucus]
  - Polyps [Adenomatous, fibrous anal, juvenile]
  - Rectal Prolapse [Mucosal or complete]
  - Anal skin tags or sentinel pile
  - Anorectal sepsis [Hyderadenitis suppuritiva, AIDS, syphilis
- **Less Common:**
  - Sacro-coccygeal pilonidal sinus disease
  - Neoplasm [Benign or malignant]
  - Condylomas

  - Connective tissue masses like papilloma, fibroma, and lipoma.
  - Antibioma [Organized abscess]
  - Inflammatory conditions [Proctitis, anal cryptitis and papillitis]
  - Inflammatory bowel disorders [Ulcerative colitis and Crohn's disease]
  - Hypertrophied anal papillae.
- **Uncommon**
  - Strictures of anal canal or rectum
  - Solitary rectal ulcer
  - Incontinence [Flatus or feces]

INVESTIGATIONS

- The patient's history, and inspection and palpation of the anorectum remain the basic, essential features of diagnosis.
- A successful interaction with the patient leads to a diagnosis and a treatment plan that is acceptable to both the physician and the patient.
- **Anoscopy [proctoscopy]** remains the mainstay in the detection of anal pathologies.
- When a more proximal lesion is suspected, a **sigmoidoscopy or colonoscopy** along with **biopsy** is needed.
- Anorectal physiology and **endoanal ultrasonography** are also regarded as essential investigative techniques in a colorectal laboratory.

MANAGEMENT OF ANORECTAL DISEASES

- Most cases can be treated by conservative medical treatment (e.g., dietary changes, sitz baths, analgesics, antibiotics, stool softeners, hemorrhoidal creams and suppositories) or nonsurgical procedures.

ANAL FISSURES

- **Acute anal fissures** are superficial and are usually multiple. They respond well to conservative therapies like warm sitz bath, application of various hemorrhoidal creams, analgesics, and dietary modifications.
- Proper anal hygiene and correction of chronic constipation or diarrhea are essential to prevent recurrence of fissures.

---

[42] *Gupta PJ. Treatment trends in anal fissures. Bratisl Lek Listy. 105: 30-34, 2004*

- **Chronic anal fissures** are mostly found on the posterior or anterior midline. They are often associated with pathologies like sentinel tags, anal papillae, fibrous polyps or hemorrhoids. Therapies useful for acute fissures may only provide short-term relief in such chronic forms. In addition, they need some sort of internal sphincter manipulation. Such manipulation may be either surgical or nonsurgical.
- Despite the initial success with these pharmacological agents in the treatment of patients with chronic anal fissures, a growing concern is developing about their use. Increases in the incidences of adverse effects and a decrease in long-term efficacy have been the major drawbacks of such nonsurgical therapies.
- Surgery remains the option to be offered to patients with relapse or therapeutic failure of pharmacological treatment already undergone.

- o   Avoidance of colonic stimulants like coffee, tea and spices
- o   Use of flavonoid derivatives [Diosmin] and calcium dobisilate
- o   Use of hemorrhoidal creams, ointments and suppositories
- o   Use of anti-pruritics
- o   Adequate local hygiene

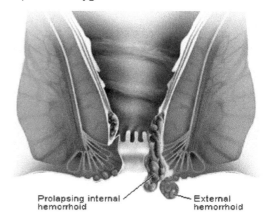

Prolapsing internal hemorrhoid — External hemorrhoid

a   b

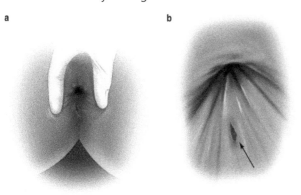

Anal fissure   Anal fissure

HAEMORRHOIDS

- It has been estimated that 50% of the population develops hemorrhoids by the age of 50[43].
- Although patients often consider the condition to be a single simple disease, it may not be so.
- Hemorrhoids share their symptoms with a whole series of other diseases and it is this lack of specificity that calls for a thorough examination to reach a precise diagnosis.

Medical treatment of haemorrhoids

- Although not constituting an etiological treatment of the disease, conservative treatment does have a role in relieving the symptoms of hemorrhoids and associated complaints[44].
- Medical treatment of haemorrhoids consists of:
  - o   Control of constipation using bran, mucilage, lactulose or bulk forming laxatives
  - o   Increasing daily intake of fiber

ANORECTAL ABCESS

- The anorectal area may be involved in several infectious and inflammatory processes. Abscesses often have their origin in an infection in the anal glands.
- The suppurative process then tracks through the various planes in the anorectal region.
- The infection can present at the anal verge as a perianal abscess. These abscesses can easily be drained in the office under local anesthesia.
- Bacterial, viral, and protozoal infections can be transmitted to the anorectum via anoreceptive intercourse.

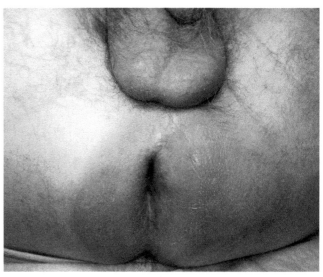

Anorectal abscess

---

43 *Orlay G. Haemorrhoids—a review. Aust Fam Physician. 2003; 32: 523-526.*

44 *Janicke DM, Pundt MR. Anorectal disorders. Emerg Med Clin North Am 14: 757-788, 1996.*

- Anorectal sepsis is a medical emergency requiring immediate hospitalization and treatment, including surgical debridement and high dosages of broad-spectrum antibiotics. Rarely, perineal sepsis can occur as a complication of rubber band ligation or sclerotherapy of internal hemorrhoids. Potential rectal complications arising out of HIV infection include infectious diarrhea, acyclovir-resistant strains of HSV2, Kaposi's sarcoma, lymphoma, and squamous cell carcinoma.

ANAL FISTULA

- Patients with fistulas are generally referred to a specialist for treatment. In addition to simple fistulotomy, treatments include cutting or draining setons, endo-anal mucosal advancement flaps, sliding cutaneous advancement flaps, fistulectomy with muscle repair and fibrin glue injection.

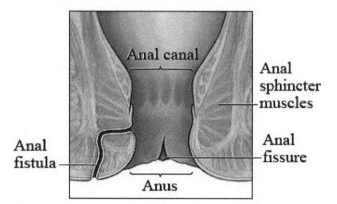

Pilonidal Abscesses and Sinuses

- Pilonidal abscesses can be drained under local anesthesia in the office. Sinuses can be laid open in a similar manner.
- The presence of hair in the wound is one of the prime causes of incomplete healing or recurrence.
- The hair should be meticulously shaved at regular intervals. Care should be taken that the wound continues to remain free of hair all the time. Multiple or recurrent sinuses should be dealt with only by specialist centers.

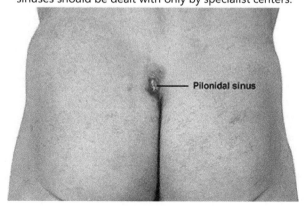

RECTAL PROLAPSE

- Rectal prolapse may be mucosal or full thickness [procedentia]. In mucosal prolapse, there is a complete eversion of the anal mucosa. On the other hand, rectal prolapse is a full-thickness evagination of the rectal wall outside the anal opening.
- Generally, a prolapsed rectum can be reduced with gentle digital pressure; an incarcerated rectal prolapse is rare. Several maneuvers to help reduce the prolapse have been described and include sedation, field block with local anesthetic, and sprinkling the prolapse with either salt or sugar to decrease the edema and to reduce the prolapse.
- Although no medical treatment is available for rectal prolapse, internal prolapse should always be first treated medically with **bulking agents, stool softeners, and suppositories or enemas**. Biofeedback may be helpful if paradoxical pelvic floor contraction also exists.

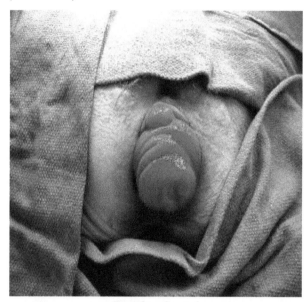

Rectal prolapsed

- Contributing factors, such as constipation and diarrhea, should be addressed and eliminated if possible.
- Supportive care should be provided according to the clinical picture, particularly in the presence of an irreducible prolapse and with gangrene or rupture of the rectal mucosa. Obtain a prompt surgical evaluation if anal incontinence is present.
- If the prolapse cannot be reduced and the viability of the bowel is in question, emergency resection is required. Rupture of the rectum also constitutes a surgical emergency. Obtain a prompt surgical consultation with a general surgeon or a colorectal surgeon.
- In cases of uncomplicated rectal prolapse, arrange surgical follow-up care for further evaluation and definitive treatment.

RECTAL POLYPS

- The commonest type is the adenomatous polyp, which may be scattered throughout the colon.
- A complete colonic evaluation is mandatory to determine the extension of the pathology. These polyps may well be a precursor to malignancy.
- A child presenting with bleeding per the rectum and the protrusion of 'something' from the anus may have a juvenile rectal polyp, which needs colonoscopy, biopsy, and removal. Occasionally, fibrous anal polyps may be found in association with anal fissures or hemorrhoids. These also have to be removed.

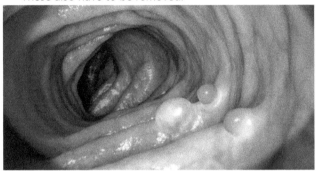

Colorectal polyps

ANORECTAL MALIGNANCY

- Treatment of malignancies of the rectum and anal canal- Cancer of the anorectum can manifest itself in many different symptoms or may be found incidentally during rectal examination. Pain in the early stages is usually absent, and the pathology may generally be considered to be and treated as 'piles' because of intermittent bleeding per the rectum. An external or internal mass may be palpable. Anal cancer can present as an ulcer, as a polyp, or as a verrucous growth.
- Most anal cancers respond well to treatment with combined chemotherapy and pelvic radiation.
- Colorectal cancers almost always need surgical treatment. Once these cancers become symptomatic, the prognosis worsens. When it is diagnosed at an early stage, 95% of patients with colorectal cancer may well survive for periods exceeding 5 years.

ANAL WARTS [CONDYLOMAS]

- These present as warty growths in or around the anus.
- There may be a single wart, or there may be a crop growth of different sizes extending in the perineum and genitals. Although common in those who engage in anal intercourse, they can also occur in patients with no such history in whom the infection is believed to occur due to the pooling of secretions in the anal area from elsewhere.

- These warts can produce pruritus, soiling and bleeding and may be a constant source of irritation. Various office procedures are available for their treatment.
- Treatment of anal warts:
  o Application of 85% trichloroacetic acid [TCA]
  o Cryotherapy (oral interferon and fluorouracil)
  o Radiofrequency (ablation, laser removal, electrodessication, surgery)

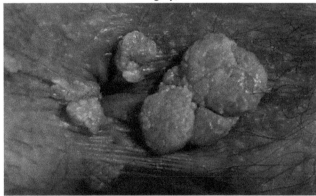

Anal warts

INFLAMMATORY BOWEL DISEASES

- The anorectal area can be involved in several infectious and inflammatory processes. They present with rectal discomfort, tenesmus, rectal discharge, and constipation/increased stool frequency.
- The rectal mucosa are often friable, and these processes are usually associated with a mucopurulent discharge.
- **Ulcerative colitis or Crohn's disease** can involve the rectal area, presenting as proctitis or fistulae.
- A fulllength colonoscopy and biopsy are needed to establish the diagnosis. Medical treatment proves beneficial in most patients.
- Drugs like sulfasalazine, 5-aminosalicylic acid and corticosteriods have often been found effective in containing the problem.
- These medicines are also used in the form of suppositories and enemas. In to case of failure of medical therapy or recurrence, surgical intervention is indicated.

EXTERNAL ANAL TAGS

- These are usually asymptomatic.
- They are mere remnants of old thrombosed external hemorrhoids.
- If these tags cause symptoms like itching, anxiety, or hygienic problems, they can be removed under local anesthesia. If they are too extensive, excision may be needed under a short general anesthesia.

ANAL STENOSIS OR STRICTURE

- A conservative approach using stool softeners, osmotic agents, and lubricants that ensure the smooth passage of the stool is effective in most cases.
- Regular anal dilatation using a metal dilator is another option in anal strictures of recent origin. If the above treatment fails, then surgical correction is needed.

SOLITARY RECTAL ULCER

- This is found less commonly, and the pathology can affect patients of all ages. Chronic solitary ulcer is usually associated with defecation disorders and is often confused with or mistaken for rectal cancer.
- The patient presents with an ulcerated mass.
- The appearance closely resembles cancer. The lesion must be biopsied to make sure that it is not neoplastic.
- Treatment includes laxatives and excision in appropriate cases.

INCONTINENCE

- Treatment is generally directed at the underlying cause and minimizing symptoms. Discrete muscle injuries are usually best treated by surgical sphincter repair.
- Fecal incontinence secondary to neuropathy is treated with bulking and antimotility agents.
- Recent approaches to the surgical therapy of incontinence include the use of an artificial bowel sphincter, and the electrical stimulation of sacral nerves to modify pelvic floor function[45].

RECTAL INJURIES

- Rectal injuries may result from penetrating or blunt trauma, iatrogenic injuries, or the presence of foreign bodies. Rectal injury should be suspected when a patient presents with low abdominal, pelvic, or perineal pain or bleeding per the rectum after sustaining trauma or undergoing an endoscopic or surgical procedure.

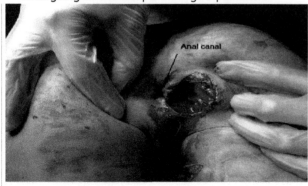

- Tetanus prophylaxis, intravenous antibiotics, and surgical intervention are indicated in all but superficial rectal tears.

CONSTIPATION

- This is a symptom that is not measurable scientifically.
- It has more emotional components than physical ones and should therefore be dealt with in a holistic manner.
- It is important to determine whether the patient is complaining of infrequent defecation, excessive straining at defecation, abdominal pain or bloating, a general sense of malaise attributed to constipation, soiling, or a combination of symptoms. It is imperative to rule out any definable abnormality as a cause of the symptoms.
- The treatment of constipation is multimodal. The patient should be reassured and asked to stop current treatment for constipation, if any.
- The patient may be made aware of the need to recognize the call for stool, to attend to it forthwith, and to not to postpone it for any reason, and should be encouraged to adopt a regular defecation schedule.
- Daily dietary fiber intake should be increased and bulking agents like ispaghula [psyllium], methyl cellulose, bran, karaya gum, and similar preparations that are useful in facilitation of the defecatory process should be prescribed.
- **Lactulose, sorbitol, and lactilol** have minimal known side effects and are considered safe in pregnancy and for children. They may also be prescribed for elderly patients.
- **Senna, bisacodyl, sodium picosulfate, and magnesium salts** should be used with caution as they can cause symptoms like bloating, colicky pain, and purging.
- **Low doses of polyethylene glycol and sodium phosphate** may be used for intermittent lavage of the bowel.
- Drugs like **cisapride, mosapride, itiopride, and docusates** are known to improve intestinal motility and may be prescribed for a prescribed duration.
- **Liquid paraffin** is perhaps one of the most widely consumed oral laxatives. However, its long-term use could lead to reduced absorption of fat-soluble vitamins.
- For patients with intractable constipation behavioral techniques to modify **pelvic floor and intestinal function** are now being considered as the mainstay of therapy. A combination of bowel training, dietary management, and regular exercise could possibly help achieve complete relief from the problem.

45 Kamm MA. Diagnostic, pharmacological, surgical, and behavioral developments in benign anorectal disease. Eur J Surg Suppl. 119- 123, 1998.

II. ACUTE LOWER GIT BLEEDING

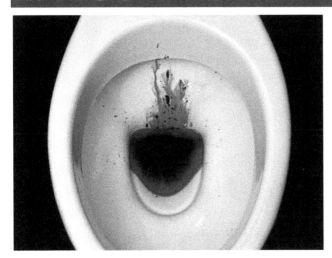

INTRODUCTION

Lower gastrointestinal bleeding (LGIB) accounts for approximately 20%-33% of episodes of gastrointestinal (GI) hemorrhage, with an annual incidence of about 20-27 cases per 100,000 population in Western countries. However, although LGIB is statistically less common than upper GI bleeding (UGIB), it has been suggested that LGIB is underreported because a higher percentage of affected patients do not seek medical attention. Indeed, LGIB continues to be a frequent cause of hospital admission and is a factor in hospital morbidity and mortality, particularly among elderly patients[46].

DEFINITION

Acute LGIB has been defined as bleeding that is of recent duration, originates beyond the ligament of Treitz, results in instability of vital signs, and is associated with signs of anemia with or without the need for blood transfusion.
LGIB is generally classified under three groups according to the amount of bleeding.
Massive hemorrhage is a life-threatening condition and requires transfusion of at least 4 units (U) of blood within 1 hour.

Massive lower GI bleeding is defined by:

*   *Passage of large volume of blood PR*
*   *Haemodynamic instability or shock*
*   *Initial decrease in haematocrit level of 6g/dL*
*   *Transfusion of at least 2 units of RCC*
*   *Bleeding that continues for 3 days*
*   *Significant re-bleeding within 1 week*

46 *Qayed E, Dagar G, Nanchal RS. Lower gastrointestinal hemorrhage.* Crit Care Clin. *2016 Apr. 32(2):241-54.*

CAUSES
These include:
*   *Diverticular disease*
*   *Inflammatory bowel disease*
*   *Neoplasia*
*   *Benign anorectal disease*
*   *Angiodysplasia*
*   *Other causes of lower GI bleeding include:*
    o   *Radiation injury*
    o   *Meckels Diverticulum*
    o   *Other small bowel pathology*
    o   *Solitary Rectal Ulcers*
    o   *Portal colopathy*
    o   *Prostate biopsy sites*
    o   *Dieulafoy lesions*
    o   *Endometriosis*
    o   *Colonic varices*

10-15% of patients with an apparent lower GI bleed will in fact have an upper GI source for their bleeding

DIVERTICULOSIS

*   Diverticulosis is the most common cause of lower gastrointestinal bleeding. Diverticula are outpouchings of the bowel wall that are composed only of mucosa, most commonly in the descending and sigmoid colon.
*   Their incidence increases with age. Diverticular disease bleeds are classically painless, whilst diverticulitis is classically painful.

HAEMORRHOIDS

*   Haemorrhoids are pathologically **engorged vascular cushions** in the anal canal that can present as a mass, with pruritus, or fresh red rectal bleeding.
*   The blood is classically on the **surface of the stool** or toilet pan, rather than mixed in with it. Large haemorrhoids can also **thrombose** which can be extremely painful.

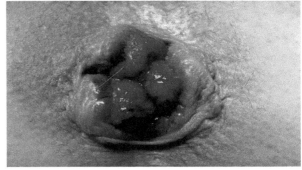

Haemorrhoids located in the 3, 7, and 11 o'clock positions

MALIGNANCY

- With any case of PR bleeding, especially in the elderly population, **malignancy should be suspected**, as this may be a colorectal cancer.
- In the assessment of any patient with haematochezia, it is important to enquire about **other lower GI symptoms**, **weight loss**, or **relevant family history**, potentially suggestive a diagnosis of malignancy.

CLINICAL Features

Key aspects to ascertain from clinical assessment include:

- **Nature of bleeding**, including duration, frequency, colour of the bleeding, relation to stool and defecation
- **Associated symptoms**, including pain (especially association with defaecation), haematemesis, PR mucus, or previous episodes
- **Family history** of bowel cancer or inflammatory bowel disease
- A **PR examination** is essential for every patient presenting with haemotochezia, allowing assessment for any rectal masses or anal fissures.

INVESTIGATIONS

- All patients presenting with rectal bleeding should have **routine bloods*** (FBC, U&Es, LFT, coagulation studies) and a **Group and Save** requested (as a minimum).
- The presence of an elevated serum urea to creatinine ratio (>30:1) suggests an **upper GI source of bleeding** being more likely.
- **Stool cultures** are also useful to exclude infective causes
- ABG, ECG, PR & FOB, CXR

*Acute bleeds may not initially show reduced Hb level due to haemoconcentration, however ongoing bleeding will show a reduced Hb

BLEED CRITERIA (HIGH RISK):

- *Ongoing bleeding*
- *Hypotension (SBP < 100mmHg)*
- *Abnormal clotting (PT > 1.2 sec)*
- *Altered mental status*
- *Significant co-morbidities*

ED MANAGEMENT OF GI BLEEDING

- Resuscitate patient – O2, IV fluids +/- blood
  - Shocked patients should receive fluid therapy to a MAP of 65 mmHg and red cells transfused after loss 30% circulating volume.
- Monitoring - include stool chart for colour and volume.

- Platelets may be required for those on antiplatelet agents. For information on massive blood ransfusion (i.e. needing platelets and FFP).
- Reverse bleeding disorders.
- Colonoscopy with haemostatic techniques like clipping/adrenaline injections.
- If bleeding continues significantly and resources available then embolization.
- If above fails/not available the surgical intervention – laparotomy.

ADMIT OR DISCHARGE FROM ED

(adapted from SIGN guidelines)

Consider for discharge with outpatient follow up if:

- age <60
- no evidence of haemodynamic compromise, and;
- no evidence of gross rectal bleeding, and;
- an obvious anorectal source of bleeding on rectal examination

Consider for admission if:

- age ≥60 years, or;
- haemodynamic disturbance, or;
- evidence of gross rectal bleeding, or;
- taking anticoagulation/antiplatelet agent.

For those admitted:

- patients with continued brisk bleeding/haemodynamic instability/significant comorbidities should be admitted to ICU.
- patients who are haemodynamically stable with minimal active bleeding are candidates for ward admission with close monitoring.
- patients who undergo intervention should not come back to the ED and should go to the ward/ICU following the procedure.

Further References and Resources

- *Scottish Intercollegiate Guidelines Network: Healthcare Improvement Scotland (2008) - Management of Acute Upper and Lower Gastrointestinal Bleeding - Guideline 105*
- *Cagir, B (2014) 'Lower Gastrointestinal Bleeding', Medscape.*
- *Raphaeli, T & Menon, R (2012) 'Current treatment of Lower Gastrointestinal Hemorrhage', Clinical Colon Rectal Surgery, December, vol. 25, no. 4, pp. 219-227.*
- *Life In The Fast Lane - Lower GI Bleeding Management Flow Chart*

6. Blackout & Syncope
I. TRANSIENT LOSS OF CONCIOUSNESS (TLoC)

1. INTRODUCTION

- **Transient loss of consciousness:** sudden onset, complete loss of consciousness of brief duration with relatively rapid recovery; distinct from persistent loss of consciousness or coma in its causes, assessment and management
- **Blackout:** synonymous with transient loss of consciousness
- **Faint:** synonymous with transient loss of consciousness
- **Syncope:** transient loss of consciousness due to global cerebral hypoperfusion caused by hypotension secondary to a fall in cardiac output (CO) and/or systemic vascular resistance (SVR). It is a common chief complaint of patients presenting to the emergency department
- **Seizure:** episode of abnormal electrical activity in the brain
- **Convulsion:** rapid, repetitive muscle contraction, which may be a feature of seizures
- **Collapse:** implies patient lost consciousness and fell over
- **Mechanical fall:** implies patient fell over but there was no preceding loss of consciousness eg due to slipping or tripping; a term disliked by geriatricians because it implies there is no medical problem and discourages people from investigating the cause of the fall; the assessment of falls will be covered elsewhere

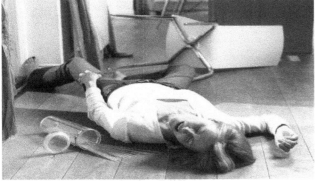

Image Source: Health Digest

- The differential diagnosis for syncope is broad and the management varies significantly depending on the underlying etiology.

- In the emergency department, determining the cause of a syncopal episode can be difficult.
- However, a thorough history and certain physical exam findings can assist in evaluating for life-threatening diagnoses.
- Risk-stratifying patients into low, moderate and high-risk groups can assist in medical decision making and help determine the patient's disposition.
- Advancements in ambulatory monitoring have made it possible to obtain prolonged cardiac evaluations of patients in the outpatient setting.

2. PATHOPHYSIOLOGY OF SYNCOPE

- Syncope is a symptom and not a diagnosis.
- Properly defined, syncope is a transient loss of consciousness with return to baseline neurological function without medical intervention.
- The pathophysiology of a syncopal episode is the same regardless of the cause. Syncope occurs due to a period of global hypoperfusion of the cerebral cortex or focal hypoperfusion of the reticular activating system that results in a loss of consciousness.
- Patients with loss of consciousness that have a persistent alteration in mental status, new neurological complaints or loss of consciousness that is related to alcohol or illicit drugs are not classified as true syncope.

SYNCOPE VS. NEAR SYNCOPE

- Near syncope is a spectrum of syncope and should be approached similarly. The key difference is that in near syncope the hypoperfusion of the brain does not result in loss of consciousness.
- The mechanism and causes of near syncope are identical to syncope[47]. In general, patients with near syncope tend to be younger and have fewer comorbidities.
- Although patients with near syncope have about half as many serious outcomes—including arrhythmias and death—the occurrence of these outcomes is still significant.

---

[47] *Quinn JV. Syncope and presyncope: same mechanism, causes, and concern. Ann Emerg Med 2015; 65:277-8.*

3. ETIOLOGY OF SYNCOPE

Classification	Definition	Causes
Neurocardiogenic	Inappropriate vasodilation ± bradycardia	Increases vagal tone (micturation, defecation); situational (prolonged standing); vagal nerve stimulation (shaving)
Orthostatic	Documented postural hypotension with symptoms	Drop in systolic blood pressure by ≥ 20 mmHg or tachycardia > 20 bpm; example : volume loss, dysfunction of autonomic nervous system, medication side effects
Neurologic	Least common, must return to baseline with no neurological defecits	Example: transient ischemic attack's, seizure, complex migraine, subclavian steal
Cardiac	Most dangerous form, can be life-threatening, multiple etiologies	Arrhythmias (tachy or brady), valvular heart disease, myocardial infarction, cardiac tamponade
Unknown	Unexplained despite thorough work-up	Rule out potential life-threatening causes

CARDIAC ETIOLOGIES OF SYNCOPE

Example of the most common causes of syncope based on underlying cardiac etiology

	Examples
Tachyarrhythmia	Ventricular tachycardia, ventricular fibrillation, WPW with SVT
Bradyarrhythmia	Sinus bradycardia, Mobitz II, 3rd degree AV block
Valvular lesion	Aortic stenosis, mitral stenosis
Myocardial infarction	Rare
Cardiac tamponade	Myocardial rupture, pericarditis, aortic dissection
Channelopathy	Brugada, prolonged QT, short QT

4. EMERGENCY DEPARTMENT APPROACH[48]

- In the ED setting, patients that present with syncope can be risk stratified to determine who needs further investigation.
- Patients with apparent neurologic or cardiac causes should be admitted.
- Patients with vagal and orthostatic syncope can be safely discharged once medically optimized.
- In the remaining patients, the question to consider is who is at risk for a lethal arrhythmia and whether this is something that can be accurately predicted.

HISTORY

- Ask the person who has had the suspected TLoC, as well as any witnesses, to describe what happened before, during, and after the event.
- Try to contact, by telephone, any witnesses who are not present at the consultation. Record details about:
  - Circumstances of the event;
  - Person's posture immediately before tloc;
  - Presence or absence of any prodromal symptoms (such as sweating or feeling warm/hot) and movement during event (for example, jerking of the limbs and duration);
  - Appearance (for example, whether eyes were open or shut) and colour of the person during the event;
  - Any biting of the tongue (record whether the side or the tip of the tongue was bitten);
  - Injury occurring during the event (record site and severity);
  - Duration of the event (onset to regaining consciousness);
  - Presence or absence during the recovery period of confusion or weakness down one side; and
  - Current medication that may have contributed to tloc (for example, diuretics).

- Ask also about details of any previous TLoC, including number of episodes and frequency, as well as the person's medical history and any family history of cardiac disease (for example, personal history of heart disease and family history of sudden cardiac death).

---

[48] *National Institute for Health and Clinical Excellence. Transient loss of consciousness ('blackouts') management in adults and young people. London: NICE; 2010. NICE clinical guideline 109. [Online]*

EXAMINATION

- Perform examination as clinically indicated. For example:
  - o Check and record vital signs (such as pulse rate, respiratory rate, and temperature) and lying and standing blood pressure, if clinically appropriate;
  - o Examine for other cardiovascular and neurological signs, such as cardiac murmurs or neurological deficit, where relevant.

ELECTROCARDIOGRAM

- It is recommended that everyone has a 12-lead electrocardiogram (ECG) recorded using automated interpretation.
- If any of the following abnormalities are present, referral within 24 hours for specialist cardiovascular assessment is recommended:
  - o conduction abnormality (for example, complete right- or left-bundle branch block or any degree of heart block);
  - o evidence of delayed atrioventricular conduction, including bundle branch block;
  - o evidence of a long or short QT interval; or
  - o any ST segment or T wave abnormalities.

- **Electrocardiogram 'red flags' that should prompt specialist cardiovascular assessment within 24 hours:**
  - o Inappropriate persistent bradycardia
  - o Any ventricular arrhythmia (including ventricular ectopic beats)
  - o Long QT (corrected QT >450 ms) and short QT (corrected QT <350 ms) intervals
  - o Brugada syndrome[a]
  - o Ventricular pre-excitation (part of Wolff-Parkinson-White syndrome)
  - o Left or right ventricular hypertrophy
  - o Abnormal T wave inversion
  - o Pathological Q waves
  - o Atrial arrhythmia (sustained)
  - o Paced rhythm

[a] *An inherited ion channel disorder, characterised by abnormal ST segment elevation in leads V1 to V3 on electrocardiogram. This predisposes the individual to ventricular arrhythmia and sudden cardiac death and may present with syncope.*

- The possibility of underlying problems that are either causing or contributing to TLoC should not be forgotten; relevant examinations and investigations may be required (for example, into blood glucose or haemoglobin levels).

4. NON-SYNCOPAL TLoC

- Seizure: Epileptic, Non-epileptic
- Hypoglycaemia
- Falls, Trauma, Head injury
- Dizziness or Vertigo without loss of consciousness.
- Cataplexy, Narcolepsy
- TIA, Stroke (very unlikely as a cause of LOC is no positive neurology on examination)
- Drop attack.
- Psychogenic pseudosyncope

EPILEPSY

- People who present with features that are strongly suggestive of epileptic seizures will require referral to a specialist in epilepsy. Features to note are:
  - o a bitten tongue;
  - o head turning to one side during TLoC;
  - o no memory of abnormal behaviour that was witnessed before, during, or after TLoC by someone else;
  - o unusual posturing;
  - o prolonged jerking of limbs (note that brief seizure-like activity can often occur during uncomplicated faints);
  - o confusion following the event;
  - o prodromal *déjà vu* (whereby an unfamiliar situation feels familiar or is recognised) or *jamais vu* (whereby a familiar situation feels totally unfamiliar or is not recognised).

SEIZURE vs SYNCOPE

CLINICAL FEATURES OF SYNCOPE		
Feature	**Seizure**	**Syncope**
Trigger	Rare	Common
Prodrome	Aura – unpleasant smell, epigastric sensation	Presyncopal features like nausea, sweating, pallor
Onset	Sudden	Gradual
Duration	1–3 minutes	1–30 seconds
Colour	Cyanosed	Usually pale
Convulsions	Tonic-clonic movements, automatism, neck turned to one side	May have movement after loss of consciousness
Tongue bite	Common, on the side	Rare, usually on the tip
Post event	Confusion, aching muscles, joint dislocations	Rapid recovery, nausea or vomiting afterwards

5. RISK STRATIFICATION

1. OESIL (Osservatorio Epidemiologico della Sincope nel Lazio) Score:

This score is based on the presence of:

- *Age over 65 years;*
- *Previous history of cardiovascular disease;*
- *Syncope without prodrome and*
- *Abnormal ECG*

It predicts 12-month mortality which rises from under 1% for patients with no risk factors to over 50% in patients with all 4 risk factors.

2. The San Francisco Rule

The San Francisco Syncope Rule: CHESS
Congestive cardiac failure history
Haematocrit < 30%
ECG abnormality; new, any non-sinus rhythm
Shortness of breath
Systolic Blood Pressure <90 mm Hg
The presence of any factor is considered sufficient for the patient to be high risk.

In the original validation study, the incidence of serious adverse events was 6.7% with the rule being 98% sensitive and 56% specific to predict adverse events.

3. The EGSYS Score:

Predictor	Score
Palpitations preceding syncope	4
Syncope during effort	3
Heart disease/ abnormal ECG	3
Syncope while supine	2
Precipitating/ Predisposing factors	-1
Autonomic prodromes	-1

This specifically identified cardiac syncope with a score of 3 or more being 99% sensitive and 65% specific for identifying cardiac syncope (positive and negative predictive values 33% and 99%).

6. INVESTIGATION STRATEGIES

Investigations are guided by the history and examination. Initial tests in primary care include:

- **Orthostatic blood pressure** measurement.
- **ECG:** there may be evidence of ischaemia or arrhythmias.
- **FBC** if anaemia or bleeding is suspected (acute anaemia will cause syncope but patients adapt in cases of chronic anaemia).
- **Fasting blood glucose**, if hypoglycaemia is a possibility.

- In most cases, the initial assessment will lead to a definite, or at least a likely, diagnosis, which will clarify the selection of further investigations and management.
- However, syncope is often multifactorial, especially in older individuals.

Arrhythmia related syncope can be diagnosed on ECG in the presence of:

- Sinus bradycardia rate under 40 bpm
- Mobitz II second degree block or above
- Alternating right and left bundle branch block
- Ventricular tachycardia or rapid supraventricular tachycardia
- Pacemaker malfunction

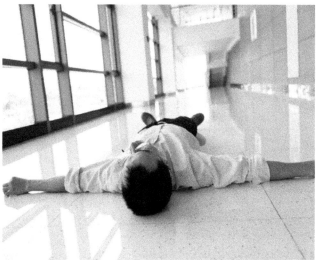

Image source: healthxchange

Further investigations

- By this stage a history, examination and limited ED-based investigations will have allowed appropriate risk stratification.
  - o **High risk patients** will require admission for further urgent investigation and appropriate intervention.
  - o **Low risk patients** can be discharged, a proportion of whom may require further investigation which can appropriately be performed as an outpatient.

- **Echocardiography**
  - o Should be performed in any patient with a cardiac murmur and should be used to diagnose and quantify heart failure when this is suspected. If aortic stenosis is suspected, echocardiography should be performed urgently.
  - o This will commonly be done as an inpatient.

- **Carotid sinus massage**
  - For 5 to 10 seconds with continuous ECG and blood pressure monitoring can be used to diagnose carotid sinus syndrome.
  - *It is considered positive if it produces a drop in systolic blood pressure of 50 mm Hg or a period of asystole of 3 seconds.*

- **Ambulatory monitoring: who to monitor**
  - Low risk patients that have a negative work up in the ED do not need ambulatory monitoring; however, it may provide reassurance especially for patients with recurrent syncopal episodes or symptoms of palpitations and lightheadedness.
  - These patients can be discharged with expedited follow-up and ambulatory monitoring as warranted. Patients that are intermediate risk may also require ambulatory monitoring but this can be guided by the clinical suspicion for an arrhythmia and the inpatient or outpatient resources available.
  - Patients that are high risk warrant in-patient admission and may also benefit from prolonged ambulatory monitoring if 24 to 48 hours of inpatient telemetry is normal.

- **Tilt table testing**
  - Involves slowly moving the patient from supine to standing with a cardioinhibitory or vasodepressor response being considered positive for neurocardiogenic or vasovagal syncope. Protocols vary and various provocative drugs may be used.

5. ED MANAGEMENT
- Management in the ED for patients who have presented with syncope is naturally limited by the fact that, by definition, they have made a full recovery from their index event.
- Intervention in the ED is essentially geared towards achieving robust risk stratification (as described previously) and confidently discharging patients at low risk with no follow-up (ie. normal examination, no risk factors), whilst identifying those who require either

  (a) admission for urgent investigation (eg. patients with cardiac failure or suspicion of aortic stenosis) or

  (b) further out-patient investigation (eg. patients with mild orthostatic or vasovagal syncope).

Cardiological causes[49]
- TLoC can occur due to an underlying cardiological problem. Referral for cardiovascular assessment within 24 hours is recommended if any of the following apply:
  - ECG abnormality;
  - Heart failure (history or physical signs);
  - TLoC occurs during exertion;
  - Family history of sudden cardiac death in people aged <40 years and/or an inherited cardiac condition;
  - New or unexplained breathlessness;
  - Heart murmur.

- TLoC occurring during exercise indicates that a cardiac arrhythmic cause is probable; it should be distinguished from TLoC that occurs shortly after stopping exercise, when a vasovagal cause is more likely.
- The episode may not be related to epilepsy if any of the following features are present:
  - prodromal symptoms that, on other occasions, have been abolished by sitting or lying down;
  - sweating before the episode or pallor during the episode; or
  - prolonged standing that appeared to precipitate the TLoC.

Uncomplicated faint, situational syncope, and orthostatic hypotension:
- Uncomplicated faint (uncomplicated vasovagal syncope) should be diagnosed when there are no features that suggest an alternative diagnosis (note that brief seizure activity can occur during uncomplicated faints and is not necessarily diagnostic of epilepsy). Features suggestive of uncomplicated faint include:
  - **P**osture (prolonged standing or similar episodes that have been prevented by lying down);
  - **P**rovoking factors (such as pain or a medical procedure); and
  - **P**rodromal symptoms (such as sweating or feeling warm/hot before TLoC).

These are known as 'the three Ps'.

---

49 *National Institute for Health and Clinical Excellence. Transient loss of consciousness ('blackouts') management in adults and young people. London: NICE; 2010. NICE clinical guideline 109. [Online]*

SITUATIONAL SYNCOPE

- Should be diagnosed when there are no features from the initial assessment that suggest an alternative diagnosis and syncope is clearly and consistently provoked by straining during micturition (usually while standing) or by coughing or swallowing.
- If a diagnosis of uncomplicated faint or situational syncope is made, no further immediate management is required.
- The mechanism of the syncope, possible triggers, and avoidance strategies should be discussed and patients reassured.

ORTHOSTATIC HYPOTENSION

- Should be suspected on the basis of the initial assessment when there are no features suggesting an alternative diagnosis and the history is typical.
- If these criteria are met, measure the patient's lying and standing blood pressure (with repeated measurements while standing for 3 minutes).
- If clinical measurements do not confirm orthostatic hypotension despite a suggestive history, refer the person for further specialist cardiovascular assessment.
- If orthostatic hypotension is confirmed, likely causes or contributing factors, such as diuretics, should be considered.

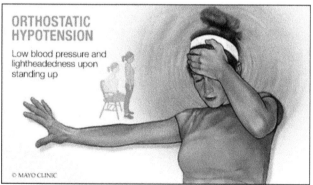

Orthostatic hypotension| Source John Saddington

Further assessment and referral

- The outcome from the initial assessment will be that all people with TLoC who do not have a firm diagnosis of uncomplicated faint, situational syncope, orthostatic hypotension, or symptoms suggestive of epilepsy should have a specialist cardiovascular assessment by the most appropriate local service.
- The aim is to categorise the TLoC as either caused by suspected structural heart disease, suspected cardiac arrhythmia, suspected neurally mediated, or unexplained.

- Specific guidance is given as to appropriate further investigation, depending on the suspected cause.
- The following tests are likely during specialist assessment:
  - An ambulatory ECG is required to diagnose a suspected cardiac arrhythmia. The type chosen will depend, in particular, on the frequency of TLoC and will require, for example, 24- or 48-hour monitoring or external or implantable event recorders.
  - People with structural heart disease may have several mechanisms for syncope and so should have investigations for arrhythmia, as well as consideration of orthostatic hypotension and neurally medicating syncope, in addition to cardiac imaging.
  - TLoC during exercise requires urgent (within 7 days) exercise testing, unless there is a possible contraindication (such as suspected aortic stenosis or hypertrophic cardiomyopathy). The patient should refrain from exercise until further assessment.
  - For people with suspected carotid sinus syncope and for those with unexplained syncope who are aged ≥60 years, carotid sinus massage is the first-line investigation.
  - For people with suspected vasovagal syncope for whom recurrent episodes of TLoC adversely affect their quality of life or represent a high risk of injury, a tilt test is recommended. This will assess whether the syncope is accompanied by a severe cardioinhibitory response (usually asystole).
  - An ambulatory ECG is recommended for all people with unexplained syncope (including after negative carotid sinus massage test in those for whom this is appropriate). A tilt test is not recommended before ambulatory ECG.
- Appropriate advice for people who experience TLoC is also included in the guidance.
- This involves advising them that they must not drive (see below) while waiting for a specialist assessment and explaining the fact that they will need to report to the Driver and Vehicle Licensing Agency[50] following diagnosis. Consideration of safety at work may also be required. In addition, patients should be told what to do if they have another event before assessment is completed.

---

[50] DVLA (March 2019). At a glance guide to the current medical standards of fitness to drive [Online]

II. DRIVING AND COMMON ED CONDITIONS

- In the UK, following a single vasovagal syncope, driving is not restricted and the Driver and Vehicle Licensing Agency (DVLA) does not need to be informed. If recurrent, on each occasion it must be due to strong **P**rovocation, associated with **P**rodromal symptoms and **P**osture, i.e. it is unlikely to occur while sitting or lying - the '3 Ps'. Greater restrictions apply if the situation is more complicated, such as cough syncope, or if diagnosis is less clear. If in doubt, contact the DVLA.

DVLA STANDARDS OF FITNESS TO DRIVE OF COMMON ED CONDITIONS

Disorder	Car or Motorcycle	Bus or Lorry
REFLEX VASOVAGAL SYNCOPE: Syncope with the 3"Ps" (**Provocation/ Prodrome/ Postural**). If recurrent, will need to check the "3 Ps" apply on each occasion.	**No driving restrictions.** (Except Cough Syncope) DVLA need not be notified.	**No driving restrictions** (Except Cough Syncope) DVLA need not be notified
LOSS OF CONSCIOUSNESS/ LOSS OF OR ALTERED AWARENESS: likely to be unexplained syncope but with a high probability of reflex vasovagal syncope	**No driving restrictions.** DVLA need not be notified.	**Can drive 3 months** after the event. (Except Cough Syncope)
LOSS OF CONSCIOUSNESS/ LOSS OF OR ALTERED AWARENESS with High Risk Factors. (Includes > 1 episode in previous 6 months)	**Licence refused/revoked for 6 months** if no cause identified. **Can drive 4 weeks after** the event if the cause has been identified and treated.	**Licence refused/revoked for 12 months** if no cause identified. **Can drive 3 months after** the event if the cause has been identified and treated.
COUGH SYNCOPE	Driving must cease for **6 months** if a single episode, **increased to 12 months** if multiple attacks.	**5 years off** driving from the date of the last attack.
FIRST UNPROVOKED EPILEPTIC SEIZURE / SOLITARY FIT	**6 months off** driving from the date of the seizure	**5 years off** driving from the date of the seizure.
PRESUMED LOSS OF CONSCIOUSNESS/loss of or altered awareness with Seizure markers.	**6 months off** driving from the date of episode. If a person suffers recurrent episodes of LOC with seizure markers, **12 months' freedom** from such episodes must be attained.	**5 years off** driving from the date of an episode if the licence holder has undergone assessment by an appropriate specialist and no relevant abnormality has been identified.
CEREBROVASCULAR DISEASE: including stroke due to occlusive vascular disease, spontaneous intracerebral haemorrhage, TIA, amaurosis fugax and intracranial venous thrombosis.	Must not drive for **1 month.** May resume driving after this period if the clinical recovery is satisfactory. There is no need to notify DVLA unless there is residual neurological deficit 1 month after the episode;	Licence refused or revoked for **1 year** following a stroke or TIA. Can be considered for licensing after this period provided that there is no debarring residual impairment likely to

	Multiple TIAs over a short period may require at **least 3 months free** from further attacks before resuming driving and should notify DVLA.	affect safe driving and there are no other significant risk factors.
ANGINA	Driving **must cease** when symptoms occur at rest, with emotion or at the wheel. Driving may recommence when satisfactory symptom control is achieved. DVLA need not be notified.	**Refusal or revocation** with continuing symptoms (treated and/or untreated) Re-licensing may be permitted thereafter provided: Free from angina for at least 6/52; The exercise or other functional test requirements can be met and there is no other disqualifying condition.
ACUTE CORONARY SYNDROMES (ACS)	If successfully treated by coronary angioplasty, driving may recommence after **1 week.** If not successfully treated by coronary angioplasty, driving may recommence after **4 weeks** provided: • There is no other disqualifying condition. **DVLA need not be notified.**	All Acute Coronary Syndromes disqualify the licence holder from driving for at **least 6 weeks**. Re/licensing may be permitted thereafter provided: • The exercise or other functional test requirements can be met. • There is no other disqualifying condition.
ARRHYTHMIA Sinoatrial disease Significant atrio-ventricular conduction defect Atrial flutter/fibrillation Narrow or broad complex tachycardia.	Driving **must cease** if the arrhythmia has caused or is likely to cause incapacity. Driving may be permitted when underlying cause has been identified and controlled for at **least 4 weeks**. DVLA need not be notified unless there are distracting/disabling symptoms.	Disqualifies from driving if the arrhythmia has caused or is likely to cause incapacity.
HYPERTENSION	Driving may continue unless treatment causes unacceptable side effects. DVLA need not be notified.	Disqualifies from driving if resting BP consistently >180/100 mm Hg.
DIABETICS with Impaired awareness of Hypoglycaemia	If confirmed, **driving must stop.** Driving may resume provided reports show awareness of hypoglycaemia has been regained, confirmed by consultant/GP report.	If confirmed, **driving must stop**. Driving may resume provided reports show awareness of hypoglycaemia has been regained, and there are no other debarring complications of DM such as a visual field defect.
PERSISTENT ALCOHOL MISUSE	Licence revocation or refusal until a **minimum 6-month** period of controlled drinking or abstinence has been attained, with normalisation of blood parameters.	Revocation or refusal of a vocational licence until at **least 1-year period** of abstinence or controlled drinking has been attained, with normalisation of blood parameters.
LIABILITY TO SUDDEN ATTACKS OF UNPROVOKED OR UNPRECIPITATED DISABLING GIDDINESS	**Cease driving** on diagnosis. Driving will be permitted when satisfactory control of symptoms achieved.	Licence **refused or revoked** if condition sudden and disabling. Must be symptom free and completely controlled for **at least 1 year** from last attack before re-application.

7. Breathlessness

INTRODUCTION

- Dyspnoea is one of the most common presenting symptoms encountered by clinicians.
- The causes of dyspnoea can be several and range from cardiac, pulmonary, anemia, obesity, hysterical/psychogenic, physical deconditioning, among others.
- As these causes are varied, it is essential to differentiate life-threatening causes causes from benign, self-limiting conditions.
- Several definitions for describing dyspnea have been postulated including "uncomfortable sensation of breathing", "difficult, laboured, uncomfortable breathing",[51] "sensation of feeling breathless or experiencing air hunger".
  - **Dyspnoea**: refers to the sensation of difficult or uncomfortable breathing.
  - **Tachypnoea** is an increase in the respiratory rate above normal;
  - **Hyperventilation** is increased minute ventilation relative to metabolic need,
  - **Hyperpnoea** is a disproportionate rise in minute ventilation relative to an increase in metabolic level. These conditions may not always be associated with dyspnea.
  - **Orthopnoea** is the sensation of breathlessness in the recumbent position, relieved by sitting or standing.
  - **Paroxysmal nocturnal dyspnoea (PND)** is a sensation of shortness of breath that awakens the patient, often after 1 or 2 hours of sleep, and is usually relieved in the upright position.
  - **Trepopnoea** is dyspnea that occurs in one lateral decubitus position as opposed to the other.
  - **Platypnoea** refers to breathlessness that occurs in the upright position and is relieved with recumbency.
  - **Bradypnoea:** an inappropriately reduced respiratory rate which can occur when a patient becomes exhausted following prolonged tachypnoea or following ingestion of certain toxins.

---

[51] *Wright GW, Branscomb BV. The origin of the sensations of dyspnea. Trans Am Clin Climatol Assoc 1954; 66:116-25.*

CAUSES AND CLASSIFICATION
CAUSES OF DYSPNOEA BASED ON ORGAN SYSTEMS
Head & neck, upper airways
- Angioedema, Anaphylaxis
- Infection of the pharynx
- Vocal cord dysfunction
- Foreign body, Trauma

Chest wall, pleura, lungs
- Rib fractures, Flail chest
- Pneumomediastinum
- Copd exacerbation, Asthma attack
- Pulmonary embolism
- Pneumothorax, Pleural effusion
- Pneumonia
- Acute respiratory failure
- Lung contusion/trauma
- Hemorrhage
- Lung cancer
- Exogenous allergic alveolitis

Heart
- Acute coronary syndrome/myocardial infarction
- Acutely decompensated congestive heart failure
- Pulmonary edema
- High-output failure
- Cardiomyopathy
- (tachy-)arrhythmia
- Valvular heart disease
- Pericardial tamponade

CNS/Neuromuscular
- Stroke
- Neuromuscular disease

Toxic/metabolic
- Organophosphate poisoning
- Salicylate poisoning
- Carbon monoxide poisoning
- Ingestion of other toxic substances
- (diabetic) ketoacidosis

Other
- Sepsis, Fever, Encephalitis
- Anemia
- Traumatic brain injury
- Acute renal failure
- Drugs (e.g., beta-blockers, ticagrelor)
- Hyperventilation, Anxiety
- Intra-abdominal process
- Ascites, Pregnancy, Obesity

CLINICAL ASSESSMENT

- Immediate evaluatoin Patients presenting with acute dyspnoea should be immediately evaluated and triaging should be done for signs of clinical instability, such as:

  (i) suspected upper airway obstruction (e.g., stridor);

  (ii) tachypnoea (> 24 breaths/minute) or apnoea;

  (iii) gasping or breathing effort without movement of air;

  (iv) chest retractions or use of accessory muscles of respiration;

  (v) presence of hypotension;

  (vi) presence of hypoxaemia;

  (vii) unilateral or absent breath sounds; and

  (viii) altered consciousness.

HISTORY

- While evaluating a patient with dyspnoea, the following should be meticulously recorded: onset, duration, pattern, progression, severity, diurnal variation, relation to exercise, exertion, aggravating and relieving factors.
- The terminology used by the patient can sometimes give a clue to the cause of dyspnoea: chest tightness or constricted breathing (bronchial asthma); smothering or suffocating sensation (heart failure, acute coronary syndromes); need to sigh (heart failure).

Onset

- In adult patients presenting with sudden onset dyspnoea, acute pulmonary thromboembolism, acute coronary syndrome or spontaneous pneumothorax, acute respiratory distress syndrome (ARDS), foreign body aspiration, psychogenic causes should be high in the list of differential diagnosis.

Duration

- Common causes of dyspnoea that is slowly progressing over hours or days include bronchial asthma, chronic obstructive pulmonary disease (COPD), pleural effusion, pneumonia, congestive heart failure, small pulmonary emboli, interstitial lung disease or malignancy; psychogenic acuses; and cardiac diseases like coronary artery disease, congestive heart failure.[52]

Pattern

- Prolonged bed rest prior to acute onset dyspnoea may indicate acute pulmonary embolism.
- Orthopnoea (dysnoea in supine position, relieved on assuming upright position) is classically seen in left heart failure but can also occur in COPD, bilateral diaphragmatic palsy, asthma triggered by gastric reflux, among others.
- Paroxysmal nocturnal dyspnea (PND) is not always diagnostic of left heart failure as nocturnal episodes of dyspnoea occur in variety of conditions. Dyspnoea and deoxygenation upon assuming upright position is termed platypnoea-orthodeoxia and is seen in right-to-left shunting of blood (e.g., large patent foramen of ovale, hepatopulmonary syndrome).
- Dyspnoea in upright position, relieved in supine position is called platypnoea and it seen in left atrial myxoma or hepatopulmonary syndrome.
- Trepopnoea is dyspnoea in lateral decubitus position and is seen in unilateral pleural effusion.

Variations

- Intermittent episodes of dyspnoea may be seen with bronchial asthma, heart failure, pleural effusion, recurrent pulmonary embolism, gastro-oesophageal reflux disease; aspiration.
- In addition to ardivascular diseases, exercise-induced dyspnoea is seen in exercise-induced asthma as well.
- Seasonal or diurnal dyspnoea is seen in bronchial asthma. Aggravation of dyspnoea during winter months may occur with COPD.

Other associated symptoms

- Dyspnoea presenting with other associated symptoms may help in localizing the system involved and understanding the nature of disease.
- Dyspnoea associated with central chest pain, points to aortic dissection, pulmonary embolism or acute coronary syndrome.
- If the pain is sharp and aggrevated by cough or deep breathing it could be due to pleural irritation.
- Fever indicates an infectious cause.
- If anxiety precedes dyspnoea it could be a panic attack or pychogenic dyspnea.
- When dyspnoea is associated with cough, haemoptysis, pedal oedema, or wheeze most probable aetiological causes are shown.

[52] Ailani RK, Ravakhah K, DiGiovine B, Jacobsen G, Tun T, Epstein D, West BC. Dyspnea differentiation index: A new method for the rapid separation of cardiac vs pulmonary dyspnea. Chest 1999; 116:1100-4.

PHYSICAL EXAMINATION

- A thorough physical examination helps the clinician to assess the severity, diagnose the cause and in prompt management of the patient.
- Whether the patient is able to complete full sentences while talking is carefully observed.
- **In acute severe asthma**, patients cannot complete full sentences while talking. Use of accessory muscles of respirations, paradoxical breathing or sitting in tripod position, signs of pallor, cyanosis, clubbing and pedal oedema are looked for. Haemodynamic stability of the patient is checked by assessing the vital signs. Further, whether the patient is able to maintain saturation on room air is assessed using pulse oximetry.
- On measuring blood pressure pulsus paradoxus should be watched for as its presence points to pericardial disease, restrictive heart disease.
- **On respiratory system examination**, the symmetry of chest wall movements with respiration is observed. Percussion (e.g., dull note in pleural effusion, hyperresonant in tension pneumothorax) and auscultation (wheeze, crepitations, decreased or hyperreasonant sounds, bronchial breath sounds) give valuable clue to the aetiological diagnosis.
- **On cardiovascular system examination** signs of heart failure should be looked for. Elevated jugular venous pressure (JVP), peripheral oedema, S3 gallop rhythm, presence of murmurs are valuable clues to the aetiological cause indicate that patient is in fluid over load secondary to heart failure. Paradoxical inward movement of abdominal muscles indicate weakness of diaphragm.

SYMPTOMS AND SIGNS

Symptoms and signs accompanying dyspnea that may be of differential diagnostic significance[53]

Additional symptoms and signs	Differential diagnostic considerations
Diminished or absent breathing sounds	COPD, severe asthma, (tension) pneumothorax, pleural effusion, hematothorax
Distention of the neck veins	
with rales in the lungs	ADHF, ARDS
with normal auscultatory	pericardial tamponade, acute

Additional symptoms and signs	Differential diagnostic considerations
findings	pulmonary arterial embolism
Dizziness, syncope	valvular heart disease (e.g., aortic valvular stenosis), hypertrophic or dilated cardiomyopathy, marked anemia, anxiety disorder, hyperventilation
Hemodynamic dysfunction:	
hypertensive	hypertensive crisis, panic attack, acute coronary syndrome
hypotensive	forward heart failure, metabolic disturbance, sepsis, pulmonary arterial embolism
Hemoptysis	lung cancer, pulmonary embolism, bronchiectasis, chronic bronchitis, tuberculosis
Hyperventilation	acidosis, sepsis, salicylate poisoning, psychogenic (incl. anxiety)
Impairment of consciousness	psychogenic hyperventilation, cerebral or metabolic disturbance, pneumonia
Orthopnea	acute congestive heart failure, toxic pulmonary edema
Pain	
on respiration	pneumothorax, pleuritis/pleuropneumonia, pulmonary embolism
independent of respiration	myocardial infarction, aortic aneurysm, Roemheld syndrome, renal or biliary colic, acute gastritis
Pallor	marked anemia
Paradoxical pulse	right-heart failure, pulmonary arterial embolism, cardiogenic shock, pericardial tamponade, exacerbation of bronchial asthma
Peripheral edema	congestive heart failure
Rales	ADHF, ARDS, pneumonia
Use of auxiliary muscles of respiration	respiratory failure/ARDS, severe COPD, severe asthma
Wheezes	(exacerbation of) bronchial asthma, COPD, ADHF, foreign body

---

[53] Berliner, Dominik et al. "The Differential Diagnosis of Dyspnea." Deutsches Arzteblatt international vol. 113,49 (2016): 834-845. [Online]

INVESTIGATION

- **Electrocardiogram** should be obtained immediately if history and physical examination are in favour of heart failure, acute coronary syndrome, cardiac arrhythmias, pulmonary embolism or pulmonary hypertension.
- Chest imaging consisting of **chest radiograph, computed tomography of the chest**, and **bedside thoracic ultrasonography** are helpful in diagnosing pleural effusions, pulmonary oedema, pneumothorax or consolidation.
- **Thoracic ultrasonography** is emerging as a point-of-care diagnostic test recently.
- It has been reported that lung ultrasonography improves diagnostic accuracy of acute dyspnoea when performed within 1 hour of admittance to emergency room (ER).[54]
- Further, it has also been observed that combination of lung ultrasonography with or without testing for N-terminal pro-brain natriuretic peptide (NT-proBNP) has high diagnostic accuracy for differentiating acute dyspnoea due to heart failure from COPD/bronchial asthma-related acute dyspnoea in prehospital/ED setting.
- FBC (anaemia), renal functions and serum electrolytes help in identifying kidney disease.
- **Arterial blood gas (ABG) analysis** will help in knowing the type of respiratory failure and also gives information about the acid-base state of the patient.
- Other laboratory tests that are useful include cardiac biomarkers like troponin, D-dimer, N-terminal pro-brain natriuretic peptide (NT-proBNP), exercise testing, pulmonary function testing including spirometry, reversibility testing, diffusion capacity of lung for carbon monoxide, among others are useful in appropriate situations.

TREATMENT

- Depending the initial aetiological clues, further diagnostic work-up is planned and the patient is administered appropriate specific treatment accordingly.

---

[54] *Cibinel GA, Casoli G, Elia F, Padoan M, Pivetta E, Lupia E, et al. Diagnostic accuracy and reproducibility of pleural and lung ultrasound in discriminating cardiogenic causes of acute dyspnea in the emergency department. Intern Emerg Med 2012; 7:65-70.*

THE USE OF PULSE OXIMETER

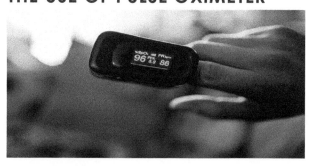

BACKGROUND

- Anoninvasive method of measuring the oxygenation level in the blood.
- Measures the amount of red and infrared light in an area of pulsatile blood flow.
- Because red light is primarily absorbed by deoxygenated blood and infrared light is primarily absorbed by oxygenated blood, the ratio of absorption can be measured.
- Because the amount of light absorbed varies with each pulse wave, the difference of measurement between two points in the pulse wave occurs in the arterial blood flow, with more than several hundred measurements per second. This is compared against baseline values, giving both the pulse oximetry oxygen saturation (SpO_2) and the pulse rate.

INDICATIONS

o Endotracheal intubation
o Cardiac arrest
o Procedural sedation
o Asthma/chronic obstructive pulmonary disease (COPD)
o Respiratory complaints
o Acute respiratory distress syndrome (ARDS)
o Sleep disorders/sleep apnea
o Shunts in cyanotic heart diseases

TECHNICAL CONSIDERATIONS

- Several situations can cause an erroneous SpO_2 reading, especially with the use of transmission probes.
- Darker skin pigments, certain nail polishes, dyshemoglobinemias (eg, carboxyhemoglobin, methemoglobin), intravenous dyes (eg, methylene blue), hypoperfusion, and hypoxia (especially with SpO_2 readings< 80%) can cause errors.
- Motion and exposure to ambient or excessive light has also been shown to cause erroneous SpO_2 readings.

INITIAL APPROACH TO THE ACUTELY BREATHLESS PATIENT IN THE ED

Adapted from RCEM Learning

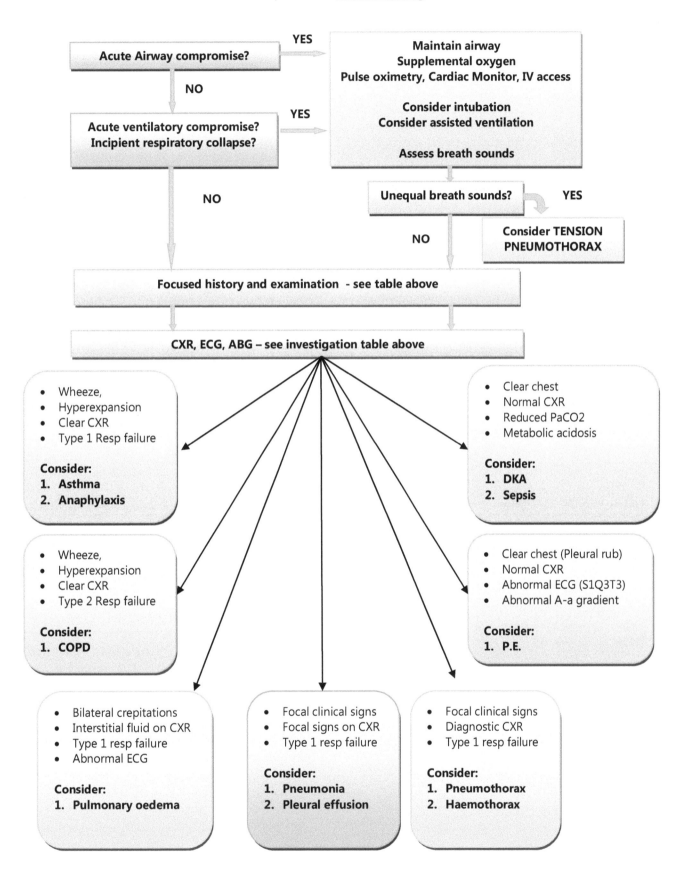

I. COVID-19 IN EMERGENCY MEDICINE

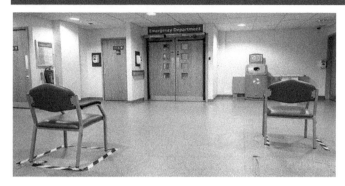

INTRODUCTION

- COVID-19 is an emerging, rapidly evolving situation. We've referenced the latest available WHO guideline & Medscape article published on Jun 09, 2020 by Dr Melissa Kohn[55].
- This indication is not exhaustive, but we will continue to add content and highlight key information, guidance regarding the COVID-19 pandemic. This chapter might be updated at later stage as new information becomes available.

BACKGROUND

- Coronavirus disease (COVID-19) is an infectious disease associated with the novel coronavirus known as severe acute respiratory syndrome coronavirus 2 (SARS-CoV-2).
- At this time, there are no specific vaccines or treatments for COVID-19. However, there are many ongoing clinical trials evaluating potential treatments. WHO will continue to provide updated information as soon as clinical findings become available[56].
- The virus that causes COVID-19 infects people of all ages. However, evidence to date suggests that two groups of people are at a higher risk of getting severe COVID-19 disease.
- These are older people (that is people over 60 years old); and those with underlying medical conditions (such as cardiovascular disease, diabetes, chronic respiratory disease, and cancer).
- The risk of severe disease gradually increases with age starting from around 40 years.
- It's important that adults in this age range protect themselves and in turn protect others that may be more vulnerable[57].

DIFFERENTIAL DIAGNOSIS

- Viral infections (which may occur simultaneously with COVID-19) in the differential diagnosis include the following:
  - Influenza
  - Parainfluenza
  - Human metapneumovirus
  - Human rhinovirus
  - Adenovirus
  - Respiratory syncytial virus
- Bacterial infections in the differential diagnosis include the following:
  - Haemophilus influenzae pneumonia
  - Streptococcus pneumoniae pneumonia
  - Moraxella catarrhalis pneumonia
- Atypical pneumonia in the differential diagnosis includes the following:
  - Legionellosis
  - Mycoplasma pneumoniae pneumonia

CLINICAL PRESENTATION

History

- Initially, a travel history was an important factor in determining which patients were at risk for COVID-19. If a patient had recently traveled to China, specifically the Hubei province, the concern was high for a COVID-19 diagnosis[58].
- Now, however, COVID-19 is spread within communities with social history having replaced travel history in the workup.
- Social history should include whether a patient has been in close contact (within 6 feet) with a known positive patient or a patient under investigation for COVID-19.
- Additionally, employment questions should include whether a patient is a healthcare worker, as such personnel are potentially at higher risk of contracting the disease, depending on their type of work and/or access to PPE.
- Reported symptoms of the illness include fever, fatigue, and nonproductive cough[59]. Other symptoms reported are body aches, shortness of breath, and diarrhea. New symptoms are continuing to be investigated and may include anosmia and dysgeusia.

[55] Melissa Kohn. Coronavirus Disease 2019 (COVID-19) in Emergency Medicine. June 09, 2020 [Medscape]

[56] World Health organisation. Coronavirus [Online]

[57] World Health organisation. Coronavirus disease 2019 (COVID-19) Situation Report – 51 [Online]

[58] Chen N, Zhou M, Dong X, et al. Epidemiological and clinical characteristics of 99 cases of 2019 novel coronavirus pneumonia in Wuhan, China: a descriptive study. Lancet. 2020 Feb 15. 395 (10223):507-513. [Medline].

[59] Huang C, Wang Y, Li X, et al. Clinical features of patients infected with 2019 novel coronavirus in Wuhan, China. Lancet. 2020 Feb 15. 395 (10223):497-506. [Medline].

- Patients are reporting onset of symptoms over a period of a week, with rapid progression to respiratory distress around day 8.
- Severe conditions that patients with COVID-19 have presented with include septic shock, diabetic ketoacidosis, acute kidney injury, acute cardiac injury, and dysrhythmias[60].
- A patient's age and comorbidities are a valuable part of history, with elderly patients, especially those with multiple comorbidities, having higher rates of complications and death.
- Once patients are admitted to the hospital, there will be more time to obtain additional history.
- In addition, a patient's family may be able to provide more information regarding travel, social, and medical history.

Physical exam

- Evaluation of vital signs will provide some initial information regarding a possible infection.
- **A high fever** may be present, but some patients develop only a low-grade fever when infected.
- **Tachycardia** can accompany a fever and may be present in the early stages of shock.
- **Tachypnea** can indicate the beginning of respiratory distress. In addition, a pulse oximeter can be used to catch a COVID-19 infection, as many patients have been found on initial assessment to be hypoxic.
- Further evaluation of a patient suspected to have COVID-19 infection should be conducted in a private room, preferably one employing negative pressure.
- The examiner should be dressed with PPE for droplet precautions, including mask, eye protection, gown, and gloves.
- The remainder of a typical physical exam on a COVID-19-infected patient may reveal increased work of breathing using accessory muscles, circumoral cyanosis, and/or confusion from hypoxia. Lung sounds initially are unremarkable, but the patient can develop a mild expiratory wheeze.
- As the disease progresses, **fine crackles** can be heard, as in early pneumonia.
- Once a patient has developed acute respiratory distress syndrome (ARDS), **course rales and diffuse rhonchi** are heard.

Asymptomatic & Pre-Symptomatic Infection

- Several studies have documented SARS-CoV-2 infection in patients who never develop symptoms (asymptomatic) and in patients not yet symptomatic (pre-symptomatic) [61].
- Since asymptomatic persons are not routinely tested, the prevalence of asymptomatic infection and detection of pre-symptomatic infection is not yet well understood. One study found that as many as 13% of reverse transcription-polymerase chain reaction (RT-PCR)-confirmed cases of SARS-CoV-2 infection in children were asymptomatic[62].

Hypercoagulability and COVID-19

- Some patients with COVID-19 may develop signs of a hypercoagulable state and be at increased risk for venous and arterial thrombosis of large and small vessels[57].

LABORATORY FINDINGS

- **Lymphopenia** is the most common laboratory finding in COVID-19, and is found in as many as 83% of hospitalized patients[63].
- Lymphopenia, neutrophilia, elevated serum alanine aminotransferase and aspartate aminotransferase levels, elevated lactate dehydrogenase, high CRP, and high ferritin levels may be associated with greater illness severity.
- **Elevated D-dimer and lymphopenia** have been associated with mortality.
- **Procalcitonin** is typically normal on admission, but may increase among those admitted to an ICU.
- Patients with critical illness had high plasma levels of inflammatory makers, suggesting potential immune dysregulation. [64]

Radiographic Findings

- Chest radiographs of patients with COVID-19 typically demonstrate bilateral air-space consolidation, though patients may have unremarkable chest radiographs early in the disease[57].
- Chest CT images from patients with COVID-19 typically demonstrate bilateral, peripheral ground glass opacities[57].

[60] Chen T, Wu D, Chen H, et al. Clinical characteristics of 113 deceased patients with coronavirus disease 2019: retrospective study. BMJ. 2020 Mar 26. 368:m1091. [Medline].

[61] Chan JF, Yuan S, Kok KH, et al. A familial cluster of pneumonia associated with the 2019 novel coronavirus indicating person-to-person transmission: a study of a family cluster. Lancet 2020;395:514-23.

[62] Lu X, Zhang L, Du H, et al. SARS-CoV-2 Infection in Children. N Engl J Med 2020;382:1663-5.

[63] Guan WJ, Ni ZY, Hu Y, et al. Clinical Characteristics of Coronavirus Disease 2019 in China. N Engl J Med 2020;382:1708-20.

[64] Huang C, Wang Y, Li X, et al. Clinical features of patients infected with 2019 novel coronavirus in Wuhan, China. Lancet 2020;395:497-506.

- Because this chest CT imaging pattern is non-specific and overlaps with other infections, the diagnostic value of chest CT imaging for COVID-19 may be low and dependent upon radiographic interpretation.

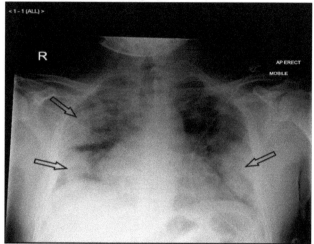

Consolidation. Anterior-posterior (AP) chest radiograph of patient B, a man in his 50s, with severe covid-19 pneumonia, showing bilateral dense peripheral consolidation and loss of lung markings in the mid and lower zones (outlined arrows) | BMJ image

- One study found that 56% of patients who presented within two days of diagnosis had a normal CT. Conversely, other studies have identified chest CT abnormalities in patients prior to the detection of SARS-CoV-2 RNA. Given the variability in chest imaging findings, chest radiograph or CT alone is not recommended for the diagnosis of COVID-19.
- The American College of Radiology also does not recommend CT for screening, or as a first-line test for diagnosis of COVID-19.

TREATMENT
- The recommendations were based on scientific evidence and expert opinion and will be updated as more data become available.

1. Mildly symptomatic patients
- Patients with only mild symptoms of fever, cough, and/or body aches are likely to be discharged from the ED rather than require admission, since treatment at home tends to be sufficient.
- Patients may use over-the-counter medications for symptomatic relief, including antipyretics, analgesics, and cough medications, along with oral hydration. Infected patients should isolate themselves from others in their home as much as possible, and common areas should frequently be disinfected to reduce the risk of virus spread. If an infected patient must leave home, he or she should wear a facemask in order to protect others from infection.

2. Severe Disease
- Some patients with COVID-19 who require hospitalisation are typically in need of **respiratory support**. In the ED, such support may mean only a need for oxygen via a nasal cannula, while other patients may be in respiratory arrest, requiring intubation and mechanical ventilation. Aerosol-generating procedures, such as high-flow oxygen and noninvasive positive-pressure ventilation, are high risk for healthcare providers, and strict isolation precautions should be taken.
- Nebulized medications can be considered in patients with acute bronchospasm who have a known diagnosis of asthma or chronic obstructive pulmonary disease (COPD). Otherwise, these agents have not been found to be useful and come with a high level of risk to providers.
- If quick improvement is not seen, more aggressive measures should be considered. While in the ED, aggressive treatment would likely include **preparation for mechanical ventilation**.
- Intubation would typically be performed with the use of rapid sequence intubation, preferably by the most qualified provider. When preoxygenating via bag-valve-mask ventilation or CPAP, precautions must be taken because both are considered aerosolizing procedures.
- **Video laryngoscopy** can aid in increasing the distance between the provider and the patient during intubation.
- **A viral filter** needs to be placed in the airway circuit once an endotracheal tube has been inserted.
- No definitive pharmacologic treatments for COVID-19.

3. Pediatric Management
- Illness among pediatric patients with COVID-19 is typically milder than among adults. Most children present with symptoms of upper respiratory infection. However, severe outcomes have been reported in children, including deaths[57].
- Data suggest that infants (<12 months of age) may be at higher risk for severe illness from COVID-19 compared with older children.
- CDC and partners are also investigating reports of multisystem inflammatory syndrome in children (MIS-C) associated with COVID-19[57].

II. ASTHMA

BTS ASTHMA ASSESSMENT

Near Fatal Asthma	↑$PaCO_2$ and/or requiring mechanical ventilation with raised inflation pressures
Life Threatening Asthma	**Any one of the following in a patient with severe asthma:**

PEF <33% best or predicted	Silent chest	Dysrhythmia
SpO_2 <92%	Cyanosis	Hypotension
PaO_2 <8 kPa	Feeble respiratory effort	Exhaustion
Normal $PaCO_2$ (4.6-6.0 kPa)	Bradycardia	Confusion/coma

Acute severe asthma	**Any one of:**	
	PEF 33-50% best or predicted	Inability to complete sentences in one breath
	Resp rate >25/min	
	Heart rate >110/min	
Moderate asthma exacerbation	Increasing symptoms	No features of acute severe asthma
	PEF >50-75% best or predicted	
Brittle asthma	**Type 1**: wide PEF variability (>40% diurnal variation for >50% of the time over a period >150 days) despite intense therapy	
	Type 2: sudden severe attacks on a background of apparently well-controlled asthma	

1. ACUTE SEVERE ASTHMA IN ADULT

Immediate management of acute severe asthma	**Subsequent management**

o High-flow oxygen.
o High-dose beta-2 agonists via oxygen driven nebulizer.
o Salbutamol 5mg, Terbutaline 10mg.
o Ipratropium bromide, 0.5mg via oxygen driven nebulizer.
o Prednisolone 40–50mg orally, or hydrocortisone 100mg IV, or both.
 	
o **Monitor**
  ▪ **PEF** 15–30min intervals.
  ▪ **Pulse oximetry:** maintain SpO_2 >92%.
  ▪ **Arterial blood gases.**
 	
o **A chest X-ray is only indicated if:**
  ▪ *There is suspected pneumothorax or pneumo-mediastinum;*
  ▪ *There is suspected consolidation;*
  ▪ *There is failure to respond to therapy;*
  ▪ *Mechanical ventilation is required.*
	o ***If the patient is improving:***
	1. Continue oxygen therapy;
	2. Give IV Hydrocortisone 100mg 6 hourly or Prednisolone 40–50mg orally daily;
	3. Give nebulized salbutamol and Ipratropium 4–6 hourly.
	o ***If the patient is not improving:***
	1. Continue oxygen therapy;
	2. Give nebulized salbutamol 5mg more frequently, every 15–30 mins or 10mg continuously hourly;
	3. Continue Ipratropium 0.5mg 4–6 hourly;
	4. Give Magnesium Sulphate 1.2–2.0g IV as slow infusion over 20mins;
	5. Consider IV beta-2 agonist or aminophylline;
	6. Consider need for tracheal intubation and Mechanical ventilation.
	o ***Discuss with Critical Care team if there is:***
	1. *Need for tracheal intubation and ventilatory support;*
	2. *Continuing failure to respond to treatment;*
	3. *A deteriorating PEF;*
	4. *Persistent or worsening hypoxia;*
	5. *Hypercapnia;*
	6. *Development of acidosis (fall in pH or increase in hydrogen ion concentration);*
	7. *Exhaustion; Drowsiness or confusion;*
	8. *Coma*
	9. *Respiratory arrest.*

MANAGEMENT OF ACUTE SEVERE ASTHMA IN ADULTS IN ED/ BTS GUIDELINE

Time | **Measure PEF and Arterial saturations**

PEF >50-75% best or predicted **MODERATE ASTHMA**	PEF 33-50% best or predicted **ACUTE SEVERE ASTHMA**	PEF < 33% best or predicted **LIFE-THREATENING ASTHMA**
$SpO_2 \geq 92\%$ PEF >50-75% best or predicted No features of acute severe asthma	**Features of severe asthma:** $SpO_2 <92\%$ PEF 33-50% best or predicted Resp rate >25/min Heart rate >110/min Inability to complete sentences in one breath	$SpO_2 <92\%$ $PaO_2 <8$ kPa normal $PaCO_2$ (4.6-6.0 kPa) Silent chest, Cyanosis, Exhaustion Hypotension, Feeble resp effort Bradycardia, Dysrhythmia, Confusion/coma

5 MINS

Give **SALBUTAMOL** (give 4 puffs initially and give a further 2 puffs, every 2 min according to response up to a maximum of 10 puffs) preferably via spacer.	Give **SALBUTAMOL** 5mg by oxygen driven nebuliser	Obtain senior/ICU help now if any life-threatening features are present

15-20 MINS

Clinically stable and **PEF >75%**	Clinically stable and **PEF <75%**	No Life-threatening features and **PEF 50-75%**	Life-Threatening features or **PEF <50%**	**IMMEDIATE MANAGEMENT** • Oxygen to maintain SpO_2 94-98% • Salbutamol 5mg • Ipratropium 0.5mg via Oxygen-driven nebuliser • Prednisolone 40-50mg orally or IV Hydrocortisone 100mg

Repeat Salbutamol 5 mg nebuliser
Give Prednisolone 40-50mg orally

MEASURE ARTERIAL BLOOD GASES:
Markers of severity;
• **Normal or raised PaCO2 (PaCO2 >4.6kPa, 35mmHg)**
• **Severe hypoxia (PaO2 <8kPa)**
• **Low pH or high H+**

60 MINS

Patient recovering and PEF >75%	No signs of severe asthma and PEF 50-75%	Signs of severe Asthma or PEF <50%	• Give/repeat Salbutamol 5mg with Ipratropium 0.5mg by Oxygen-driven nebuliser after 15 minutes • Consider continuous salbutamol nebuliser 5-10mg/hr • Consider IV Magnesium sulphate 1.2-2g over 20min • Correct fluid/electrolytes, especially K+ disturbances • CXR • Repeat ABG

OBSERVE AND MONITOR:
• SpO_2
• Heart rate
• Respiratory rate

120 MINS

Patient stable and PEF >50%	Signs of severe Asthma or PEF <50%	**ADMIT** Patient accompanied by a Nurse or Doctor at all times

POTENTIAL DISCHARGE:
- *In all patients who received nebulised β2 agonists prior to presentation, consider an extended observation period prior to discharge.*
- *If PEF <50% on presentation, give prednisolone 40-50mg/day for 5 days*
- *In all patients ensure treatment supply of inhaled steroid and β2 agonist and check inhaler technique*
- *Arrange GP follow up within 2 working days post-discharge*
- *Fax or email discharge letter to GP*
- *Refer to asthma liaison nurse/chest clinic*

III. COPD EXACERBATIONS

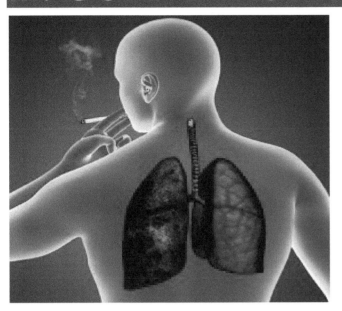

INTRODUCTION

- COPD is a preventable and treatable disease state characterised by airflow limitation that is not fully reversible. It encompasses both emphysema and chronic bronchitis. The airflow limitation is usually progressive and is associated with an abnormal inflammatory response of the lungs to noxious particles or gases.
- It is primarily caused by cigarette smoking.
- Although COPD affects the lungs, it also has significant systemic consequences. Exacerbations and comorbidities are important contributors to the overall condition and prognosis in individual patients.[65]
- A diagnosis of COPD should be considered in a patient over the age of **35** who presents with exertional breathlessness, cough, sputum production, wheeze or frequent winter bronchitis **in the presence of risk factors.**

CLINICAL PRESENTATION

- The classic presentation of a patient with a COPD exacerbation includes wheezing, productive cough, dyspnea on exertion, hypoxia, and tachycardia.
- The patient may relate increased use of inhalers, sputum change, or a new requirement of an upright sleeping position (eg, chair).
- However, these symptoms have a significant overlap with other causes of dyspnea and a wide differential diagnosis should be entertained initially.

---

[65] *Global Initiative for Chronic Obstructive Lung Disease (GOLD). Global strategy for the diagnosis, management, and prevention of chronic obstructive pulmonary disease. 2018*

- Typical Symptoms of COPD
  - Cough
  - Wheezing
  - Chest congestion
  - Fatigue
  - Sputum change in color or quantity
  - Fever/chills
- The spectrum of symptoms can range from mild to severe.
- The mildly affected patient may note mild dyspnea on exertion. More symptomatic patients may complain of mild to severe dyspnea at rest. Some may only be able to speak one sentence due to breathlessness: "I can't breathe." The most severely affected will not be able to speak at all.
- **RISK FACTORS**
  - **Smoking** is by far the largest risk factor for COPD
  - Occupational exposure to fumes or dust
  - Occupational exposure to tobacco smoke
  - Alpha 1 antitrypsin deficiency.

AETIOLOGY OF EXACERBATIONS

- Most COPD exacerbations are due to viral or bacterial infections of the respiratory tract, however in some cases they are caused by environmental pollution.
- Up to 30% have an unknown aetiology.

INVESTIGATIONS

- Investigations that should be performed in the ED when a patient is presenting with an exacerbation of COPD include:
  - **Arterial blood gas analysis**: to evaluate evidence of acidosis, hypercapnia and hypoxaemia
  - **CXR:** A chest radiograph is the most common study necessary in evaluating the COPD patient. A typical chest x-ray will show increased AP diameter, flattening of the diaphragm, decreased lung markings and the absence of another acute abnormality, such as pneumothorax, pulmonary edema or infiltrate. Significant abnormalities such as pneumonia, pulmonary edema or pneumothorax will require a change in therapy.
  - **ECG:** rarely specific in COPD, but frequently necessary in the evaluation of elderly patients with multiple co-morbidities to help exclude other disease processes. The EKG may diagnose a significant arrythymia, STEMI, or show acute ischemic changes suggestive of an acute coronary syndrome. A rare, but specific finding in COPD patients is multifocal atrial tachycardia

- **FBC:** This may identify anaemia as a cause of breathlessness or show evidence of secondary polycythaemia.
- **Urea and electrolytes**
- **Theophylline level** if the patient is already on theophylline therapy
- **Sputum analysis:** if sputum is purulent a sample should be sent for microscopy, culture and sensitivity.
- **Blood cultures** if pyrexia present

DIAGNOSIS OF COPD
Clinical factors that may help differentiate asthma & COPD

FEATURE	COPD	ASTHMA
Smoker or ex-smoker	Nearly all	Possible
Symptoms aged < 35 years	Rare	Often
Chronic productive cough	Common	Uncommon
Breathlessness	Persistent & progressive	Variable
Night waking with SOB/Wheeze	Uncommon	Common
Diurnal or day to day variability of symptoms	Uncommon	Common

ED MANAGEMENT OF COPD
- **Bronchodilators and oxygen therapy:**
  - The most commonly used bronchodilators in the ED are **Beta 2 agonists such as salbutamol and terbutaline,** and anticholinergics such as **ipratropium bromide**
  - If a patient is **acidotic or hypercapnic** nebulisers should be **driven by air not oxygen.**
  - Oxygen should be given to maintain saturations in a targeted range which should normally be **88-92%.**
- **Steroids:**
  - Oral corticosteroids should be used in all patients admitted to hospital
  - **Prednisolone 30mg for 7 to 14 days**
- **Antibiotics:**
  - Antibiotics should be given to those with purulent sputum or those with clinical signs of pneumonia or CXR changes.
  - Empirical antibiotic therapy should be with **aminopenicillin, macrolide or tetracycline** unless local microbiological policy states otherwise.
- **Theophylline / Aminophylline:**
  - Intravenous aminophylline should be considered **only if there is an inadequate response to nebulised bronchodilators**.

- The loading dose of aminophylline should be omitted in patients taking oral theophylline.
- The dose of oral theophylline should be reduced at the time of an exacerbation if the patient needs concurrent macrolide or fluoroquinolone antibiotics.

- **NON-INVASIVE VENTILATION:**
  - Non-invasive ventilation should be used as the treatment of choice for **hypercapnic respiratory failure** if optimal medical therapy has not been successful.
  - **Optimal Medical Therapy:** The Royal College of Physicians guideline states that maximum medical treatment includes:
    - Controlled **oxygen** therapy to maintain **SaO_2 88-92%**
    - **Nebulised salbutamol** 2.5-5 mg
    - **Nebulised Ipratropium** 500 micrograms
    - **Prednisolone** 30 mg
    - **Antibiotic** agent when indicated
  - **NIV** should be considered **within 60 minutes** of arrival to hospital in all patients with an exacerbation of COPD and a persistent respiratory acidosis in whom the above treatment has been unsuccessful.
  - Non-invasive ventilation used as an adjunct to standard care has been found to be associated with lower mortality, lower need for intubation, lower likelihood of treatment failure and shorter duration of stay in hospital.
- **Other therapy:**
  - **Hospital at home** and **assisted discharge schemes** are safe, effective and should be considered in patients who would otherwise require hospital admission.
  - **Smoking cessation**

PROGNOSIS
- A UK audit has shown death in 14% of patients admitted to hospital within 3 months of admission. The most important prognosticators for death in this group were:
  - Poor performance status*
  - Low arterial pH on admission*
  - Presence of bilateral leg oedema*
  - Age >70
  - Home circumstances, particularly in the patient is in a nursing home
  - Unrecordable peak flow on admission
  - Pulse oximetry showing oxygen saturation under 86%
  - Intervention with assisted ventilation
- The 3 marked with * were the 3 major independent predictors of mortality.

IV. PNEUMONIA

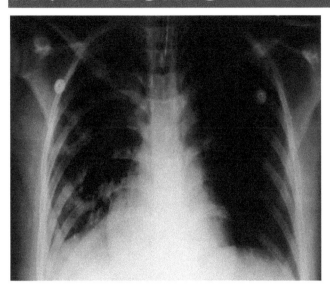

INTRODUCTION

- Community-acquired pneumonia (CAP) is defined as pneumonia acquired outside hospital or healthcare facilities. Clinical diagnosis is based on a group of signs and symptoms related to lower respiratory tract infection with presence of fever >38ºC, cough, expectoration, chest pain, dyspnoea, and signs of invasion of the alveolar space. However, older patients in particular are often afebrile and may present with confusion and worsening of underlying diseases.
- Emergency medicine physicians need to be able to identify and differentiate community-acquired pneumonia (CAP) from healthcare-associated pneumonia (HCAP) in order to effectively manage patients and provide the appropriate antibiotic treatment.
- Pneumonia is categorized based on whether a patient is coming from the community, has significant healthcare system contact, or is hospitalized.
- This distinction is important because contact with the healthcare system or developing pneumonia in-hospital increases the patient's risk of having pathogens that would be inadequately treated with the antibiotics used for patients coming from the community, especially multi-drug resistant pathogens.

COMMUNITY-ACQUIRED PNEUMONIA (CAP)

- Occurs in a patient from the community or general population that does not have any significant contact with the healthcare system.
- CAP may occur due to:
  - Typical pathogens: Streptococcus pneumoniae, Haemophilus influenzae, Moraxella catarrhalis.
  - Atypical pathogens: Mycoplasma pneumonia, Chlamydophila pneumonia, Legionella species, and respiratory viruses.
  - S. pneumoniae is the single most common pathogen causing CAP and is responsible for 20-50% of infections.
- **Typical pathogens:**
  - Streptococcus pneumoniae, Haemophilus influenzae, Moraxella catarrhalis
  - Seen on gram stain
  - Can be inhibited or killed using beta-lactam antibiotics
- **Atypical pathogens:**
  - Mycoplasma pneumonia, Chlamydophila pneumonia, Legionella species, and respiratory viruses
  - Cannot be visualized on gram stain and require special culture methods
  - Are not killed or inhibited by penicillins or other beta-lactam antibiotics

HEALTHCARE-ASSOCIATED PNEUMONIA (HCAP)

- Occurs in patients that have had significant exposure or contact with the healthcare system.
- This includes patients residing in nursing homes, patients that have been recently hospitalized, or those that receive dialysis, IV medications, or home wound care.
- HCAP Criteria:
  - Hospitalization for ≥2 days in the preceding 90 days
  - Residence in a nursing home/facility
  - In the past 30 days:
    - Attendance at a hospital or hemodialysis clinic
    - Home or clinic IV therapy (antibiotics and chemotherapy)
    - Home wound care
- Healthcare-associated pneumonia (HCAP) may be due to pathogens such as Pseudomonas aerugunosa, Escherichia coli Klebsiella pneumonia, Acinebacter, and Staphylococcus aureus. These gram negative aerobes and gram positive cocci are not inhibited or killed by the antibiotics used to treat CAP.

HOSPITAL-ACQUIRED PNEUMONIA (HAP)

- Develops in patients ≥48 hours after hospitalization and is not incubating at the time of admission, a subtype of HAP, ventilator-associated pneumonia (VAP) develops >48-72 hours after intubation.
- HAP patients are at an increased risk of multi-drug resistant infections, have poorer prognoses, and high mortality.

- Although these patients aren't usually treated in the emergency department, it is from this patient population that the HCAP category was derived, with the goal of identifying patients at increased risk for multi-drug resistant pathogens coming from community settings.

SIGNS AND SYMPTOMS

- Patients with pneumonia may present with signs and symptoms such as fever, chills, productive cough, pleuritic pain, chest pain, and shortness of breath or malaise.
- The differential diagnosis includes other respiratory entities such as bronchitis, viral upper respiratory infections, influenza, pulmonary embolus, tuberculosis, pleural effusion, and other cardiac-pulmonary pathologies.

PRESENTATION

Community-acquired Pneumonia

- Historical features are not helpful in distinguishing typical from atypical CAP. Several prospective studies have shown that the history and physical are neither sensitive nor specific in identifying pneumonia.
- Classically the "typical" CAP caused by Streptococcus pneumonia is described as presenting with the sudden onset of fever or chills, productive cough, and pleuritic chest pain.
- Atypical CAP may have a more protracted course beginning with upper respiratory symptoms, slowly worsening cough, malaise and fatigue. Historically, these symptoms were nonresponsive to initial penicillin treatment. Although these are considered classic presentations of typical and atypical pneumonias, these classic presentations are not considered to be sensitive or specific for pneumonia.

"Classic" findings:

- **Typical Pneumonias**
  - Streptococcus pneumonia – bloody or rust colored sputum
  - Haemophilus influenzae – fever, muscle pain, fatigue
- **Atypical Pneumonias**
  - Mycoplasma pneumonia – "walking pneumonia;" upper respiratory symptoms, gradually worsening over weeks or even months
  - Chlamydiophila pneumonia – pharyngitis, laryngitis and sinusitis, associated with outbreaks in close-contact settings (dorms, prisons)
  - Legionella – respiratory and gastrointestinal symptoms

Healthcare-associated Pneumonia

- Staphylococcus aureus risk factors include vent-dependence, intravenous drug use, immunocompromised, recent influenza infection, and aspiration

- Pseudomonas aeruginosa risks factors include high-dose steroid use, prolonged hospitalization or nursing home residence, and preexisting lung disease

Special Population

- **Aspiration Pneumonia**
  - Aspiration occurs when there is inhalation of oropharyngeal or gastric contents into the larynx or respiratory tract.
  - It should be differentiated from aspiration pneumonitis, which is a chemical injury from inhalation of gastric contents due to regurgitation that can occur with drug overdose, seizures, cerebrovascular accident, or use of anesthesia.
  - Patients at risk for aspiration include patients with dysphagia due to neurologic disorder, nursing home residents, and patients who abuse alcohol.
  - Aspiration of oropharyngeal secretions may result in respiratory tract pathogens that include Enterobacteriaceae, Pseudomonas aerguinosa and Staphylococcus aureus.
  - Antibiotics with activity against gram-negative organisms such as third-generation cephalosporins, fluoroquinolones and piperacillin are recommended for treatment.

- **Immunocompromised Patients**
  - Immunocompromised patients represent a special subset of pneumonia given the increased susceptibility to a spectrum of potential pathogens.
  - Patients comprising this population include those with solid organ transplants, cystic fibrosis, HIV/AIDS, hematopoietic cell transplants, pregnant women, and patients with immune defects.
  - General considerations include obtaining a thorough past medical history, as well as asking about medications such as chemotherapy, immunomodulating agents, and steroids. Leukopenia and CD4 count may guide evaluation and treatment considerations.
  - Pneumocystis jirovecii (previously classified as Pneumocystis carinii) is typically found in immunocompromised patients with such as HIV/AIDS.
  - Symptoms include dyspnea, nonproductive cough, and fever. Chest x-ray usually shows bilateral infiltrates, but may also present with a lobar consolidation.
  - Treatment for PCP is trimethoprim-sulfamethoxazole (TMP-SMX). Tuberculosis is another important consideration in immunocompromised patients as well as patients with a history of prior tuberculosis infection, night sweats, weight loss, or exposure from shelters, prisons, or recent travel to endemic areas.

PHYSICAL EXAM, BEYOND THE ABCS

- A full physical exam is important to both evaluate for alternative diagnoses as well as clues related to a particular pneumonia. The physical exam starts with initial vitals and inspection of the patient for respiratory distress.
- Patients sitting upright or in the "tripod position" with nasal flaring, chest retractions, and abdominal breathing exhibit an increased work of breathing and may have impending respiratory failure.
- Review of vital signs may show tachypnea, tachycardia, hypotension, hypoxia, and fever.
- Examination of the chest involves a four-step process: including inspection, palpation, percussion, and auscultation of the chest.
- The positive predictive value of abnormal breath sounds in acute respiratory illness is 55% further illustrating the difficulty in diagnosing pneumonia with the physical exam. There are no individual or combination of clinical findings that rule in the diagnosis of pneumonia (Metlay et al. 1999).
- Examiners should look for other signs of dyspnea such as congestive heart failure, pericardial effusions, pleural effusions, pulmonary embolus, and neoplasms.
- Lastly it is important to evaluate the head, ears and throat as many of these patients may initially had an upper respiratory infection that developed into a bacterial pneumonia and concomitant bacterial infections.

DIAGNOSTIC TESTING

1. Blood Studies

The following laboratory tests may not be useful for diagnostic purposes but are useful for classifying illness severity and site-of-care/admission decisions [66]:

- **Serum chemistry panel** (Na, potassium, Bicarbonate, blood urea nitrogen [BUN], creatinine, glucose)
- **Arterial blood gas** (ABG) determination (serum pH, arterial oxygen saturation, arterial partial pressure of oxygen and carbon dioxide) – Hypoxia and respiratory acidosis may be present.
- **Venous blood gas** determination (central venous oxygen saturation)
- **Full blood cell** (FBC) count with differential
- **Serum free cortisol value**
- **Serum lactate level**

A pulse oximetry finding of less than 90-92% indicates significant hypoxia, and an elevated C-reactive protein (CRP) level may be predictive of more serious disease.

However, CRP has not been clearly shown to differentiate bacterial versus viral illness.[67]

- **Blood cultures**
  - Prior to January 2014 blood cultures were recommended for all CAP patients admitted to the hospital, with reimbursement tied to this metric, despite a lack of evidence suggesting that obtaining blood cultures in CAP patients leads to changes in treatment that improve outcomes.
  - In fact, multiple studies have demonstrated that in CAP, both the yield of blood cultures and how often they result in a change in management is very low.
  - Additionally, studies have demonstrated that false positive blood cultures lead to increased length of stay, inappropriately broad antibiotic coverage, and expose patients to the risks associated with both.
  - As of January 2014, obtaining blood cultures in routine CAP patients admitted to the floor is no longer a reportable metric and is not required by most hospitals; however, consult your institutional guidelines and protocols.
  - Blood cultures should be obtained in any patient ill enough to require ICU admission or mechanical ventilation, all septic patients, as well patients with CAP that are at increased risk for bacteremia and resistant organisms.
  - These risk factors for CAP patients include:
    - Cavitary lesions
    - Leukopenia
    - Severe liver disease
    - Asplenia
    - Pleural effusion
    - Alcohol abuse
    - Severe CAP
  - Of note, blood culture yield increases directly with volume.

Sputum

- Sputum induction for gram stain and culture should not be routinely performed in the emergency department, as it poses an infection risk to both providers and other patients and is unlikely to change ED management.

2. Imaging studies
Chest radiography

- The main diagnostic modality for both community and hospital acquired pneumonia is **chest radiography**.

---

[66] van der Poll T, Opal SM. Pathogenesis, treatment, and prevention of pneumococcal pneumonia. Lancet. 2009 Oct 31. 374(9700):1543-56.

[67] Kang YA, Kwon SY, Yoon HI, Lee JH, Lee CT. Role of C-reactive protein and procalcitonin in differentiation of tuberculosis from bacterial community acquired pneumonia. Korean J Intern Med. 2009 Dec. 24(4):337-42.

- Some studies have shown that the absence of abnormal vital signs or abnormalities on chest examination reduces the likelihood of pneumonia and the need for further diagnostic studies (Metlay et al. 1999).
- Factors that predict pneumonia on chest x-ray include temperature >37.8°C, tachycardia >100bpm, absence of asthma, rales, and locally decreased breath sounds on auscultation. Pulmonary infiltrates on chest x-ray may confirm the clinical diagnosis.
- Lobar consolidation is typical of Streptococcus pneumoniae or Klebsiella pneumoniae while multi-lobar infiltrates are more consistent with Staphylococcus aureus and Pseudomonas aeruginosa.

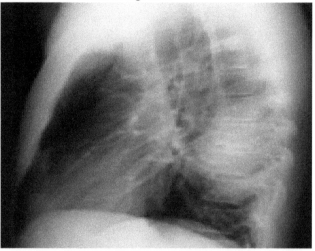

Lateral chest x-ray demonstrating a pneumonia

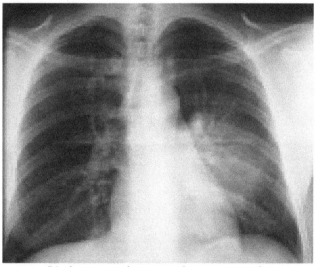

PA chest x-ray demonstrating a pneumonia

- Atypical infections such as Mycoplasma pneumonia, Chlamydophila, and Legionella may reveal patchy infiltrates on radiography.
- Despite these patterns on chest radiography, it is important to note that typical pathogens can present with diffuse infiltrates and atypical pathogens with discrete consolidations.

- Radiographic evidence of pneumonia may not be evident on initial chest radiography in patients with early aspiration pneumonias or severe dehydration; however infiltrates develop on subsequent studies.

Bedside Ultrasound
- More recently, several studies have demonstrated the utility of bedside ultrasound as a reliable, noninvasive diagnostic tool for the detection of pneumonia in children, adolescents and adults, having a sensitivity of 86% and specificity of 89% and LR 7.8 (95% CI, 5.0-12.4) (Shah et al. 2013).
- Emergency physicians with advanced sonography skills may be able to identify consolidation; however, ultrasound is operator dependent and therefore its use in identifying pneumonia is operator dependent as well.

Computer Tomography
- The gold standard for the identification of pneumonia is Computer Tomography of the chest; however, the majority of outpatient community acquired pneumonias will be diagnosed with chest x-ray. CT is more sensitive than plain films of the chest and may be used with patients with an equivocal chest x-ray, or when other etiologies for the patient's presentation are suspected.

ECG
- An ECG should be ordered on patients with pneumonia, especially those with tachycardia. Patients with congestive heart failure, cardiothoracic disease, and severe sepsis/septic shock may develop cardiac ischemia and infarction secondary to a severe pneumonia.

CURB-65 SCORE

Symptom	Points
Confusion	1
Urea >7 mmol/l	1
Respiratory Rate≥30	1
BP: SBP<90mmHg, DBP≤60mmHg	1
Age ≥ 65	1

0 to 1 (<5% mortality)	0-1: Treat as an outpatient
2 to 3 (< 10% mortality)	2: Consider a short stay in hospital or watch very closely as an outpatient
4 to 5 (15-30% mortality)	3-5: Requires hospitalization with consideration as to whether they need to be in the intensive care unit

- **Other factors suggesting a need for admission irrespective of their CURB-65 score:**
  1. Hypoxaemia (SaO$_2$ <94% or PaO$_2$ <8 kPa) regardless of FiO$_2$.
  2. Bilateral or multi-lobe involvement on the chest radiograph.

3. Presence of a co-existing disease e.g. CCF, chronic renal failure
4. Age over 50 years
5. Social admissions in elderly with no adverse factors (other than age).

5. MANAGEMENT OF CAP IN THE ED
INITIAL ACTIONS AND PRIMARY SURVEY
- All patients should have a set of vital signs including temperature, pulse, blood pressure, pulse oximetry, and respiratory rate.
- The emergency physician should start with the "ABCs" approach.
- Acutely ill patients will need peripheral access, monitoring and supplemental oxygen.
- Patients in respiratory distress may require a non-rebreather for oxygenation, noninvasive ventilation, or endotracheal intubation for those with imminent respiratory failure.

- **GENERAL MANAGEMENT**
  - o Patients should be given the following advice: **Rest, Drink plenty of fluids, Stop smoking.**
  - o Patients discharged from the ED should be advised to see their GP for review **within 48 hours** or sooner if clinically indicated.
  - o **Oxygen:** if the oxygen saturations < 94% on air or PaO2 < 8kPa.
  - o **Steroids:** not recommended in the routine treatment of pneumonia of any severity.

- **SPECIFIC MANAGEMENT**
  1. ANTIBIOTIC THERAPY
  - Offer antibiotic therapy as soon as possible after diagnosis, and certainly **within 4 hours**, to patients with **hospital-acquired pneumonia.**

1. LOW-SEVERITY CAP
- o Offer a **5-day course of a single antibiotic** to patients with low-severity community-acquired pneumonia.
  - ▪ **Amoxicillin 500mg Po Tds X5/7 (IV if PO not possible)**
  - ▪ **Penicillin allergic**: **Clarithromycin 500 mg PO bid** or **Doxycycline 200 PO mg stat** then **100 mg PO.**
- o Consider extending the course of the antibiotic for longer than 5 days as a possible management strategy for patients with low-severity CAP whose symptoms do not improve as expected after 3 days.
- ⊥ *Do not routinely offer patients with low-severity community-acquired pneumonia:*
  - o *A fluoroquinolone*
  - o *Dual antibiotic therapy.*

2. MODERATE- SEVERITY CAP
- o Consider a **7- to 10-day course** of antibiotic therapy for patients with moderate- or high-severity community-acquired pneumonia.
- o Consider **dual antibiotic therapy** with **Amoxicillin and a Macrolide** for patients with moderate-severity community-acquired pneumonia.
  - ▪ **Amoxicillin 500mg-1g Po Tds + Clarithromycin 500 mg PO bid (IV if PO not possible)**

3. HIGH-SEVERITY CAP
- o **Co-amoxiclav 1.2g IVI tds + Clarithromycin 500mg bid IV**
- o *Add **Levofloxacin 500mg PO/IV OD**: if Legionella suspected.*
- o **Penicillin allergy:**
  - ▪ **Not IgE mediated reaction/Anaphylaxis:** Cefuroxime 750mg-1.5g TDS IV + Clarithromycin 500mg bid IV
  - ▪ **Severe IgE mediated reaction:** Levofloxacin 500mg PO/IV OD (12 hly if severe)

4. GLUCOCORTICOSTEROID TREATMENT
- o *Do not routinely offer a glucocorticosteroid to patients with CAP unless they have other conditions for which glucocorticosteroid treatment is indicated.*

- **PATIENT INFORMATION**
  - o Explain to patients with community-acquired pneumonia that after starting treatment their symptoms should steadily improve, although the rate of improvement will vary with the severity of the pneumonia, and most people can expect that by:
    - ▪ **1 week:** fever should have resolved
    - ▪ **4 weeks**: chest pain and sputum production should have substantially reduced
    - ▪ **6 weeks:** cough and breathlessness should have substantially reduced
    - ▪ **3 months:** most symptoms should have resolved but fatigue may still be present
    - ▪ **6 months:** most people will feel back to normal.
  - o Advise patients with community-acquired pneumonia to consult their healthcare professional if they feel that their condition is deteriorating or not improving as expected.

V. SPONTANEOUS PNEUMOTHORAX

INTRODUCTION

- Spontaneous pneumothorax is classified into primary and secondary spontaneous pneumothorax.
- **Primary spontaneous pneumothorax (PSP)**
  - Occurs in healthy individuals without a coexisting lung disease, usually as a result of rupture of a pulmonary bleb.
  - Risk factors for PSP include tall-and-thin body shape, maleness, and smoking.[68]
- **Secondary spontaneous pneumothorax (SSP)**
  - Occurs in people with a wide variety of parenchymal lung diseases. These individuals have underlying pulmonary pathology that alters normal lung structure enters the pleural space via distended, damaged, or compromised alveoli.
  - The presentation of these patients may include more serious clinical symptoms and sequelae due to comorbid conditions.
- **Recognised causes of a secondary pneumothorax:**
  - **Obstructive airway disease:** Asthma, COPD
  - **Lung and pleural malignancy**
  - **Infection**: Pneumonia (particularly pneumocystis jiroveci [formerly PCP]), TB
  - **Suppurative lung disease:** Cystic Fibrosis, Bronchiectasis, Lung abscess
  - **Interstitial lung disease:** Sarcoidosis, Idiopathic Pulmonary Fibrosis, Hypersensitivity pneumonitis, Pneumoconiosis, Catamenial.
- The symptoms will vary depending on the cause e.g. fever, weight loss, night sweats but the primary complaint is that of **breathlessness** which is often out of proportion to the size of the pneumothorax radiologically.
- Unlike symptoms, the examination findings in primary spontaneous pneumothoraces are affected by the size of the pneumothorax. A small pneumothorax can be impossible to identify on clinical examination.
- If the pneumothorax is large, then some of the following features may be present:
  - Tachycardia and Tachypnoea
  - Reduced breath sounds on the affected side
  - Reduced chest expansion on the affected side as the patient splints the chest wall
  - Hyper-resonance on the affected side

- Decreased tactile / vocal fremitus on the affected side.
- The diagnosis is usually confirmed radiologically, following which specific information should be sought in order to guide management, advice and appropriate patient disposition/ follow-up.
- **Tension Pneumothorax**
  - If the pleural leak exerts a one-way valve effect, then a tension pneumothorax can develop.
  - This recognition and management of this complication is discussed later in the session.

CLINICAL EVALUATION

- The typical symptoms of chest pain and dyspnoea may be relatively minor or even absent[69], so that a high index of initial diagnostic suspicion is required.
- Many patients (especially those with PSP) therefore present several days after the onset of symptoms.[70]
- The longer this period of time, the greater is the risk of re-expansion pulmonary oedema (RPO).
- In general, the clinical symptoms associated with SSP are more severe than those associated with PSP, and most patients with SSP experience breathlessness that is out of proportion to the size of the pneumothorax.[71] [72]
- These clinical manifestations are therefore unreliable indicators of the size of the pneumothorax. When severe symptoms are accompanied by signs of cardiorespiratory distress, tension pneumothorax must be considered.
- The physical signs of a pneumothorax can be subtle but, characteristically, include reduced lung expansion, hyper-resonance and diminished breath sounds on the side of the pneumothorax. Added sounds such as 'clicking' can occasionally be audible at the cardiac apex. The presence of observable breathlessness has influenced subsequent management in previous guidelines.[73]
- In association with these signs, cyanosis, sweating, severe tachypnoea, tachycardia and hypotension may indicate the presence of tension pneumothorax (see later section).

---

[68] Hsu H.-H., Chen J.-S. The etiology and therapy of primary spontaneous pneumothoraces. Expert Review of Respiratory Medicine. 2015;9(5):655–665.doi: 10.1586/17476348.2015.1083427.

[69] BTS guidelines. Management of spontaneous pneumothorax: British Thoracic Society pleural disease guideline 2010 [Online]

[70] O'Hara VS. Spontaneous pneumothorax. Milit Med 1978;**143**:32–5. (**3**).

[71] Wait MA, Estrera A. Changing clinical spectrum of spontaneous pneumothorax. Am J Surg 1992;**164**:528–31. (**2+**).

[72] Tanaka F, Itoh M, Esaki H, et al. Secondary spontaneous pneumothorax. Ann Thorac Surg 1993;**55**:372–6. (**2–**).

[73] Miller AC, Harvey JE. Guidelines for the management of spontaneous pneumothorax. BMJ 1993;**307**:114–16. (**4**).

- Arterial blood gas measurements are frequently abnormal in patients with pneumothorax, with the arterial oxygen tension (PaO2) being <10.9 kPa in 75% of patients, but are not required if the oxygen saturations are adequate (>92%) on breathing room air.
- The hypoxaemia is greater in cases of SSP, the PaO2 being <7.5 kPa, together with a degree of carbon dioxide retention in 16% of cases in a large series. Pulmonary function tests are poor predictors of the presence or size of a pneumothorax and, in any case, tests of forced expiration are generally best avoided in this situation.
- The diagnosis of pneumothorax is usually confirmed by imaging techniques (see below) which may also yield information about the size of the pneumothorax, but clinical evaluation should probably be the main determinant of the management strategy as well as assisting the initial diagnosis.

INVESTIGATION STRATEGIES

Standard erect PA chest x-ray
- This has been the mainstay of clinical management of primary and secondary pneumothorax for many years, although it is acknowledged to have limitations such as the difficulty in accurately quantifying pneumothorax size.
- Major technological advances in the last decade have resulted in the advent of digital chest imaging, so that conventional chest films are no longer easily available in clinical practice in the UK or in many other modern healthcare systems.
- Since then there have been technological advances, such that digital imaging may now be as reliable as more conventional chest x-rays in pneumothorax diagnosis, but there have been no more recent studies to confirm this.

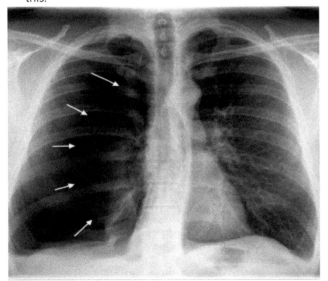

- The diagnostic characteristic is displacement of the pleural line. In up to 50% of cases an air-fluid level is visible in the costophrenic angle, and this is occasionally the only apparent abnormality.
- The presence of bullous lung disease can lead to the erroneous diagnosis of pneumothorax, with unfortunate consequences for the patient.
- If uncertainty exists, then CT scanning is highly desirable (see below).

Lateral x-rays
- These may provide additional information when a suspected pneumothorax is not confirmed by a PA chest film but, again, are no longer routinely used in everyday clinical practice.

Ultrasound scanning
- Specific features on ultrasound scanning are diagnostic of pneumothorax[74] but, to date, the main value of this technique has been in the management of supine trauma patients.

CT scanning
- This can be regarded as the 'gold standard' in the detection of small pneumothoraces and in size estimation.[75]
- It is also useful in the presence of surgical emphysema and bullous lung disease and for identifying aberrant chest drain placement or additional lung pathology. However, practical constraints preclude its general use as the initial diagnostic modality.

SIZE OF PNEUMOTHORAX
- The size of pneumothoraces does not correlate well with the clinical manifestations.
- The clinical symptoms associated with secondary pneumothoraces are more severe in general than those associated with primary pneumothoraces, and may seem out of proportion to the size of the pneumothorax[76].
- The clinical evaluation is therefore probably more important than the size of the pneumothorax in determining the management strategy.
- Commonly, the plain PA chest x-ray has been used to quantify the size of the pneumothorax. However, it tends to underestimate the size because it is a two-dimensional image while the pleural cavity is a three-dimensional structure.

[74] Warakaulle DR, Traill Z. Imaging of pleural disease. Imaging 2004;**16**:10–21. (**4**)

[75] Kelly A-M, Weldon D, Tsang AYL, et al. Comparison between two methods for estimating pneumothorax size from chest x-rays. Respir Med 2006;**100**:1356–9. (**2+**).

[76] BTS guidelines. Management of spontaneous pneumothorax: British Thoracic Society pleural disease guideline 2010 [Online]

- The 2003 BTS guidelines[77] advocated a more accurate means of size calculation than its predecessor in 1993, using the cube function of two simple measurements, and the fact that a **2 cm radiographic pneumothorax approximates to a 50% pneumothorax by volume**.
- There are difficulties with this approach, including the fact that some pneumothoraces are localised (rather than uniform), so that measurement ratios cannot be applied.
- The shape of the lung cannot be assumed to remain constant during collapse. The choice of a 2 cm depth is a compromise between the theoretical risk of needle trauma with a more shallow pneumothorax and the significant volume and length of time to spontaneous resolution of a greater depth of pneumothorax.
- Assuming a symmetrical pattern of lung collapse, then this measure is normally taken from the chest wall to the outer edge of the lung at the level of the hilum.

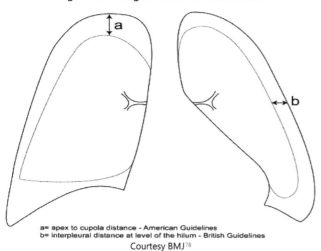

a= apex to cupola distance - American Guidelines
b= interpleural distance at level of the hilum - British Guidelines
Courtesy BMJ[78]

INFORMATION REQUIRED FOR PLANNING MANAGEMENT AND FOLLOW UP FOR A PATIENT WITH A SPONTANEOUS PNEUMOTHORAX

1. Age of the patient
2. Does the patient feel breathless?
3. Determine if the pneumothorax is primary or secondary by reviewing the patients:
   - Past medical history and Medication
   - History of presenting complaint (specifically ask about trauma)
   - Chest radiograph
4. History of previous pneumothorax (side, size and treatment)

5. Classify the size of the pneumothorax from the chest radiograph
   - Small ≤2cm
   - Large >2cm
6. Duration of symptoms
7. Smoker (and how many cigarettes they smoke per day)
8. Family history of pneumothorax
9. Vocation
10. Plans for holidays/ hobbies involving flying or SCUBA diving

EMERGENCY DEPARTMENT MANAGEMENT OF SPONTANEOUS PNEUMOTHORAX

- Management depends upon whether the patient is **symptomatic**, whether the pneumothorax is **primary or secondary** and its **size** on the PA radiograph.

Management of PSP

- Patients with PSP or SSP and significant breathlessness associated with any size of pneumothorax should undergo active intervention.
- Chest drains are usually required for patients with tension or bilateral pneumothorax who should be admitted to hospital.
- Observation is the treatment of choice for small PSP without significant breathlessness.
- Selected asymptomatic patients with a large PSP may be managed by observation alone.
- Patients with a small PSP without breathlessness should be considered for discharge with early outpatient review. These patients should also receive clear written advice to return in the event of worsening breathlessness.

Management of SSP

- All patients with SSP should be admitted to hospital for at least 24 h and receive supplemental oxygen in compliance with the BTS guidelines on the use of oxygen.
- Most patients will require the insertion of a small-bore chest drain.
- All patients will require early referral to a chest physician.
- Those with a persistent air leak should be discussed with a thoracic surgeon at 48 h.

SUPPLEMENTAL OXYGEN

o A pneumothorax will resolve up to **4 times faster** if high flow oxygen is administered.
o Symptomatic patients and those admitted for observation should have high flow oxygen administered (**15l/min via a non-rebreathe mask with a reservoir**).

---

[77] Henry M, Arnold T, Harvey. BTS guidelines for the management of spontaneous pneumothorax. Thorax 2003;**58**(Suppl II):39–52. (**4**).

[78] BTS guidelines. Management of spontaneous pneumothorax: British Thoracic Society pleural disease guideline 2010 [Online]

- **Entonox** diffuses into air spaces and **can convert an uncomplicated pneumothorax into a tension pneumothorax.**
- Its use as an analgesic is contraindicated in this setting.

IMPORTANT ADVICES

- *Smokers* should be advised to quit and seek assistance from their GP to successfully achieve this.
- *Patients should not fly* until a week has elapsed since complete resolution of the pneumothorax has been demonstrated on a chest radiograph or until they have recovered from a definitive surgical procedure aimed to prevent pneumothorax recurrence.
- *Patients should never dive* after a pneumothorax unless bilateral surgical pleurectomy has been performed.

SPECIALIST REFERRAL

- Referral to a respiratory physician should be made within 24 h of admission.
- Complex drain management is best effected in areas where specialist medical and nursing expertise is available.
- *Failure of a pneumothorax to re-expand or a persistent air leak should prompt early referral to a respiratory physician, preferably within the first 24 h.*
- *Such patients may require prolonged chest drainage with complex drain management (suction, chest drain repositioning) and liaison with thoracic surgeons.*
- *Drain management is also best delivered by nurses with specialist expertise. Surgical referral is discussed in a later section.*

REFER TO CARDIOTHORACIC SURGEON IF[76]:

1. Second ipsilateral pneumothorax
2. First contra-lateral pneumothorax
3. Bilateral spontaneous pneumothorax
4. Persistent air leak or failure of lung re-expansion 5 days after chest drain insertion
5. Spontaneous haemothorax
6. Professions at risk (e.g. pilots, divers)
7. Pregnancy

DISCHARGE AND FOLLOW-UP

- Patients should be advised to return to hospital if increasing breathlessness develops.
- All patients should be followed up by respiratory physicians until full resolution.
- Air travel should be avoided until full resolution.
- Diving should be permanently avoided unless the patient has undergone bilateral surgical pleurectomy and has normal lung function and chest CT scan postoperatively.

KEY LEARNING POINTS
Adapted from RCEM Learning

- **Smoking** is strongly associated with pneumothorax recurrence.
- **Breathless patients** require intervention regardless of pneumothorax size.
- **All** patients with **secondary pneumothoraces** require admission.
- **Oxygen** should be applied to all patients with a pneumothorax if they are breathless or require admission.
- Without supplemental oxygenation, spontaneous pneumothoraces resolve at a rate of approximately 2% of the hemi-thorax volume per day.
  - **A 1cm pneumothorax** (~25% pneumothorax) would be expected to fully resolve in approximately 12 days.
  - **A 2cm pneumothorax** (~30-50% pneumothorax) may take 3-4 weeks to fully resolve.
- Aspiration should be performed until the patient **coughs**; **no more can be aspirated** or when **2.5L have been aspirated**.
- Simple (needle) aspiration should be considered the first-line treatment for primary spontaneous pneumothoraces that require intervention.
- It should only be used for secondary pneumothoraces when the pneumothroax is small (1-2cm) and the patient is not breathless.
- Small drains are as effective as large drains in treating spontaneous pneumothoraces and their use is preferred.
- Patients discharged from the ED following a spontaneous pneumothorax should ideally be reviewed by a **respiratory physician after 2 weeks**.
- In practice, it may be impossible to access specialist clinics in the recommended timeframe.
- If this is the case, then the patient should be advised to initially return to the ED, at 2 weeks, **for a repeat chest radiograph and senior doctor review pending specialist review.**
- If the pneumothorax is recurrent, or the patient has a high-risk vocation, referral for a cardiothoracic outpatient appointment is appropriate.

ED APPROACH TO SPONTANEOUS PNEUMOTHORAX
Adapted from RCEM Learning

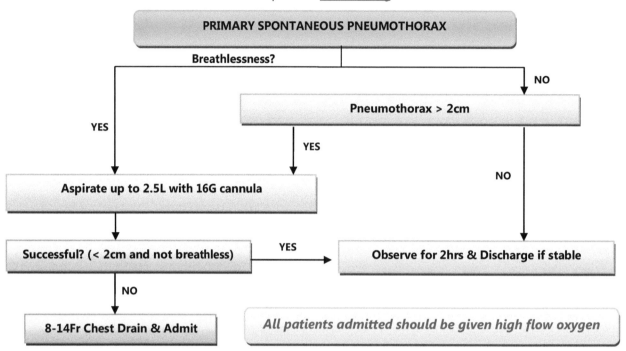

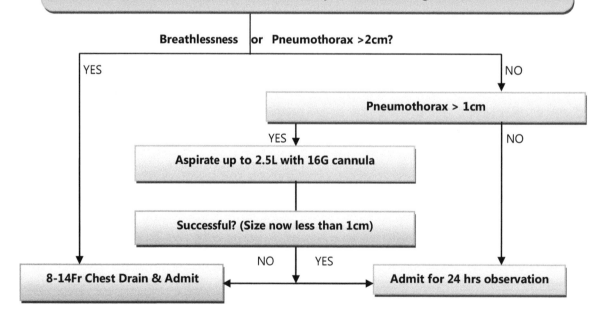

VI. PLEURAL EFFUSION

INTRODUCTION

- A pleural effusion is an abnormal collection of fluid in the pleural space resulting from excess fluid production or decreased absorption.[79]
- It is the most common manifestation of pleural disease. The pleural space is bordered by the parietal and visceral pleurae. The parietal pleura covers the inner surface of the thoracic cavity, including the mediastinum, diaphragm, and ribs.
- The visceral pleura envelops all lung surfaces, including the interlobar fissures. The right and left pleural spaces are separated by the mediastinum.

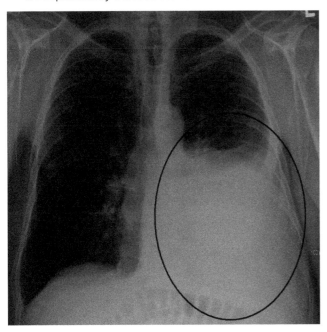

- The pleural space plays an important role in respiration by coupling the movement of the chest wall with that of the lungs in two ways.
  - First, a relative vacuum in the space keeps the visceral and parietal pleurae in close proximity.
  - Second, the small volume of pleural fluid, which has been calculated at 0.13 mL/kg of body weight under normal circumstances, serves as a lubricant to facilitate movement of the pleural surfaces against each other in the course of respirations.
- This small volume of fluid is maintained through the balance of hydrostatic and oncotic pressure and lymphatic drainage, a disturbance of which may lead to pathology.

AETIOLOGY

- The most common causes of pleural effusion are: Congestive heart failure, cancer, pneumonia, and pulmonary embolism.
- Pleural fluid puncture (pleural tap) enables the differentiation of a transudate from an exudate, which remains, at present, the foundation of the further diagnostic work-up.
- When a pleural effusion arises in the setting of pneumonia, the potential development of an empyema must not be overlooked.
- Lung cancer is the most common cause of malignant pleural effusion, followed by breast cancer.

Differentiating Exudate From Transudate

- **An exudate** tends to suggest a local process adjacent to or involving the pleura, whereas a transudate suggests a systemic process. As a consequence, with few exceptions, patients who present with a new pleural effusion should undergo a diagnostic thoracentesis.
- Subsequent testing is aimed at further identifying the underlying etiology or grading the severity of disease. Depending on the clinical setting, this evaluation may be completed in the emergency department (ED) or initiated in the ED and completed in an inpatient service.[80]
- The distinction between transudate and exudate is generally made by measurement of serum and pleural fluid lactate dehydrogenase (LDH) and protein concentrations.
  - A **transudate** contains **less than 25 g/l of protein**
  - An **exudate** contains **more than 35 g/l of protein**
- If the pleural fluid contains protein at levels between **25 g/l and 35 g/l**, then **Lights Criteria** should be used to decide whether the effusion is a transudate or an exudate.

LIGHTS CRITERIA

- *States that **the fluid is an exudate** if one or more of the following criteria are met:*
  - *Pleural fluid Protein: Serum protein ratio is greater than 0.5 (PfP/SP>0.5)*
  - *Pleural fluid LDH: Serum LDH is greater than 0.6 (PfLDH/SLDH>0.6)*
  - *Pleural fluid LDH is greater than two thirds the upper limit of normal serum LDH. (PfLDH>2/3 upper limit SLDH)*

---

[79] Diaz-Guzman E, Dweik RA. Diagnosis and management of pleural effusions: a practical approach. Compr Ther. 2007 Winter. 33(4):237-46.

[80] Yinon Y, Kelly E, Ryan G. Fetal pleural effusions. Best Pract Res Clin Obstet Gynaecol. 2008 Feb. 22(1):77-96.

CLINICAL ASSESSMENT

- **Classical symptoms and signs**
  - o Dyspnoea, stony dullness to chest percussion, reduced breath sounds, reduced tactile fremitus, and asymmetric chest expansion.
- **Non-specific features**
  - o Chest pain, upper abdominal pain, shoulder tip pain, peripheral oedema, haemoptysis, evidence of malignancy.
  - o *Patients with chest pain and pleural effusion* *are more likely to have an exudative aetiology such as pleural infection, pulmonary infarction (PE) or malignancy.*

INVESTIGATION STRATEGIES

- o **Chest Radiograph**: to identifying the size and location of the effusion and any underlying aetiology.
- o **Blood:**
  - ▪ ABG, FBC, U&E,
  - ▪ Serum Protein,
  - ▪ Serum LDH,
  - ▪ Serum Glucose,
  - ▪ Serum Amylase
- o **Pleural fluid analysis: The gross appearance of the fluid** should be noted as this may suggest a specific diagnosis
  - ▪ Protein content, LDH level, Cytology,
  - ▪ Cell count and differential, Fluid pH
  - ▪ Fluid glucose, Gram staining and culture

ADVANCED IMAGING STUDIES

- **Ultrasound**: The BTS strongly recommends the use of ultrasound to guide pleural aspiration. *If US is not employed and the aspiration fails, no subsequent attempts should be made until imaging has been performed.*
- **CT Scanning**: useful in differentiating benign from malignant pleural effusion.

ED MANAGEMENT OF PLEURAL EFFUSION

- On the basis of presentation in the ED, patients with pleural effusions may be:
  (1) stable and require hospital admission,
  (2) stable and not require hospital admission, or
  (3) unstable.
- Generally, any patient who requires thoracentesis in the ED should be admitted to the hospital.
- Stable patients who do not require admission include those in whom the clinical circumstances clearly explain the effusion, prior investigations of the cause were performed, effusions are typical of their disease and are asymptomatic, and diagnostic or therapeutic thoracentesis is not required.

- In such patients, thoracentesis is not indicated emergently and can be deferred. Therapy for the specific cause of the effusion, if indicated, should be initiated.
- If the patient does not improve after a few days, diagnostic thoracentesis should be performed. This assumes that the patient is reliable, has a stable social situation, and has a physician with whom to follow-up.
- Stable patients requiring admission include those with no prior history of pleural effusion, patients with parapneumonic effusions who do not appear to be septic, and patients with a prior history of pleural effusion whose condition has deteriorated.
- Although these patients are not in acute respiratory distress, diagnostic thoracentesis is warranted. This need not be performed in the ED if it can be performed promptly by the accepting inpatient service. When the cause of the pleural effusion is obvious, appropriate medical therapy should be initiated in the ED.
- For suspected parapneumonic effusions, appropriate antibiotics should be administered in the ED, including coverage for anaerobic organisms.
- Simple parapneumonic effusions have the potential to become complicated effusions or empyemas. Antimicrobial therapy alone is not sufficient for complicated parapneumonic effusions or empyemas. In these cases, prompt tube thoracostomy and antibiotics are required.
- Unstable patients include those in septic shock or respiratory distress or with hemodynamic compromise due to the effusion. The initial treatment focus should be on stabilization of the patient.
- Patients with dyspnea or severe respiratory distress should be placed on the gurney in an upright position, as this will increase tidal volume and decrease the work of breathing and may improve symptoms of congestive heart failure and/or pulmonary edema.
- Life-threatening traumatic or medical conditions (eg, tension hydropneumothorax, massive effusion with contralateral mediastinal shift, pulmonary embolism, esophageal perforation, traumatic rupture of the thoracic duct, strangulated diaphragmatic hernia) must be ruled out. These patients require immediate diagnostic and therapeutic thoracentesis.

  ↳ *No more than 1.5 litres of fluid should be drained in the first hour as* **re-expansion pulmonary oedema** (which as a significant mortality risk) can result when greater volumes are drained.

VII. CARDIOGENIC PULMONARY OEDEMA

INTRODUCTION

- Cardiogenic pulmonary edema (CPO) is defined as pulmonary edema due to increased capillary hydrostatic pressure secondary to elevated pulmonary venous pressure.
- CPO reflects the accumulation of fluid with a low-protein content in the lung interstitium and alveoli as a result of cardiac dysfunction

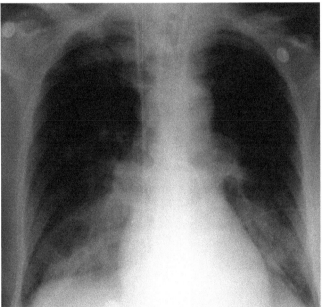

Radiograph shows acute pulmonary edema in a patient who was admitted with acute anterior myocardial infarction. Findings are vascular redistribution, indistinct hila, and alveolar infiltrates.

- Pulmonary edema can be caused by the following major pathophysiologic mechanisms:
  - **Imbalance of Starling forces** - Ie, increased pulmonary capillary pressure, decreased plasma oncotic pressure, increased negative interstitial pressure
  - **Damage to the alveolar**-capillary barrier
  - **Lymphatic obstruction**
  - **Idiopathic (unknown) mechanism**
  - **Increased hydrostatic pressure** leading to pulmonary edema may result from many causes, including excessive intravascular volume administration, pulmonary venous outflow obstruction (eg, mitral stenosis or left atrial [LA] myxoma), and LV failure secondary to systolic or diastolic dysfunction of the left ventricle. CPO leads to progressive deterioration of alveolar gas exchange and respiratory failure. Without prompt recognition and treatment, a patient's condition can deteriorate rapidly.

ETIOLOGY

- CPO is caused by elevated pulmonary capillary hydrostatic pressure leading to transudation of fluid into the pulmonary interstitium and alveoli.
- Increased LA pressure increases pulmonary venous pressure and pressure in the lung microvasculature, resulting in pulmonary edema.

CLINICAL ASSESSMENT

HISTORY

- Patients with cardiogenic pulmonary edema (CPO) present with the dramatic clinical features of left heart failure. Patients develop a sudden onset of extreme breathlessness, anxiety, and feelings of drowning. Clinical manifestations of acute CPO reflect evidence of hypoxia and increased sympathetic tone (increased catecholamine outflow).
- Patients most commonly complain of shortness of breath and profuse diaphoresis. Patients with symptoms of gradual onset (eg, over 24 h) often report dyspnea on exertion, orthopnea, and paroxysmal nocturnal dyspnea.
- Cough is a frequent complaint and may provide an early clue to worsening pulmonary edema in patients with chronic LV dysfunction. Pink, frothy sputum may be present in patients with severe disease. Occasionally, hoarseness may be present as a result of compression of the recurrent laryngeal nerve palsy from an enlarged left atrium, such as in mitral stenosis **(Ortner sign).**
- Chest pain should alert the physician to the possibility of acute myocardial ischemia/infarction or aortic dissection with acute aortic regurgitation, as the precipitant of pulmonary edema.

PHYSICAL EXAMINATION

- **Airway**
  - Usually Patent, patients may be sitting upright, they may demonstrate air hunger, and they may become agitated and confused.
- **Breathing**
  - Tachypnoea with use of accessory muscles
  - The saturation is usually low (below 90% on room air)
  - Auscultation of the lungs usually reveals fine, crepitant rales, but rhonchi or wheezes may also be present. Rales are usually heard at the bases first; as the condition worsens, they progress to the apices.
- **Circulation**
  - Sinus tachycardia.
  - Skin mottling at presentation is an independent predictor of an increased risk of in-hospital mortality.

- o **Hypertension** is often present, because of the hyperadrenergic state.
- o **Hypotension** indicates severe LV systolic dysfunction and the possibility of cardiogenic shock.
- o **Cool extremities** may indicate low cardiac output and poor perfusion.
- o Auscultation of murmurs can help in the diagnosis of acute valvular disorders manifesting with pulmonary edema.
  - ▪ *Aortic stenosis is associated with a harsh crescendo-decrescendo systolic murmur, which is heard best at the upper sternal border and radiating to the carotid arteries. In contrast, acute aortic regurgitation is associated with a short, soft diastolic murmur.*
  - ▪ *Acute mitral regurgitation produces a loud systolic murmur heard best at the apex or lower sternal border.*
  - ▪ *In the setting of ischemic heart disease, this may be a sign of acute MI with rupture of mitral valve chordae.*
  - ▪ *Mitral stenosis typically produces a loud S_1, opening snap, and diastolic rumble at the cardiac apex.*
- o Another notable physical finding is skin pallor or mottling resulting from peripheral vasoconstriction, low cardiac output, and shunting of blood to the central circulation in patients with poor LV function and substantially increased sympathetic tone.
- o Patients with concurrent right ventricular (RV) failure may present with hepatomegaly, hepatojugular reflux, and peripheral edema.

- **Disability**
  - o Patient ppears anxious and diaphoretic.
  - o Severe CPO may be associated with a change in mental status, which can be caused by hypoxia or hypercapnia.
  - o Although CPO is usually associated with hypocapnia, hypercapnia with respiratory acidosis may be seen in patients with severe CPO or underlying chronic obstructive pulmonary disease (COPD).

- **Exposure**
  - o Afebrile
  - o The skin might be cold and clammy.

INVESTIGATION STRATEGIES
- **ECG**
  - o It will often show a **tachycardia** and **possible left ventricular hypertrophy**.
  - o It may reveal precipitating causes such as **ST segment changes** associated with an ACS (STEMI or NSTEMI) or an **arrhythmia** e.g. atrial fibrillation.
- **CXR**
  - o Helpful in excluding other causes of breathlessness, such as pneumonia or pneumothorax.

- o A normal CXR in the acutely short of breath patient would be more likely to suggest a pulmonary embolus or COPD/asthma.
- o **The chest X-ray in CPO can show (images below):**
  - ♣ Cardiomegaly and Upper lobe blood diversion,
  - ♣ KERLEY B septal lines,
  - ♣ Fluid in the interlobar fissures and Pleural effusions,
  - ♣ Bat's wing hilar shadowing

- **Arterial Blood Gas**
  - o **Hypoxaemia**: **Type 1 respiratory failure**; this contrasts with COPD patients in extremis (**who have type 2 respiratory failure**).

- **Other Blood Tests:**
  - o Baseline bloods including **FBC, U&Es, LFT, Troponin, BNP and INR**

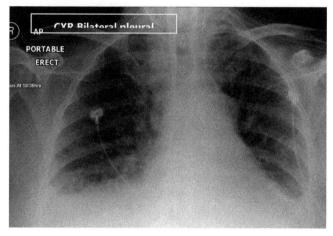

ED MANAGEMENT OF CPO
Treatment Should Consist of:
- **Sitting the Patient Up**,
- Administering **High Flow O$_2$**,
- **Intravenous Nitrates** And
- Instituting **NIV** If Appropriate.

A	Sit the patient Up
B	**High flow O$_2$**: 15L/minute with a reservoir bag **NIV:** • **CPAP** Commence PEEP at 5-7.5 cm H$_2$O & increase up to 10cm as tolerated • **BiPAP**
C	• **Nitrates 10-20mcg/min;** Increase the nitrate infusion every 3-5 min by 5-10 mcg/min as BP allows until improvement. • **Nitroprusside**: Cautious infusion at **0.3 mcg/Kg/min** • **Dobutamine** Infusion commenced at **2-3mcg/kg/min** • **Furosemide 20-40mg IV**
D	**Morphine** (Only small boluses) **2.5-5mg IV**

VIII. VALVULAR HEART DISEASE

INTRODUCTION

- The diagnosis of valvular heart disease is a difficult problem in everyday clinical practice. There is a wide spectrum of presentation – in some cases **murmurs** are found incidentally and in others, patients present very late with dire haemodynamic consequences of neglected valve lesions that may preclude them from definitive surgery.
- With the decline in rheumatic heart disease and the ageing population in the developed world, there has been a change in the disease patterns of valve lesions over the last few decades. Western populations are experiencing greater numbers of degenerative valve disease. In the developing world, however, rheumatic heart disease remains an important cause of valve pathology. Sliwa et al.,[81] in the Heart of Soweto Study, showed an incidence of new cases of rheumatic heart disease of 23.5/100 000 cases per annum.
- **An electrocardiogram (ECG)** and a **chest radiograph (CXR)** are seen as important adjuncts to clinical evaluation and may provide important diagnostic clues to confirming pathology.

1. AORTIC STENOSIS

- Haemodynamically significant obstruction usually occurs when the valve area is Patients are asymptomatic for many years. Once symptoms occur, however, there is a rapid decline in life expectancy.

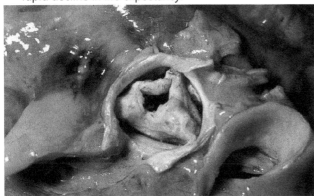

Aortic Stenosis

- Aortic stenosis (AS) is the most common valve lesion in western countries and mainly a disease of the elderly. Common causes of AS include:

---

[81] Sliwa K, Carrington M, Mayosi BM, Zigiriadis E, Mvungi R, Stewart S. Incidence and characteristics of newly diagnosed RHD in urban African adults: Insights from the Heart of Soweto Study. Eur Heart J 2010;31:719-727.

Commonest cause in young adults.

Congenital	The valve can be bi- or unicuspid. In pure AS in the under 70s who require surgery 50% had a calcified bicuspid valve.

- **Rheumatic:** Commonest cause worldwide.
- **Calcific (degenerative):** Commonest cause in the UK. 50% of surgical cases in the over 70s.

Acquired

- **Rare causes:**
  - o Rheumatoid involvement,
  - o Irradiation and
  - o Obstruction due to infected vegetations.

❖ *Hypertension, smoking and raised cholesterol are all risk factors for aortic valve calcification*

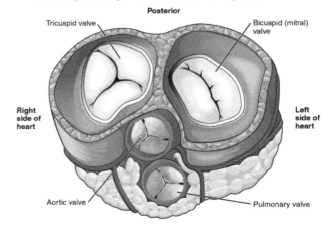

CLINICAL, ECG AND CXR FINDINGS ASSOCIATED WITH AORTIC STENOSIS

Pulse	Slow rising small volume with a sustained peak. (pulsus parvus et tardus) Often absent in the elderly due to loss of aortic compliance.
Cardiac impulse	Sustained heaving apical impulse with a precordial thrill. Laterally displaced apex beat indicates onset of heart failure.
Auscultation	**Harsh systolic ejection murmur, 2nd intercostal space left sternal edge and radiating to the carotids.** The murmur softens and becomes prolonged as the severity of AS increases Single second heart sound (S2) in moderate AS. Paradoxical splitting of S2 or soft/ obscured by murmur in severe AS. Fourth heart sound "gallop rhythm"

ECG	LVH criteria (or strain pattern) but may be absent despite severe obstruction: 10-15% of severe AS have normal ECGs May show RBBB or LBBB AF usually in association with simultaneous Mitral Valve Disease
CXR	Seldom helpful. May show normal sized heart and a dilated proximal ascending aorta. Late signs are of LV/LA dilatation and pulmonary oedema. Calcium in the aortic valve of a patient <45 is indicative of AS

MANAGEMENT IN THE ED
The management of the critically ill aortic stenosis patient can be very challenging.
These patients need a valve replacement, so **consulting cardiothoracic surgery** as soon as possible is prudent.

EMERGENCY MANAGEMENT
1. The crashing aortic stenosis patient in cardiogenic shock should be resuscitated with fluids and inotropic medications such as **dopamine and dobutamine.**
2. The hypertensive aortic stenosis patient with acute pulmonary edema, should be managed cautiously. **Nitroprusside** can be considered, but it has **only** been studied in patients undergoing invasive hemodynamic monitoring in the ICU setting. Based on recent data, **Nitroglycerin** may be safe in the ED setting, but this should be used with caution, and it is unknown if this even improves outcomes.
3. All patients with AS need **antibiotic cover** for certain surgical procedures to protect against infective endocarditis.

2. AORTIC REGURGITATION
- Aortic regurgitation may occur as a result of leaflet pathology or secondary to aortic root pathology.
- **Acute regurgitation** is poorly tolerated and constitutes a medical and surgical emergency. It is commonly caused by infective endocarditis or aortic root dissection.
- **Chronic regurgitation** is well tolerated and patients are often asymptomatic for many years.
- Common causes of primary valve lesions are rheumatic heart disease, infective endocarditis, congenital bicuspid valves, and rheumatoid arthritis.
- Conditions primarily affecting the root, and hence causing regurgitation, are Marfan's syndrome, syphilis, sero-negative spondyloarthritides, aortic dissection and osteogenesis imperfecta.

AETIOLOGY OF ACUTE AND CHRONIC AR

Acute AR (PARI)		• **P**rosthetic valve dysfunction • **A**ortic dissection • **R**upture of an aortic valve leaflet (e.g. trauma) • **I**nfective endocarditis
Chronic AR	Congenital	Usually a bicuspid valve or supravalvular stenosis (suspect if isolated lesion in a chronic presentation.

	Acquired	• Calcific degeneration
		• Aortic root dilatation
		• Rheumatic fever
		• Previous infective endocarditis
		• Rare causes:
		  ○ Connective tissue diseases : - Marfan's syndrome, Ehlers-Danlos ;
		  ○ Autoimmune diseases: - rheumatoid arthritis, systemic lupus erythematous, ankylosing spondylitis; Syphilis;
		  ○ Appetite suppressant drug: Fenfluramine.

PATHOPHYSIOLOGY
- Regurgitation of blood into the left ventricle during diastole causes volume overloading.
- The pathophysiology of acute and chronic AR is different:
  ○ **In acute AR** there is a sudden increase in the volume of blood in the LV during diastole. The left ventricle volume can only increase marginally in response to this acute change so left ventricular end diastolic pressure rises sharply. LA and pulmonary venous pressure rises and results in acute heart failure.
  ○ **In chronic AR** there is time for compensation and the LV progressively dilates and hypertrophies to maintain the ejection fraction. Tachycardia decreases the diastolic filling time and so reduces the regurgitant volume. During early stages of the disease the heart is able to respond to exertion with an appropriate increase in cardiac output. As a result, AR can be tolerated for years.

CLINICAL FEATURES
CHRONIC AORTIC REGURGITATION
Patients may be asymptomatic for years although a murmur may have been previously noted.

Common symptoms:
- Awareness of the heart beat /palpitations especially at rest (because of the hyperactive dilated LV).
- Chest pain
- Fatigue

As the disease progresses:
- Heart failure
- Angina (as in AS this can occur despite normal coronary arteries)

ACUTE AORTIC REGURGITATION
- In acute AR, the clinical presentation will depend on the underlying cause. If the regurgitation is mild the predominant symptoms may relate to the underlying cause; for example, acute tearing chest pain radiating to the back suggests aortic dissection, or the peripheral signs and symptoms of sepsis in infective endocarditis.
- AR associated with aortic dissection means that the dissection involves the ascending aorta down to the annulus.

CLINICAL, ECG, CXR FINDINGS ASSOCIATED WITH ACUTE AND CHRONIC AORTIC REGURGITATION

	Chronic AR	**Acute AR**
Pulse	Rapid rise and quick collapse (water hammer pulse), double impulse, wide pulse pressure • **Corrigan's sign**- visible carotid pulsation • **Traube's sign= 'pistol shot'**- sound heard over the femoral artery • **Quincke's pulse**- capillary pulsation visible on shining a light through the fingertips	Tachycardia Rapid rate of rise of arterial pulse
Cardiac impulse	Hyperdynamic, maybe visible	Normal or hyperkinetic
Auscultation	Soft blowing diastolic murmur LSE. Best heard with the patient sitting forward in fully held expiration Duration of the murmur in	Early blowing diastolic murmur

diastole correlates with severity of AR. **Austin Flint murmur**- apical diastolic murmur caused by obstruction of mitral flow produced by the partial closure of the mitral valve by the regurgitant jet and rapid rising LV diastolic pressure.

ECG	In moderate/ severe disease- LVH with or without strain pattern	Non-specific ST-T changes and sinus tachycardia or may be normal or show changes consistent with the underlying cause
CXR	Cardiomegaly with LV prominence and possibly dilated aorta	'normal' heart size and pulmonary oedema

MANAGEMENT IN THE ED
- In acute severe AR secondary supportive management is needed while the underlying cause is being treated.
- **Blood cultures** should be taken unless there is an obvious underlying cause (e.g. aortic dissection or AMI)

EMERGENCY MEASURES
- Contact specialist services
- In acute AR supportive measures are directed at reducing pulmonary venous pressure and increasing cardiac output.
- They will include the use of vasodilators, intubation and positive pressure ventilation.
- Inotropic support may be needed but can worsen the AR. Nitrates and diuretics have little effect and the intra-aortic balloon pump is contraindicated.
- Any patient with known AR presenting in heart failure will need admission for evaluation and consideration of aortic valve replacement.
- In an acute presentation of a patient with chronic AR adjustment of medical therapies such as diuretics, vasodilators, rate and rhythm control is needed acutely.

OTHER MANAGEMENT ISSUES

↓ *AR patients have an increased risk of developing endocarditis and should receive appropriate antibiotic prophylaxis.*

MITRAL VALVE DISEASE

There are three types of mitral valve dysfunction:
- *Mitral Stenosis (MS)*
- *Mitral Regurgitation (MR)*
- *Mitral Valve prolapse (MVP)*

3. MITRAL STENOSIS

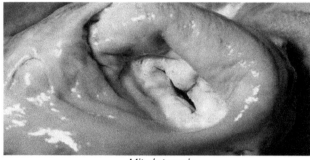

Mitral stenosis

- Mitral stenosis (MS) is almost exclusively caused by **chronic rheumatic heart disease.**
- The rheumatic process leads to inflammation, resulting in commissural fusion, thickening and fibrosis of both the leaflets and subvalvular apparatus.

AETIOLOGY OF MITRAL STENOSIS

Acquired	Other rare causes are:
Rheumatic heart disease (commonest cause worldwide)	• *Infective endocarditis* • *Calcification of the mitral annulus* • *SLE* • *Carcinoid Syndrome* • *Left atrial myxoma can cause left atrial obstruction and mimic MS*

PATHOPHYSIOLOGY OD MS

- The obstruction to atrial emptying in MS causes an elevation in left atrial and pulmonary venous pressure, leading to reduced lung compliance and breathlessness on exertion.
- Reactive pulmonary arterial hypertension causes right ventricular hypertrophy and failure.
- Progressive stenosis cause left atrial dilatation and consequent atrial fibrillation which will further impair the function of the atrium.
- Left ventricular filling becomes impaired and cardiac output becomes compromised.

CLINICAL FEATURES

The main clinical presentations are:
- **Exertional breathless, Orthopnoea, PND** (Paroxysmal Nocturnal Dyspnoea), Breathlessness on exertion is often the first symptom noticed.
- **Acute pulmonary oedema** – Hyperdynamic states with an associated tachycardia such as pregnancy, infection, uncontrolled AF and anaemia may result in a worsening of symptoms
- **Atrial fibrillation** – Onset is associated with a marked deterioration of the patient's clinical state. – Risk of left atrial thrombus and systemic embolism
- **Haemoptysis** – This used to be the second most common presentation but is rarer now that the disease is recognized sooner.
- **Fatigue** (due to reduced cardiac output)

CLINICAL, ECG AND CXR FINDINGS ASSOCIATED WITH MITRAL STENOSIS

Pulse	Small volume, irregular (usually AF)
Cardiac impulse	'Tapping' apex due to "palpable" first heart sound (S1)
Auscultation	Loud first heart sound (S1) (in sinus rhythm), Opening snap and rumbling mid-diastolic murmur. Early diastolic murmur of pulmonary regurgitation (Graham Steell murmur)
ECG	Broad or biphasic P-wave best seen in Lead-II indicating LA hypertrophy. R axis deviation. AF common, RV hypertrophy in later stages
CXR	Straightening of the left heart border indicating a dilated LA ('double atrial shadow'). Pulmonary congestion
Other features	Mitral facies: peripheral cyanosis of the cheeks

EMERGENCY MEASURES IN THE ED

- Close attention to fluid balance.
- Antipyretics as appropriate.
- Find and treat underlying infection if suspected.
- Diuretics may be needed to relieve pulmonary congestion but addressing the shortened diastolic filling caused by any tachycardia will be of most benefit in the emergency setting.
- Rate control with **beta blockers, digoxin or calcium channel blockers** will be required for rapid atrial fibrillation.

- *Any consideration of cardioversion must recognize the significant incidence of atrial thrombus and the risks of embolisation.*
- Acute haemoptysis is relatively rare but can be severe. It is caused by vessel rupture due to venous congestion and may require referral to a cardiothoracic surgeon.
- All MS patients in atrial fibrillation should be on long term anticoagulants. There is little benefit to those in sinus rhythm. Systemic embolisation may be due to sub-therapeutic anticoagulation therapy. Patients may also present with complications of over anticoagulation.

4. MITRAL REGURGITATION

- MR may be classified depending on the clinical presentation (acute or chronic) or leaflet pathology (functional versus organic).
- Acute MR is a medical emergency presenting with acute pulmonary oedema and hypotension and is usually caused by endocarditis, myocardial infarction with papillary muscle rupture or spontaneous rupture of the chordae.

Mitral Regurgitation

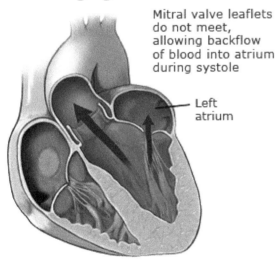

Mitral valve leaflets do not meet, allowing backflow of blood into atrium during systole

Left atrium

AETIOLOGY OF ACUTE AND CHRONIC MITRAL REGURGITATION

Acute MR	Chronic MR
• Ruptured chordae tendinae • Partial or complete papillary muscle rupture (e.g. due to acute myocardial infarction, trauma or infective endocarditis)	• Rheumatic heart disease • LV dilatation secondary to ischaemic heart disease or cardiomyopathy • Myxomatous degeneration • Mitral valve prolapse

PATHOPHYSIOLOGY OF MR

- During systole, a portion of the ejection fraction regurgitates into the left atrium. The portion is known as **the regurgitant volume**. This can also be expressed as the regurgitant fraction which is the regurgitant volume/ejection volume.
- Moderate MR is said to be present when the regurgitant fraction is in the range of **30 to 50%**; **severe MR is defined as a regurgitant fraction >50%.**

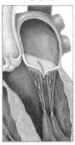 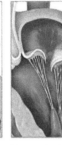 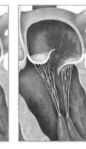 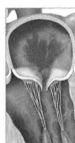

Normal mitral valve | Degenerative MR caused by mitral valve prolapse | Degenerative MR caused by flail leaflet | Functional MR

CLINICAL FEATURES

A. CHRONIC MITRAL REGURGITATION

- With progressive leaking of the mitral valve the left side of the heart has time to adapt. Both the LA and LV will enlarge to cope with the increase in blood volume and the LV will hypertrophy to deliver the increase in stroke volume needed to maintain cardiac output. Dilatation of the LA may result in AF and marked symptoms.

B. ACUTE MITRAL REGURGITATION

- The patient will be acutely unwell with signs and symptoms of acute pulmonary oedema as well as signs of the underlying cause such as acute myocardial infarction or infective endocarditis.
- An echocardiograpy should be obtained urgently to rule out VSD, diagnose MR and assess LV function.

CLINICAL, ECG & CXR FINDINGS ASSOCIATED WITH ACUTE & CHRONIC MR

	Acute MR	Chronic MR
Pulse	Tachycardia	Tachycardia / AF common (Prominent 'a' wave in JVP in SR)
Cardiac impulse	Hyperdynamic	Diffuse and displaced laterally. Systolic thrill at apex

Auscultation	Pansystolic murmur radiating to the axilla and back 3rd Heart Sound May be difficult to hear in the acutely breathless and tachycardic patient	Pansystolic murmur radiating to the axilla and back 3rd Heart Sound
ECG	No changes or acute MI	LA and LV hypertrophy AF common
CXR	Pulmonary oedema with a normal sized heart or minimally enlarged LA	Increased LA and LV size Pulmonary venous congestion
ECHO	Urgent – to rule out ventricular septal defect, diagnose MR and assess LV function	

MANAGEMENT IN THE ED

- *Blood cultures* should be taken in any patient with acute MR and no obvious infarct.
- *Acute MR associated with myocardial infarction is a cardiovascular emergency and may require surgical intervention*

EMERGENCY MEASURES

- **Contact specialist services** as may need surgical intervention as an emergency.
- **Treat acute myocardial infarction** if underlying cause.
- **Treat pulmonary oedema**. This may be difficult if the patient is in cardiogenic shock.
- Intubation and positive pressure ventilation should be considered early.
- CPAP can be helpful. Reduce preload and afterload with nitrate infusion and ACE inhibitors if tolerated. Diuretics and inotropes may also be needed. Patients with cardiogenic shock with acute MR may benefit from intraaortic balloon pump.

Acute presentations of chronic MR are usually related to the onset of AF.
Therapy is directed at reducing afterload to reduce LV work and controlling AF.
Acute presentation of a patient with known chronic MR may indicate they require surgical intervention.

5. MITRAL VALVE PROLAPSE
(Floppy mitral valve, Barlow's syndrome)

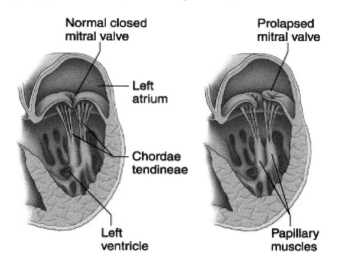

- MVP is prolapse of a portion of the valve leaflets into the left atrium during systole associated with a small amount of regurgitation of blood.
- The condition is found in between 2-5% of the population and occurs more commonly in women. Most cases are idiopathic.
- It can be acquired secondary to IHD, Rheumatic heart disease and hypertrophic cardiomyopathy.

PATHOPHYSIOLOGY

- One or both of the mitral valve leaflets show fibromyxomatous changes. At the end of diastole, the valve closes normally but as the pressure in the LV rises the leaflet proplases back into the LA.
- Strain on the papillary muscles can lead to mitral regurgitation.

CLINICAL FEATURES

- Although most patients are asymptomatic, a wide variety of symptoms have been associated with MVP such as chest pain, breathlessness and palpitations.
- MVP may progress to clinically significant MR and there is an increased risk of infective endocarditis and cerebrovascular events.
- Men, those aged >45 and patients with significant MR are at high risk for complications. The association with sudden death is uncertain and is usually in the high-risk group.
- Some patients have been noted to have long QT intervals.

CLINICAL, ECG AND CXR FINDINGS ASSOCIATED WITH MITRAL VALVE PROLAPSE

Pulse	normal
Cardiac impulse	normal
Auscultation	Midsystolic click – a high pitched sound caused by sudden tensing of the mitral valve apparatus as the leaflet prolapse
ECG	Most cases no abnormality
CXR	No abnormality unless significant MR

ACUTE PROBLEMS
- Attribution of symptoms to MVP is controversial.
- A patient with significant associated MR may have symptoms and signs related to this.
- Otherwise, when MVP has previously been diagnosed or is suspected, the role of emergency care is to exclude another acute cause for presenting symptoms.
- In the absence of another cause needing immediate treatment, the patient should be referred back to their own doctor for follow up or further investigation. Normal antibiotic prophylaxis precautions should be followed.

RIGHT SIDED VALVE LESIONS
- Both the tricuspid and pulmonary valves can be stenotic or regurgitant.
- In the emergency setting, the most important presentation is **tricuspid regurgitation** secondary to either **infective endocarditis in intravenous drug abusers** or **chronic obstructive pulmonary disease (COPD) with pulmonary hypertension** and subsequent right ventricular failure/dilatation.

6. TRICUSPID REGURGITATION
AETIOLOGY OF TRICUSPID REGURGITATION

Congenital	Acquired
Ebstein's anomaly	• RV dilatation mitral valve disease, • RV infarction, • Pulmonary hypertension • Infective endocarditis (IVDA) • Marfan's syndrome

- Tricuspid stenosis (TS) is rare and usually rheumatic in origin. Most patients with rheumatic tricuspid valve (TV) disease present with tricuspid regurgitation (TR) or a combination of TR and TS.

- Isolated rheumatic TS is uncommon, but usually accompanies MV disease.
- Less common and unusual causes of obstruction to right atrial (RA) emptying include congenital tricuspid atresia, RA tumours, carcinoid syndrome, endomyocardial fibrosis, TV vegetations, pacemaker leads or extracardiac tumours.[82]
- TS is found at autopsy in 15% of patients with rheumatic heart disease, but is of clinical significance in

CLINICAL FEATURES
- Patients are usually asymptomatic unless right heart failure develops and the patient complains of oedema, ascites and abdominal pain from liver congestion.
- Intravenous drug abusers may present acutely unwell with a **staphylococcal endocarditis**.

CLINICAL, ECG AND CXR FINDINGS ASSOCIATED WITH TRICUSPID REGURGITATION

Pulse	AF common Large 'v' waves in JVP
Auscultation	Soft pansystolic murmur at LSE louder on inspiration Third heart sound (S3) often heard
ECG	No specific changes
CXR	Cardiomegaly, pleural effusion
Other features	Tender enlarged pulsatile liver

ACUTE PROBLEMS
- *Tricuspid endocarditis in a drug abuser needs blood cultures and aggressive antibiotic therapy covering staphylococcal infection.*
- *Early surgery may be needed.*

7. PROSTHETIC VALVES
- There are two types of prosthetic valves: mechanical valves and bioprosthetic (tissue) valves. The major differences between the two relate to risk of thromboembolism (higher with mechanical valves) and structural deterioration (higher with bioprostheses)[83]
- Mechanical valves are classified into three groups: bileaflet, tilting disc and ballcage. Bileaflet mechanical valves are most commonly implanted.
- Patients with mechanical valves require long-term anticoagulation.

[82] Bruce CJ, Connolly HM. Right-sided valve disease deserves a little more respect. Circulation 2009;119(20):2726-2734. [http://dx.doi.org/10.1161/CIRCULATIONAHA.108.776021]

[83] Pibarot P, Dumesnil JG. Prosthetic heart valves: Selection of the optimal prosthesis and long-term management. Circulation 2009;119(7):1034-1048. [http://dx.doi.org/10.1161/CIRCULATIONAHA.108.778886]

- The risk of thromboembolism is about 6 times higher without anticoagulants, and the risk of de novo valve thrombosis is also higher. Warfarin is the anticoagulant of choice and the international normalised ratio should be between 2.5 and 3.5.

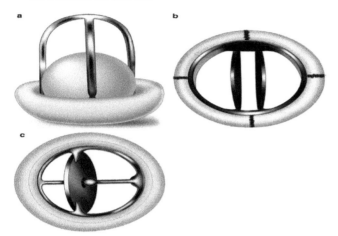

- Antiplatelet agents such as aspirin do not provide adequate protection and are not recommended without the use of anticoagulants. Bioprostheses were developed to overcome the challenges of long-term anticoagulation and increased risk of thromboembolism associated with mechanical valves.
- A stented tissue valve consists of three tissue leaflets mounted on a ring with semi-rigid stents that facilitate implantation. Because stents add to obstruction and increase stress on the leaflets, stentless tissue valves were developed for the aortic position and are particularly useful for patients with small aortic roots.
- More recently, a transcatheter bioprosthesis has been developed, which can be implanted via a catheter at the aortic valve position.[84]
- Homograft aortic valves are harvested from cadavers, sterilised with antibiotics and cryopreserved at −196° for long periods before implantation.
- Pulmonary autografts (Ross procedure) involve removal of a patient's native pulmonary valve and reimplantation to replace the diseased aortic valve.

ACUTE PROBLEMS WITH PROSTHETIC VALVES
4.1. VALVE THROMBUS AND EMBOLISATION

- Prosthetic valves may become obstructed due to thrombosis, pannus formation, or a combination of both. Valve thrombosis may be obstructive or non-obstructive. Thrombosis may occur slowly as a chronic progressive worsening of function or may occur more acutely.

- Inadequate anticoagulation is almost always associated with left-sided heart valve thrombosis[85] A patient may present in cardiogenic shock, with systemic embolisation (cerebral infarction) or with sudden death.
- The diagnosis should be suspected if the patient is known to have a mechanical valve and the distinctive crisp click sound is reduced on auscultation. Echocardiography is needed to confirm the diagnosis. In a cerebral vascular event a CT scan should be performed to exclude a bleed. Heparin anticoagulation or as necessary thrombolysis, thrombectomy or valve replacement.

4.2. ENDOCARDITIS

- One of the deadliest complications of prosthetic valves is infectious endocarditis. In addition to the presence of a foreign body, patients with prosthetic valves have frequent hematogenous exposures through multiple arterial or venous puncture sites. Multiple blood cultures should be considered during febrile illnesses prior to the administration of antibiotics (ideally, the first and last samples should be drawn from different sites at least one hour apart).[86]

4.3. PROSTHETIC VALVES & ACUTE HAEMORRHAGE

- In acute haemorrhage the risk of causing valve thrombosis is outweighed by the risk of on-going bleeding.
- Warfarin should be reversed (in consultation with Haematology services). When stable the patient should receive heparin and warfarin restarted.

---

[84] O'Gara PT, Bonow RO, Otto CM. In: Otto CM, Bonow RO, eds. Valvular Heart Disease: A Companion to Braunwald's Heart Disease. Philadelphia, PA: Saunders/Elsevier, 2009:383-398.

[85] Butany J, Ahluwalia MS, Munroe C, et al. Mechanical heart valve prostheses: Identification and evaluation. Cardiovasc Pathol 2003;12:1-22.

[86] Dunmire SM. Infective Endocarditis and Valvular Heart Disease. In: Marx JA, ed. Rosen's Emergency Medicine: Concepts and Clinical Practice. Philadelphia: Mosby Elsevier; 2006:1300-1309.

IX. PULMONARY EMBOLISM

Recognised clinical features found in patients with a PE are:
1. Dyspnoea (70% of patients)
2. Tachypnoea (RR>20)
3. Pleuritic chest pain
4. Apprehension
5. Tachycardia (>100bpm)
6. Cough
7. Haemoptysis
8. Leg pain
9. Clinically evident DVT (10% of patients)

WELLS CRITERIA FOR P.E.

WELLS' CRITERIA	SCORE
Clinically suspected DVT	3.0
PE at least as likely or more likely than alternative diagnosis	3.0
Pulse rate >100	1.5
Immobilisation >3 days	1.5
Surgery last 4 weeks	1.5
Previous VTE	1.5
Haemoptysis	1.0
Malignancy	1.0

Clinical probability simplified scores

PE likely	**> 4 points**
PE unlikely	**4 points or less**

INVESTIGATIONS

- **ECG changes in Pulmonary Embolism:**
  - Sinus Tachycardia
  - RBBB
  - P Pulmonale
  - Extreme right axis deviation (+180 degrees)
  - S1 Q3 T3
  - T-wave inversions in V1-4 and lead III
- Clockwise rotation with persistent S wave in V6

PULMONARY EMBOLUS RULE-OUT CRITERIA

All answers to the following questions must be yes:

Low risk by Gestalt or other criteria?

Age <50?

Pulse <100?

Oxygen saturations on room air >94%?

No unilateral leg swelling?

No haemoptysis?

No recent trauma or surgery?

No previous VTE?

No oral hormone use?

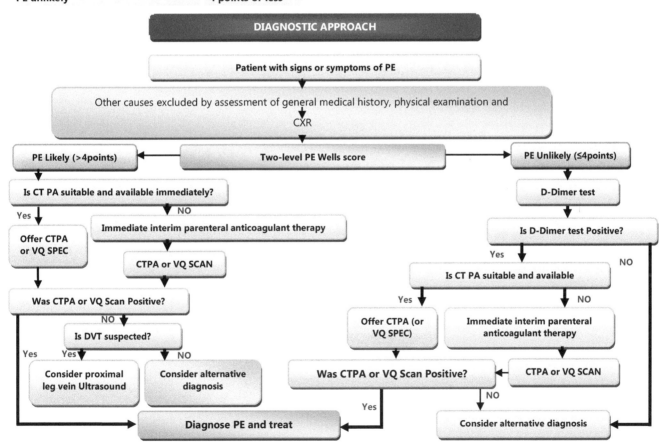

Moussa Issa | www.moussaissabooks.com

- o Wells' Clinical Decision Rule **(CDR)** to predict pre-test probability - two scores with **≤ 4 = 'unlikely'**, and **> 4 = 'likely'.**
    - If CDR score is unlikely (≤ 4), perform D-dimer:
        - If negative, rules out = no PE.
        - If D-Dimer positive, perform CTPA.
            - o If CTPA negative rules out,
            - o If positive, treat.
    - If CDR score likely (> 4), do CTPA:
        - If negative, rules out.
        - If positive, treat.

All pregnant / post-partum women with suspected DVT or PE are at high risk and need definitive imaging; there is no role for a D-dimer assay.

- **Imaging**
    - o **Low and intermediate risk patients** with a **positive D-dimer** and **high-risk patients** require further imaging.
    - o Imaging techniques include the following:
        - **CT pulmonary angiogram (CTPA)**
        - **Isotope lung scanning (V/Q scanning)**
        - **Echocardiography**
        - **Ultrasound**

CTPA is the investigation of choice due to its greater sensitivity and specificity for PE than V/Q scanning and its ability to identify alternate diagnoses.

MANAGEMENT OF PE IN THE ED

- The pathophysiological processes occurring in acute PE have recently been described.
- Supportive therapy includes oxygen and, in some patients, analgesia.
- In hypotensive patients it is common practice to use plasma expanders and inotropic support.[87]
- The effects of acute PE on right heart function due to arterial obstruction by thrombus are exacerbated by concomitant pulmonary vasoconstrictors, and animal studies on the effect of antagonists to these and of direct pulmonary vasodilators suggest that such agents have a potential future role in massive PE.[88]

1. PATIENTS AWAITING INVESTIGATION

- o All patients in the PE likely subgroup and those in the PE unlikely subgroup who have a positive D-dimer need to receive **anticoagulation** (usually with low molecular weight heparin) whilst awaiting further investigation (e.g. via CTPA).
- o Only if CTPA is immediately available can such anticoagulation be deferred until results are available.
- o For patients who have an **allergy to contrast media**, or **who have renal impairment**, or whose risk from irradiation is high: – Assess the suitability of a ventilation/perfusion single photon emission computed tomography (V/Q SPECT) scan or, if a V/Q SPECT scan is not available, a V/Q planar scan, as an alternative to CTPA. – If offering a V/Q SPECT or planar scan that will not be available immediately, offer interim parenteral anticoagulant therapy.

2. STABLE PATIENTS WITH CONFIRMED PE

- o **OXYGEN**: Oxygen should be administered to any patient with oxygen saturations of <94% on room air.
- o **ANTICOAGULATION**
    - All patients with confirmed PE require **anticoagulation**.
    - The 2012 NICE Guidelines advocate anticoagulation for **3 months for all patients in the first instance.**
    - The decision to continue beyond 3 months needs to be evaluated based on the individuals risk of recurrences compared to risk of bleeding.
    - If there have been **multiple episodes or continuing risk factors** such as malignancy **lifelong anticoagulation** should be recommended.
    - Most centres anticoagulate patients initially with low-molecular weight heparin LMWH whilst loading with warfarin.
    - The LMWH should be continued for a minimum of **5 days** and until the **INR is 2 or greater** for at least 24 hours, whichever is longer.
    - There are some groups in whom warfarin may not be appropriate such as **IV drug misusers, pregnant patients** and patients with **liver disease or cancer**.
    - In these groups anticoagulation is usually achieved solely with **LMWH injections.**
    - **Fondaparinux,** a newer alternative to LMWH, may be considered for certain religious groups (part of the production process of LMWH uses pigs) and patients who have had previous problems with heparin such as thrombocytopenia.

---

[87] **Vieillard-Baron A**, Page B, Augarde R, et al. Acute cor pulmonale in massive pulmonary embolism: incidence, echocardiographic pattern, clinical implications and recovery rate. Intensive Care Med2001;**27**:1481–6.

[88] **Smulders YM**. Contribution of pulmonary vasoconstriction to haemodynamic instability after acute pulmonary embolism. Implications for treatment? Neth J Med2001;**58**:241–7.

3. UNSTABLE PATIENTS WITH SUSPECTED OR CONFIRMED PE
o **THROMBOLYSIS**
- *100 mg Alteplase infusion over 2hrs (10mg given as a bolus stat)*
- It is indicated for patients with **severe circulatory compromise** or a picture of **massive PE**.
- Prior proof of PE is not needed if the patient is peri-arrest and thrombolysis should be administered immediately in such patients.
- **Unfractionated heparin 80 units/kg** should be given 3 hours after thrombolysis if the patient remains alive.
- *In the setting of massive PE: only active internal bleeding or recent intracranial bleed are absolute contraindications to thrombolysis.*
- *In patients with non-massive PE: there is no benefit from routine thrombolysis as they normally have a good prognosis.*
- *NICE 2012 suggests that haemodynamically stable patients should not be given thrombolysis.*

PE IN SPECIAL CIRCUMSTANCES
1. PE AND ACTIVE CANCER
- In patients with cancer initial treatment with heparin and warfarin is given in the standard manner, but the relative risk of recurrence is 3 and of bleeding is 6 compared with other patients.[89] In the absence of evidence from randomised trials in this population, duration of treatment is arbitrary.
- For those with recurrence in spite of adequate anticoagulation, options include:
(a) aiming for a higher INR of 3.0-3.5 (which further increases the risks of bleeding), (b) switching to long term LMWH while continuing anticoagulation, or (c) inserting an IVC filter, the value of which is questionable.

2. PE AND PREGNANCY
o Women presenting with symptoms and signs of an acute PE should have an electrocardiogram (ECG) and a chest X-ray (CXR) performed. [New 2015]
o **In women with suspected PE who also have symptoms and signs of DVT:**
- **Compression duplex ultrasound** should be performed. If compression ultrasonography confirms the presence of DVT, no further investigation is necessary and treatment for VTE should continue. [New 2015]

o **In women with suspected PE without symptoms and signs of DVT:**
- Do CXR
- **When the CXR is normal:** Only a Perfusion part of V/Q scan is preferred.
- **When the chest X-ray is abnormal:** CTPA should be performed in preference to a V/Q scan.
o Anticoagulant treatment should be continued until PE is definitively excluded.
o Women with suspected PE should be advised that, compared with CTPA, V/Q scanning may carry a slightly increased risk of childhood cancer but is associated with a lower risk of maternal breast cancer; in both situations, the absolute risk is very small.

TREATMENT OF PE IN PREGNANCY
- Warfarin is teratogenic and should be avoided until after delivery; its use does not preclude breast feeding.
- Treatment during pregnancy should therefore be with therapeutic doses of LMWH[90] or subcutaneous calcium heparin. Approaching delivery, UFH should be substituted because its anticoagulant effect can more easily be reversed if necessary; there are different views about whether it should be discontinued or the dose reduced 4-6 hours before the expected time of delivery.
- It is advised that anticoagulation should continue for 6 weeks after delivery or for 3 months after the initial episode, whichever is the longer.
- **LMWH: Enoxaparin SC 1mg/kg bd.**
- **Unfractionated Heparin:** reserved for cases of massive PE (where it may be used in combination with thrombolysis). UFH is associated with osteoporosis and thrombocytopenia and is not recommended for prolonged use.
- **A temporary IVC filter** may be inserted prior to delivery as anticoagulation will need to be stopped due to the risk of haemorrhage.
- *When VTE occurs in the antepartum period, delivery should be delayed, if possible, to allow maximum time for anticoagulation rather than putting in a filter.*

3. PE AND IV DRUG MIS-USERS
- **LMWH: Enoxaparin SC 1mg/kg bd for 3-6months**
- **Antibiotics** given that PE in this group is often associated with sepsis.
- **IVC filters** may be useful in patients with persistent risks for DVT and PE in whom long term anticoagulation is unacceptable.

[89] *Joung S*, Robinson B. Venous thromboembolism in cancer patients in Christchurch, 1995-1999. NZ Med J2002;**115**:257-60.

[90] *Laurent P*, Dussarat GV, Bonal J, et al. Low molecular weight heparins: a guide to their optimum use in pregnancy. Drugs2002;**62**:463-77.

8. Bruising & Spontaneous Bleeding in the ED

I. THE OVER-ANTICOAGULATED PATIENT

INTRODUCTION

- Non-Vitamin K antagonist oral anticoagulants (NOAC) are now widely used in patients with non-valvular atrial fibrillation (AF) and for the treatment and prevention of venous thromboembolism (VTE) in NHS Health facilities.
- NOACs include dabigatran, (direct thrombin inhibitor), apixaban and rivaroxaban (Factor Xa inhibitors). There are conditions in which NOAC treatment is contraindicated, notably, in patients with a mechanical heart valve[91].
- NOAC use has not been studied in the following conditions: cerebral venous sinus thrombosis, portal and splenic vein thrombosis and non-lower limb DVT. NOACs are not suitable for use in patients with hemodynamically significant valvular heart disease. Unfractionated heparin (UFH) and warfarin are the oldest most widely used anticoagulants and both have specific antidotes for the reversal of anticoagulation.

Clotting Factors Involved in Coagulation

- In the coagulation cascade, chemicals called **clotting factors** (or coagulation factors) prompt reactions that activate still more coagulation factors. The process is complex, but is initiated along two basic pathways:
  - ○ **The extrinsic pathway,** which normally is triggered by trauma.
  - ○ **The intrinsic pathway,** which begins in the bloodstream and is triggered by internal damage to the wall of the vessel.
- Both of these merge into a third pathway, referred to as the common pathway.
- All three pathways are dependent upon the 12 known clotting factors, including Ca^{2+} and vitamin K.
- Clotting factors are secreted primarily by the liver and the platelets.

- The liver requires the fat-soluble vitamin K to produce many of them. Vitamin K (along with biotin and folate) is somewhat unusual among vitamins in that it is not only consumed in the diet but is also synthesized by bacteria residing in the large intestine.
- The calcium ion, considered factor IV, is derived from the diet and from the breakdown of bone. Some recent evidence indicates that activation of various clotting factors occurs on specific receptor sites on the surfaces of platelets.
- The 12 clotting factors are numbered I through XIII according to the order of their discovery. Factor VI was once believed to be a distinct clotting factor, but is now thought to be identical to factor V.
- Rather than renumber the other factors, factor VI was allowed to remain as a placeholder and also a reminder that knowledge changes over time.

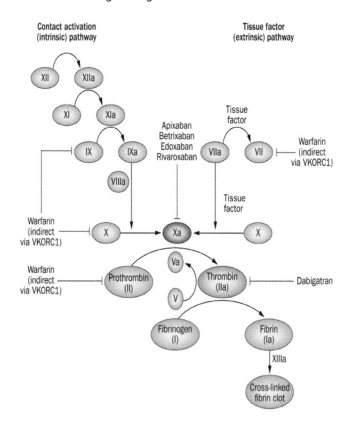

[91] Boehringer Ingelheim Pty Limited. *Product Information Pradaxa® (dabigatran etexilate). Therapeutic Goods Administration Website [updated 28 February 2017]; [Online]*

ANTICOAGULANTS-MECHANISM OF ACTION

	Mechanism	Drugs
Anticoagulants Rx: arterial & venous Thrombosis	Direct thrombin inhibitor	• Dabigatran • Argatroban

	Indirect thrombin inhibitor	• **Heparin (UFH)**
		• **LMWH**
		  ○ Enoxaparin
		  ○ Tinzaparin
		  ○ Dalteparin
		• **Direct Xa inhibitor**
		  ○ Rivaroxaban
		  ○ Apixaban
		  ○ Fondaparinux

	Vit K antagonist	• Warfarin
Antiplatelet Drugs Rx: arterial disease	Cox-1 inhibitors	• Aspirin
	Glycoprotein IIb/IIIa inhibitors	• Abciximab • Eptifibatide • Tirofiban
	ADP inhibitors	• Clopidogrel • Prasugrel • Ticagrelor
	Phosphodiesterase inhibitor	• Dipyridamole • Cilostazol
Thrombolytics Rx: arterial & venous Thrombosis	Plasminogen activators	• Streptokinase • Reteplase • Tenecteplase • Alteplase

- **Vitamin K antagonists (VKA)-** inhibit the synthesis of Vitamin K dependant clotting factors II, VII, IX, X, Protein C and S:
  - Warfarin (Coumarins)

- **Indirect thrombin inhibitors:**
  - **Heparin (unfractionated heparin-UFH)**
  - **Low molecular weight heparin (LMWH):**
    - Dalteparin
    - Tinzaparin
    - Enoxaparin
  - **Factor Xa inhibitors:**
    - Fondaparinux
    - Rivaroxaban

- **Direct thrombin inhibitors-** bind directly to thrombin and block its interaction with its substrates.
  - Dabigatran

CLINICAL ASSESSMENT & RISK STRATIFICATION

- **Major bleeding can be described as:**
  - "Bleeding that is associated with hemodynamic compromise and a significant risk of death occurs in an anatomically critical site, requires transfusion (≥ 2 U of packed red blood cells), or results in a hemoglobin drop ≥ 2 g/dL such as:
    - Intracerebral bleeding,
    - Uncontrollable epistaxis,
    - Catastrophic gastrointestinal bleeding and
    - Catastrophic genitourinary bleeding.
  - Bleeding associated with long-term morbidity
    - Intraocular bleeding
    - Intraarticular,
  - Bleeding requiring surgical intervention, or
  - Bleeding requiring blood transfusion.

- **Minor bleeding can be regarded as**
  - Any bleeding that is not major such as:
    - Haemoptysis,
    - Purpura,
    - Epistaxis
    - Mild haematuria and Unexplained or excessive haematomas.

INVESTIGATIONS

- In all cases of anticoagulation associated adverse events, the following tests are needed:
  - FBC,
  - U&Es,
  - LFTs
  - Cross match / Group&Save
  - Coagulation profile (PT, aPTT, d-dimer)
  - Platelet count
  - CT scan of the head: ?intracranial bleeding
  - Echocardiogram: ?valve thrombosis
  - Other studies depend on patient presentation.

ED MANAGEMENT

The general principles for the management of over-coagulation can be committed to memory using the mnemonic: **HASH-TI**

1. **H**old further doses of the anticoagulant
2. Consider using an **A**ntidote
3. **S**upportive treatment – volume resuscitation and inotropic support
4. Local or surgical **H**aemostatic measures – also agents like tranexamic acid
5. **T**ransfusion - packed red cells, platelets, etc
6. **I**nvestigate for the bleeding source

1. PARENTERAL ANTICOAGULANTS

Agent	Lab test & monitoring	Half-life	Reversing agent	Dose management
UFH	APTT/APTTr	45-90 mins	Protamine	1mg/100iu
LMWH	Anti-factor Xa assay	3-6hrs	Protamine	1mg/100iu (1 mg enoxaparin =100 iu)
Fonda-parinux	Anti-factor Xa assay	17 hrs	Recombin ant factor VIIa	90 g/kg

BLEEDING WITH IV UNFRACTIONATED HEPARIN (PUMP-HEP)

- STOP heparin pump
- Check APTT ratio and a FBC (if APTT ratio >3.0 INR may be unreliable)
- Consider reversal by administration of protamine sulphate injection by slow intravenous injection (max rate 5 mg/min) over a period of >5 minutes
- Reversal effect can be monitored by APTT

BLEEDING ON LOW MOLECULAR WEIGHT HEPARIN, E.G. DALTEPARIN OR ENOXAPARIN

- Bleeding is rare even if Anti-Xa level high
- Check FBC, coagulation screen and request freeze 'plasma'
- If within 8h of LMWH adminstration consider reversal with protamine sulphate over a period of >5 mins (1mg per 100 antiXa units)
- If ineffective, consider further protamine sulphate 0.5 mg per 100 anti-Xa units
- Consider rFVIIa if there is continued lifethreatening bleeding despite protamine sulphate and the time frame suggests LMWH may be contributing to bleeding. (2C)

BLEEDING ON FONDAPARINUX SODIUM

- Doses above the recommended regimen may increase risk of bleeding
- There is no antidote to Fondaparinux - manage through cessation of drug and haemostatic measures. Consider rFVIIa if there is continued life-threatening bleeding

BLEEDING ON DANAPAROID SODIUM

- Patient on DANAPAROID? (half-life of Anti-Xa activity of approx 24hours, can be monitored by anti-Xa assay)
- There is no antidote to Danaparoid - manage through cessation of drug and haemostatic measures. Consider plasmapheresis if there is continued lifethreatening bleeding

2. ORAL ANTICOAGULANTS

2.1. VITAMIN K ANTAGONISTS

2.1.1. Warfarin

INTERACTIONS OF WARFARIN	
Liver enzymes inducers (INR Reduction) = **PC BRAS**	Liver Enzyme Inhibitors (INR Elevation) = **AO DEVICES**
Phenytoin **C**arbamazepine **B**arbiturates **R**ifampicin **A**lcohol excess **S**ulphonurea	**A**miodarone and **A**llopurinol **O**meprazole **D**isulfiram (Metronidazole) **E**rythromycin **V**alproate **I**soniazid **C**imetidine (and **C**iprofloxacin) Acute **E**thanol intoxication **S**ulphonamide

VITAMIN K ANTAGONISTS – REVERSAL

ACTIONS TO BE TAKEN FOR HIGH INR (WITH NO BLEEDING)

- **INR >8.0**
  - Stop VKA
  - Give Vitamin K **orally** using the IV preparation
  - Recheck INR at 24 hours
  - Repeat Vit K administration orally if INR remains high
  - Restart Warfarin when INR <5.0

- **INR 5.0-8.0**
  - *Stop VKA* for 1-2 doses
  - Restart when INR <5.0 with reduced maintenance dose
  - INR should correct to <5.0 in 24-72hours
  - The cause of elevated INR should be investigated

ACTIONS TO BE TAKEN FOR HIGH INR (MINOR BLEEDING ONLY)

- **INR >8.0**
  - Stop VKA
  - Give Vitamin K **Intravenously** using the IV preparation
  - Recheck INR at 24 hours
  - Repeat Vit K administration **Intravenously** if INR remains high
  - Restart Warfarin when INR<5.0

- **INR 5.0-8.0**
  - *Stop VKA*
  - Give Vitamin K Intravenously using the IV preparation
  - Restart when INR <5.0 with reduced maintenance dose
  - The cause of elevated INR should be investigated

MANAGEMENT OF BLEEDING WITH WARFARIN OR OTHER VITAMIN K ANTAGONIST ORAL ANTICOAGULANTS[92]

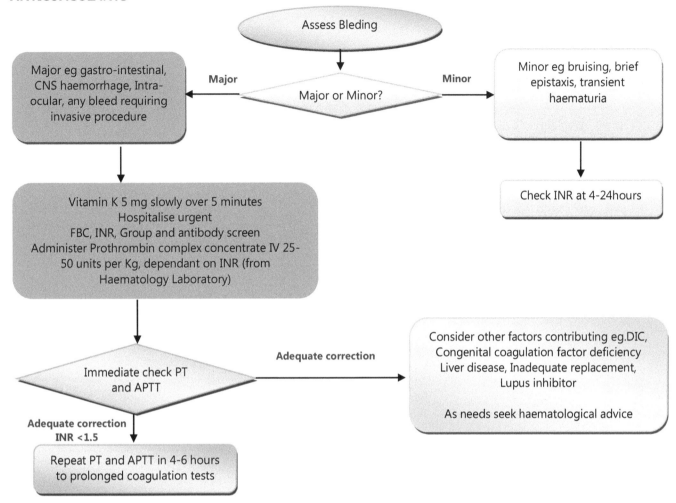

THE USE AND DOSAGE OF BERIPLEX® P/N PROTHROMBIN COMPLEX CONCENTRATE (FACTORS II, VII, IX AND X) IN MAJOR BLEEDING IN COUMARIN ANTICOAGULATED PATIENTS

Standard Operating Procedure

- Request from Haematology Laboratory
- Dose as 25-50 units of FIX per Kg, titrated against INR (Each bottle of Beriplex® P/N 500 contains 500 units FIX in 20mls.)
- Reconstitute as per manufacturer's instruction eg 500 units in 20ml water for injection warmed to maximum 37oC.
- Maximum single dose 5000 UNITS FIX (200mls).
- Administer infusion: first 1ml over 1 minute in case of reaction, then 8ml/min (max equivalent to approx 210 units/min)
- Patients may have reactions, commonly chills, as with other blood products.
- Administer vitamin K 5mg IV, as the PCC only has a half-life of some 6 hours, compared to 30-40 hours for warfarin.
- See nomograms for guide for given Kg body weight range and INR

Initial INR	2.0 – 3.9	4.0 – 6.0	>6.0
Approximate dose units (Factor IX)/kg body weight	25	35	50
Approximate dose ml/kg body weight	1	1.4	2
Maximum Single Dose for patients weighing 100kg or over	2500 units	3500 units	5000 units

NB: Check INR immediately after infusion to demonstrate correction, as per protocolRepeated dosing with prothrombin complex concentrate (Beriplex® P/N) for patients requiring urgent reversal of Vitamin K antagonist treatment is not supported by clinical data and therefore not recommended

---

[92] *Royal Conwal Hospitals, Anticoagulation Related Bleeding - Guideline Summary* [online]

BLEEDING WITH THROMBOLYTIC THERAPY

- Patient bleeding POST-THROMBOLYSIS?
    - Check FBC and Coagulation screen
    - Consider tranexamic acid 10mg/kg IV and/or cryoprecipitate (which is rich in fibrinogen)
    - Seek advice if needed from on call CoE consultant (in cases of stroke)

BLEEDING WITH DABIGATRAN EXETILATE

- Patient on DABIGATRAN?
    - In life threatening bleed administer Idarucizumab (Praxbind ®) Available in the emergency drug fridge and given as a 5g IV Bolus (2x2.5g vials)
    - In non life-threatening bleed apply standard haemostatic measures, add oral activated charcoal if drug taken within last 2 hours

ASSESSMENT OF BLEEDING WITH RIVAROXABAN, APIXABAN OR EDOXABAN (ANTI-XA THERAPIES)

- Patient on ANTI-XA THERAPY?
    - There is no specific antidote to these drugs
    - Determine time since last dose
    - Initiate resuscitation with IV fluids, blood transfusion and other general haemostatic supportive measures as necessary
    - Check FBC, U&E's and a coagulation screen (If within the normal reference ranges, then there is likely to be only a low level of the anticoagulant present)
    - If platelets <50 consider platelet transfusion
    - In patients with ongoing life-threatening bleeding, not controlled by the above measures, administer prothrombin complex concentrate (PCC) at 25units/kg

MANAGEMENT OF BLEEDING WITH THE ANTI-XA ANTICOAGULANTS [93]

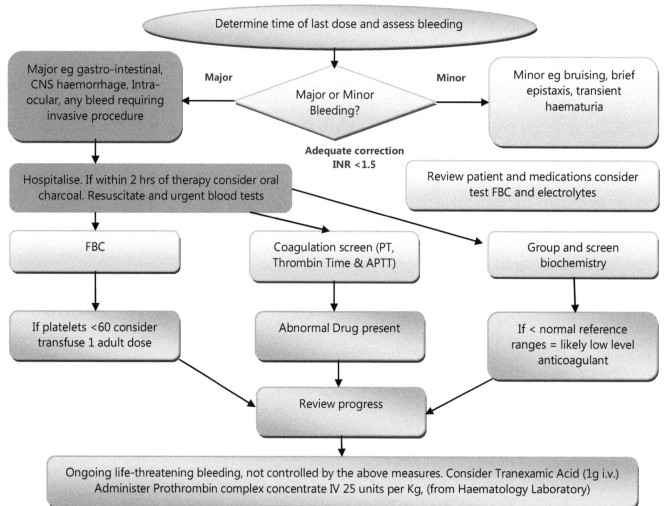

II. EASY BRUISING IN THE ED

1. INTRODUCTION

- Easy bruising is a common complaint in medical practice for both primary care clinicians and hematologists.
- Easy bruising implies that no significant trauma has occurred to the skin or soft tissue to cause the bruise, and the bruises are larger and/or more frequent than what would normally be seen.
- It is a common complaint of patients seen in a medical practice. Surveys of normal healthy individuals report the frequency of easy bruising to range from 12% to 55%.[94]
- These conditions are often referred to as disorders of primary hemostasis or the purpuric disorders since they are characteristically associated with mucosal and cutaneous bleeding. Mucosal bleeding may be manifest as epistaxis and/or gingival bleeding, and large bullous hemorrhages may appear on the buccal mucosa due to the lack of vessel protection afforded by the submucosal tissue. Bleeding into the skin is manifested as **petechiae or superficial ecchymoses.**
- Patients with platelet abnormalities tend to bleed immediately after vascular trauma and rarely experience delayed bleeding, which is more common in the coagulation disorders. The following are the types of bleeding most often associated with these disorders:

1. PETECHIAE

- Petechiae are small capillary hemorrhages. They characteristically develop in crops in areas of increased venous pressure, such as the dependent parts of the body.
- As a result, they are most dense on the feet and ankles, fewer are present on the legs.

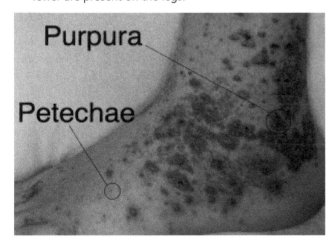

- Petechiae are not found on the sole of the foot where the vessels are protected by the strong subcutaneous tissue. They are asymptomatic and not palpable, and should be distinguished from small telangiectasias, angiomas, and vasculitic purpura.
- **Purpura** is the name given to the discolouration of the skin or mucous membranes due to haemorrhage from small blood vessels.
- **Telangiectasia** is a condition in which there are visible small linear red blood vessels (broken capillaries). Visible small blood vessels that are blue in colour (spider veins) are called **venulectasia**, because venules are involved.

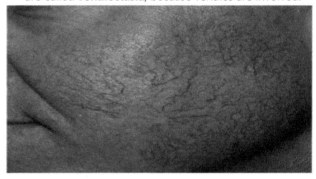

2. ECCHYMOSES

- Ecchymotic lesions characteristically are purple in color and are small, multiple, and superficial in location.
- Ecchymoses or bruises are larger extravasations of blood.
- They usually develop without noticeable trauma and do not spread into deeper tissues.

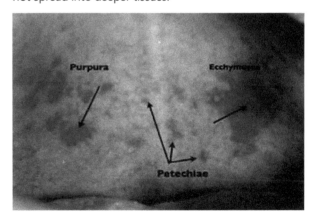

3. MENORRHAGIA

- **Menorrhagia** (menstrual flow that does not taper after more than three days) and **metrorrhagia** (bleeding in between periods) are common in women with bleeding disorders; up to 15 to 20 percent of women presenting with menorrhagia may have some type of bleeding diathesis, such as von Willebrand disease, immune thrombocytopenia (ITP), platelet function defect.

---

[94] Srámek A, Eikenboom JC, Briët E, et al. *Usefulness of patient interview in bleeding disorders. Arch Intern Med. 1995;155:1409-1415.*

2. PATHOPHYSIOLOGY

A bruise (ecchymosis) is a collection of blood beneath the skin, resulting from extravasation of blood from surrounding vessels. Easy bruising can result from abnormalities affecting the blood vessels themselves, the surrounding skin and subcutaneous structures, platelet number and function, or coagulation cascade function. Physical injury to a blood vessel normally triggers a vigorous physiologic response. Damage to endothelial tissue causes activation and adhesion of circulating platelets with the assistance of von Willebrand factor. This in turn results in the rapid formation of a platelet plug at the site of injury. Stabilization of the plug via fibrin deposition subsequently results from activation of the coagulation cascade. A problem or defect at any step of this process will increase the risk of abnormal bruising and bleeding, regardless of the degree of trauma.

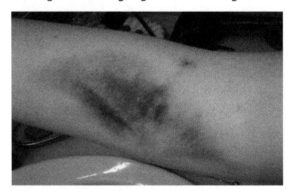

3. CAUSES OF ABNORMAL BRUISING

- Abnormal bruising is not exclusively a result of haemostatic disorders.
- In addition to nonaccidental injury, collagen disorders, though rare, should be considered in the differential diagnoses.

Common

- Senile purpura
- Medications (antiplatelet agents, anticoagulants, and Non-Steroidal Anti-inflammatories Drugs)
- Excess alcohol use and liver cirrhosis
- von Willebrand disease (prevalence 1%-2% of general population)
- Purpura simplex or easy bruising syndrome
- Vitamin C and vitamin K deficiencies
- Vasculitis
- Gastrointestinal diseases

Rare

- Haemophilia and rare coagulation factor (I, II, V, VII, XI) deficiencies
- Acquired haemophilia or von Willebrand disease (older individuals

1. THROMBOCYTOPENIA

- **Immune thrombocytopenic purpura (ITP)** is the commonest haemostatic disorder of childhood to present with easy bruising, usually associated with petechiae, purpura, and mucosal bleeding.
- The diagnosis is of exclusion, and made on the basis of an otherwise well patient, without lymphadenopathy or organomegaly, with isolated thrombocytopenia and a normal blood film and clotting screen.
- The latter two in a well child excludes leukaemia, meningococcal septicaemia, and haemolytic uraemic syndrome. Persistence of thrombocytopenia beyond a few months from presentation should trigger referral to a specialist for further investigations.
- These should be directed towards exclusion of rare congenital causes of isolated thrombocytopenia (such as **May–Hegglin syndrome** and other **giant platelet familial thrombocytopenia syndromes, Fanconi's anaemia, and amegakaryocytic thrombocytopenia**), before concluding that the patient has chronic ITP.
- Although investigations at this stage may include examination of the bone marrow, if this has not already been performed, careful reexamination of the blood film and parental blood counts may be the simplest way to exclude some of these rare conditions.

2. PLATELET FUNCTION DISORDERS

- Poor platelet aggregability is caused by a variety of acquired and inherited disorders, the commonest being NSAID use.
- Inherited disorders of platelet function are rare, but should be suspected in a patient with symptoms of thrombocytopenia but a normal platelet count, or mild thrombocytopenia relative to the severity of haemorrhagic symptoms.
- The best known, and easiest to diagnose, are **Glanzmann's thrombasthenia** and **Bernard Soulier syndrome**, which result from a measurable (by flow cytometry) lack of expression of platelet membrane receptors essential for activation and aggregation.
- **Storage pool deficiency** is harder to diagnose, as few patients have the classical clinical and laboratory features, and the laboratory tests required to exclude it are difficult to perform and interpret.
- Inheritance of most platelet function disorders is autosomal recessive, so it may not be apparent without testing the extended family.
- Given the difficulties in diagnosis, it is probably best to refer patients suspected of a platelet function defect to a specialist.

3. DISORDERS OF COAGULATION FACTORS

- Inherited Autosomal dominantly inherited **Von Willebrand's disease (VWD)** is the commonest congenital disorder of haemostasis, affecting up to 1% of the population; it often presents with easy bruising as the sole symptom, although mucosal bleeding is also common. Purpura and petechiae are not common despite the abnormal platelet aggregation, which is a feature of this condition along with a variable reduction in concentrations of von Willebrand factor (VWF) and factor VIII. Post-pubertal females may have menorrhagia. Family history is frequently positive, but may be silent and only uncovered on parental testing. The majority of cases are mild with concentrations just below the normal range. This may cause diagnostic difficulty, as the venepuncture ordeal can stimulate release of factor VIII and VWF from endothelial stores, often pushing marginally sub-normal concentrations to within the normal range. Where suspicion is strong, and concentrations borderline normal, repeat tests may be justified, but should be postponed until a management decision rests on the diagnosis (for example, impending surgery), or venepuncture is being undertaken for another purpose.
- **Mild haemophilia A (factor VIII deficiency) or B (factor IX deficiency)** are much less common, but can present with symptoms similar to those of VWD. X linked recessively inherited, female carriers can be affected as a result of skewed lyonisation. Moderate and severe haemophilia A or B presents in infancy with atypical bruising, and haemarthroses later on when it should be easy to diagnose, although the latter is not infrequently misdiagnosed as pyogenic arthritis. Family history is absent in the 30% of sporadic haemophilia cases arising from a new mutation in maternal or grandparental germ line. Congenital deficiencies of other coagulation factors are much rarer and variably associated with a risk of bleeding, except for factor XII deficiency, which is always asymptomatic.
- **Acquired Sick neonates** bruise easily, usually as a result of a low platelet count. Bruising in infants younger than 9 months is rare, and should always prompt a search for a cause. **Physical abuse** should be suspected at this age, more than any other, if another explanation for bruising is not found. An uncommon cause of bruising at this age is **haemorrhagic disease of the newborn (HDN),** which occurs when prophylactic vitamin K has not been administered at birth, or has been given orally to subsequently breast-fed infants without the one- and three-month boosters.

- Unrecognized, it can result in catastrophic intracranial haemorrhage. Once recognized it is easily treated with intravenous vitamin K.
- Outside infancy, vitamin K deficiency is usually caused by malabsorption, liver disease, or a combination of the two.
  - **Coeliac disease** may present with easy bruising as the sole symptom, although most patients will have other signs of malabsorption.
  - Similarly, **inflammatory bowel disease and chronic liver disease** may have easy bruising as a dominant presenting symptom.

4. COLLAGEN DISORDERS

- Vascular integrity is essential for primary haemostasis to be effective. Defective collagen compromises capillary and skin elasticity, thereby manifesting symptoms similar to those of thrombocytopenia or platelet function defect.
- Not all patients have the classic features of *Ehler–Danlos syndrome, Marfan's syndrome, or acquired autoimmune disorders.* A simple test of thumb hyperflexibility is claimed to identify patients with a mild inherited bleeding diathesis without abnormalities of haemostasis or other features of a collagen disorder.

5. NON-ACCIDENTAL INJURY

- An atypical pattern of bruising in the absence of other haemorrhagic symptoms and a normal count and clotting screen should prompt a review of other indicators to exclude nonaccidental injury.
- It is important to remember that non-accidental injury and a bleeding disorder are not mutually exclusive.

INVESTIGATION APPROACH

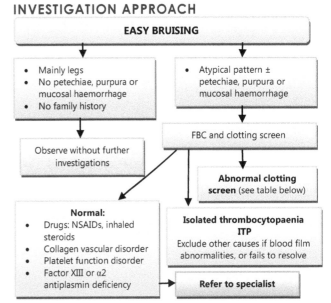

If the blood count and clotting screen are normal, a significant disorder of haemostasis is unlikely.

ABNORMALITIES OF CLOTTING SCREEN

Abnormality	Cause
Isolated prolongation of PT (Extrinsic Pathway)	1. Vit K deficiency (HDN, malabsoption) 2. Liver failure 3. Warfarin *
Isolated prolongation of aPPT (Intrinsic Pathway)	1. VWD or 2. Coagulation factor deficiencies: • Factors VIII, IX and X-clinically significant • Factor XII_ not significant 3. Lupus anticoagulant-DRVVT 4. Heparin*
Combined abnormalities (Common Pathway)	1. Liver failure 2. Vit K deficiency 3. DIC* 4. Rare- afibrinogenaemia or dysfibrinogenaemia

* Suspect in certain circumstances as described in text.

- Further investigations of screening test abnormalities are dictated by the specific abnormality.
- **Thrombocytopenia** raises suspicion of ITP, although, if the bruising history is of insidious onset and the thrombocytopenia is associated with a raised mean cell volume, **Fanconi's anaemia** should be excluded.
- **An isolated prolongation of the PT** is most likely to be a result of vitamin K deficiency or liver disease, and should be investigated further by performing a **factor VII assay.**
- **Isolated prolongation of the APTT** may be caused by a deficiency of any of the intrinsic pathway coagulation factors, or heparin if the sample has been taken from a heparinised catheter or cannula. If the latter is suspected, a **TT** and **reptilase time** (RT) should be performed before undertaking coagulation factor assays:
  - **Prolongation of the TT with a normal RT** is suggestive of heparin contamination.
  - **If both the RT and TT are prolonged**, the most likely cause is a **low fibrinogen concentration, or dys- fibrinogenaemia** if this is normal.
  - If heparin contamination is not suspected, or is excluded, **an isolated prolongation of APTT** requires factor assays to exclude **VWD or coagulation factor deficiency.**

- It is sensible to start with factor VIII "complex" studies, including VWF antigen and function (ristocetin co-factor assay), and a factor IX assay, as these are clinically significant abnormalities that are important to exclude.
- If these are normal, factor XI and XII concentrations should be checked. If these too are normal, a **lupus anticoagulant** should be suspected. Usually this results in a prolonged APTT uncorrected by addition of normal plasma to the test, but this is not always the case. A **Dilute Russell Viper Venom Time (DRVVT)** is the diagnostic test for lupus anticoagulant. If positive, it usually has no clinical significance in children, as it is most often a result of transient antiphospholipid antibodies after a viral infection that can persist for months to years causing no clinical problems. In adults it is associated with an **increased risk of arterial and venous thrombosis.**
- The APTT is often prolonged without an apparent cause on detailed investigations and is most often a result of clinically insignificant factor XII deficiency.
- **Combined abnormalities of the PT and APTT** are often a result of moderate to severe vitamin K deficiency or liver failure.
- Although unlikely in children, warfarin overdose can produce the same abnormality, and should be suspected in cases of **Munchausen syndrome** by proxy or accidental poisoning caused by certain types of rat poisons, which contain coumarin analogues.
- The most common cause of combined PT and APTT abnormalities is **Disseminated Intravascular Coagulopathy**, but this is usually not a differential diagnosis for easy bruising.
- Inherited deficiencies of factors V or X also produce similar laboratory abnormalities but are very rare.
- **Platelet function defects** cannot be excluded on the basis of a normal count and clotting screen, but require specific tests for diagnosis, including bleeding time, **platelet aggregometry**, and **nucleotide release assays**.
- Bleeding times are operator dependent and are difficult to perform in very young children.
- Although yet to be fully validated, new methods of in vitro bleeding time assay such as the **PFA-100** may in time supersede these, and provide an easy method to exclude platelet function disorders.
- The PFA-100 instrument measures the time it takes flowing blood to block an aperture coated with collagen and adrenaline or ADP.

III. IMMUNE THROMBOCYTOPENIC PURPURA

OVERVIEW

- Immune thrombocytopenic purpura (ITP) is a clinical syndrome in which a decreased number of circulating platelets (thrombocytopenia) manifests as a bleeding tendency, easy bruising (**purpura**), or extravasation of blood from capillaries into skin and mucous membranes (**petechiae**). Although most cases of acute ITP, particularly in children, **are mild and self-limited,** intracranial hemorrhage may occur when the platelet count drops below $10 \times 10^9/L$[95]; this occurs in 0.5-1% of children, and half of these cases are fatal[96]. Peripheral blood smear from a patient with immune thrombocytopenic purpura (ITP) shows a decreased number of platelets, a normal-appearing neutrophil, and normal-appearing erythrocytes.

- ITP is diagnosed by excluding other diseases; therefore, the absence of other findings from the peripheral smear is at least as important as the observed findings.

- This smear demonstrates the absence of immature leukocytes (as in leukemia) and fragmented erythrocytes (as in thrombotic thrombocytopenic purpura) and no clumps of platelets (as in pseudothrombocytopenia).

SIGNS AND SYMPTOMS

- ITP is a primary illness occurring in an otherwise healthy person. Signs of chronic disease, infection, wasting, or poor nutrition indicate that the patient has another illness. Splenomegaly excludes the diagnosis of ITP.

- An initial impression of the severity of ITP is formed by examining the skin and mucous membranes, as follows:
  - Widespread petechiae and ecchymoses, oozing from a venipuncture site, gingival bleeding, and hemorrhagic bullae indicate that the patient is at risk for a serious bleeding complication. If the patient's blood pressure was taken recently, petechiae may be observed under and distal to the area where the cuff was placed and inflated.
  - Suction-type electrocardiograph (ECG) leads may induce petechiae. Petechiae over the ankles in ambulatory patients or on the back in bedridden ones suggest mild thrombocytopenia and a relatively low risk for a serious bleeding complication

Findings suggestive of intracranial hemorrhage include:

- Headache, blurred vision, somnolence, or loss of consciousness

- Hypertension and bradycardia, which may be signs of increased intracranial pressure

- On neurologic examination, any asymmetrical finding of recent onset. On fundoscopic examination, blurring of the optic disc margins or retinal hemorrhage

DIAGNOSIS

- FBC: isolated thrombocytopenia is the hallmark of ITP. Anemia and/or neutropenia may indicate other diseases.
- Peripheral blood smear
- Bone marrow aspiration and biopsy

MANAGEMENT

ITP has **no cure**, and relapses may occur years after seemingly successful medical or surgical management. Most children with acute ITP do not require treatment, and the condition resolves spontaneously. Treatment is as follows:

- **Corticosteroids** remain the drugs of choice for the initial management of acute ITP: Oral prednisone, IV methylprednisolone, or high-dose dexamethasone.
- **IV immunoglobulin (IVIG)** has been the drug of second choice for many years
- For **Rh(D)-positive patients** with intact spleens, **IV Rho immunoglobulin (RhIG)** offers comparable efficacy, less toxicity, greater ease of administration, and a lower cost than IVIG
- **Rituximab** is third-line therapy
- **Platelet transfusions** may be required to control clinically significant bleeding but are not recommended for prophylaxis
- If 6 months of medical management fails to increase the platelet count to a safe range (about 30,000/μL), splenectomy becomes an option
- **Thrombopoietin receptor agonists** (i.e., eltrombopag, romiplostim) may maintain platelet counts at safe levels in adults with chronic ITP refractory to conventional medical management or splenectomy

Pregnant women require special consideration for delivery, as follows:

- **If the Platelet > $50 \times 10^9/L$**: the risk of serious hemorrhage is low, but beginning oral prednisone a week before delivery is a reasonable precaution
- **If the platelet < $50 \times 10^9/L$** before delivery, treatment with oral prednisone and IVIG is recommended
- Avoiding the use of IV RhIG in this situation until safety data are available is advisable.
- Rarely, splenectomy may be required to manage acute hemorrhage

---

[95] *Butros LJ, Bussel JB. Intracranial hemorrhage in immune thrombocytopenic purpura: a retrospective analysis. J Pediatr Hematol Oncol. 2003 Aug. 25(8):660-4.*

[96] *Fogarty PF, Segal JB. The epidemiology of immune thrombocytopenic purpura. Curr Opin Hematol. 2007 Sep. 14(5):515-9.*

IV. HAEMOPHILIA

1. HEMOPHILIA A

- **Hemophilia A** is an inherited bleeding disorder in which the blood does not clot normally.[97] People with hemophilia A will bleed more than normal after an injury, surgery, or dental procedure.
- This disorder can be severe, moderate, or mild. In severe cases, heavy bleeding occurs after minor injury or even when there is no injury (spontaneous bleeding).
- Bleeding into the joints, muscles, brain, or organs can cause pain and other serious complications. .

ETIOLOGY

- Hemophilia A is caused by genetic changes (mutations) in the *F8* gene. This gene is responsible for making the Factor VIII protein, an important protein that helps start the formation of blood clots.
- Mutations in the *F8* gene lead to reduced or absent levels of Factor VIII in the blood, making it hard for the body to form blood clots.[98]

SIGNS AND SYMPTOMS

- Depending on the level of FVIII activity, patients with hemophilia may present with easy bruising; inadequate clotting of traumatic or even mild injury; or, in the case of severe hemophilia, spontaneous hemorrhage.
- **Signs of hemorrhage include the following:**
  - **General:** Weakness, orthostasis, tachycardia, tachypnea
  - **Musculoskeletal (joints):** Tingling, cracking, warmth, pain, stiffness, and refusal to use joint (children)
  - **CNS:** Headache, stiff neck, vomiting, lethargy, irritability, and spinal cord syndromes
  - **Gastrointestinal:** Hematemesis, melena, frank red blood per rectum, and abdominal pain
  - **Genitourinary:** Hematuria, renal colic, and post circumcision bleeding
  - **Other:** Epistaxis, oral mucosal hemorrhage, hemoptysis, dyspnea (hematoma leading to airway obstruction), compartment syndrome symptoms, and contusions; excessive bleeding with routine dental procedures

DIAGNOSIS

- Laboratory studies for suspected hemophilia include:
  - FBC
  - Normal values for FVIII assays are 50-150%.
  - Screening coagulation studies (prothrombin time [PT], activated partial thromboplastin time [aPTT])
  - FVIII assay
  - FVIII inhibitor assay (Bethesda assay, Nijmegen modified Bethesda assay)

Expected laboratory values are as follows:

- Hemoglobin/hematocrit: Normal or low
- Platelet count: Normal
- Bleeding time and PT: Normal
- APTT: Significantly prolonged in severe hemophilia, but may be normal or minimally prolonged in mild or even moderate hemophilia
- Imaging studies for acute bleeds are chosen on the basis of clinical suspicion and anatomic location of involvement, as follows:
  - **CT Brain without contrast** are used to assess for spontaneous or traumatic intracranial haemorrhage
  - **MRI scans** of the head and spinal column are used for further assessment of spontaneous or traumatic hemorrhage. MRI is also useful in the evaluation of the cartilage, synovium, and joint space
  - **Ultrasonography** is useful in the evaluation of joints affected by acute or chronic effusions

ED MANAGEMENT OF HEMOPHILIA A

- There is no cure for hemophilia A, but current treatments can prevent many of the symptoms of hemophilia A.
- Treatment may include medications and replacing the missing clotting factor (replacement therapy).
- This type of replacement therapy is done by slowly injecting or dripping concentrated factor VIII into a vein (intravenous infusion). The type and frequency of treatment often depends on the severity of the disorder in each person.
- People with mild or moderate hemophilia A may be treated with replacement therapy as needed (for example, when a bleeding episode occurs). This is called 'on-demand' therapy.
- Some people with mild hemophilia A may be treated with **desmopressin (DDAVP)**[99]. Desmopressin raises the levels of factor VIII in the blood and may be given directly into a vein or through a nasal spray.
- Drugs known as **antifibrinolytics,** which slow the breakdown of clotting factors in the blood, can also be used to treat a mild form of the disorder.

97 Konkle BA, Huston H, Fletcher SN. Hemophilia A. GeneReviews. June 22, 2017. [Online]

98 Hemophilia. Genetics Home Reference. August, 2012; [Online]

99 Robert A Zaiden. Hemophilia A. Medscape. November 7, 2014; [Online]

- Some people with severe hemophilia A may receive regular factor VIII replacement therapy to prevent bleeding episodes and other complications such as joint damage. This is referred to as prophylactic or preventative therapy. These factor VIII infusions may be done as often as necessary depending on the severity.
- The immune system of some people with the severe form of hemophilia A may start to make antibodies (inhibitors) that prevent the replacement factor VIII from working.[100]
- Treatment for these people includes larger doses of replacement factor VIII and/or medications that may help block the inhibitors. Infusions of replacement Factor VIII can be given at home. This is especially important for people with severe disease because the infusion works the best within one hour of a bleeding episode.
- In general, prompt treatment is important because it reduces pain and damage to the joints, muscles, or other affected tissues or organs.

2. HEMOPHILIA B

- Hemophilia B, or **Christmas disease**, is an inherited, X-linked, recessive disorder that results in deficiency of functional plasma coagulation factor IX.
- Spontaneous mutation and acquired immunologic processes can result in this disorder as well.
- Hemophilia B constitutes about 20% of hemophilia cases, and about 50% of these cases have factor IX levels greater than 1%.

SIGNS AND SYMPTOMS

- The hallmark of hemophilia is hemorrhage into the joints. This bleeding is painful and leads to long-term inflammation and deterioration of the joint (typically the ankles in children, and the ankles, knees, and elbows in adolescents and adults), resulting in permanent deformities, misalignment, loss of mobility, and extremities of unequal lengths.
- With mild hemophilia, hemorrhage is most likely to occur with trauma or surgery. A traumatic challenge relatively late in life may have to occur before mild or moderate hemophilia is suspected.

Signs and symptoms of moderate and severe hemophilia include the following:

- **Neonates:** Prolonged bleeding and/or severe hematoma following procedures such as circumcision, phlebotomy, and/or immunizations; intracranial hemorrhage
- **Toddler:** Trauma-related soft-tissue hemorrhage; oral bleeding during teething

- **Children:** Hemarthrosis and hematomas with increasing physical activity; chronic arthropathy (late complication); traumatic intracranial hemorrhage (life threatening)
- There may also be signs and symptoms of infectious disease related to HIV/AIDS or hepatitis.

DIAGNOSIS
Laboratory tests
Laboratory studies for suspected hemophilia B include the following:

- **FBC:** Normal or low hemoglobin/hematocrit levels; normal platelet count
- **Coagulation studies:** Do not delay coagulation correction pending test results; normal bleeding and prothrombin times; normal or prolonged activated partial thromboplastin time
- **Factor IX (FIX) assay:** Mild disease, result is over 5%; moderate, 1-5%; severe, below 1%
- **von Willebrand factor (vWF) and factor VIII levels:** To exclude vWF deficiency as primary diagnosis (low vWF and low FVIII)
- Screening tests for HIV and hepatitis
- Genetic carrier and fetal testing

IMAGING STUDIES
- **CT BRAIN (without contrast):** To assess for spontaneous or traumatic intracranial hemorrhage
- **MRI:** To further evaluate spontaneous/traumatic hemorrhage in the head or spinal column; also, to assess cartilage, synovia, and joint spaces
- **Ultrasonography:** To assess joints affected by acute or chronic effusions
- **Joint radiography:** Of limited value in acute hemarthrosis; to evaluate untreated or inadequately treated disease; in those with recurrent joint hemorrhages, chronic degenerative joint disease may be evident

ED MANAGEMENT OF HEMOPHILIA B
- **Factor IX** is the treatment of choice for acute hemorrhage or presumed acute hemorrhage in patients with hemophilia B. **Recombinant factor IX** is the preferred source for replacement therapy. Ideally, patients with hemophilia should be treated at a comprehensive hemophilia care center.
- Management of hemophilia B includes the following:
  - Control of hemostasis
  - Treatment of bleeding episodes
  - Administration of factor replacement products and medications
  - Use of factor inhibitors
  - Rehabilitation of patients with hemophilia synovitis
  - Primary and/or secondary prophylaxis

---

[100] *Hemophilia A. NORD. Updated 2015 [Online].*

- Treatment may also vary with site-specific locations (eg, joints, mouth, gastrointestinal region, head).

PHARMACOTHERAPY

- The following medications are used in the management of hemophilia B:
  - Factor IX-containing products (eg, factor IX, recombinant factor IX, factor IX complex)
  - Recombinant coagulation factor VIIa
  - Recombinant coagulation factor IX
  - Antifibrinolytics (eg, epsilon aminocaproic acid, tranexamic acid)
  - Antihemophilic agents (eg, desmopressin, anti-inhibitor coagulant complex, human antihemophilic factor, recombinant human antihemophilic factor, plasma-derived prothrombin complex concentrates/factor IX complex concentrates, plasma-derived coagulation factor IX concentrate)
  - Monoclonal antibodies (eg, rituximab). Analgesics (eg, narcotic agents, NSAIDS, acetaminophen with codeine or synthetic codeine analogs)

3. VON WILLEBRAND DISEASE

- Von Willebrand disease (vWD) is a common, inherited, genetically and clinically heterogeneous hemorrhagic disorder caused by a deficiency or dysfunction of the protein termed von Willebrand factor (vWF).
- Consequently, defective vWF interaction between platelets and the vessel wall impairs primary hemostasis.
- vWF, a large, multimeric glycoprotein, circulates in blood plasma at concentrations of approximately 10 mg/mL.
- In response to numerous stimuli, vWF is released from storage granules in platelets and endothelial cells.
- It performs two major roles in hemostasis.
  - First, it mediates the adhesion of platelets to sites of vascular injury.
  - Second, it binds and stabilizes the procoagulant protein factor VIII (FVIII).

- vWD is divided into three major categories, as follows[101]:
  - **Type 1 VWD** is the most common form. Around 80% of all people with VWD have this form. In type 1 VWD, the von Willebrand Factor (VWF) works normally, but there is not enough of it. Symptoms are usually mild, depending on the level of VWF in the blood.
  - **In type 2 VWD**, the amount of VWF in people's blood is often normal but the VWF doesn't work properly.

- Type 2 VWD is divided into subtypes 2A, 2B, 2M and 2N. Certain subtypes may be treated differently, which makes knowing the exact type of VWD you have very important.
- **Type 3 VWD** is very rare. People with type 3 VWD have very little or no VWF in their blood. Symptoms are more severe and can also include joint and muscle bleeding. Bleeding can occur more often.

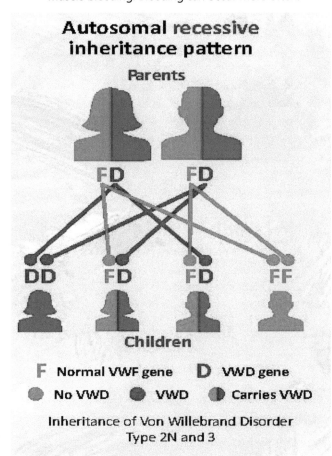

Inheritance of Von Willebrand Disorder Type 2N and 3

Screening tests typically include the following:

- Prothrombin time (PT)
- Activated partial thromboplastin time (aPTT)
- Factor VIII coagulant activity
- Ristocetin cofactor (RCoF) activity
- Concentration of vWF antigen (vWF:Ag)

- The main treatment options for patients with vWD are:
  - Desmopressin (DDAVP),
  - Recombinant vWF, and
  - vWF/factor VIII (vWF/FVIII) concentrates.
  - In addition, antifibrinolytic drugs (i.e., aminocaproic acid, tranexamic acid) can be used orally or intravenously to treat mild mucocutaneous bleeding

---

[101] Haemophilia Foundation Australia. A guide for people living with von Willebrand disorder. [online]

V. DISSEMINATED INTRAVASCULAR COAGULATION

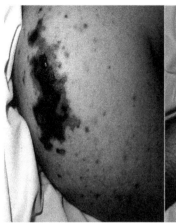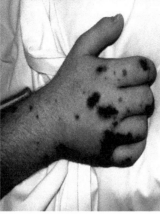

OVERVIEW

- DIC results from pathological overactivation of the coagulation cascade, leading to the consumption of **clotting factors** as well as of **fibrinogen and platelets**.
- It is seen in association with a number of well-defined clinical situations, including **sepsis, major trauma, malignancy and obstetric emergencies**.
- The resultant widespread intravascular clotting causes:
  - Blood vessel occlusion, leading to tissue ischaemia
  - End-organ damage depletion of clotting factors, fibrinogen and platelets, leading to profuse and uncontrollable bleeding haemolysis of passing red cells by fibrin strands in the small vessels, leading to a microangiopathic haemolytic anaemia

CLINICAL FINDINGS

- Clinically, DIC is characterized by bleeding from any site.
- Bleeding into the skin gives petechiae and/or widespread ecchymoses. Intracranial, pulmonary and gastrointestinal bleeding may be life-threatening.
- Early evidence of DIC is often seen at sites of iatrogenic trauma: as excessive bleeding from venepuncture sites or from the oropharynx after intubation or as haematuria following catheterization. Despite greater understanding and more aggressive therapy, the mortality from severe DIC remains high, and early recognition and treatment is vital for any chance of survival.

DIAGNOSIS

- Diagnosis of DIC requires the presence of clinical manifestations of DIC – either haemorrhagic or thrombotic – and the following laboratory investigations:
  - Thrombocytopenia on the FBC
  - Reduced fibrinogen
  - Raised INR, PT & APTT
  - Elevated D-dimer

- Raised fibrinogen degradation products (FDPs)
- Remember that the:
  - **INR (PT) and APTT are raised** because of the depletion of clotting factors required for both the extrinsic and intrinsic coagulation pathways.
  - **The platelet count is low**, owing to consumption of platelets in the myriad blood clots forming throughout the microvasculature.
  - **D-dimer** is a fibrin degradation product (FDP) that, along with other FDPs, is elevated owing to excess fibrinolysis of the pathological clots.
  - At the end of the clotting cascade, activated thrombin cleaves fibrinogen to give fibrin, which, in polymer form, is the essential molecular ingredient of blood clots; thus, the **low fibrinogen level in DIC** indicates the pathological overactivity of the clotting cascade.

ED MANAGEMENT OF DIC

- Management is treatment of the underlying disorder, since this is the only way to halt the overactivation of the clotting cascade. However, once DIC is recognized, aggressive supportive measures are required and, where appropriate, should be initiated in the ED:
  - Attend to life-threatening issues such as airway compromise or severe haemorrhage requiring resuscitation and aggressive blood transfusion.
  - Determine the underlying cause of the patient's DIC and initiate therapy.
  - Once DIC is suspected, draw blood for coagulation studies, D-dimer, fibrinogen and FDPs to confirm the diagnosis.
  - Cross-match blood in preparation for transfusion.
  - Replace platelets with platelet concentrates as guided by platelet counts.
  - Replenish clotting factors with fresh frozen plasma (FFP), cryoprecipitate and/or antithrombin III concentrate as guided by a haematologist.
  - The patient will certainly need ITU care.
  - Involve a haematologist early.
- ***Treat cause!***
- ***FFP*** *for APTT and INR*
- ***Cryoprecipitate*** *for fibrinogen (> 1.0)*
- ***Platelets*** *for thrombocytopaenia (aim > 50)*
- *Consider **FIIa***
- *Consider **heparin** if not bleeding (in chronic DIC)*

VI. LEUKAEMIA

DEFINITION

- Acute leukaemia is the commonest malignancy of childhood. In the United Kingdom, one in 2 000 children develop the disorder, with around 450 new cases being diagnosed annually.[102]
- In people with leukaemia, the bone marrow produces large numbers of abnormal white blood cells that grow and multiply "out of control".
- These abnormal cells may not function properly and may affect the ability of normal blood cells to perform their usual functions.
- There are many types of leukaemia, some of which are more common in children, while others are more common in adults.

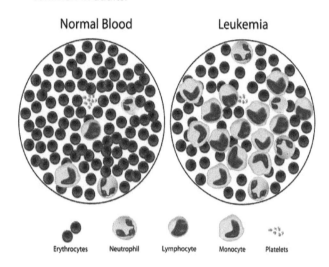

- The different types of leukaemia are classified according to how quickly the disease develops and worsens:
  - Either chronic or acute
  - Lymphoid cells or Myeloid cells.

- The four most common types of leukaemia are:
  - Chronic lymphocytic leukaemia (CLL): occurs mainly in adults and almost never in children.
  - Chronic myeloid leukaemia (CML): occurs mainly in adults.
  - Acute lymphoblastic leukaemia (ALL): occurs more commonly in children but also affects adults.
  - Acute myeloid leukaemia (AML): occurs in both adults and children.

102 Draper GJ, Stiller CA, O'Connor CM, Vincent TJ, Elliott P, McGale P, et al. The geographical epidemiology of childhood leukaemia and non-Hodgkin lymphomas in Great Britain, 1966-83. OPCS studies on medical and population subjects, no 53. London: OPCS, 1991.

RISK FACTORS

The precise cause of leukaemia is not known. However, some genetic, environmental and lifestyle factors that increase the likelihood of developing leukaemia have been identified. The risk factors, which differ for different types of leukaemia, include the following:

- **Radiation:** exposure to very high levels of radiation increases the risk of acute myeloid leukaemia, chronic myeloid leukaemia, and acute lymphocytic leukaemia
- **Smoking:** cigarette smoking increases the risk of acute myeloid leukaemia
- **Benzene:** exposure to benzene can lead to the development of acute myeloid leukaemia, chronic myeloid leukaemia, and acute lymphocytic leukaemia
- **Previous cancer treatment:** cancer patients treated with certain types of chemotherapy and radiation therapy may later develop acute myeloid leukaemia or acute lymphocytic leukaemia
- **Family history:** some people have a genetic susceptibility to developing leukaemia
- **Chromosomal abnormalities:** people with certain genetic conditions, such as Down syndrome, have a higher risk of developing leukaemia.

SIGNS, SYMPTOMS, AND DIAGNOSIS

- The symptoms of leukaemia are typically vague and non-specific and may be overlooked early in the disease because they resemble symptoms of influenza and other common illnesses. Additionally, some forms of chronic leukaemia produce no symptoms initially and can go unnoticed and hence untreated for many years.
- Depending on the type of leukaemia, symptoms may include:
  - Fever or chills
  - Fatigue and weakness
  - Frequent infections, which may be severe
  - Weight loss for no apparent reason
  - Swollen lymph nodes and an enlarged liver or spleen
  - Bone and joint pain
  - Excessive sweating, particularly at night
  - Bleeding and bruising easily
  - Tiny red spots on the skin.
- A diagnosis of leukaemia is based on a full medical history, physical examination, and blood and bone marrow tests. **Blood tests** are done to determine whether white blood cell counts are abnormally high, which is suggestive of leukaemia. **Bone marrow tests** are done to help determine treatment options.

TREATMENT

- Treatment of leukaemia depends on the type of leukaemia, the extent of the disease, prior treatment, and the age and health of the patient.
- The aim of treatment is to destroy the leukaemia cell and make the symptoms go away.
- The types of treatment used for leukaemia include:
  - **Chemotherapy:** the main form of treatment for leukaemia. It involves the use of drugs that kill leukaemia cells. Depending on the type of leukaemia, a single drug or a combination of drugs may be used.
  - **Biological therapy:** this includes the use of drugs called monoclonal antibodies, such as **rituximab,** which work by attaching to the surface of some types of leukaemia cells, thereby helping the immune system to recognise and kill the leukaemia cells.
  - **Targeted therapy:** uses drugs that target specific vulnerabilities within leukaemia cells to inhibit their growth. For example, the drug imatinib blocks the action of a specific enzyme that is required for the growth of leukaemia cells in people with chronic myeloid leukaemia.
  - **Radiation therapy:** uses high-energy beams to damage leukaemia cells and stop their growth. Radiation therapy may be used to prepare for a stem cell transplantation.
  - **Stem cell transplantation:** a procedure in which diseased bone marrow is replaced with healthy bone marrow. Prior to a stem cell transplantation, high doses of chemotherapy or radiation therapy are given to destroy diseased bone marrow. An infusion of blood-forming stem cells that help to rebuild bone marrow is then given. Transplants may be the patient's own stem cells (autologous transplant) or stem cells from another person (allogeneic transplant).
- Many people with acute leukaemia can be cured with immediate treatment.
- Achieving cure in chronic leukaemia is more difficult. Chronic leukaemia without symptoms may not need immediate treatment – a watchful waiting approach may be taken and treatment started once symptoms start to appear.
- When treatment for chronic leukaemia is given, its goal may be to control the disease and symptoms.
- Chronic leukaemia is not often cured with chemotherapy but stem cell transplantation may achieve cure in some people.
- Outcome (prognosis) depends on several factors. These include the patient's age, type of leukaemia, extent to which the leukaemia has spread, and when in the course of the disease treatment is started.

VII. BONE MARROW FAILURE

INTRODUCTION

- **Bone marrow failure** is the reduction or cessation of blood cell production affecting one or more cell lines.
- **Pancytopenia** or decreased numbers of circulating red blood cells (RBCs), White blood cells (WBCs) and platelets is seen in most cases of bone marrow failure, particularly in severe or advanced stages.

PATHOPHYSIOLOGY

- The Pathophysiology of bone marrow failure includes the following mechanisms;
  1. Destruction of hematopoietic stem cells due to injury by drugs, chemicals, radiation, viruses or autoimmune mechanisms.
  2. Premature senescence and apoptosis of stem cells due to inherited mutations.
  3. Ineffective hematopoiesis owing to stem cell mutations or vitamin B12 or folate deficiency.
  4. Disruption of the bone marrow microenvironment that supports hematopoiesis.
  5. Decreased production of hematopoietic growth factors or related hormones.
  6. Loss of normal hematopoietic tissue due to infiltration of the marrow space with abnormal cells.

COMPLICATIONS OF BONE MARROW FAILURE

- The clinical consequences of bone marrow failure vary depending on the extent and duration of the cytopenias.
  - Severe pancytopenia can be rapidly fatal if untreated.
  - Some patients may present initially with no symptoms and their cytopenia is inadvertently detected during a routine examination.
  - Thrombocytopenia can result in clinically significant bleeding.
  - The decreased in RBCs and Hemoglobin (Hb) leads to symptoms of anemia including fatigue, pallor and cardiovascular complications sustained neutropenia increases the risk of bacterial or fungal infections that can be life-threatening.
- Because there are many mechanisms involved in the various bone marrow failure syndromes, accurate diagnosis is essential so that the appropriate treatment can be instituted.

APLASTIC ANEMIA

- Aplastic anemia is a syndrome of bone marrow failure characterized by peripheral pancytopenia and marrow hypoplasia.
- Although the anemia is often normocytic, mild macrocytosis can also be observed in association with stress erythropoiesis and **elevated fetal hemoglobin levels.**
- Low power, H and E showing a hypocellular bone marrow with increased adipose tissue and decreased hematopoietic cells in the marrow space.

SIGNS AND SYMPTOMS

- The clinical presentation of patients with aplastic anemia includes symptoms related to the decrease in bone marrow production of hematopoietic cells.
- The onset is insidious, and the initial symptom is frequently related to **anemia or bleeding**, although fever or infections may be noted at presentation.
- Signs and symptoms of aplastic anemia may include the following:
  - Pallor
  - Headache
  - Palpitations
  - Dyspnea
  - Fatigue
  - Foot swelling
  - Gingival bleeding, petechial rashes
  - Overt and/or recurrent infections
  - Oropharyngeal ulcerations
- A subset of patients with aplastic anemia present with jaundice and evidence of clinical hepatitis.

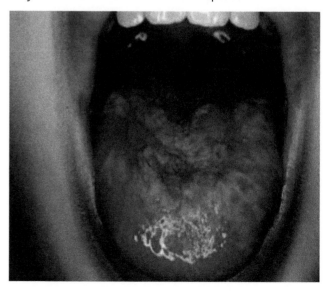

RISK FACTORS

1. Drug or toxin exposure
2. Paroxysmal nocturnal haemoglobinuria (PNH)
3. Recent hepatitis
4. Pregnancy

DIAGNOSIS

- Aplastic anaemia (AA) is defined by pancytopenia with hypocellular marrow and no abnormal cells.
- At least 2 of the following peripheral cytopenias must be present: haemoglobin <100 g/L (<10 g/dL), platelets <50 × 10^9/L, absolute neutrophil count <1.5 × 10^9/L.
- Bone marrow should show hypocellularity without evidence of significant dysplasia, blasts, fibrosis, or other abnormal infiltrate.

- **Testing**
  - Laboratory testing for suspected aplastic anemia includes the following:
    - FBC, U&Es, LFT
    - Hb electrophoresis and blood-group testing
    - Peripheral blood smears
    - Biochemical profile
    - Serology for hepatitis and other viral entities
    - Autoimmune-disease evaluation for evidence of collagen-vascular disease
    - Fluorescence-activated cell sorter profiling
    - Fluorescent-labeled inactive toxin aerolysin testing
    - Diepoxybutane incubation
    - Histocompatibility testing

- **Procedures**
  - **Bone marrow biopsy** is performed in addition to aspiration to assess cellularity qualitatively and quantitatively.
  - **Bone marrow culture** may be useful in diagnosing mycobacterial and viral infections; however, the yield is generally low.

ED MANAGEMENT

- Severe or very severe aplastic anemia is a hematologic emergency, and care should be instituted promptly.
- Clinicians must stress the need for patient compliance with therapy.
- The specific medications administered depend on the choice of therapy and whether it is supportive care only, immunosuppressive therapy, or hematopoietic cell transplantation.

- **Pharmacotherapy**
  - The following medications are used in patients with aplastic anemia:
    - Immunosuppressive agents (eg, cyclosporine, methylprednisolone, equine antithymocyte globulin, rabbit antithymocyte globulin, cyclophosphamide, alemtuzumab)
    - Hematopoietic growth factors (eg, eltrombopag, sargramostim, filgrastim)
    - Antimetabolite (purine) antineoplastic agents (eg, fludarabine)
    - Chelating agents (eg, deferoxamine, deferasirox)

- **Nonpharmacotherapy**
- Nonpharmacologic management of aplastic anemia includes the following:
  - Supportive care
  - Blood transfusions with blood products that have undergone leukocyte reduction and irradiation
  - Hematopoietic cell transplantation

- **Surgical option**
  - Central venous catheter placement is required before the administration of hematopoietic cell transplantation.

9. Chest Pain

I. CHEST PAIN SYNDROMES

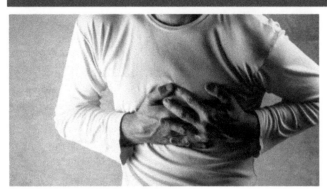

1. THE SPECTRUM OF PATHOLOGY PRESENTING WITH CHEST PAIN

System	CVS	Pulmonary	GIT
Life-threatening	AMI Aortic dissection PE	Tension pneumothorax	Oesophageal rupture
Urgent	Unstable angina Coronary vasospasm Pericarditis Myocarditis	Simple pneumothorax	Pancreatitis
Non-urgent	Stable angina Valvular heart disease Hypertrophic cardiomyopathy	Viral pleurisy Pneumonia	Cholecystitis Oesophageal reflux Biliary colic Peptic ulcer
		Musculoskeletal	**Other**
Urgent			Mediastinitis
Non-urgent		Costochondritis Chest wall injury	Postherpetic neuralgia Herpes zoster Malignancy Psychological/ anxiety

2. CARDIAC & NON-CARDIAC CAUSES OF CHEST PAIN

CHEST PAIN	
Cardiac	
Ischaemic	**Non-ischaemic**
• Angina • Unstable Angina • Myocardial Infarction	• Pericarditis • Myocarditis
Non-cardiac	
Gastro-oesophageal	**Non-Gastro-oesophageal**
• GOR • Oesophageal spasm • PUD	• Aortic Dissection • PE • Pneumonia • Pneumothorax • Musculoskeletal

3. CHARACTERISTIC DESCRIPTION OF SYMPTOMS ASSOCIATED WITH MAJOR CAUSES OF CHEST PAIN

CONDITION	DESCRIPTION OF SYMPTOMS
Ischaemic cardiac pain	• Retrosternal 'pressure', 'tightness', 'constricting' • Radiation to shoulders, arms, neck and jaw, Crescendo in nature, related to exertion, • Associated with diaphoresis, sweating, nausea, pallor
Pericarditis	• Atypical, retrosternal, sometimes pleuritic • Positional **relieved on sitting forward**
Gastro-oesophageal	• Retrosternal, **'burning'** • Associated with ingestion
Aortic dissection	• **'Tearing'** pain, sudden in onset, Radiation to back
Pulmonary embolism	• Atypical, may be pleuritic • Associated with breathlessness; occasional haemoptysis
Pneumothorax	• Atypical, may be pleuritic • Associated with cough, sputum, fever
Musculoskeletal	• Sharp, Positional, Pleuritic • Aggravated by movement, deep inspiration and coughing

4. RISK FACTORS ASSOCIATED WITH MAJOR LIFE-THREATENING CAUSES OF CHEST PAIN

CONDITION	RISK FACTORS
Acute coronary syndromes	• Previous known coronary artery disease (previous myocardial infarction, angioplasty, etc.) • Positive family history • Advanced age, Male gender • Diabetes, Hypertension, • Hypercholesterolaemia • Active smoker, • Obesity, Sedentary Lifestyle • Aspirin usage
Aortic dissection	• Chronic hypertension • Inherited connective tissue disorder, e.g. Marfan syndrome, Ehlers-Danlos syndrome • Bicuspid aortic valve • Coarctation of the aorta • Pregnancy • Inflammatory aortic disease, e.g. Giant Cell Arteritis

Pulmonary embolism	• Previous history of venous thromboembolic disease • Pregnancy or puerperium • Positive family history of venous thromboembolic disease (two or more family members) • Recent prolonged immobilisation (>3 days) • Major surgery within previous 12 weeks • Fracture of lower limb within previous 12 weeks • Active cancer (within previous 6 months, recent treatment, palliation) • Lower extremity paralysis

5. PHYSICAL FINDINGS ASSOCIATED WITH CHEST PAIN CONDITIONS

DIAGNOSIS	PHYSICAL FINDINGS
ACS	• Diaphoresis, • Pallor • Tachycardia, Tachypnoea,
Complications of acute MI	• **Hypotension,** • **Third heart sound,** • **Pulmonary crepitations**, • Elevated JVP, bradycardia, new murmur
Aortic dissection	• Diaphoresis, hypotension, • Hypertension, tachycardia, **differential blood pressures and/or pulses,** • **New murmur** (aortic regurgitation), • **Focal neurological findings**
Pulmonary embolism	• Acute respiratory distress, diaphoresis, • Hypotension, tachycardia, hypoxaemia, • Elevated JVP, pleural rub
Pneumonia	• **Fever, signs of pulmonary collapse/consolidation**, • Tachycardia, tachypnoea
Oesophageal rupture	• Diaphoresis, hypotension, • Tachycardia, **Fever, Hamman's sign*,** • **Subcutaneous emphysema**, • Epigastric tenderness
Simple pneumothorax	• Tachypnoea, tachycardia, **unilateral diminished air entry and breath sounds**, subcutaneous emphysema
Tension pneumothorax	• Tachypnoea, • Hypotension, • Tachycardia, • Hypoxaemia, **elevated JVP,** • **Unilateral diminished air entry and breath sounds**, • Subcutaneous emphysema, • **Tracheal deviation**

Pericarditis	• Tachycardia, **Fever,** • **Pericardial rub**
Myocarditis	• Hypotension, tachycardia, • Fever, **third heart sound,** • Pulmonary crepitations, • **Displaced apex beat**
Mediastinitis	• Tachycardia, **fever,** • **Hamman's sign*,** • Subcutaneous emphysema, • Hypotension
Cholecystitis	• Diaphoresis, Fever, • Tachycardia, • **Right upper quadrant tenderness**

Certain physical signs, or combinations of signs, are highly suggestive of certain diagnoses and are highlighted in bold.
** **Hammans sign:** audible systolic noise on cardiac auscultation*

6. ECG FINDINGS ASSOCIATED WITH NON-ISCHAEMIC CHEST PAIN CONDITIONS

ECG FINDING	CONTEXT	DIAGNOSIS
Diffuse concave-upward ST segment elevation	Positional pain Pericardial rub	**Pericarditis**
Right ventricular strain pattern	Pleuritic pain Hypoxia Pleural rub	**P.E.**
Diffuse ST/T wave changes	Atypical pain Heart failure	**Myocarditis**
Inferior ST elevation	Tearing chest pain Radiation to back Differential pulses Differential blood pressures New diastolic murmur	**Aortic dissection**

7. RADIOGRAPHIC FINDINGS IN CONDITIONS PRESENTING WITH CHEST PAIN

CONDITION	RADIOGRAPHIC FINDING
ACS	• No specific radiographic finding
Aortic dissection	• Mediastinal widening • Abnormal aortic contour • Globular heart shadow • Pleural effusion (haemothorax)
Pneumothorax	• Absence of pulmonary vascular markings
Tension pneumothorax	• Absence of pulmonary vascular markings • Mediastinal displacement
Pneumonia	• Localised or diffuse pulmonary infiltration

	• Localised pulmonary atelectasis • Localised Consolidation
Pulmonary embolism	• Normal chest radiograph • Localised pulmonary atelectasis • Small pleural effusion
Oesophageal rupture	• Pneumomediastinum
Mediastinitis	• Pneumomediastinum
Pericarditis	• Globular heart shadow
Myocarditis	• Enlarged cardiac shadow

8. ANCILLARY INVESTIGATIONS

- The history, physical examination, ECG and CXR will normally allow the emergency physician to be fairly confident to achieve a diagnosis in a patient with chest pain presenting to the ED.

- **ACS:**
  o Cardiac markers (e.g. troponin) and
  o Possible exercise testing.

- **PULMONARY EMBOLISM**
  o For patients at low risk: **D-dimer assay.**
  o For patients at intermediate or high risk: **Ventilation perfusion (V/Q) scan or CT Pulmonary Angiogram (CTPA).**

- **AORTIC DISSECTION**:
  o **CT Mediastinum** (to definitively exclude aortic dissection)

LEARNING BITE

- *Pulmonary embolism* will rarely be definitively diagnosed without ancillary investigations (D-Dimer, V/Q scan, or CTPA)
- *Aortic dissection* is a diagnosis that should be strongly suspected if the appropriate features are present upon clinical assessment: the history (tearing pain), examination (new murmur of aortic regurgitation, differential blood pressures), ECG (inferior ischaemic changes) and CXR (widened mediastinum) will, when present in combination, be pathognomonic of aortic dissection. However, due to the potentially catastrophic nature of aortic dissection if undiagnosed, this condition will need to be definitively excluded even if the index of suspicion is low (e.g. if only one of the characteristic clinical features is present).
- In patients in whom the diagnosis is virtually certain from the clinical presentation, the anatomical extent of the dissection will need to be defined.

- In either case, a **CT mediastinum** will need to be performed and this will be diagnostic and define the anatomical extent.
- CT mediastinum will be required to definitively exclude aortic dissection and/or to define its anatomical extent

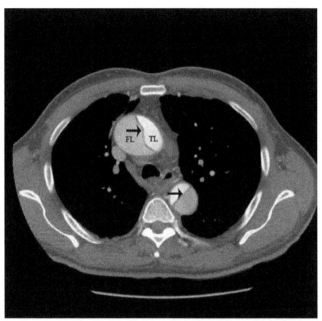

Aortic dissection The arrows demonstrate the intimal flaps in both the ascending aorta (anterior) and the descending aorta (posterior). TL= is the true lumen as this has contrast within it whilst the darker false lumen (FL) does not.

II. ST ELEVATION WITHOUT INFARCTION

INTRODUCTION

- Acute myocardial infarction resulting from an occlusive thrombus is recognized on an electrocardiogram by ST-segment elevation.[103] Early reperfusion therapy has proved beneficial in such infarctions.

- The earlier the reperfusion, the greater the benefit, and the time to treatment is now considered to indicate the quality of care. These days, when thrombolytic treatment and percutaneous intervention are carried out so readily, it is important to remember that acute infarction is not the only cause of ST-segment elevation.

NORMAL ST-SEGMENT ELEVATION AND NORMAL VARIANTS

- The level of the ST segment should be measured in relation to the end of the PR segment, not the TP segment.[104]

- In this way, ST-segment deviation can still be detected accurately, even if the TP segment is not present because the P wave is superimposed on the T wave during sinus tachycardia or if the PR segment is depressed or there is a prominent atrial repolarization (Ta) wave.

- Since the majority of men have ST elevation of 1 mm or more in precordial leads, it is a normal finding, not a normal variant, and is designated as a male pattern; ST elevation of less than 1 mm is designated as a female pattern.[105] In these patterns, the ST segment is concave.

- The deeper the S wave, the greater the ST-segment elevation – a relation that is often observed in patients with left ventricular hypertrophy.

- Since the QRS vector loop is swung posteriorly in these patients, often resulting in a QS pattern in leads V1 through V3, ST-segment elevation in these leads can be deceiving. In some healthy young people, especially in black men, the ST segment is elevated by 1 to 4 mm in the midprecordial leads as a normal variant.

- This pattern is commonly referred to as early repolarization,[106] even though clinical studies have failed to demonstrate an earlierthan-normal onset of ventricular recovery.

---

[103] DeWood MA, Spores J, Notske R, et al. Prevalence of total coronary occlusion during the early hours of transmural myocardial infarction. N Engl J Med 1980;303:897-902.

[104] Fletcher GF, Balady GJ, Amsterdam EA, et al. Exercise standards for testing and training: a statement for healthcare professionals from the American Heart Association. Circulation 2001;104:1694-740.

[105] Surawicz B, Parikh SR. Prevalence of male and female patterns of early ventricular repolarization in the normal ECG of males and females from childhood to old age. J Am Coll Cardiol 2002;40:1870-6.

[106] Kambara H, Phillips J. Long-term evaluation of early repolarization syndrome (normal variant RS-T segment elevation). Am J Cardiol 1976;38:157-61.

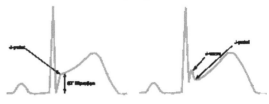

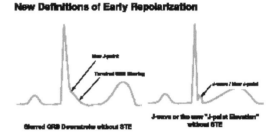

An example of the early-repolarization pattern.

- In most instances of early repolarization, the ST-segment elevation is most marked in V4, there is a notch at the J point (the junction between the QRS complex and the ST segment), and the ST segment is concave.

- The T waves are tall and are not inverted. Early repolarization of atrial tissue is also present, resulting in PR-segment depression. However, the PR-segment depression is not as marked as that in patients with acute pericarditis.

- If this early-repolarization pattern involves limb leads, the ST segment is more elevated in lead II than in lead III and there is reciprocal ST segment depression in lead aVR but not in aVL, whereas in most patients with inferior infarctions, the ST segment is more elevated in lead III than in lead II and there is reciprocal ST-segment depression in lead aVL. In most cases of this normal variant, the QT interval is short, whereas it is not short in acute infarction or pericarditis.

- This normal variant differs from the early-repolarization pattern in that the T waves are inverted and the ST segment tends to be coved.

- Thus, normally, in the precordial leads there can be no ST-segment elevation (or an elevation of lessthan 1 mm, which is the female pattern) or there can be normal ST-segment elevation (1 mm or more, the male pattern), an early-repolarization pattern as a normal variant, or ST elevation of the normal variant.

- The ST segment represents completed ventricular myocardial depolarization. This segment can be FLAT or can be sloping.

- The European Society of Cardiology defines the height of ST elevation in AMI as being measured at the J point.

Three questions are important in evaluating the ST segment:
1. Where is the baseline?
2. What is the J point?
3. Where along the ST segment do we measure?

1. Baseline

- **ST segment elevation** is defined as deviation of the ST segment by greater than 0.1mV above a line joining 2 successive TP segments; if the TP segment is not clearly identifiable then the PR segment can be used.

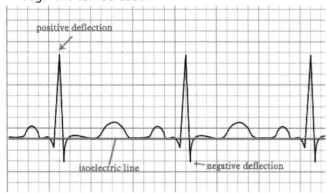

Demonstrating the baseline

2. J point

- This is be defined as the junction between the QRS complex and the ST segment.

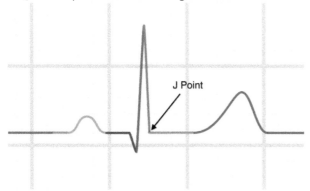

Identification of the J point

3. MEASUREMENT OF ST ELEVATION

- An **ST elevation** is considered significant if the vertical distance inside the ECG trace and the baseline at a point 0.04 seconds after the J-point is at least 0.1 mV (usually representing 1 mm or 1 small square) in a limb lead or 0.2 mV (2 mm or 2 small squares) in a precordial lead.

RECOGNITION OF ST SEGMENT ELEVATION WITHOUT INFARCTION

1. ST SEGMENT MORPHOLOGY:

- **BER** produces widespread ST-segment elevation that may mimic pericarditis or acute MI.
- BER can be difficult to differentiate from pericarditis because both conditions are associated with concave ST elevation.
- Using the ST-segment elevation (from the end of the PR segment to the J point) compared with the amplitude of the T wave in V6 can distinguish between these two conditions.
- An ST-segment–T-wave ratio greater than 0.25 suggests pericarditis, but if the ratio is less than 0.25, it is consistent with BER.

ST SEGMENT MORPHOLOGY

- Acute STEMI may produce ST elevation with either concave, convex or obliquely straight morphology.
- A convex ST segment shape is more likely to be associated with AMI than a concave shape. However, do not assume that because ST segment elevation is not convex that it cannot be a STEMI.

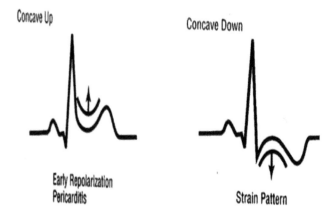

2. DISTRIBUTION OF ST SEGMENT ELEVATION

- ST segment elevation due to STEMI follows a coronary artery "territorial" distribution which is not typically seen in other conditions.
- It may also be accompanied by reciprocal changes.
- ST segment elevation due to BER is typically evident in the precordial leads: 74% in V1-V2, 73% in V3-V4 and 37% in inferior leads.
- ST segment elevation is more diffuse in pericarditis.

Distribution of ST segment changes and association with cause

Cause	ST elevation site	Reciprocal changes
STEMI	Coronary artery distribution	Common
Pericarditis	Diffuse	In aVR not AVL
BER	Chest leads	In aVR in 50%
BRUGADA	V1 and V2	No
Ventricular Aneurysm	Mostly anterior	No

3. MAGNITUDE OF ST SEGMENT ELEVATION
- The magnitude of ST segment elevation can help to differentiate BER from STEMI.

4. "NOTCH" OR "SLUR" AT THE END OF THE QRS (AT THE J POINT):
- An upward sloping notch at the end of the QRS segment is one of the features seen in BER more visible in the precordial leads in BER.
- This is not a feature of pericarditis.

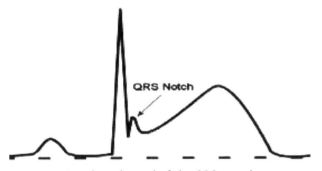

Notch at the end of the QRS complex

(v) ST SEGMENT ELEVATION TO T WAVE HEIGHT RATIO
- Both BER and pericarditis can have ST segments and T waves that look morphologically similar making distinguishing between them difficult.
- Comparing the height of the ST segment to that of the T wave can aid in this process. This can be expressed as a ratio.
- **The most useful place to measure this is in V6.** When this ratio is **greater than 0.25** it indicates the diagnosis of pericarditis is more likely with a positive predictive value of 90%. It can be done in other leads but with less accuracy.[107]

⤋ *The ST:T wave ratio in V6 of > 0.25 makes Pericarditis more likely.*

---

[107] *Leilah J Dare. RCEM Learning. ST Segment elevation without infarction. [Online]*

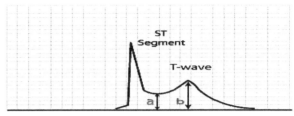

Where a is the height of the ST Segment and b is the height of the T Wave

$$\frac{a}{b} > 0.25$$

Demonstration of ST/T wave ratio measurement- Courtesy RCEM learning

PATHOLOGICAL CAUSES OF ST ELEVATION

Cardiac	• STEMI
	• Pericarditis
	• Ventricular Aneurysm
	• Brugada syndrome
	• LBBB
Intracranial	• Stroke
	• Raised ICP
	• Intracranial haemorrhage
Abdominal	• Peritonitis
Drugs	• Digoxin
	• Isoprenaline
	• Quinidine
	• Procainamide
Metabolic	• Hypothermia
	• Hyperventilation
	• Hyperkalaemia
Other	• Spinal cord injury
	• PE

IMPORTANT CAUSES OF ST ELEVATION WITHOUT INFARCTION
1. CARDIAC CAUSES

(i) BENIGN EARLY REPOLARISATION

Benign early repolarisation (BER: AKA 'high-take off; J-point elevation) is an ECG pattern most commonly seen in young, healthy patients < 50 years of age.
- It produces widespread ST segment elevation that may mimic pericarditis or acute MI.
- Up to 10-15% of ED patients presenting with chest pain will have BER on their ECG, making it a common diagnostic challenge for clinicians.
- The physiological basis of BER is poorly understood. However, it is generally thought to be a normal variant that is not indicative of underlying cardiac disease.
- BER is less common in the over 50s, in whom ST elevation is more likely to represent myocardial ischaemia.
- It is rare in the over 70s.

(ii) PERICARDITIS

- In patients with acute pericarditis, the ST segment is elevated diffusely in the precordial leads as well as in the limb leads, indicating involvement of more than one coronary vascular territory, which rarely happens in acute myocardial infarction. In addition, the PR segment is depressed, and such depression is the atrial counterpart of ST-segment elevation. Diffuse pericarditis involves not only the subepicardial layer of the ventricular wall, which is responsible for the ST-segment elevation, but also the subepicardial layer of the atrial wall, which causes an atrial injury pattern.
- Depression of the PR segment, however, is not specific for acute pericarditis, since early repolarization or atrial infarction can also cause the depression.
- In patients with diffuse pericarditis, the ST-segment axis is often close to 45 degrees in the frontal plane,[108] which falls into the positive zone of both leads III and aVL, and the ST segment is elevated in both these leads and is also more elevated in lead II than in lead III.
- In patients with acute inferior infarction, which is most often due to occlusion of the right coronary artery, the ST-segment axis is close to the axis of lead III, which is opposite the axis of lead aVL; therefore, the ST-segment elevation in lead III is always associated with reciprocal ST-segment depression in leads aVL and I.
- In addition, the ST segment is more elevated in lead III than in lead II. In acute inferior infarction due to occlusion of the circumflex coronary artery, which accounts for about 20 percent of acute inferior infarctions, the axis of the ST segment is often close to that of aVF.

CAUSES OF PERICARDITIS

- *Idiopathic*
- *Viral*
- *Non-viral infections*
- *Transmural infection*
- *Trauma*
- *Neoplasms*
- *Uraemia*
- *Systemic inflammatory disorders*

85% of patients have an **audible friction rub** during the course of their disease. 15% of patients with idiopathic pericarditis and up to 60% of patients with neoplastic, TB or purulent pericarditis have clinical evidence of **tamponade.**

- ❖ 85% of patients with pericarditis have a pericardial friction rub at some point during their illness
- ❖ **ECG findings** include widespread concave ST elevation, ST depression in lead aVR and widespread PR depression. The ST segment to T wave height ratio in lead V6 is normally > 0.25
- ❖ Troponin levels are elevated in 35-50% of patients with pericarditis.
- ❖ Other blood tests (e.g. full blood count, viral serology) are of little help in finding a cause.
- ❖ **Echocardiography** should be performed to aid diagnosis, evaluate the size of any associated effusion and to look for other poor prognostic indicators.

PROGNOSTIC CRITERIA

Poor prognostic indicators associated with pericarditis:

- *Temperature > 38*
- *Subacute onset (severe weeks)*
- *Immunosuppressed*
- *Associated with trauma*
- *Oral anticoagulant therapy*
- *Myopericarditis*
- *Large pericardial effusion (20mm width on echo)*
- *Cardiac tamponade*

ED MANAGEMENT

- The treatment for uncomplicated pericarditis is non-steroidal anti-inflammatory medication **(NSAIDs)** to relieve discomfort.
- **Steroids** are not to be used in the first instance for idiopathic pericarditis as they may increase the risk of recurrence. They may be used in pericarditis associated with systemic inflammatory disorders.
- **Colchicine** can be considered in conjunction with the NSAIDs.

- ❖ Avoid steroids as first line treatment in idiopathic uncomplicated pericarditis
- ❖ Discharging someone from ED without an echocardiogram means that not all poor prognostic indicators have been excluded and that an incomplete assessment has been made.
- ❖ Following a normal echocardiogram, a patient may be discharged with NSAIDs if otherwise well.

---

[108] *Hurst JW, Logue RB, Schant RC, Wenger NK, eds. The heart, arteries, and veins. 4th ed. New York: McGraw-Hill, 1978:1182.*

(iii) BRUGADA SYNDROME

- The disorder, known as the Brugada syndrome, accounts for 40 to 60 percent of all cases of idiopathic ventricular fibrillation.[109]
- The syndrome has been linked to mutations in the cardiac sodium-channel gene, which result in a depression or a loss of the action-potential dome in the right ventricular epicardium but not in the endocardium, creating a transmural voltage gradient that is responsible for the ST-segment elevation in the right precordial leads and the genesis of ventricular fibrillation.
- The ST-segment elevation is primarily limited to leads V1 and V2 and can have a **saddleback shape**, but in typical cases the ST segment begins from the top of the R' wave, is downsloping, and ends with an inverted T wave.
- This pattern is so distinctive that it should not be mistaken for acute infarction.
- In anteroseptal infarction complicated by right bundle-branch block, the downstroke of the R' wave and the beginning of the ST segment have a distinct transition, and the ST segment is horizontal or upsloping, not downsloping.
- The ST-segment elevation in the Brugada syndrome may be present continuously or intermittently.
- Sodium-channel blockers such as ajmaline, flecainide, procainamide, and cocaine can unmask or induce this electrocardiographic pattern.[110]

CLINICAL FEATURES INCLUDE

- Episodes of arrhythmia (usually rapid polymorphic VT), Collapse or sudden death.
- The episodes are more common in the night or the early hours of the morning.
- There may be a family history of sudden death.
- It has a male predominance (ratio 8:1).
- There are 3 types, each with specific ECG appearances.
- These ECG findings can be dynamic and can be unmasked or exaggerated by **sodium channel blockers** such as **flecainide**.
- Brugada Syndrome is not associated with identifiable structural cardiac abnormalities.
- ST segment elevation occurs in the right precordial leads V_1 to V_3.
- The exact morphology of the ST segment gives rise to the 3 types.

[109] Chen Q, Kirsch GE, Zhang D, et al. Genetic basis and molecular mechanism for idiopathic ventricular fibrillation. Nature 1998; 392:293-6.

[110] Littmann L, Monroe MH, Svenson RH. Brugada-type electrocardiographic pattern induced by cocaine. Mayo Clin Proc 2000; 75:845-9.

DIAGNOSTIC CRITERIA

Type 1

- Coved ST segment elevation >2mm in >1 of V1-V3 followed by a negative T wave.
- This is the only ECG abnormality that is potentially diagnostic.
- It is often referred to as **Brugada sign.**

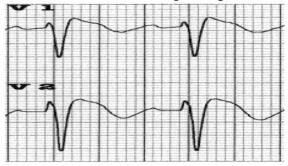

Brugada sign

This ECG abnormality must be associated with one of the following clinical criteria to make the diagnosis:

- Documented ventricular fibrillation (VF) or polymorphic ventricular tachycardia (VT).
- Family history of sudden cardiac death at <45 years old.
- Coved-type ECGs in family members.
- Inducibility of VT with programmed electrical stimulation.
- Syncope.
- Nocturnal agonal respiration.

	ST elevation characteristic	T wave characteristic
Type 1	ST elevation slopes downward	Goes into inverted T wave
Type 2	High take off ST elevation > 2mm Saddle shape	Goes into upward Biphasic T wave remaining 1 mm above baseline
Type 3	Less ST elevation Saddle shape	Upward T wave

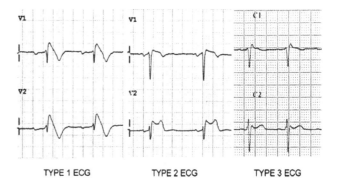

TYPE 1 ECG   TYPE 2 ECG   TYPE 3 ECG

- The other two types of Brugada are non-diagnostic but possibly warrant further investigation.
- If Type 1 ECG morphology is demonstrated there is no need for drug testing but this is not the case in **Types 2 and 3 where sodium channel blockers are used to confirm the diagnosis.**

Type 2

- Brugada Type 2 has >2mm of saddleback shaped ST elevation.

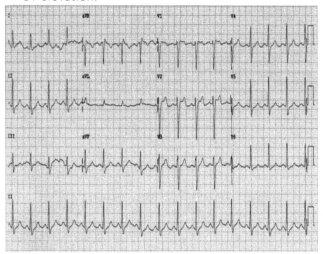

Type 3

- Brugada type 3: can be the morphology of either type 1 or type 2, but with <2mm of ST segment elevation.

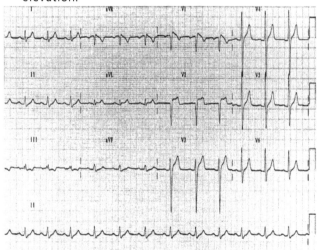

ED MANAGEMENT OF BRUGADA SYNDROME

- The only proven therapy is an **Implantable Cardioverter Defibrillator (ICD).**
- Quinidine has been proposed as an alternative in settings where ICD's are unavailable or where they would be inappropriate (eg: neonates).

(iv) VENTRICULAR ANEURYSM

- The majority of ventricular aneurysms are seen after large anterior myocardial infarctions.
- This diagnosis may be indicated by the clinical history and the presence of previously recorded discharge ECGs.
- The commonest site of ST segment elevation is in the anterior leads reflecting the most likely site of the original STEMI. Clinical and ECG features will be static unlike those of a patient presenting with an acute STEMI.
- The other ECG characteristics can be seen below.

ECG characteristics associated with ventricular aneurysm

Ventricular aneurysm	
Height of ST elevation	1mm - 3mm
ST morphology	Any shape
ST site	More common anteriorly
T wave	Diminished in size
Q waves	Present in the STEMI distribution

(v) DRESSLER SYNDROME

- It is a secondary form of pericarditis that occurs in the setting of injury to the heart or the pericardium. It consists of fever, pleuritic pain, pericarditis and/or a pericardial effusion.
- The symptoms tend to occur 2-3 weeks after myocardial infarction, but can also be delayed for a few months. It tends to subside in a few days, and very rarely leads to pericardial tamponade.
- An **elevated ESR** is an objective laboratory finding.

Causes:

- It is believed to result from an autoimmune inflammatory reaction to myocardial neo-antigens formed as a result of the MI.
- A similar pericarditis can be associated with any pericardiotomy or trauma to the pericardium or heart surgery.

Differentials:

- Pulmonary embolism,
- other causes of pleuritic chest pain.

Treatment:

- Aspirin for 4-6 weeks
- NSAIDS (to be avoided in patients with known coronary artery disease, aspirin is preferred)
- Colchicine
- Prednisolone (if the above aspirin and NSAIDs fail to respond

(vi) Prinzmetal's variant angina

- When an epicardial artery is completely "pinched off" as a result of spasm, the ST segment becomes elevated in the leads facing the affected area, reflecting transmural ischemia.
- In this condition, called Prinzmetal's angina, the spasm is usually brief and the ST segment returns to normal, with no resultant myocardial damage.
- The ST-segment elevations in Prinzmetal's angina and in acute infarction are indistinguishable, since they reflect the same pathophysiological process: transmural ischemia from occlusion of an epicardial artery by transient spasm in the first condition and by persistent thrombus in the second. If the spasm lasts long enough, infarction results.
- Prinzmetal's variant angina (PVA) is characterized by recurrent episodes of chest pain (angina) that usually occur when a person is at rest, between midnight and early morning.
- "Typical" angina, by contrast, is often triggered by physical exertion or emotional stress.
- Episodes of PVA can be very painful, and may last from several minutes to thirty minutes.
- In some cases the pain may spread from the chest to the head, shoulder, or arm. The pain associated with PVA is caused by a **spasm in the coronary arteries.**
- This results in an obstruction of blood flow. In some people, persistent spasms increase the risk for serious complications such as a life-threatening arrhythmia or heart attack.

RISK FACTORS

- PVA most commonly occurs in people who smoke and people who have high cholesterol or high blood pressure.
- In many cases it occurs for unknown reasons in otherwise healthy people. In some cases it may be triggered by alcohol withdrawal, stress, exposure to cold, certain medications, or use of stimulants such as cocaine.
- The diagnosis of PVA involves findings on an ECG, evidence of the spasms on angiogram, and relief of sudden symptoms with medicines called nitrates.

Treatment

- Sublingual nitroglycerin (a nitrate).
- Calcium channel blockers or long-acting nitrates.
- For people with PVA who smoke, quitting smoking can lead to a significant decrease in the frequency of episodes.

(vii) LEFT BUNDLE BRANCH BLOCK

- Making the diagnosis of acute infarction in the presence of left bundle-branch block can be problematic, since the ST segment is either elevated or depressed secondarily, simulating or masking an infarction pattern.
- These secondary ST-T changes are shifted to the opposite direction from the major component of the QRS complex (i.e., discordant).
- When these changes are concordant, they are specific for acute myocardial infarction.[111] However, in left bundle-branch block, the QRS complexes are mostly negative in leads V1 to V3, and the ST-segment elevation from an anteroseptal infarction cannot be manifested as a concordant ST-segment shift.
- At times, replacement of the secondary concave ST segment with a convex ST segment may indicate an associated anteroseptal infarct.
- Another criterion that has been proposed for recognizing an associated anteroseptal infarct is ST-segment elevation of 5 mm or more.
- Madias et al. found that 6 percent of 128 patients with left bundle-branch block had STsegment elevation of at least 5 mm in one or more of leads V1 through V3 in the absence of infarction.[112]

SGARBOSSA CRITERIA FOR AMI IN LBBB

1. *ST segment elevation of 1mm or more concordant with (in the same direction as) the QRS complex in leads V5 or V6*
2. *ST segment depression of 1mm or more concordant with the QRS complex in leads V1, V2 or V3.*
3. *ST segment elevation of 5mm or more that was discordant with (in the opposite direction from) the QRS complex.*

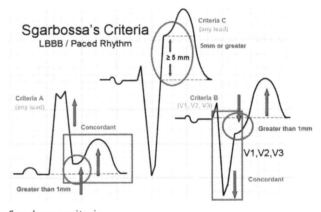

Sgarbossa criteria

[111] Hands ME, Cook EF, Stone PH, et al. Electrocardiographic diagnosis of myocardial infarction in the presence of complete left bundle branch block. Am Heart J 1988; 116:23-31.

[112] Madias JE, Sinha A, Agarwal H, Ashtiani R. ST-segment elevation in leads V1-V3 in patients with LBBB. J Electrocardiol 2001;34: 87-8.

2. NON CARDIAC CAUSES
(i) PULMONARY EMBOLISM (PE)

- ECG changes associated with significant PE reflect right ventricular strain (due to outflow obstruction) and are mainly in the inferior and anteroseptal leads.
- In addition to ST segment elevation (which is an unusual finding in PE), there are other ECG findings that are associated with PE.

ECG FEATURES ASSOCIATED WITH PE

- Sinus tachycardia
- Right Axis deviation
- RBBB (Complete or incomplete)
- S1Q3T3 pattern
- Positive T wave in lead V1
- T wave inversion in inferior or anteroseptal leads

(ii) HYPERKALAEMIA

- Hyperkalemia as a cause of ST-segment elevation is well recognized. In 1956, Levine et al. reported four cases of ST-segment elevation due to hyperkalemia resembling acute myocardial infarction or pericarditis, and they coined the term "dialyzable currents of injury."[113]
- Other electrocardiographic features of hyperkalemia that are often, but not always, present are widened QRS complexes; tall, pointed, and tented T waves; and low-amplitude or no P waves.
- Even though the pseudoinfarction pattern of hyperkalemia is well known, the ST-segment elevation is so striking at times that one cannot help agonizing over the possibility of coexistent acute infarction.

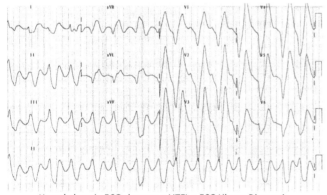

Hyperkalaemia ECG changes • LITFL • ECG Library Diagnosis

- In patients with hyperkalemia, the elevated ST segment is often downsloping, a finding that is somewhat unusual in acute myocardial infarction, which is more likely to be characterized by an ST segment that has a plateau or a shoulder or is upsloping.
- An echocardiogram can be extremely useful in this situation.

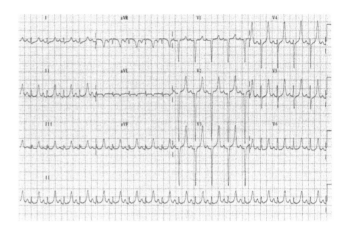

(iii) SUBARACHNOID HAEMORRHAGE

- QT prolongation, T inversion, and ST-segment abnormalities are the most common ECG changes detected in patients with SAH.
- Cardiac troponin I elevation is seen in 20% to 40% of patients with SAH[114]. However, these increases are generally under the diagnostic value for myocardial infarction.
- It should be considered that, in patients with neurologic signs or in patients without chest pain, ECG abnormalities may be related to an intracranial event in addition to cardiac ischemia.

[113] Levine HD, Wanzer SH, Merrill JP. Dialyzable currents of injury in potassium intoxication resembling acute myocardial infarction or pericarditis. Circulation 1956; 13:29-36.

[114] Tung P, Kopelnik A, Banki N, Ong K, Ko N, Lawton MT, et al. Predictors of neurocardiogenic injury after subarachnoid hemorrhage. Stroke 2004;35:548-51.

III. ACUTE CORONARY SYNDROMES

INTRODUCTION

- Acute coronary syndrome (ACS) refers to a spectrum of clinical presentations ranging from those for ST-segment elevation myocardial infarction (STEMI) to presentations found in non–ST-segment elevation myocardial infarction (NSTEMI) or in unstable angina[115]. It is almost always associated with rupture of an atherosclerotic plaque and partial or complete thrombosis of the infarct-related artery.

PATHOPHYSIOLOGY OF ACS

- Four diverse mechanisms cause acute coronary syndromes (ACS):
  - Plaque rupture, also referred to as fissure, traditionally considered the dominant substrate for ACS, usually associates with both local inflammation, as depicted by the blue monocytes, and systemic inflammation, as indicated by the gauge showing an increase in blood C-reactive protein (CRP; measured with a high-sensitivity [hsCRP] assay).
  - In some cases, plaque rupture complicates atheromata that do not harbor large collections of intimal macrophages, as identified by optical coherence tomography criteria, and do not associate with elevations in circulating CRP. Plaque rupture usually provokes the formation of fibrin-rich red thrombi.
  - Plaque erosion appears to account for a growing portion of ACS, often provoking non–ST-segment-elevation myocardial infarction. The thrombi overlying patches of intimal erosion generally exhibit characteristics of white platelet-rich structures.
  - Vasospasm can also cause ACS, long recognized as a phenomenon in the epicardial arteries but also affecting coronary microcirculation.

CLINICAL ASSESSMENT

- **History**
- The classic presenting symptom of ACS is **chest pain,** which is traditionally described as having a characteristic nature:
  - *Heavy, aching or tight*
  - *Central chest or left sided*
  - *Not related to respiration or movement*
  - *May radiate to one or both arms, neck, or jaw*

- Atypical presentations of ACS are common, occurring in up **to 33% of patients**, mostly in the elderly, diabetics and women.
- Advanced age, co-morbid factors, delay in diagnosis, delayed or reduced use of reperfusion therapy, and reduced use of adjuvant therapies all contribute to the increased mortality in this population.

CLASSIFICATION OF ACS
STEMI (S-T SEGMENT ELEVATION MYOCARDIAL INFARCTION)

- Presentation with clinical symptoms consistent with an acute coronary syndrome together with S-T segment elevation on ECG. New LBBB may be included in this sub-heading as the treatment approach is similar to STEMI[116]

NSTEACS (NON S-T SEGMENT ELEVATION ACUTE CORONARY SYNDROME)

- As UA and NSTEMI often have identical clinical presentation, they are collectively termed non-ST elevation acute coronary syndrome (NSTE-ACS) in the latest guidance from the American College of Cardiology (ACC) and American Heart Association (AHA) [117]
- NSTEACS refers to any acute coronary syndrome which does not show S-T segment elevation. The ECG may show S-T segment depression or transient S-T segment elevation, but often will be normal

NON-STEMI (NON S-T SEGMENT ELEVATION MYOCARDIAL INFARCTION)

- NSTEMI is diagnosed in patients determined to have symptoms consistent with ACS and troponin elevation but without ECG changes consistent with STEMI.

UNSTABLE ANGINA

- Unstable angina and NSTEMI differ primarily in the presence or absence of detectable troponin leak.
- A small but still significant proportion (< 4 %) of patients presenting with possible cardiac chest pain in whom biomarkers and ECGs are normal will have unstable angina due to underlying coronary artery disease
- Note that **"unstable angina"** is measured against a patient's usual pattern of **"stable angina"**. New onset angina should be considered unstable in the first instance.

---

[115] David L Coven. Acute Coronary Syndrome. [Medscape online]

[116] Chris Nickson. Acute Coronary Syndrome. [litfl online]

[117] Amsterdam EA, Wenger NK, Brindis RG et al. AHA/ACC guideline for the management of patients with non–ST-elevation acute coronary syndromes: a report of the American College of Cardiology/American Heart Association Task Force on Practice Guidelines

CLINICAL PRESENTATION AND IMMEDIATE ASSESSMENT

- Patients with suspected acute coronary syndrome should be assessed immediately by an appropriate healthcare professional and a 12 lead electrocardiogram should be performed
- Repeat 12 lead electrocardiograms should be performed if there is diagnostic uncertainty or a change in the clinical status of the patient, and at hospital discharge
- Patients with persisting bundle branch block or st segment change should be given a copy of their electrocardiogram to assist their future clinical management should they represent with a suspected acute coronary syndrome.

BIOCHEMICAL DIAGNOSIS

- In patients with suspected acute coronary syndrome, serum troponin concentration should be measured on arrival at hospital to guide appropriate management and treatment
- To establish a diagnosis in patients with an acute coronary syndrome, a serum troponin concentration should be measured 12 hours from the onset of symptoms
- To establish a diagnosis in patients with an acute coronary syndrome when symptom onset is uncertain, serum troponin concentration should be measured 12 hours from presentation
- When considering a diagnosis of acs, serum troponin concentrations should not be interpreted in isolation but with regard to the clinical presentation of the patient

ECG LOCALISATION OF CORONARY ARTERY TERRITORIES

Location of MI	Leads affected	Vessels involved
Septal wall	V1-V2	LAD (septal branch)
Anterior wall	V2-V4	LAD (Diagonal branch)
Lateral wall	I, aVL, V5, V6	LCX
Inferior wall	II, III, aVF	RCA (posterior descending branch)
Posterior wall	V1-V4 (V7-V9)	LCX RCA
Right Ventricle MI	V1, V4R	RCA
Atrial MI	PTa in I, V5, V6	RCA

Left Anterior Descending (LAD), Left Circumflex (LCx) and Right Coronary Artery (RCA)

1. ST-SEGMENT ELEVATION MI

- Presents with central chest pain that is classically heavy in nature, like a sensation of pressure or squeezing. Examination is variable, and findings range from normal to a critically ill patient in cardiogenic shock.
- ST-elevation myocardial infarction (STEMI) is suspected when a patient presents with persistent ST-segment elevation in 2 or more anatomically contiguous ECG leads in the context of a consistent clinical history.
- Creatine kinase-MB and cardiac-specific troponins confirm diagnosis.
- Treatment should, however, be started immediately in patients with a typical history and ECG changes, without waiting for laboratory results.
- Immediate and prompt revascularization can prevent or decrease myocardial damage and decrease morbidity and mortality.
- About 15% of patients in the US who have an acute MI will die of it. Survivors of acute MI should be closely followed up for adequate modification of risk factors and development of complications.

A. ACUTE INFERIOR MYOCARDIAL INFARCTION

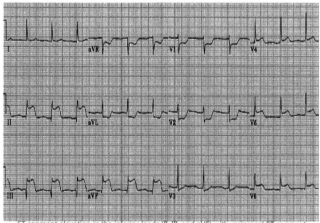

ST segment elevation in the inferior leads (II, III, and aVF) with reciprocal ST segment depression in the anterior leads (V1, V2, and V3), possibly representing posterior extension of the infarct.

B. ACUTE ANTERIOR MYOCARDIAL INFARCTION

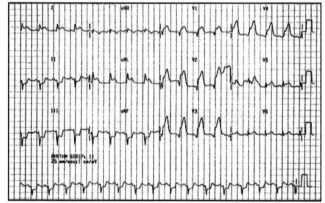

ST segment elevation across the

1. ANTERIOR STEMI

- An **anterior** wall myocardial infarction – also known as **anterior** wall **MI**, or AWMI, or **anterior** ST segment elevation **MI**, or **anterior** **STEMI** – occurs when **anterior** myocardial tissue usually supplied by the left **anterior** descending coronary artery suffers injury due to lack of blood supply[118].

How to Recognise Anterior STEMI

- ST segment elevation in the anterior leads (V3 and V4) at the J point and sometimes in the septal or lateral leads, depending on the extent of the MI. This ST segment elevation is concave downward and frequently overwhelms the T wave. This is called "tombstoning" for obvious reasons; the shape is similar to that of a tombstone.
- Reciprocal ST segment depression in the inferior leads (II, III and aVF).

Patterns of Anterior Infarction

- The nomenclature of anterior infarction can be confusing, with multiple different terms used for the various infarction patterns
- The following is a simplified approach to naming the different types of anterior MI:
- The precordial leads can be classified as follows:
  - Septal leads = V1-2
  - Anterior leads = V3-4
  - Lateral leads = V5-6
- The different infarct patterns are named according to the leads with maximal ST elevation:
  - Septal = V1-2
  - Anterior = V2-5
  - Anteroseptal = V1-4
  - Anterolateral = V3-6, I + aVL
  - Extensive anterior / anterolateral = V1-6, I + aVL
- (NB. While these definitions are intuitive, there is often a poor correlation between ECG features and precise infarct location as determined by imaging or autopsy.)

Clinical Pearls[119]

Other important ECG patterns to be aware of:

- **Anterior-inferior STEMI** due to occlusion of a "wraparound" LAD simultaneous ST elevation in the precordial and inferior leads due to occlusion of a variant LAD that wraps around the cardiac apex to supply both the anterior and inferior walls of the left ventricle.
- **Left main coronary artery occlusion:** widespread ST depression with ST elevation in aVR ≥ V1

- **Wellen's syndrome:** deep precordial T wave inversions or biphasic T waves in V2-3, indicating critical proximal LAD stenosis (a warning sign of imminent anterior infarction)
- **De Winter T waves:** upsloping ST depression with symmetrically peaked T waves in the precordial leads; a "STEMI equivalent" indicating acute LAD occlusion.

ECG Examples
Example 1

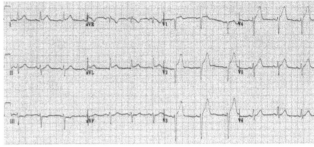

Courtesy-Life in the Fast lane Online

Hyperacute Anteroseptal STEMI, ST elevation is maximal in the anteroseptal leads (V1-4). Q waves are present in the septal leads (V1-2). There is also some subtle STE in I, aVL and V5, with reciprocal ST depression in lead III. There are hyperacute (peaked) T waves in V2-4. These features indicate a **hyperacute anteroseptal STEMI**

Example 2

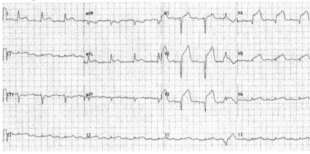

Courtesy-Life in the Fast lane Online

There is ST elevation and Q wave formation in V2-5
ST elevation is now also present in I and aVL.
There is some reciprocal ST depression in lead III. This is an **acute anterior STEMI** - this patient needs urgent reperfusion!

Example 3

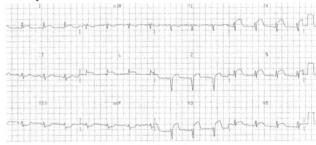

Courtesy-Life in the Fast lane Online

ST elevation in V2-6, I and aVL.
Reciprocal ST depression in III and AVF.
Extensive Anterolateral STEMI (acute)

---

[118] Anterior STEMI. *OOHCPD Online*

[119] Ed Burns. Anterior STEMI. *Life in the Fast lane Online*

Example 4

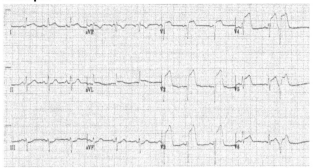

Courtesy-Life in the Fast lane Online

ST elevation in V1-6 plus I and aVL (most marked in V2-4). Minimal reciprocal ST depression in III and aVF. Q waves in V1-2, reduced R wave height (a Q-wave equivalent) in V3-4. There is a premature ventricular complex (PVC) with "R on T" phenomenon at the end of the ECG; this puts the patient at risk for malignant ventricular arrhythmias. **Extensive Anterior STEMI (acute)**

Example 5

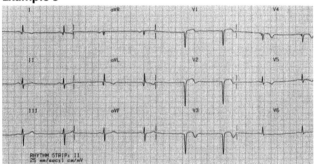

Courtesy-Life in the Fast lane Online

Deep Q waves in V1-3 with markedly reduced R wave height in V4. Residual ST elevation in V1-3 ("left ventricular aneurysm" morphology). Biphasic/inverted T waves in V1-5. Poor R wave progression (R wave height < 3mm in V3). Abnormal Q waves and T-wave inversion in I and aVL. The pattern indicates prior infarction of the anteroseptal and lateral walls. **Prior Anteroseptal / Lateral MI**

Example 6

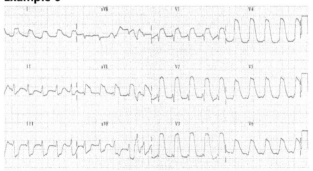

Courtesy-Life in the Fast lane Online

Massive ST elevation with **"tombstone"** morphology is present throughout the precordial (V1-6) and high lateral leads (I, aVL). This pattern is seen in proximal LAD occlusion and indicates a large territory infarction with a poor LV ejection fraction and high likelihood of cardiogenic shock and death. **Extensive anterior MI ("*tombstoning*" pattern)**

Example 7

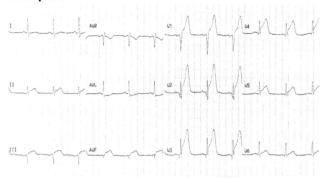

Courtesy-Life in the Fast lane Online

ST elevation is present throughout the precordial and inferior leads. There are hyperacute T waves, most prominent in V1-3. Q waves are forming in V1-3, as well as leads III and aVF. This pattern is suggestive of occlusion occurring in "type III" or "wraparound" LAD (i.e. one that wraps around the cardiac apex to supply the inferior wall). **Anterior-inferior STEMI**

Example 8

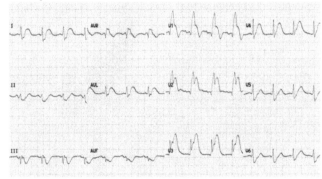

Courtesy-Life in the Fast lane Online

This patient's ECG shows several signs of a very proximal LAD occlusion (Ostial LAD occlusion (septal STEMI)): ST elevation maximal in V1-2 (extending out to V3). There is a new RBBB with marked ST elevation (> 2.5 mm) in V1 plus STE in aVR – these features suggest occlusion proximal to S1. **Septal STEMI**

Example 9

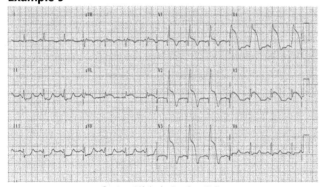

Courtesy-Life in the Fast lane Online

ST elevation maximal in V1-4. The following signs of proximal LAD occlusion are present: RBBB, ST elevation in aVR, STE in aVL and > 1 mm ST depression in the inferior leads. **Acute anteroseptal STEMI**

2. INFERIOR STEMI

- An inferior wall myocardial infarction occurs when inferior myocardial tissue supplied by the right coronary artery, or RCA, is injured due to thrombosis of that vessel[120].
- Up to 40% of patients with an inferior STEMI will have a concomitant right ventricular infarction[121]. These patients may develop severe hypotension in response to nitrates and generally have a worse prognosis. Up to 20% of patients with inferior STEMI will develop significant bradycardia due to second- or third-degree AV block. These patients have an increased in-hospital mortality (>20%). Inferior STEMI may also be associated with posterior infarction, which confers a worse prognosis due to increased area of myocardium at risk.

How to recognise an inferior STEMI

- ST segment elevation in the inferior leads (II, III and aVF)
- Reciprocal ST segment depression in the lateral and/or high lateral leads (I, aVL, V5 and V6)

Which Artery is the Culprit?

Inferior STEMI can result from occlusion of all three coronary arteries:

1. The vast majority (~80%) of inferior STEMIs are due to occlusion of the dominant **right coronary artery (RCA).**
2. Less commonly (around 18% of the time), the culprit vessel is a dominant **left circumflex artery (LCx).**
3. Occasionally, inferior STEMI may result from occlusion of a "type III" or **"wraparound" left anterior descending artery (LAD)**. This produces the unusual pattern of concomitant inferior and anterior ST elevation.

While both RCA and circumflex occlusion may cause infarction of the inferior wall, the precise area of infarction in each case is slightly different:

o The RCA territory covers the medial part of the inferior wall, including the inferior septum.
o The LCx territory covers the lateral part of the inferior wall and the left posterobasal area.

RCA occlusion is suggested by:

- ST elevation (STE) in lead III > lead II
- Presence of reciprocal ST depression in lead I
- Signs of right ventricular infarction: STE in V1 and V4R

Circumflex occlusion is suggested by:

- ST elevation in lead II = lead III
- Absence of reciprocal ST depression (STD) in lead I
- Signs of lateral infarction: STE in the lateral leads I and aVL or V5-6

---

[120] Anterior STEMI. *OOHCPD Online*

[121] Ed Burns. Anterior STEMI. *Life in the Fast lane Online*

ECG Examples[122]
Example 1

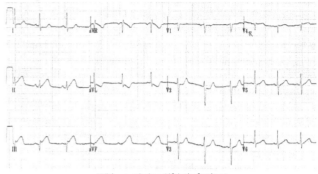

With permission-Lifeinthefastlane

Hyperacute (peaked) T waves in II, III and aVF with relative loss of R wave height. Early ST elevation and Q-wave formation in lead III.
Reciprocal ST depression and T wave inversion in aVL.
ST elevation in lead III > lead II suggests an RCA occlusion; the subtle ST elevation in V4R would be consistent with this.
Early inferior STEMI

Example 2

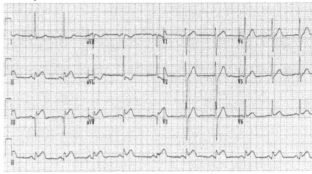

Courtesy-Life in the Fast lane Online

ST elevation in II, III and aVF. Q-wave formation in III and aVF.
Reciprocal ST depression and T wave inversion in aVL
ST elevation in lead II = lead III and absent reciprocal change in lead I (isoelectric ST segment) suggest a **circumflex artery occlusion**
Inferior STEMI

Example 3

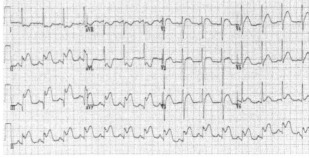

Courtesy-Life in the Fast lane Online

Marked ST elevation in II, III and aVF with early Q-wave formation.
Reciprocal changes in aVL. ST elevation in lead III > II with reciprocal change present in lead I and ST elevation in V1-2 suggests RCA occlusion with associated RV infarction: *This patient should have right-sided leads to confirm this.*
Inferior STEMI

---

[122] Ed Burns. Anterior STEMI. *Life in the Fast lane Online*

Example 4

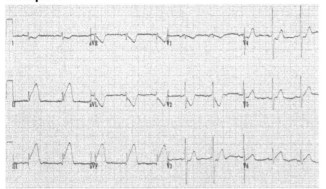

Courtesy-Life in the Fast lane Online

Hyperacute T waves in II, III and aVF. Early ST elevation and loss of R wave height in II, III and aVF. Reciprocal change in aVL and lead I. **Hyperacute inferior STEMI**

Example 5

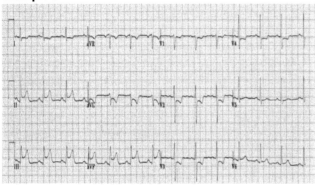

Courtesy-Life in the Fast lane Online

The concave ST elevation in II, III and aVF may be mistaken for pericarditis. However, the fact that the ST elevation is localised to the inferior leads with reciprocal changes in aVL confirms that this is an inferior STEMI. **Inferior STEMI**

Example 6

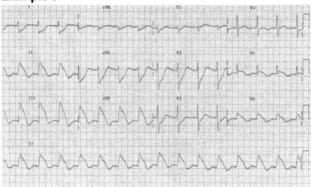

Courtesy-Life in the Fast lane Online

Marked ST elevation in II, III and aVF with a "tombstone" morphology. Reciprocal change in aVL.
ST elevation is also present in the lateral leads V5-6, indicating an extensive infarct of the inferior and lateral walls.
In patients with inferior STEMI, ST elevation of 2mm or more in leads V5 and V6 is predictive of extensive coronary artery disease and a **large area of infarction. Massive inferolateral STEMI**

Example 7

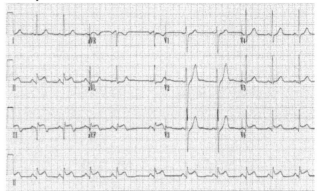

Courtesy-Life in the Fast lane Online

Well-formed Q waves in III and aVF suggest that this STEMI is not acute. The T waves in III and aVF are beginning to invert.
There is still some residual ST elevation in the inferior (II, III, avF) and lateral (V5-6) leads. ST elevation may take 2 weeks to resolve after an acute inferior MI (even longer for an anterior STEMI).
NB. If this patient had ongoing chest pain you would still treat them as an acute STEMI! **Recent inferolateral STEMI**

Example 8

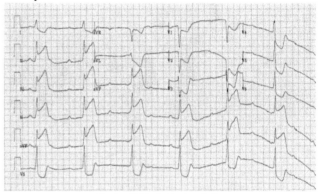

Courtesy-Life in the Fast lane Online

Inferior STEMI with third degree heart block and slow junctional escape rhythm.

Example 9

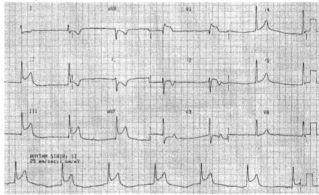

Courtesy-Life in the Fast lane Online

Inferior STEMI with sinus node dysfunction (either sinus arrest or extreme sinus bradycardia) and a slow junctional escape rhythm.

3. POSTERIOR STEMI
Clinical Significance[123]
Posterior infarction accompanies 15-20% of STEMIs, usually occurring in the context of an inferior or lateral infarction. Isolated posterior MI is less common (3-11% of infarcts).

Posterior extension of an inferior or lateral infarct implies a much larger area of myocardial damage, with an increased risk of **left ventricular dysfunction and death.** Isolated posterior infarction is an indication for emergent coronary reperfusion. However, the lack of obvious ST elevation in this condition means that the diagnosis is often missed.

How to spot Posterior Infarction
As the posterior myocardium is not directly visualised by the standard 12-lead ECG, reciprocal changes of STEMI are sought in the **anteroseptal leads V1-3.**

Posterior MI is suggested by the following changes in V1-3:
* Horizontal ST depression
* Tall, broad R waves (>30ms)
* Upright T waves
* Dominant R wave (R/S ratio > 1) in V2

In patients presenting with ischaemic symptoms, horizontal ST depression in the anteroseptal leads (V1-3) should raise the suspicion of posterior MI.

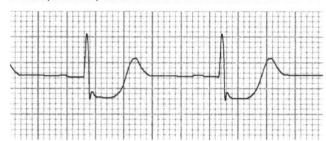

Typical appearance of posterior infarction in V2

Posterior infarction is confirmed by the presence of ST elevation and Q waves in the posterior leads (V7-9).

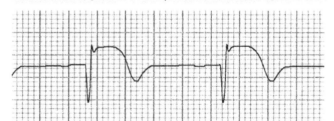

This picture illustrates the reciprocal relationship between the ECG changes seen in STEMI and those seen with posterior infarction. The previous image (depicting posterior infarction in V2) has been inverted. See how the ECG now resembles a typical STEMI!

---
[123] Ed Burns. Posterior Myocardial Infarction. *Life in the Fast lane Online*

Posterior leads
Leads V7-9 are placed on the posterior chest wall in the following positions (see diagram below):
* V7: Left posterior axillary line, in the same horizontal plane as V6.
* V8: Tip of the left scapula, in the same horizontal plane as V6.
* V9: Left paraspinal region, in the same horizontal plane as V6.

The degree of ST elevation seen in V7-9 is typically modest – note that only 0.5 mm of ST elevation is required to make the diagnosis of posterior MI!

Example ECGs
Example 1
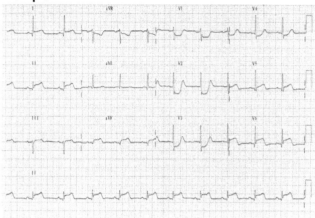
Cortesy-Life in the Fast lane Online

Posterior extension is suggested by: Horizontal ST depression in V1-3, Tall, broad R waves (> 30ms) in V2-3, Dominant R wave (R/S ratio > 1) in V2 and Upright T waves in V2-3
Inferolateral STEMI

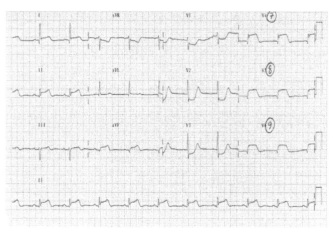
Cortesy-Life in the Fast lane Online

The same patient, with posterior leads recorded.
Marked ST elevation in V7-9 with Q-wave formation confirms involvement of the posterior wall, making this an **inferior-lateral-posterior STEMI (= big territory infarct!).**

Example 2

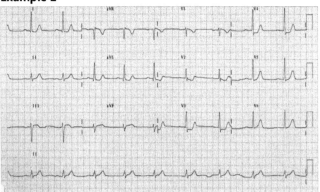

Cortesy-*Life in the Fast lane Online*

In this ECG, **posterior MI** is suggested by the presence of:
ST depression in V2-3, Tall, broad R waves (> 30ms) in V2-3
Dominant R wave (R/S ratio > 1) in V2
Upright terminal portions of the T waves in V2-3. (The ECG changes extend out as far as V4, which may reflect superior-medial misplacement of the V4 electrode from its usual position).

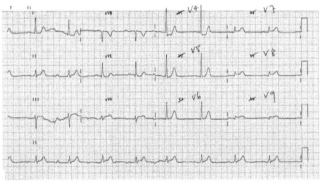

Cortesy-*Life in the Fast lane Online*

The same patient, with posterior leads recorded. Posterior infarction is diagnosed based on the presence of ST segment elevation >0.5mm in leads V7-9. Note that there is also some inferior STE in leads III and aVF (but no Q wave formation) suggesting early inferior involvement.

Example 3

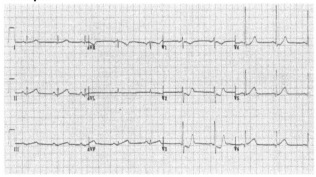

Cortesy-*Life in the Fast lane Online*

The ST depression and upright T waves in V2-3 suggest posterior MI. There are no dominant R waves in V1-2, but it is possible that this ECG was taken early in the course of the infarct, prior to pathological R-wave formation. There are also some features suggestive of early inferior infarction, with hyperacute T waves in II, III and aVF.

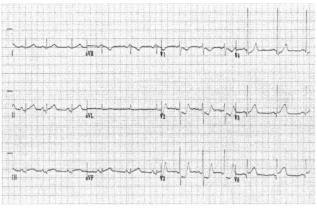

Cortesy-*Life in the Fast lane Online*

An ECG of the same patient taken 30 minutes later: there is now some ST elevation developing in V6. With the eye of faith there is perhaps also some early ST elevation in the inferior leads (lead III looks particularly abnormal).

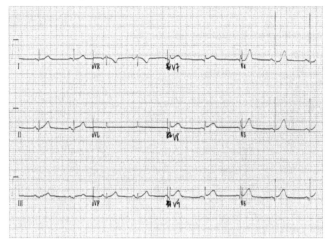

Cortesy-*Life in the Fast lane Online*

The same patient with posterior leads recorded. **Posterior infarction** is confirmed by the presence of ST elevation >0.5mm in leads V7-9.

4. LATERAL STEMI

Clinical Significance of lateral STEMI[124]

The lateral wall of the LV is supplied by branches of the **left anterior descending (LAD)** and **left circumflex (LCx) arteries**. Infarction of the lateral wall usually occurs as part of a larger territory infarction, e.g. **anterolateral STEMI.**

Isolated lateral STEMI is less common, but may be produced by occlusion of smaller branch arteries that supply the lateral wall, e.g. the **first diagonal branch** (D1) of the LAD, the **obtuse marginal branch** (OM) of the LCx, or **the ramus intermedius.**

Lateral STEMI is a stand-alone indication for emergent reperfusion. Lateral extension of an anterior, inferior or posterior MI indicates a larger territory of myocardium at risk with consequent worse prognosis.

How to recognise a lateral STEMI

- ST elevation in the lateral leads (I, aVL, V5-6).
- Reciprocal ST depression in the inferior leads (III+ aVF).
- ST elevation primarily localised to leads I and aVL is referred to as a **high lateral STEMI.**

NB. Reciprocal change in the inferior leads is only seen when there is ST elevation in leads I and aVL. This reciprocal change may be obliterated when there is concomitant inferior ST elevation (i.e. an inferolateral STEMI)

Patterns of lateral infarction

Three broad categories of lateral infarction:

- **Anterolateral STEMI** due to LAD occlusion.
- **Inferior-posterior-lateral STEMI** due to LCx occlusion.
- **Isolated lateral infarction** due to occlusion of smaller branch arteries such as the D1, OM or ramus intermedius.

ECG Examples

Example 1

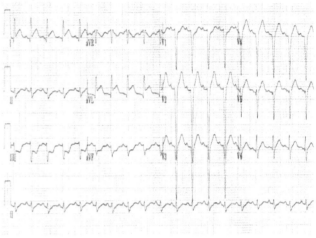

With permission-Lifeinthefastlane

---

[124] Ed Burns. Lateral STEMI. *Life in the Fast lane Online*

ST elevation is present in the high lateral leads (I and aVL).

There is also subtle ST elevation with hyperacute T waves in V5-6.

There is reciprocal ST depression in the inferior leads (III and aVF) with associated ST depression in V1-3 (which could represent anterior ischaemia or reciprocal change).

This pattern is consistent with an acute infarction localised to the superior portion of the lateral wall of the left ventricle. The culprit vessel in this case was an occluded **first diagonal branch of the LAD. High Lateral STEMI**

Example 2

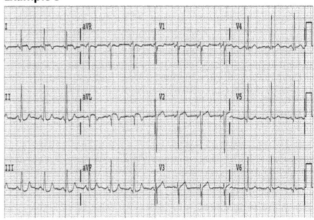

Cortesy- Life in the Fast lane Online

ST elevation is present in the high lateral leads (I and aVL).

There is reciprocal ST depression in the inferior leads (III and aVF).

QS waves in the anteroseptal leads (V1-4) with poor R wave progression indicate prior anteroseptal infarction.

This pattern suggests proximal LAD disease with an acute occlusion of the first diagonal branch (D1). **High Lateral STEMI**

Example 3

Cortesy- Life in the Fast lane Online

There is subtle ST elevation in the high lateral leads (I and avL).

There is a pathological Q wave in aVL plus inverted T waves in both I and aVL.

This pattern is diagnostic of a recent ("completed") high lateral MI.

The patient in this case had a 90% occlusion of his obtuse marginal artery (= a branch of the LCx supplying the lateral wall of the LV). **Recent High Lateral MI**

Example 4

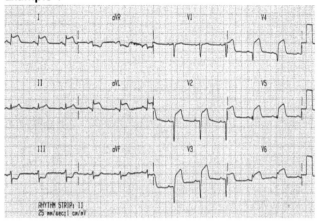

Cortesy- Life in the Fast lane Online

ST elevation is present in the anterior (V2-4) and lateral leads (I, aVL, V5-6). Q waves are present in both the anterior and lateral leads, most prominently in V2-4.

There is reciprocal ST depression in the inferior leads (III and aVF). This pattern indicates an extensive infarction involving the anterior and lateral walls of the left ventricle.

ST elevation in the precordial leads plus the high lateral leads (I and aVL) is strongly suggestive of an acute proximal **LAD occlusion** (this combination predicts a proximal LAD lesion 87% of the time).

Anterolateral STEMI

Example 5

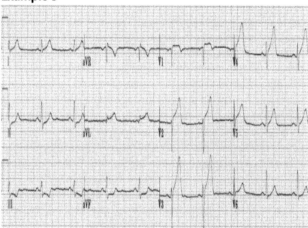

Cortesy- Life in the Fast lane Online

There is early ST elevation with hyperacute T waves in the anteroseptal leads (V1-4).

There is also subtle ST elevation in the high lateral leads (I and aVL); this may be easily missed.

However, the presence of reciprocal ST depression in the inferior leads (III and aVF) makes the **lateral ST elevation more obvious.**

This ECG represents the early stages of a large anterolateral infarction.

As with the previous case, the combination of ST elevation in the precordial and high lateral leads is indicative of proximal LAD occlusion.

Tip: ST depression localised to the inferior leads should prompt you to scrutinise the ECG for evidence of high lateral infarction

Hyperacute Anterolateral STEMI

Example 6

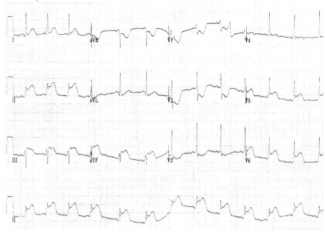

Cortesy- Life in the Fast lane Online

There is ST elevation in the inferior (II, III, aVF) and lateral (I, V5-6) leads. The precordial ST elevation extends out as far as V4, however the maximal STE is in V6.

ST depression in V1-3 is suggestive of associated posterior infarction (the R/S ratio > 1 in V2 is consistent with this).

This is an **acute inferolateral STEMI** with probable posterior extension.

This constellation of ECG abnormalities is typically produced by occlusion of the proximal circumflex artery.

Inferolateral STEMI

Example 7

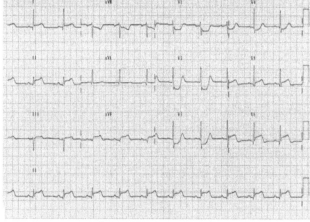

Cortesy- Life in the Fast lane Online

ST elevation is present in the inferior (II, III and aVF) and lateral leads (I, V5-6).

ST depression in V1-3 with tall, broad R waves and upright T waves and a R/S ratio > 1 in V2 indicate concomitant posterior infarction (this patient also had ST elevation in the posterior leads V7-9).

These changes are consistent with a massive infarction involving the inferior, lateral and posterior walls of the left ventricle.

The culprit vessel is again very likely to be an occluded proximal circumflex artery.

Inferoposterolateral STEMI

5. STEMI MANAGEMENT[125]

Initial management
- Move to **resuscitation**
- **IV access**, and **blood** tests taken
- **Oxygen therapy:** Use when the SaO2 is below 93 % or if the patient is shocked
- **Analgesia:** Opioid analgesia is preferred to nitrates for the initial control of pain in the setting of STEMI: e.g. IV morphine boluses titrated to clinical effect: 2.5 to 5mg IV as an initial dose, then titrated to effect every 5 to 10 minutes with further incremental doses of 2.5 to 5mg IV. If morphine is contraindicated, consider **fentanyl** at 25 to 50 micrograms IV as initial equivalent dose.
- **Anti-emetic** as required: IV 10 mg metoclopramide or IV 12.5 mg prochlorperazine

NICE GUIDELINES CG167
1. Assess eligibibility of coronary reperfusion therapy:
- Immediately assess eligibility (irrespective of age, ethnicity or sex) for coronary reperfusion therapy (either primary percutaneous coronary intervention [PCI] or fibrinolysis) in people with acute ST-elevation myocardial infarction (STEMI).
- Do not use level of consciousness after cardiac arrest caused by suspected acute STEMI to determine whether a person is eligible for coronary angiography (with follow-on primary PCI if indicated).

2. Treatment Options:
- Deliver coronary reperfusion therapy (either primary PCI or fibrinolysis) as quickly as possible for eligible people with acute STEMI.
- Offer coronary angiography, with follow-on primary PCI if indicated, as the preferred coronary reperfusion strategy for people with acute STEMI if:
  o presentation is within 12 hours of onset of symptoms **and**
  o primary PCI can be delivered within 120 minutes of the time when fibrinolysis could have been given.
- Offer fibrinolysis to people with acute STEMI presenting within 12 hours of onset of symptoms if primary PCI cannot be delivered within 120 minutes of the time when fibrinolysis could have been given.
- When treating people with fibrinolysis, give an antithrombin at the same time.
- Offer medical therapy to people with acute STEMI who are ineligible for reperfusion therapy.

- Consider coronary angiography, with follow-on primary PCI if indicated, for people with acute STEMI presenting more than 12 hours after the onset of symptoms if there is evidence of continuing myocardial ischaemia.
- Do not offer routine glycoprotein IIb/IIIa inhibitors or fibrinolytic drugs before arrival at the catheter laboratory to people with acute STEMI for whom primary PCI is planned.
- Offer coronary angiography, with follow-on primary PCI if indicated, to people with acute STEMI and cardiogenic shock who present within 12 hours of the onset of symptoms of STEMI.
- Consider coronary angiography, with a view to coronary revascularisation if indicated, for people with acute STEMI who present more than 12 hours after the onset of symptoms and who have cardiogenic shock or go on to develop it.
- Offer unfractionated heparin or low molecular weight heparin to people with acute STEMI who are undergoing primary PCI and have been treated with prasugrel or ticagrelor.
- Consider thrombus aspiration during primary PCI for people with acute STEMI.
- Do not routinely use mechanical thrombus extraction during primary PCI for people with acute STEMI.
- Consider radial (in preference to femoral) arterial access for people undergoing coronary angiography (with follow-on primary PCI if indicated).

3. For people treated with fibrinolysis:
- Offer an electrocardiogram to people treated with fibrinolysis, 60-90 minutes after administration. For those who have residual ST-segment elevation suggesting failed coronary reperfusion:
  o offer immediate coronary angiography, with follow-on PCI if indicated
  o do not repeat fibrinolytic therapy.
- If a person has recurrent myocardial ischaemia after fibrinolysis, seek immediate specialist cardiological advice and, if appropriate, offer coronary angiography, with follow-on PCI if indicated.
- Consider coronary angiography during the same hospital admission for people who are clinically stable after successful fibrinolysis.

4. General
- Offer people who have had an acute STEMI written and oral information, advice, support and treatment on related conditions and secondary prevention (including lifestyle advice), as relevant, in line with published NICE guidance (see table 1).

---

[125] *Noce Clinical guidance. Myocardial infarction with ST-segment elevation: acute management. NICE CG167*

INITIAL MANAGEMENT OF THE STEMI PATIENT

Adapted NHS Heart of England[126]

INITIAL WORKING DIAGNOSIS OF STEMI IF:

- History of ischaemic sounding chest pain/discomfort
- Persistent ST-segment elevation or (presumed) new left bundle-branch block (LBBB).
- (Confirmed by elevated markers of myocardial necrosis (eg. CK-MB, troponins) But DO NOT wait for the blood results to initiate reperfusion treatment).

MAKE SAFE

- ECG monitoring is initiated as soon as possible to detect lifethreatening arrhythmias in an area where defibrillation is immediately available
- IV access for administration of drugs

MAKE COMFORTABLE

- Pain relief with opioid analgesia (eg. morphine 5-10mg slow iv or diamorphine 2.5 - 5mg slow iv) given with antiemetic (eg. metoclopramide 10mg iv)
- Oxygen if breathless, if signs of heart failure/shock or if low oxygen saturations (Sats < 94%)
- Anxiolytic if required (opioid is usually enough, but can use additional benzodiazepine if required eg. Diazemuls 2.5 - 5mg iv)*

REFER FOR EMERGENCY REPERFUSION THERAPY

- Contact Cardiac Pathway team (local) for direct cardiac cath lab admission for Primary PCI**

*BEWARE respiratory depression particularly in combination

GIVE ANTIPLATELET THERAPY

- Aspirin 300mg po STAT (if not already given)
- PLUS 2nd antiplatelet agent ie. Prasugrel 60mg po OR clopidogrel 600mg po or Ticagralor 180mg for patients going directly to Cardiac Cath lab for Primary PCI

---

[126] Management of ST Elevation Myocardial Infarction Guidelines (Version 2, Update 2016). NHS Online

6. COCAINE ASSOCIATED CHEST PAIN

PATHOPHYSIOLOGY

- **Cocaine is a powerful sympathomimetic and increases O_2 demand:**
  - Blocking re-uptake of norepinephrine and dopamine at the pre-synaptic adrenergic terminals.
  - Cocaine causes increased heart rate and blood pressure in a dose-dependent fashion.
  - By ↑ HR, BP, and contractility, cocaine leads to ↑ myocardial demand.
- **Cocaine is a potent coronary vasoconstrictor:**
  - Vasoconstriction worse with pre-existing CAD - particularly smokers.
- **Cocaine is pro-thrombotic:**
  - It increases platelet count, activation and platelet hyper-aggregability.

CLINICAL MANIFESTATIONS

- **Cardiac**
  - Coronary vasoconstriction/spasm = acute coronary syndrome, Exacerbated by increased myocardial oxygen demand, smoking and enhanced platelet aggregation, Ventricular arrhythmias and Hypertension with risk of aortic dissection
- **CNS**
  - Severe hypertension and focal cerebral vasospasm (enhanced by lactic acidosis,
  - increased platelet aggregation and hyperpyrexia),
  - Cerebral infarction or haemorrhage,
  - Euphoria and sense of alertness,
  - Occasionally acute psychosis
  - Generalised complex epilepsy
- **Pulmonary**
  - Pulmonary oedema -? Catecholamine mediated.
  - Pneumonitis, asthma and bronchiolitis - due to immunological effects or due to adulterants in cocaine,
  - Barotrauma with smoking crack cocaine due to Valsalva manoeuvres thought to enhance the drug effect
- **Renal**
  - Rhabdomyolysis-induced renal failure- exacerbated by vasoconstriction
- **Obstetric**
  - Increased risk of spontaneous abortion,
  - Placental abruption
  - Intrauterine growth retardation - due to disruption of uteroplacental blood flow due to vasoconstriction and maternal hypertension

DIAGNOSIS

- **Presentation**
  - Chest pain (often "cardiac sounding") is the commonest (56%) presenting complaint amongst cocaine users.
  - Dyspnoea and shortness of breath are commonly associated.
  - Beware - up to half of cocaine associated AMIs do NOT report chest pain (palpitations or SOB etc).
  - Cocaine associated chest pain may be due to *Aortic Dissection, Pneumothorax or Pneumomediastinum.*
- **Physical**
  - Tachycardia, Hypertension +/- Arrhythmias
  - Tachypnoea, Hyperthermia
  - Altered mental state leading to coma +/- fits
  - Mydriasis, Diaphoresis
  - **Consider occult trauma and associated drug use**

INVESTIGATIONS

- **Electrocardiogram**
  - An abnormal ECG has been reported in 56% to 84% of patients with cocaine-associated chest pain.
  - ECG sensitivity in revealing ischaemia or MI to predict a true MI is only 36%.
- **Cardiac Biomarkers**
  - Cocaine may cause rhabdomyolysis (raised myoglobin and total **CK** in up to 75% of patients).
  - **Cardiac troponins** are the most sensitive and specific markers.

ED MANAGEMENT OF COCAINE INDUCED CHEST PAIN

- ABCDE Approach
- Rule out aortic dissection
- Sedation with **benzodiazepines** which decrease central sympathetic outflow
- Aggressive **cooling** for hyperthermia
- Aggressive **fluid resuscitation** to maintain urine output
- **Treat seizures with benzodiazepines** and further Rx as necessary
- **Urgent CT brain for all seizures** as high incidence of primary intracranial pathology
- Treat myocardial ischaemia with **Aspirin, Nitrates and/or Benzodiazepines. Heparin, Opiates** (MONAH).
- Treat ventricular tachyarrhythmias and QTc prolongation with **Bicarbonate +/- Magnesium**
- Treat severe hypertension with **Nitroprusside.**
- **Early PCI** is particularly preferred over **fibrinolysis** in patients with cocaine-associated MI

CONTRAINDICATED DRUGS

- **B-blockers contraindicated** (unopposed alpha stimulation worsens coronary and peripheral vasoconstriction).
  - **Avoid Labetalol** as despite alpha and beta blockade the predominant effect is beta-blockade.
- **Avoid anti-arrhythmics (including amiodarone)**
- **Avoid Epinephrine** if cardiac arrest occurs
- **Prolonged neuromuscular blockade** occurs with **suxamethonium** due to acquired pseudocholinesterase deficiency. *Blockade rarely lasts more than 20 minutes*

IV. ENDOCARDITIS

INTRODUCTION

- Infective endocarditis (IE) is defined as an infection of the endocardial surface of the heart, which may include one or more heart valves, the mural endocardium, or a septal defect.
- Its intracardiac effects include severe valvular insufficiency, which may lead to intractable congestive heart failure and myocardial abscesses.
- IE also produces a wide variety of systemic signs and symptoms through several mechanisms, including both sterile and infected emboli and various immunological phenomena.[127]
- IE currently can be described as infective endocarditis in the era of intravascular devices, as infection of intravascular lines has been determined to be the primary risk factor for *Staphylococcus aureus* bloodstream infections (BSIs).
- *S aureus* has become the primary pathogen of endocarditis.
- Vegetation on valves does not always represent an infective process.
- **Loefflers endocarditis** is a part of the hypereosinophilic syndrome, and responds well to treatment with steroids, hydroxyurea and anticoagulation.
- **Non-Bacterial Thrombotic Endocarditis (NBTE)** is associated with endocardial damage due to high pressure jets or with hypercoagulable states and though it is usually sterile, it is a site for subsequent infection.

AETIOLOGY

- The following are the main underlying causes of NVE:
  - Rheumatic valvular disease (30% of NVE) - Primarily involves the mitral valve followed by the aortic valve
  - Congenital heart disease (15% of NVE) - Underlying etiologies include a patent ductus arteriosus, ventricular septal defect, tetralogy of Fallot, or any native or surgical high-flow lesion.
  - Mitral valve prolapse with an associated murmur (20% of NVE)
  - Degenerative heart disease - Including calcific aortic stenosis due to a bicuspid valve, Marfan syndrome, or syphilitic disease

CLASSIFICATION

Subacute bacterial endocarditis

- SBE, although aggressive, usually develops insidiously and progresses slowly (ie, over weeks to months). Often, no source of infection or portal of entry is evident.
- SBE is caused most commonly by streptococci (especially viridans, microaerophilic, anaerobic, and nonenterococcal group D streptococci and enterococci) and less commonly by S. aureus, Staphylococcus epidermidis, Gemella morbillorum, Abiotrophia defective (formerly, Streptococcus defectivus), Granulicatella species, and fastidious Haemophilus species.
- SBE often develops on abnormal valves after asymptomatic bacteremia due to periodontal, gastrointestinal, or genitourinary infections.

Acute bacterial endocarditis

- ABE usually develops abruptly and progresses rapidly (ie, over days). A source of infection or portal of entry is often evident.
- When bacteria are virulent or bacterial exposure is massive, ABE can affect normal valves.
- It is usually caused by S. aureus, group A hemolytic streptococci, pneumococci, or gonococci.

Prosthetic valvular endocarditis

- PVE develops in 2 to 3% of patients within 1 year after valve replacement and in 0.5%/year thereafter.
- It is more common after aortic than after mitral valve replacement and affects mechanical and bioprosthetic valves equally.
- Early-onset infections (< 2 months after surgery) are caused mainly by contamination during surgery with antimicrobial-resistant bacteria (eg, S. epidermidis, diphtheroids, coliform bacilli, Candida species, Aspergillus species).
- Late-onset infections are caused mainly by contamination with low-virulence organisms during surgery or by transient asymptomatic bacteremias, most often with streptococci; S. epidermidis; diphtheroids; and the fastidious gram-negative bacilli, Haemophilus species, Actinobacillus actinomycetemcomitans, and Cardiobacterium hominis.

---

[127] *Brusch JL. Infective endocarditis and its mimics in the critical care unit. Cunha BA, ed. Infectious Diseases in Critical Care. 2nd ed. New York, NY: Informa Healthcare; 2007. 261-2.*

IVDA infective endocarditis

- Diagnosis of endocarditis in IV drug users can be difficult and requires a high index of suspicion. Two thirds of patients have no previous history of heart disease or murmur on admission.
- A murmur may be absent in those with tricuspid disease, owing to the relatively small pressure gradient across this valve.
- Pulmonary manifestations may be prominent in patients with tricuspid infection: one third have pleuritic chest pain, and three quarters demonstrate chest radiographic abnormalities.

Adults and children with structural cardiac conditions Cardiac Conditions predisposing to Endocarditis, NICE CG641[128]

Regard people with the following cardiac conditions as being at risk of developing infective endocarditis:
- ❖ Acquired valvular heart disease with stenosis or regurgitation
- ❖ Valve replacement
- ❖ Structural congenital heart disease, including surgically corrected or palliated structural conditions, but excluding isolated atrial septal defect, fully repaired ventricular septal defect or fully repaired patent ductus arteriosus, and closure devices that are judged to be endothelialised
- ❖ Hypertrophic cardiomyopathy
- ❖ Previous infective endocarditis

PATHOPHYSIOLOGY

- Endocarditis has local and systemic consequences.

Local consequences
- Local consequences of infective endocarditis include
  - o Myocardial abscesses with tissue destruction and sometimes conduction system abnormalities (usually with low septal abscesses)
  - o Sudden, severe valvular regurgitation, causing heart failure and death (usually due to mitral or aortic valve lesions)
  - o Aortitis due to contiguous spread of infection
- Prosthetic valve infections are particularly likely to involve valve ring abscesses, obstructing vegetations, myocardial abscesses, and mycotic aneurysms manifested by valve obstruction, dehiscence, and conduction disturbances.

Systemic consequences
- Systemic consequences are primarily due to:
  - o Embolization of infected material from the heart valve
  - o Immune-mediated phenomena (primarily in chronic infection)

---

[128] CG64 Prophylaxis against infective endocarditis, NICE, March 2008

- Right-sided lesions typically produce septic pulmonary emboli, which may result in pulmonary infarction, pneumonia, or empyema.
- Left-sided lesions may embolize to any tissue, particularly the kidneys, spleen, and central nervous system. Mycotic aneurysms can form in any major artery.
- Cutaneous and retinal emboli are common.
- Diffuse glomerulonephritis may result from immune complex deposition.

CLINICAL ASSESSMENT
Symptoms and Signs
- Symptoms and signs vary based on the classification but are nonspecific.

Subacute bacterial endocarditis
- Initially, symptoms of subacute bacterial endocarditis are vague: low-grade fever (< 39° C), night sweats, fatigability, malaise, and weight loss.
- Chills and arthralgias may occur. Symptoms and signs of valvular insufficiency may be a first clue. Initially, ≤ 15% of patients have fever or a murmur, but eventually almost all develop both.
- Physical examination may be normal or include pallor, fever, change in a preexisting murmur or development of a new regurgitant murmur, and tachycardia.
- Retinal emboli can cause round or oval hemorrhagic retinal lesions with small white centers (**Roth spots).**
- Cutaneous manifestations include petechiae (on the upper trunk, conjunctivae, mucous membranes, and distal extremities), painful erythematous subcutaneous nodules on the tips of digits (**Osler nodes**), nontender hemorrhagic macules on the palms or soles (**Janeway lesions**), and **splinter hemorrhages** under the nails.
- About 35% of patients have central nervous system (CNS) effects, including transient ischemic attacks, stroke, toxic encephalopathy, and, if a mycotic CNS aneurysm ruptures, brain abscess and subarachnoid hemorrhage. Renal emboli may cause flank pain and, rarely, gross hematuria. Splenic emboli may cause left upper quadrant pain. Prolonged infection may cause splenomegaly or clubbing of fingers and toes.

Acute bacterial endocarditis and prosthetic valvular endocarditis
- Symptoms and signs of acute bacterial endocarditis and prosthetic valvular endocarditis are similar to those of subacute bacterial endocarditis, but the course is more rapid.
- Fever is almost always present initially, and patients appear toxic; sometimes septic shock develops.
- Heart murmur is present initially in about 50 to 80% and eventually in > 90%. Rarely, purulent meningitis occurs.

Right-sided endocarditis

- Septic pulmonary emboli may cause cough, pleuritic chest pain, and sometimes hemoptysis.
- A murmur of tricuspid regurgitation is typical.

EXAMINATION FINDINGS

1. Roth spots:

- Roth spots are white centered retinal hemorrhage and are associated with multiple systemic illnesses, most commonly bacterial endocarditis
- The **Litten sign** represents cotton-wool exudates.

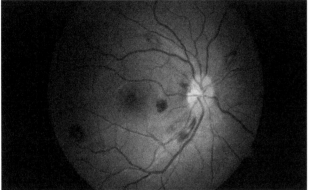

Roth's spots may be seen in leukemia, diabetes, collagen-vascular diseases, and other conditions that predispose to hemorrhage in the retina.

2. Osler's nodes:

- Osler nodes are smallish tender nodules that range from red to purple and are located primarily in the pulp spaces of the terminal phalanges of the fingers and toes, soles of the feet, and the thenar and hypothenar eminences of the hands.

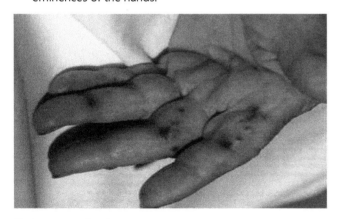

3. Janeway Lesions:

- Janeway lesions are non-tender, small erythematous or haemorrhagic macular, papular or nodular lesions on the palms or soles only a few millimeters in diameter that are often associated with infective endocarditis.
- They are however rare and frequently indistinguishable from Osler's nodes. Unlike Osler's nodes, these present early in the disease and are non-tender in nature.

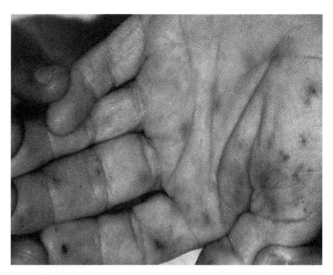

4. Splinter Haemorrhages:

- Subungual hemorrhages (ie, splinter hemorrhages) are linear and red. They are usually caused by workplace trauma to the hands and feet rather than by valvular infection. Hemorrhages that do not extend for the entire length of the nail are more likely the result of infection rather than trauma.

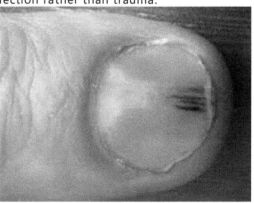

INVESTIGATION STRATEGIES[129]

- **Diagnosis**
  - Blood cultures
  - Echocardiography and sometimes other imaging modalities
  - Clinical criteria
- Because symptoms and signs are nonspecific, vary greatly, and may develop insidiously, diagnosis requires a high index of suspicion.
- Endocarditis should be suspected in patients with fever and no obvious source of infection, particularly if a heart murmur is present.

---

[129] *Habib G, Lancellotti P, Antunes MJ, et al: 2015 ESC Guidelines for the management of infective endocarditis: The Task Force for the Management of Infective Endocarditis of the European Society of Cardiology (ESC). Endorsed by: European Association for Cardio-Thoracic Surgery (EACTS), the European Association of Nuclear Medicine (EANM). Eur Heart J 36:3075–3123, 2015.*

- Suspicion of endocarditis should be very high if blood cultures are positive in patients who have a history of a heart valve disorder, who have had certain recent invasive procedures, or who abuse IV drugs. Patients with documented bacteremia should be examined thoroughly and repeatedly for new valvular murmurs and signs of emboli.
- Other than positive blood cultures, there are no specific laboratory findings. Established infections often cause a normocytic-normochromic anemia, elevated white blood cell count, increased erythrocyte sedimentation rate, increased immunoglobulin levels, and the presence of circulating immune complexes and rheumatoid factor, but these findings are not diagnostically helpful.
- Urinalysis often shows microscopic hematuria and, occasionally, red blood cell casts, pyuria, or bacteriuria.

Identification of organisms
- Identification of the organism and its antimicrobial susceptibility is vital to guide treatment.
- If endocarditis is suspected, 3 blood samples for culture (20-mL each) should be obtained within 24 hours (if presentation suggests acute bacterial endocarditis, 2 cultures within the first 1 to 2 hours).
- Each set of cultures should be obtained from a separate, fresh venipuncture site (ie, not from preexisting vascular catheters). Blood cultures do not need to be done during chills or fever because most patients have continuous bacteremia. When endocarditis is present and no prior antibiotic therapy was given, all 3 blood cultures usually are positive because the bacteremia is continuous; at least one culture is positive in 99%. Premature use of empiric antibiotic therapy should be avoided in patients with acquired or congenital valvular or shunt lesions to avoid culture-negative endocarditis. If prior antimicrobial therapy was given, blood cultures should still be obtained, but results may be negative.
- Blood cultures may require 3 to 4 weeks of incubation for certain organisms; however, some proprietary, automated culture monitoring systems can identify positive cultures within a week.
- Other organisms (eg, *Aspergillus*) may not produce positive cultures. Some organisms (eg, *Coxiella burnetii*, *Bartonella* species, *Chlamydia psittaci*, *Brucella* species) require serodiagnosis; others (eg, *Legionella pneumophila*) require special culture media or polymerase chain reaction (eg, *Tropheryma whippelii*).
- Negative blood culture results may indicate suppression due to prior antimicrobial therapy, infection with organisms that do not grow in standard culture media, or another diagnosis (eg, noninfective endocarditis, atrial myxoma with embolic phenomena, vasculitis).

Imaging studies
- **Echocardiography**, typically transthoracic (TTE) rather than transesophageal (TEE), should be done initially. TEE is more sensitive (ie, capable of revealing vegetations too small to be seen on TTE). Transesophageal echocardiography should be done when
  - Patients have a prosthetic valve
  - Transthoracic echocardiogram is nondiagnostic
  - Diagnosis of infective endocarditis has been established clinically (done to detect perforations, abscesses, and fistulas)
- **CT** is used occasionally when TEE fails to fully define paravalvular abscesses and for detection of mycotic aneurysms. Positron emission tomography (PET) scanning is an emerging tool for the diagnosis of endocarditis originating in prosthetic and intracardiac devices. CT and PET abnormalities are now included as major criteria in the European guidelines.

Diagnostic criteria
- Infective endocarditis is definitively diagnosed when microorganisms are seen histologically in (or cultured from) endocardial vegetations obtained during cardiac surgery, embolectomy, or autopsy.
- Because vegetations are not usually available for examination, there are various clinical criteria for establishing a diagnosis. They include the revised Duke Criteria (with a sensitivity and specificity > 90%—see below) and the European Society of Cardiology (ESC) 2015 modified criteria[130].
- The ESC criteria are similar to the modified Duke criteria but include expanded imaging results as major criteria as follows:
  - Vegetation, abscess, pseudoaneurysm, intracardiac fistula, valvular perforation or aneurysm, or new partial dehiscence of prosthetic valve identified by echocardiography
  - Abnormal activity around a prosthetic valve (implanted > 3 months earlier) detected by PET/CT or single-photon emission computed tomography (SPECT)/CT with radiolabeled leukocytes
  - Paravalvular lesions identified by cardiac CT
- The ESC also differs from the modified Duke minor criteria by specifying that detecting silent vascular phenomena by imaging only is sufficient.

---

[130] *Habib G, Lancellotti P, Antunes MJ, et al: 2015 ESC Guidelines for the management of infective endocarditis: The Task Force for the Management of Infective Endocarditis of the European Society of Cardiology (ESC). Endorsed by: European Association for Cardio-Thoracic Surgery (EACTS), the European Association of Nuclear Medicine (EANM). Eur Heart J 36:3075–3123, 2015.*

DUKE CRITERIA FOR IE

The **Duke criteria** are a set of clinical criteria set forward for the diagnosis of infective endocarditis.
For diagnosis the requirement is:

- **Definite:** 2 major and 1 minor criteria or 1 major and 3 minor criteria or 5 minor criteria
- **Possible:** 1 major and 1 minor, or 3 minor criteria
- **Rejected:** None of the above, or full resolution of symptoms with antibiotics in 4 days, or firm alternate diagnosis.

MAJOR CRITERIA

- **Positive blood cultures for IE**
- **Typical microorganism for IE from 2 separate blood cultures**
  - Viridans streptococci, Streptococcus bovis, and HACEK group or
  - Community-acquired Staphylococcus aureus or enterococci in the absence of a primary focus or
  - Persistently positive blood cultures, defined as recovery of a microorganism consistent with infective endocarditis from:
    - 2 blood cultures drawn 12 hours apart or all of 3 or most of 4 or more separate blood cultures, with first and last drawn at least 1 hour apart

- **Evidence of endocardial involvement**
  - Positive echocardiogram for infective endocarditis
    - Oscillating intracardiac mass on valve or supporting structures or in the path of regurgitant jets or on implanted material in the absence of an alternative anatomical explanation or
    - Abscess or
    - New partial dehiscence of prosthetic valve or
  - **New valvular regurgitation**

MINOR CRITERIA

- **Predisposing heart condition or intravenous drug use**
- **Fever:** 38°C
- **Vascular phenomena:** major arterial emboli, septic pulmonary infarcts, mycotic aneurysm, intracranial hemorrhage, conjunctival hemorrhages, and Janeway lesions
- **Immunologic phenomena:**
  - Glomerulonephritis
  - Osler nodes
  - Roth spots
  - Rheumatoid Factor
- **Microbiologic evidence:** positive blood culture but not meeting major criterion as noted previously or serologic evidence of active infection with organism consistent with infective endocarditis
- **Echocardiography findings** consistent with infective endocarditis but not meeting major criterion as noted previously

OTHER INVESTIGATIONS

1. **Cardiac catheterisation** is useful for pre-surgical evaluation but is not recommended routinely.
2. **ECG and chest X-ray** will be required to refine the diagnosis, exclude other causes for the clinical presentation and evaluate potential complications (eg cardiac failure and ischaemia).
3. **Ultrasound and CT / MRI scans** may be required to detect peripheral manifestation due to embolisation. This may include imaging the CNS to look for cerebral abscess or ischaemic stroke. Continued fever and positive blood cultures despite adequate treatment should prompt visualisation of abdominal viscera for detection of abscess, especially in the spleen.

INJECTABLE DRUG USERS

- Injectable drug use increases rate of infection as much as 200-fold. Obviously, this population presents a specific risk and should be evaluated with special care in the ED.
- The majority of cases involve the right side of the heart, with the **tricuspid valve being particularly prone**. A tricuspid murmur is difficult to appreciate due to its soft nature and lack of quiet consultation rooms in a busy emergency department.
- **Staphylococcus** is the main organism involved in right sided infections and incidence of MRSA is significant. Due to repeated exposure, there is high recurrence in this group nearing 40%. Recurrent infections are likely to involve the left side and may have varied organisms including *Pseudomonas, Bacillus, Lactobacillus, Corynebacterium* and *Candida*.
- Occasionally poly-microbial disease is identified; however, HIV does not seem to increase incidence of Endocarditis in this group of patients. Left untreated infective endocarditis is rapidly fatal with very high mortality rates.

EMERGENCY MANAGEMENT

- Treatment consists of a prolonged course of antimicrobial therapy. Surgery may be needed for mechanical complications or resistant organisms.
- Typically, antimicrobials are given IV.
- Because they must be given for 2 to 8 weeks, home IV therapy is often used.
- Any apparent source of bacteremia must be managed: necrotic tissue debrided, abscesses drained, and foreign material and infected devices removed. People with infective endocarditis should be evaluated by a dentist and treated for oral diseases that could cause bacteremia and subsequent endocarditis.
- Existing IV catheters (particularly central venous ones) should be changed. If endocarditis persists in a patient with a newly inserted central venous catheter, that catheter should also be removed.

ANTIBIOTIC REGIMENS

- **Investigate and treat promptly** any episodes of infection in people at risk of infective endocarditis to reduce the risk of endocarditis developing.
- **Offer** an antibiotic that covers organisms that cause infective endocarditis if a person at risk of infective endocarditis is receiving antimicrobial therapy because they are undergoing a GIT or GU procedure at a site where there is a suspected infection.[131]
- *Antibiotics should not be given until adequate blood cultures (2 or 3 samples from different sites over 1 hour) have been obtained.*
- Antibiotics should be broad spectrum to cover all likely organisms, typically including sensitive and resistant staphylococci, streptococci, and enterococci. Empiric antibiotic regimens should reflect local patterns of infection and antibiotic resistance; however, typical examples of broad-spectrum antibiotic coverage may include
- **Native valves:** Vancomycin 15 to 20 mg/kg IV every 8 to 12 hours (not to exceed 2 g per dose)
- **Prosthetic valve:** Vancomycin 15 to 20 mg/kg IV every 8 to 12 hours (not to exceed 2 g per dose) plus gentamicin 1 mg/kg 8 hourly plus either cefepime 2 g IV 8 hourly or imipenem 1 g IV every 6 to 8 hours (maximum dose 4 g per day). As soon as possible, the empiric drug regimen should be adjusted based on culture results.
- **IV drug abusers** frequently do not adhere to treatment, abuse IV access lines, and tend to leave the hospital too soon. For such patients, short-course IV or (less preferably) oral therapy may be used.
- **For right-sided endocarditis** caused by methicillin-sensitive *S. aureus*, nafcillin 2 g IV every 4 hours plus gentamicin 1 mg/kg IV every 8 hours for 2 weeks is effective, as is a 4-week oral regimen of ciprofloxacin 750 mg twice a day plus rifampin 300 mg twice a day.
- **Left-sided endocarditis** does not respond to 2-week courses. Current guidelines recommend 6 weeks of parenteral antibiotic therapy . However, a recent multi-center, randomized, non-blinded study of uncomplicated left-sided endocarditis found that switching to oral antibiotics (after a minimum of 10 days of parenteral therapy) to be non-inferior to continued parenteral therapy. In addition, length of hospital stay was shortened in the patients switched to oral therapy. This approach has the potential to reduce the psychologic stress and some of the risks inherent to prolonged inpatient parenteral therapy[132].

ANTIBIOTIC PROPHYLAXIS

- Traditionally prophylaxis has been offered to all people undergoing invasive procedures, both dental and non-dental, who have pre-existing endocardial defects.
- NICE (National Institute of Clinical Excellence)[133], after a thorough review, found no evidence to support this practice and recommends that routine antibiotic prophylaxis is not used.
- The current recommendation is to use prophylaxis only in cases where there is a procedure involving an area with active infection, and to promptly treat infections in patients who are at risk of developing infective endocarditis.

NICE GUIDELINE ON PROPHYLAXIS FOR ENDOCARDITIS, CG64
When to offer prophylaxis:
- **Do not offer** antibiotic prophylaxis against infective endocarditis:
  - To people undergoing dental procedures
  - To people undergoing non-dental procedures at the following sites:
    - Upper and lower GIT
    - Genitourinary tract, this includes urological, Gynaecological and obstetric procedures, and childbirth
    - Upper and lower respiratory tract, this includes ENT procedures and bronchoscopy
- **Do not offer** Chlorhexidine mouthwash as prophylaxis against infective endocarditis to people at risk undergoing dental procedures

ADVICE FOR PATIENTS AT RISK OF ENDOCARDITIS, NICE CG64
- Offer people at risk of IE clear and consistent information about prevention including:
  - The benefits and risks of antibiotic prophylaxis, and an explanation of why antibiotic prophylaxis is no longer routinely recommended
  - The importance of maintaining good oral health
  - Symptoms that may indicate IE and when to seek expert advice
  - The risks of undergoing invasive procedures, including non-medical procedures such as body piercing and tattooing.

+ Routine antibiotic prophylaxis is no longer recommended

[131] CG64 Prophylaxis against infective endocarditis, NICE, March 2008

[132] Cahill TJ, Baddour LM, Habib G, et al: Challenges in infective endocarditis. J Am Coll Cardiol 69(3):325–344, 2017.

[133] CG64 Prophylaxis against infective endocarditis, NICE, March 2008

V. MYOCARDITIS

INTRODUCTION

- Myocarditis is inflammation of the myocardium with necrosis of cardiac myocytes.
- Myocarditis may be caused by many disorders (eg, infection, cardiotoxins, drugs, and systemic disorders such as sarcoidosis) but is often idiopathic. Symptoms can vary and can include fatigue, dyspnea, edema, palpitations, and sudden death. Diagnosis is based on symptoms and clinical findings of abnormal electrocardiography (ECG), cardiac biomarkers, and cardiac imaging in the absence of cardiovascular risk factors. Endomyocardial biopsy confirms clinical diagnosis of myocarditis.
- Treatment depends on the cause, but general measures include drugs to treat heart failure and arrhythmias and rarely surgery (eg, intra-aortic balloon pump, left ventricular assist device, transplantation).
- Immunosuppression is of use in certain types of myocarditis (eg, hypersensitivity myocarditis, giant cell myocarditis, myocarditis caused by sarcoidosis)

PATHOPHYSIOLOGY

- Myocarditis is inflammation of myocardium with necrosis of cardiac myocyte cells. Biopsy-proven myocarditis typically demonstrates inflammatory infiltrate of the myocardium with lymphocytes, neutrophils, eosinophils, giant cells, granulomas, or a mixture.
- The pathophysiology of myocarditis remains a subject of research. Potential mechanisms that lead to myocardial injury include
- Direct cardiomyocyte injury caused by an infectious or other cardiotoxic agent
- Myocardial injury caused by an autoimmune reaction to an infectious or other cardiotoxic agent
- Myocardial inflammation can be diffuse or focal. Inflammation can extend into the pericardium causing myopericarditis. The extent of myocardial involvement and extension into adjacent pericardium can determine the type of symptoms.
- Diffuse involvement can lead to heart failure, arrhythmias and sometimes sudden cardiac death. Focal involvement is less likely to cause heart failure but can lead to arrhythmias and sudden cardiac death.
- Involvement of the pericardium leads to chest pain and other symptoms typical of pericarditis. Some patients remain asymptomatic whether myocardial involvement is focal or diffuse.

ETIOLOGY

- Myocarditis may result from infectious or noninfectious causes. Many cases are.
- Infectious myocarditis is most often viral in the US and other developed nations. The most common viral causes in the US are parvovirus B19 and human herpes virus 6. In developing nations, infectious myocarditis is most often associated with rheumatic carditis, Chagas disease, or AIDS.
- Noninfectious causes include cardiotoxins, certain drugs, and some systemic disorders. Myocarditis caused by drugs is termed hypersensitivity myocarditis.

Virus:
- Cocksackie & Adenovirus
- Influenza & Parainfluenza
- Varicella zoster & Epstein Barr
- Polio & Rabies
- Mumps & Rubella
- Cytomegalovirus & Herpes
- HIV & Hepatitis A, B, C and D

Parasitic
- Trypanosoma cruzi Chagas disease
- Toxoplasmosis
- Schistosomiasis
- Trichinosis

Other aetiological agents
Bacteria:
- Lyme disease
- Mycobacteria
- Mycoplasma
- Legionella
- Streptococcus species
- Chlamydia pneumonia

Fungi:
- Aspergillus
- Cryptococcus
- Candida

Immunologic illnesses:
- Diabetes mellitus
- Thyrotoxicosis
- Inflammatory bowel disease
- Systemic lupus erythematosus
- Giant cell myocarditis

GIANT CELL MYOCARDITIS

- Giant cell myocarditis is a rare form of myocarditis with a fulminant course. The etiology is unclear but may include an autoimmune mechanism. Biopsy shows characteristic multinucleated giant cells.
- Patients with giant cell myocarditis present in cardiogenic shock and frequently have intractable ventricular arrhythmias or complete heart block.
- Giant cell myocarditis has a poor prognosis but is important to rule out in the setting of an otherwise healthy patient presenting in fulminant heart failure or with intractable arrhythmias because immunosuppressive therapy can help improve survival.

SYMPTOMS AND SIGNS

- The clinical presentation of myocarditis is variable. Patients may be minimally symptomatic or have fulminant heart failure and fatal arrhythmias.
- Symptoms depend on the etiology of the myocarditis as well as the extent and severity of myocardial inflammation.
- Heart failure symptoms may include fatigue, dyspnea, and edema. Patients may show signs of fluid overload with crackles, elevated jugular venous pulses, and edema. Cardiac examination may be significant for a third (S3) or fourth (S4) heart sound.
- Systolic murmurs of mitral regurgitation and tricuspid regurgitation may be present in patients with ventricular enlargement.
- Sudden cardiac death due to a fatal arrhythmia is sometimes the presenting feature.
- Patients may experience preceding palpitations or syncope.
- When patients have concomitant pericardial inflammation, they may present with chest pain typical of pericarditis. Dull or sharp precordial or substernal pain may radiate to the neck, trapezius ridge (especially the left), or shoulders. Pain ranges from mild to severe. Unlike ischemic chest pain, pain due to pericarditis is usually aggravated by thoracic motion, cough, breathing, or swallowing food; it may be relieved by sitting up and leaning forward. A pericardial friction rub may be auscultated in patients with a pericardial effusion.
- Certain clinical findings may be indicative of a specific cause of myocarditis. Infectious myocarditis may be preceded by symptoms of fever, myalgias, and other symptoms depending on the exact pathogen. Drug-related or hypersensitivity myocarditis may be accompanied by a rash. Enlarged lymph nodes may be indicative of sarcoidosis as the underlying etiology. Fulminant heart failure and arrhythmias may be indicative of giant cell myocarditis.

- Myocarditis can be acute, subacute, or chronic. There are no set time-frames for each phase.
- The acute phase lasts a few days while the subacute phase lasts weeks to months. If myocarditis does not resolve after a few months, it is called chronic myocarditis. In some cases, myocarditis can lead to dilated cardiomyopathy.

DIFFERENTIAL DIAGNOSIS

- Ischaemic Heart Disease,
- Alcoholic Cardiomyopathy
- Cardiac Tamponade
- Cardiogenic Shock
- Chagas Disease (American Trypanosomiasis)
- Cocaine-Related Cardiomyopathy
- Coronary Artery Atherosclerosis
- Dilated Cardiomyopathy
- Hypertrophic Cardiomyopathy
- Peripartum (Postpartum) Cardiomyopathy (PPCM)
- Restrictive Cardiomyopathy
- Rheumatic Fever,
- Primary Cardiac Arrhythmia,
- Endocarditis, Pericarditis,
- PE
- Septic Shock.

DIAGNOSIS

- Laboratory studies may include the following:
  - Full blood count (FBC) - Leukocytosis (may demonstrate eosinophilia)
  - Elevated erythrocyte sedimentation rate (and other acute phase reactants, such as C-reactive protein)
  - Rheumatologic screening - To rule out systemic inflammatory diseases
  - Elevated cardiac enzymes - Creatine kinase or cardiac troponins
  - Serum viral antibody titers - For viral myocarditis

ECG

- ECG can be normal or abnormal in patients with myocarditis. ST segment abnormalities are common and can mimic myocardial ischemia.
- ST segment elevation is sometimes seen but more common findings include nonspecific ST-T wave changes. Patients may experience conduction delays and atrial or ventricular arrhythmias, including sinus tachycardia, ventricular tachycardia, and ventricular fibrillation. The ECG most commonly demonstrates a **sinus tachycardia with or without non-specific ST segment and T wave changes.**
- A finding of an unexplained sinus tachycardia with no other likely cause should prompt consideration of a diagnosis of myocarditis.

- **Possible ECG abnormalities in myocarditis:**
  - ST segment depression or elevation
  - Atrioventricular or intraventricular block
  - Non-specific T wave changes
  - Q-T prolongation
  - P-R segment depression

Cardiac enzymes

- Can be abnormal in patients with acute myocarditis. Cardiac troponin and CK-MB (creatine kinase muscle band isoenzyme) can both be elevated due to necrosis of cardiac myocytes.

- **Echocardiogram** can be normal in early or mild myocarditis. Segmental wall motion abnormalities (mimicking myocardial ischemia) can be seen. Left ventricular dilation and systolic dysfunction can also be seen as in dilated cardiomyopathy. Diastolic relaxation parameters are often abnormal on echocardiography. Possible abnormalities:
  - Decreased left ventricular ejection fraction
  - Right ventricular dysfunction
  - Multichamber dilatation (see Image)
  - Pericardial effusion
  - Wall motion abnormality focal or global

- **Transthoracic echocardiography (TTE)** is currently recommended in the initial evaluation of all patients with suspected myocarditis.

- **Cardiac MRI** is becoming increasingly important in the diagnosis of myocarditis. Cardiac MRI of patients with myocarditis may show a characteristic pattern of late gadolinium enhancement in the subepicardial and mid-myocardial walls (in contrast to ischemia where late gadolinium enhancement is usually subendocardial with extension to mid-myocardial and epicardial walls). Other diagnostic features of myocarditis on cardiac MRI are the presence of myocardial edema and myocardial hyperemia relative to skeletal muscle.

- **A CXR** may be normal or it may show cardiomegaly or features of cardiac failure. Possible abnormalities on CXR:
  - Normal
  - Pulmonary oedema
  - Cardiomegaly
  - Pleural or pericardial effusions

- Cardiac biomarkers such as **troponin or creatinine kinase** may be elevated but normal levels do not rule out a diagnosis of myocarditis

MANAGEMENT

ABC

- Supportive care is the initial treatment for patients with myocarditis.
- A rapid assessment of the ABC should be made.
- Some patients may require resuscitation with urgent initiation of invasive ventilation whilst others may not require any supplemental oxygen and are haemodynamically stable on initial presentation.
- Adequate perfusion pressures should be maintained which may require maximising preload with cautious fluid administration and/or the use of vasopressors and inotropes to maximise cardiac function. This will mandate invasive monitoring and central venous access.

HEART FAILURE

- Treatment of heart failure includes diuretics and nitrates for symptomatic relief.
- In cases of fulminant heart failure, intraaortic ballon pump (IABP), left ventricular assist device (LVAD), or transplantation may be necessary.
- Long-term drug treatment of heart failure involves ACE inhibitors, beta-blockers, aldosterone antagonists, angiotensin II receptor blockers (ARBs), or angiotensin receptor/neprilysin inhibitors (ARNIs).

ARRYTHMIAS

- Atrial and ventricular arrhythmias are treated with antiarrhythmic therapy.
- Heart block can be treated with temporary pacing but may require insertion of permanent pacemaker if conduction abnormalities persist.

ADDITIONAL FACTORS

- Other factors or co-morbidities which may exacerbate physiological compromise, (e.g. anaemia, intercurrent infection and poor glycaemic control) should be promptly identified and treated. Some patients may not maintain an adequate cardiac output despite these measures and the use of intra-aortic balloon pump or extra-corporeal membrane oxygenation may be required.

INFECTIOUS MYOCARDITIS

- Infectious myocarditis is generally treated with supportive therapy for associated heart failure and arrhythmias. Antiviral therapy has not been shown to be helpful in the treatment of viral etiologies.
- Bacterial etiologies may be treated with antibiotics, but this has not been shown to be effective except possibly in the acute infectious phase.
- Parasitic infection should be treated with appropriate antiparasitic drugs.

10. Cyanosis
I. CENTRAL & PERIPHERAL CYANOSIS

- **Cyanosis** is defined as a bluish discoloration, especially of the skin and mucous membranes, due to excessive concentration of deoxyhaemoglobin in the blood caused by deoxygenation. Cyanosis occurs as a result of an absolute amount of desaturated haemoglobin rather than a percentage; anemic patients exhibit cyanosis at a lower PaO2 than those with normal haemoglobin levels.
- **Methaemoglobin** has a chocolate brown color, even when exposed to room air. The pulse oximeter for patients with methaemoglobinemia typically reads 85%, regardless of the PaO2 or SaO2.
- **Congenital heart disease** is a prime diagnostic consideration in all infants presenting with cyanosis.
- Toxic exposures, particularly to aniline dyes and local anesthetics, are considered in acute cyanosis.
- **Sulfhaemoglobin** is reported as methaemoglobin on CO-oximetry; patients with methaemoglobinemia on CO-oximetry who do not respond to **methylene blue** treatment likely have sulfhaemoglobinemia.
- Clinical improvement of the cyanotic patient with supplemental oxygen suggests a diffusion impairment as the cause. All patients with a first episode of cyanosis or an uncertain cause require hospitalization.
- Cyanosis is divided into two main types: **Central** (around the core, lips, and tongue) and **Peripheral** (only the extremities or fingers).

1. CENTRAL CYANOSIS
- Central cyanosis is often due to a circulatory or ventilatory problem that leads to poor blood **oxygenation** in the lungs. It develops when **arterial oxygen saturation drops to ≤ 85% or ≤75%.**
- Acute cyanosis can be a result of **asphyxiation or choking,** and is one of the surest signs that respiration is being blocked.
- Central cyanosis may be due to the following causes:
  - *Central nervous system (impairing normal ventilation):*
    - *Intracranial Haemorrhage*
    - *Drug overdose (e.g. Heroin)*
    - *Tonic–clonic seizure (e.g. Grand Mal seizure)*
  - *Respiratory system*
    - *Pneumonia, Bronchiolitis,*
    - *Asthma, COPD*
    - *Pulmonary hypertension, PE, Hypoventilation*
  - *Cardiovascular diseases*
    - *Congenital heart disease (e.g. Tetralogy of Fallot, right to left shunts in heart or great vessels)*
    - *Heart failure,*
    - *Valvular heart disease,*
    - *Myocardial infarction*
  - *Haematological*
    - *Methemoglobinemia*
    - *Polycythaemia*
    - *Congenital cyanosis (HbM Boston)*
  - *Others*
    - *High altitude: cyanosis may develop in ascents to altitudes >2400 m.*
    - *Hypothermia,*
    - *Obstructive sleep apnea*

2. PERIPHERAL CYANOSIS
- Peripheral cyanosis is the blue tint in fingers or extremities, due to inadequate or obstructed circulation.
- The blood reaching the extremities is not oxygen rich and when viewed through the skin a combination of factors can lead to the appearance of a **blue color**.
- All factors contributing to central cyanosis can also cause peripheral symptoms to appear, however peripheral cyanosis can be observed in the absence of heart or lung failures.
- Small blood vessels may be restricted and can be treated by increasing the normal oxygenation level of the blood.
- Peripheral cyanosis may be due to the following causes:
  - *All common causes of central cyanosis*
  - *Heart failure*
  - *Hypovolaemia*
  - *Cold exposure*
  - *Peripheral Vascular Disease*
  - *Raynaud Phenomenon*
  - *Deep Vein Thrombosis*

II. METHAEMOGLOBINAEMIA

DEFINITION

- Methaemoglobinaemia is a rare but potentially fatal condition. It occurs when the haem molecule of haemoglobin is oxidized from ferrous to ferric form[134].
- Methaemoglobin has decreased oxygen carrying capacity. It also causes leftward shift of the oxygen dissociation curve, thus impairing tissue oxygenation. Methaemoglobinaemia can be congenital or, more commonly, acquired[3]. Many toxins have been implicated in acquired methaemoglobinaemia including local anaesthetics, metoclopramide, cocaine and volatile nitrites[135].
- In health, **MetHb is < 1%** (of total haemoglobin)

CAUSES OF METHAEMOGLOBINAEMIA

- *The most common cause of methaemoglobinaemia is toxin exposure taking a thorough history is essential.*
- *In young children, congenital causes should also be considered*

Common causes of Methemoglobinemia:

- **Idiopathic**
- **Hereditary (Innate)**
  - Hemoglobin M
  - Cytochrome-b5-reductase deficiency
  - Pyruvate kinase deficiency
  - G6PD deficiency

- **ACQUIRED**
  - **Medications**
    - Amyl nitrite
    - Antineoplastics (eg, cyclophosphamide, ifosfamide, flutamide)
    - Dapsone
    - Local anesthetics (eg, benzocaine, lidocaine, prilocaine)
    - Nitroglycerin, Nitroprusside
    - Phenacetin, Phenazopyridine (Pyridium)
    - Quinones (eg, chloroquine, primaquine)
    - Sulfonamides (eg, sulfanilamide, sulfathiazide, sulfapyridine, sulfamethoxazole)

  - **Chemical Agents**
    - Aniline dye derivatives (eg, shoe dyes, marking inks)
    - Butyl nitrite, Isobutyl nitrite
    - Chlorobenzene
    - Fire (heat-induced denaturation)
    - Food adulterated with nitrites
    - Food high in nitrates
    - Naphthalene (mothballs)
    - Nitrophenol
    - Nitrous gases (seen in arc welders)
    - Paraquat, Silver nitrate
    - Trinitrotoluene, Well water (nitrates)
  - **Pediatric Cases**
    - Reduced NADH methemoglobin reductase activity in infants (<4 mo)
    - Seen in association with low birth weight, prematurity, dehydration,
    - Acidosis, Diarrhea, And hyperchloremia

CLINICAL ASSESSMENTS
The patient presents with:

MetHb as % of total Hb*	Typical Symptoms+
3-15%	A slight discoloration (eg, pale, gray, blue) of the skin may be present.
15-20%	• Asymptomatic, • Apart from mild cyanosis
25-50%	• Headache • Dyspnea • Lightheadedness, even syncope • Weakness • Confusion • Palpitations, • chest pain
50-70%	• Cardiovascular - Abnormal cardiac rhythms • CNS - Altered mental status; delirium, seizures, coma • Metabolic - Profound acidosis
>70%	• Death usually results

- Symptom severity does not always reliably correlate to MetHb level but is affected by individual factors including pre-existing co-morbidities

---

[134] *Hunter L, Gordge L, Dargan PI, Wood DM. Methaemoglobinaemia associated with the use of cocaine and volatile nitrites as recreational drugs : a review. Br J Clin Pharmacol. 2011;72(1):18–26.*

[135] *Cassidy N, Duggan E. Potential Pitfalls with the Treatment of Acquired Methaemoglobinaemia. Ir Med J. 2015;108(1):27–8.*

- Cyanosis is usually the first sign and patients can initially appear very well for the level of cyanosis.
- This is because cyanosis secondary to methaemoglobinaemia appears at **1.5 g/dL** of MetHb,
- Whereas cyanosis secondary to hypoxaemia appears **at 5 g/dL** of deoxygenated haemoglobin, which represents a much greater reduction in oxygen carrying capacity.
- Patients often have a low SpO2 on pulse oximetry but again appear well for the degree of hypoxia.

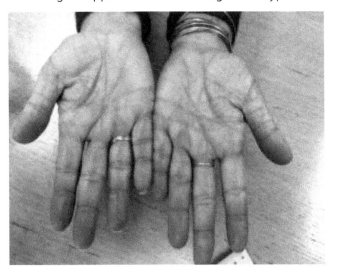

CLINICAL ASSESSMENT

- The characteristic history in the congenital (hereditary) form of the condition is the presence of diffuse, persistent, slate-gray cyanosis, often present from birth.
- There is no evidence of cardiopulmonary disease.
- Patients with hereditary methemoglobinemia are asymptomatic despite the presence of cyanosis.
- The failure of 100% oxygen to correct cyanosis is very suggestive of methemoglobinemia.
- Acute methemoglobinemia can be life-threatening and usually is acquired as a consequence of exposure to toxins or drugs. Therefore, obtaining a detailed history of exposure to methemoglobinemia-inducing substances is important. Such history may not always be forthcoming, but it should always be sought actively since long-term or repeated exposure may occur.
- Consultation with a toxicologist may be necessary, especially with exposure to a new medication, because the list of medications known to cause methemoglobinemia changes constantly.
- The most important part of the history is to elicit any **history of exposure** to account for the methaemoglobinaemia. It is also necessary to identify **co-morbidities** and any **history of cyanosis** or **haematological abnormality**.

- Examination should look for evidence of compromise (i.e. signs of hypoxia) and any clues as to the cause including presence of sepsis
- Initial assessment should follow an ABCDE approach as for every hypoxic patient, supporting ventilation and circulation and identifying and treating other causes of cyanosis or other effects of toxin exposure. Anaesthetics or ITU input may be required.

BEDSIDE TESTS

- **Chocolate Blood:** Arterial blood with elevated methemoglobin levels has a characteristic **chocolate-brown color** as compared to normal bright red oxygen containing arterial blood.

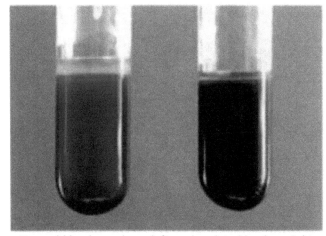

Normal blood sample on left vs chocolate blood on right

- **Point-of-care ABG** is a useful bedside test for methemoglobinemia.
- **Co-oximetry:** Co-oximetry should be performed if available. The co-oximeter is an accurate device for measuring methemoglobin and is the key to diagnosing methemoglobinemia
- **Pulse oximetry** is used extensively in the evaluation of patients with cyanosis and respiratory distress. However, findings of bedside pulse oximetry in the presence of methemoglobinemia may be misleading. Pulse oximetry measurements with low-levels of methemoglobinemia often result in falsely low values for oxygen saturation and are often falsely high in those with high-level methemoglobinemia. The reason for these inaccuracies is as follows.
  - **SaO2** will be extremely high (typically >>100 mm), because the patient is being "treated" with high levels of supplemental oxygen. This immediately excludes true hypoxemia.
  - There is an obvious mis-match between the PaO2 versus the pulse oximetry (which is typically ~80-90% saturated).

o This is known as **SaO2-saturation gap,** and it's indicative of some sort of hemoglobinopathy (most often methemoglobinemia).

Saturation Gap= SaO2 – SpO2

*The presence of a **saturation gap** of 5% or more, which is a disparity between the measured oxyhemoglobin **saturation** of the pulse oximeter and the calculated oxyhemoglobin **saturation** of the arterial blood gas is an essential clue for the diagnosis of methemoglobinemia and other dyshemoglobinemias*

INVESTIGATIONS

- Investigations to rule out hemolysis (Full blood count [FBC], reticulocyte count, peripheral smear review, lactate dehydrogenase [LDH], bilirubin, haptoglobin and Heinz body preparation) and end-organ dysfunction or failure (liver function tests, electrolytes, renal function tests) should be included in the workup.
- Urine pregnancy tests should be performed in females of childbearing age

MANAGEMENT (GENERAL AND SPECIFIC)

- Acute toxic methemoglobinemia with methemoglobin levels above 30% (or lower if symptomatic from hypoxia) is a medical emergency with potentially life-threatening complications.
- The following is appropriate in any individual with suspected or confirmed methemoglobinemia due to a toxic exposure:
  - o Discontinue the offending drug or medication
  - o Institute appropriate supportive care as needed:
    - ▪ Intravenous access,
    - ▪ Hydration for hypotension,
    - ▪ Ventilator support for respiratory compromise, or
    - ▪ Treatments targeted to neurologic complications (antiseizure medications).
- Institute additional treatment for individuals with methemoglobin levels >30 percent or those with levels of 20 to 30 percent who are symptomatic, especially if they have underlying cardiac or pulmonary disease:
  - o Individuals with any symptoms of concern (eg, more than mild headache or lethargy) and/or a methemoglobin level >30% are usually treated with **Methylene blue 1% solution (10mg/mL) at 1-2 mg/kg iv over 3-5 minutes.**
  - o MB acts faster than ascorbic acid (vitamin C) and thus is the treatment of choice for symptomatic acute toxic

methemoglobinemia.

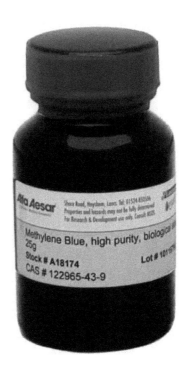

- Methylene blue should be avoided in individuals
  - o with G6PD deficiency (can precipitate hemolysis) and
  - o those taking serotonergic medications (in whom MB can precipitate serotonergic syndrome); in these cases ascorbic acid is used instead.
- **Exchange transfusion** and **hyperbaric oxygen** have been reported to be beneficial in severe disease according to case reports, but there are no controlled trials of these approache For individuals who have persistent methemoglobinemia, blood transfusion may be used, especially if the patient is anemic.
- Methylene blue or ascorbic acid often are not needed for those who are asymptomatic (or only mildly symptomatic) and have methemoglobin levels <20 percent.

11. Dental Emergencies
I. DENTAL INFECTION

INTRODUCTION

- Patients with dental infections frequently present to Emergency Departments, on weekend and after-hours access is available and many patients have no regular dentist.
- Such practitioners, however, often have little formal training in dental conditions and may not feel confident in assessing and managing these patients.[136]
- It is important to understand the principles of management, including avenues for referral and potential complications, as dental infections can be life threatening.

PATHOPHYSIOLOGY

- Dental infections arise when the hard outer coating of the tooth, the enamel, is compromised and the inner dentin is exposed, which exposes microtubules to the pulp chamber.
- These microtubules form a direct path for bacteria to invade from the oral cavity into the vascularised pulp, resulting in pulpitis and causing acute pain.
- At this stage the inflammation is contained within the tooth structure. If not treated by a dentist, the infection may spread into and destroy the local alveolar bone and form a small periapical abscess.
- Subsequent erosion of the cortical plate in the jaw allows bacteria to spread along tissue planes into potential spaces of the face and neck, depending on the specific tooth or teeth involved and the site of erosion.[137]
- Most dental infections will decompress through the gingiva or mucosa into the buccal space but deep extension is more likely when the mandibular molars are involved, as their root structures lie close to the cervical fascia. Extension from these teeth can be laterally into the submasseteric space or medially into the submandibular space.
- Further progression along these planes will lead to the submental and sublingual spaces and ultimately result in airway compromise by entering the parapharyngeal spaces and mediastinum.

- Maxillary teeth generally do not cause such problems but, instead, infection may extend infraorbitally causing peri-orbital cellulitis and, in severe cases, enter the cavernous sinus, causing cavernous sinus thrombosis and visual loss. Additionally, infection from maxillary teeth can spread into the cranial vault and cause encephalitis or meningitis.[138]

CLINICAL ASSESSMENT

- Assessment of patients with a presumed dental infection is no different from that required for other conditions.
- Following a primary survey to assess airway, breathing and circulation the clinician should take a detailed history, perform a physical examination and order relevant investigations.
- Symptoms of early dental infections include localised pain, facial swelling, halitosis and general malaise.
- There is often a long history of dental pain and the patient may have had prior dental treatment such as root canal therapy.[139] As the infection progresses, the patient may complain of the much more serious features of trismus, dysphagia, dyspnea, inability to protrude the tongue or swallow saliva, hoarse voice and stridor. The patient may lean forward in an effort to open their own airway. The most important feature on examination is the patency of the airway. If there is any doubt, the patient should be placed in an environment, such as an emergency department, where an unstable airway can be appropriately managed and the oral and maxillofacial unit should be informed.
- The face should be examined for swelling and induration. If present, the extent of these features and whether they have crossed the lower border of the mandible should be determined.
- Ask the patient to open their mouth as wide as they can and measure the distance between the medial incisors: a distance of <20-30 mm means that it will be difficult to intubate the patient and nasal intubation or a surgical airway may be required.

---

[136] Lewis C, Lynch H, Johnston B. Dental complaints in emergency departments: a national perspective. Ann Emerg Med 2003;42:93–99. Search PubMed

[137] Gonzalez-Beicos A, Nunez D. Imaging of acute head and neck infections. Radiol Clin North Am 2012;50:73–83. Search PubMed

[138] Bridgeman A, Wiesenfeld D, Newland S. Anatomical considerations in the diagnosis and management of acute maxillofacial bacterial infections. Aust Dent J 1996;41:238–45. Search PubMed

[139] Seppanen L, Lemberg KK, Lauhio A, Lindqvist C, Rautemaa R. Is dental treatment of an infected tooth a risk factor for locally invasive spread of infection? J Oral Maxillofac Surg 2011;69:986–93. Search PubMed

- Ask the patient if they can protrude their tongue and swallow, as the inability to do so may be due to an infection in the sublingual space that is raising the floor of the mouth and posteriorly displacing the tongue.

Dental	Non-Dental
Trauma	Referred sinus pain
Gingivitis	Cardiac angina felt in jaw
Dental abscess	Trigeminal neuralgia
Cervicofacial space abscess	Referred ear pain
Ludwigs angina	Parotid inflammation and infection
	Retropharyngeal abscess

- The oral cavity should be examined using a light source, looking for buccal swelling or a visible punctum. Each tooth should be examined individually for appearance, mobility and percussion tenderness.
- It is useful to understand the different numbering systems for teeth when referring to dentists or oral and maxillofacial surgeons. The most common system involves two numbers: the first number denotes the quadrant, 1 being the upper right and progressing clockwise to 4 as the lower right; the second number, 1–8, denotes medial to lateral.
- The examination should include other causes of the presenting complaint as it may not be dental in origin; for example, tonsillar and salivary gland infections may cause lower facial swelling and dysphagia, and acute sinusitis or ear infections can cause upper facial swelling.

Worrying Features in the History and Examination

- During the course of the history and examination, the clinician may identify features that suggest a more serious problem. If any of these features are present consider seeking advice from a senior colleague, anaesthetist or maxillofacial specialist as appropriate.

History	Examination
Systemic upset e.g. pyrexia, vomiting	Sublingual or pharyngeal swelling
Immunocompromised patient	Stridor
Dysphagia	Dysphonia
Rapid progression of illness	Dyspnoea
Progression of illness despite current antibiotic treatment	

The presence of any of the following may indicate actual or impending airway compromise and should prompt an urgent senior anaesthetic assessment:

- *Stridor*
- *Dyspnoea*
- *Dysphagia*
- *Dysphonia*

INVESTIGATIONS

- Relevant investigations include simple blood tests, such as **a FBC and U&Es, and an orthopantomogram** (OPG) to assess the dentition
- If the patient has generalised symptoms, **blood cultures** should be taken. Blood tests such as **C-reactive protein** do not often change the patient's management.

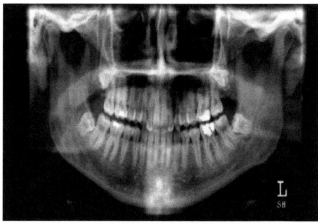

Orthopantomogram

- **A contrast computed tomography (CT)** scan of the neck and lower face should only be performed if the patient's presentation warrants it, for example, to identify a deep space infection.
- If the patient is not stable enough for a CT or the assessment does not warrant a CT, an OPG may be sufficient. If there is doubt as to the type of imaging required, it is prudent to consult the oral and maxillofacial team.

MANAGEMENT

- If the patient has airway compromise, significant facial swelling or trismus, is systemically unwell or has significant medical comorbidities, they will require admission for incision and drainage of the abscess, extraction of unrestorable teeth and possible placement of external drains.
- If the patient does not require admission they should be referred to a dental practitioner for prompt evaluation and consideration of tooth-saving techniques or buccal incision, drainage and extraction of unrestorable teeth.
- Many patients and clinicians assume that antibiotics alone are definitive treatment. This is not the case.
- Definitive treatment can be administered only by the dental practitioner.

- If the patient cannot attend the dentist that day, it is advisable to commence antibiotics and ensure the referral is completed as soon as possible.
- Dental infections are often caused by the normal oral flora and are polymicrobial, including a mixture of anaerobic and aerobic bacteria. The antibiotic chosen must target these groups of organisms and, for outpatients, a combination of a penicillin and beta-lactamase inhibitor or metronidazole provides appropriate cover.
- A widely believed myth is that a course of antibiotics is necessary before extraction of an infected tooth to prevent seeding into the cervicofacial spaces. Waiting for the infection to settle before extracting the tooth can result in life-threatening consequences as the infection spreads along the tissue planes. Teeth can be extracted in the presence of an acute infection; indeed, extraction of the offending tooth is often curative. It is a pitfall to assume that a course of antibiotics will definitively treat an established infection and this attitude often leads to prolonged morbidity and the potential for the infection to progress into a life-threatening condition.
- An appointment with a dentist should be organised for the patient as this increases compliance. This should be carefully recorded in the patient's record. Unfortunately, for many patients, Medicare does not cover dental services unless the patient holds a healthcare card.

SPECIFIC CONDITIONS

A. DENTAL ABSCESS

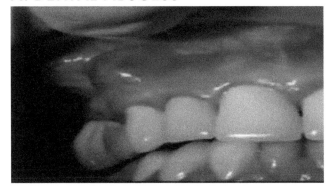

- This is one of the most common dental problems presenting to the ED. Common symptoms and signs include pain, localised erythema, periodontal and facial swelling and direct tenderness to palpation of the responsible tooth.
- A dental abscess is the final product of an inflammatory process, a suppurative collection associated with the structures surrounding the teeth.
- It is a type of odontogenic infection (i.e., an infection that originates within a tooth).

- An abscess may remain localized (damaging only the adjacent tissues) or it may develop into a diffuse cellulitis, which can lead to the development of potentially life-threatening systemic complications.
- The vast majority of otherwise healthy patients have localized infections which can be managed on an outpatient basis. The most common types of dental abscess are periapical, periodontal, and pericoronal. Other less common types include gingival or combined periodontal-endodontic. This topic primarily deals with the most common types of dental abscess.
- The type of antibiotic prescribed also varies greatly; 90% of prescriptions in one study were for either amoxicillin, metronidazole or penicillin V.
- The clinical spectrum of dental abscess ranges from minor well-localized infection to severe life-threatening complications involving multifascial spaces.
- The vast majority of otherwise healthy patients presenting with a dental infection can be managed on an outpatient basis.
- Common presenting symptoms include dental pain/toothache; intraoral and/or extraoral edema, erythema, or discharge; and thermal hypersensitivity.
- A major consideration is the potential for airway obstruction as a consequence of extension of the infection into fascial spaces surrounding the oropharynx.
- Panoramic dental x-ray reveals the source of infection in most cases; however, a periapical x-ray may also be helpful. **CT scan** is recommended if there is suspicion of a fascial space infection or if panoramic or periapical x-rays are not available.

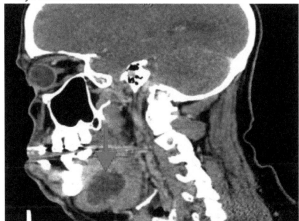

- Prompt operative intervention to identify and eliminate the source of infection and provide a path for drainage, along with antibiotic therapy and supportive care, is required. Operative treatment is considered the cornerstone of successful management.
- Immunocompromised patients must be treated in a timely fashion as tooth-related infections may spread rapidly.

B.LUDWIGS ANGINA

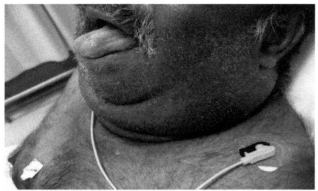

Courtesy-life in the fast lane

- Ludwig's angina is a rapidly progressive gangrenous cellulitis of the submandibular space, which can further be divided into the sublingual space and the submylohyoid space.
- The sublingual space is bounded by the oral mucosa superiorly and the mylohyoid muscle inferiorly. In Ludwig's angina, the submandibular space is the primary site of infection.[140]
- The submylohyoid space is bounded by the mylohyoid muscle superiorly and the skin and superficial fascia of the neck inferiorly. Swelling and edema in these spaces cause the floor of the mouth to feel woody and subsequently causes the tongue to elevate and protrude upward and outward. The infection also can spread laterally and posteriorly to occlude the airway, the most serious complication.
- The causes include:
  o Dental abscess/caries
  o Fracture of the mandible,
  o Trauma to the mucosal floor of the mouth,
  o Peritonsillar abscess,
  o Oral malignancies with secondary infection,
  o Salivary gland infections,
  o Infected thyroglossal cysts, and
  o Osteomyelitis.
- The most common organism isolated from wound cultures is **viridans streptococci** although infections may be polymicrobial.
- Other pathogens include:
  o *Staphylococcus aureus,*
  o *Staphylococcus epidermidis,*
  o *Bacteroides sp.,*
  o *Hemophilus influenzae,*
  o *Klebsiella pneumoniae, and*
  o *Pseudomonas aeruginosa.*

RISK FACTORS
- The majority of cases of Ludwig's angina occur in healthy patients with no comorbid diseases. Nevertheless, there are several conditions that have been shown to predispose patients to Ludwig's angina.
- These conditions include diabetes mellitus, alcoholism, acute glomerulonephritis, systemic lupus erythematosus, aplastic anemia, neutropenia, and dermatomyositis.[141]

CLINICAL PRESENTATION
- Ludwig's angina is a clinical diagnosis. The majority of patients report dental pain, or a history of recent dental procedures, and neck swelling. Less common complaints include neck pain, dysphonia, dysphagia, and dysarthria. Less than one third of adults will present in respiratory distress with dyspnea, tachypnea, or stridor.
- On physical examination, over 95% of patients have bilateral submandibular swelling and an elevated or protruding tongue. The submandibular swelling is often characterized as brawny and tense, with overlying erythema. Patients are often febrile and may be tachypneic, tachycardic, and hypoxic, all signs of impending airway collapse.
- Patients may assume an upright position and sit forward with the neck extended. There may be drooling.

INVESTIGATION
- **FBC & Blood culture.**
- **CT scan with IV contrast:** if patient is hemodynamically stable and with minimal complaints. Because airway compromise may develop rapidly, patients should be accompanied by an appropriate health care provider and monitored at all times.
- **A lateral neck radiograph** may demonstrate soft tissue swelling, subcutaneous air, and occlusion of the airway.

MANAGEMENT
- The most important feature in the management of Ludwig's angina is **maintaining a patent airway.** Airway management is the foundation of treatment for patients with Ludwig's angina. Patients should be placed on the cardiac monitor with continuous pulse oximetry and given supplemental oxygen.
- **IV antibiotic:** Ampicillin-sulbactam or Piperacillin-tazobactam in addition to metronidazole for anaerobic coverage is sufficient. Clindamycin alone may be used in patients allergic to penicillin.
- The role of corticosteroids is controversial.
- ENT/Dental Surgeon referral for simple I&D.

[140] Spitalnic SJ, Sucov A J Emerg Med. 1995 Jul-Aug; 13(4):499-503.

[141] Bansal A, Miskoff J, Lis RJ. Otolaryngologic critical care. Crit Care Clin. 2003;19:55-72.

II. DENTAL TRAUMA

INTRODUCTION

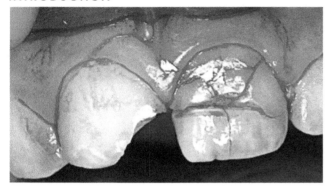

- Dental trauma is highly prevalent.[142] It can affect children and teenagers at home, at school, or outdoors. Dental trauma most frequently occurred in the home, and enamel trauma was the most common type.
- The maxillary central incisors were the most commonly affected, followed by the maxillary lateral incisors and canines.[143]
- These injuries are often seen in conjunction with facial trauma, which poses esthetic concerns to patients.
- The severity of traumatic dental injuries can range from minor cases of enamel chip to extensive injuries involving the supporting structures or dental avulsion.
- Inflammatory root resorption and eventual exodontia could result from the degeneration of the periodontal ligament cells and pulp necrosis if the above-mentioned factors are unfavorable.
- Not only does anterior tooth trauma have a negative esthetic effect, but it also threatens the capabilities for pronunciation and mastication.
- Dental trauma can be classified as:

Term	Meaning
Concussion	An injury to the tooth-supporting structures with no increase in tooth mobility, and no displacement of the tooth. The tooth however is tender to touch.
Subluxation	An injury to the tooth-supporting structures with an increase in tooth mobility. However, tooth position remains correct

Intrusion	An injury resulting in apical displacement of the tooth (i.e., the tooth has become displaced into the tooth socket)
Extrusion	Coronal displacement of the tooth (the tooth has moved out of the socket but has not come out completely)
Lateral luxation	Movement of a tooth in any direction that isn't axial. For example, the tooth may be displaced buccally or palatally
Avulsion	The tooth has been completed displaced out of the socket
Enamel fracture	Damage to the enamel of a tooth resulting in the loss of tissue, isolated to enamel only
Enamel and dentine fracture	Fracture of a tooth extending through both enamel and dentine, resulting in the loss of both tissues, not extending into the dental pulp
Complicated crown fracture	Fracture through the tooth extending into the dental pulp of a tooth. Also known as an enamel-dentine-pulp fracture
Root fracture	Fracture of the apical portion of the tooth which involved dentine, pulp and cementum
Alveolar bone fracture	Fracture of the alveolar process of the maxilla or mandible, which may or may not involve the socket itself. Note this is not the same as a fracture to the mandible or maxilla itself, and treatment between these two conditions is different.
Periodontia	Structures that are the supporting structures present around the teeth, including gingiva, bone, cementum and periodontal ligament

3. CLINICAL EVALUATION

- Initial evaluation of a patient with dental trauma should include the following:
  - o Full physical examination of the head, neck, and face
  - o Assessment of possible injuries to adjacent areas and structures (eg, facial fractures or head and neck trauma)

Imaging modalities that may be considered include the following:
  - o CT of the head, neck, and maxillofacial bones
  - o Periapical radiography
  - o Panoramic radiography of the teeth

[142] Azami-Aghash S, Azar F, Azar F, et al. Prevalence, etiology, and types of dental trauma in children and adolescents: systematic review and meta-analysis. Iran Univ Med Sci. 2015;29(40):234.

[143] Enabulele J, Oginni A, Sede M, Oginni F. Pattern of traumatised anterior teeth among adult Nigerians and complications from late presentation. BMC Res Notes. 2016;9(1). doi:10.1186/s13104-016-1871-3

Ellis and Davey classification for dental traumas

Ellis Class 1:

Simple fracture of crown, involving little or no dentin.

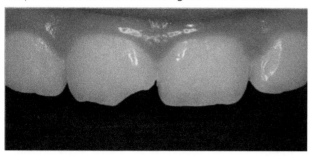

Ellis Class 2:

Extensive fracture of crown, involving considerable dentin, but no dental pulp.

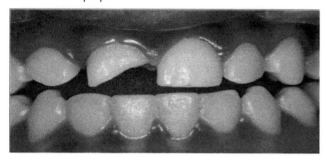

Ellis Class 3:

Extensive fracture of crown, involving considerable dentin and exposing pulp.

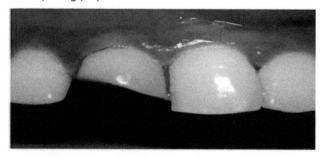

Ellis Class 4:

The traumatized tooth becomes non-vital with or without loss of crown structure.

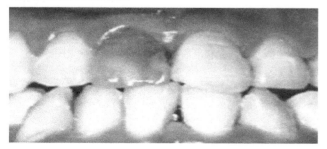

Discoloured traumatized tooth (Ellis Class 4)

Ellis Class 5:

Tooth lost as a result of trauma.

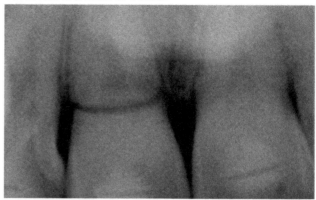

Ellis 5: Root fracture

Ellis Class 6:

Fracture of root with or without fracture of crown.

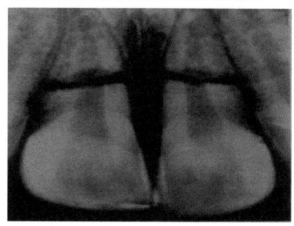

Radiograph showing horizontal root fracture

Ellis Class 7:

Displacement of tooth without fracture of crown or root.

Ellis Class 8:

Fracture of crown enmasse.

Ellis Class 9:

Traumatic injury to deciduous tooth.

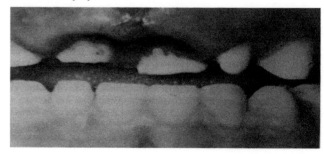

It is important to differentiate between adult and deciduous (baby) teeth. This is important in trauma cases, as it has an effect on the management of the trauma.

4. INVESTIGATIONS

Special test	Rationale
Chest X-ray	Used to exclude aspiration risk when patient is unaware of where a missing tooth or tooth fragment is.
Soft tissue view	Useful to exclude fragments of teeth becoming lodged within deep lacerations to the lips, cheeks and face
Orthopantomogram (OPT or OPG)	Assessment of dental structures. Can be useful if doubt exists over whether tooth is a deciduous (baby) or adult tooth, and useful to assess degree of damage to dental and periodontal structures. This type of x-ray can also be beneficial to assess if a tooth has fractured at crown level, or have been intruded, as in both scenarios only a very small tip of a tooth can be seen.

5. EMERGENCY DEPARTMENT CARE

Treatment of dental trauma varies according to the type of injury involved:

o Fracture
o Avulsion
o Luxation (tooth displacement)

Tetanus booster and antibiotics should be administered whenever a dental injury is at risk for infection. Arrangements should be made for prompt follow-up with a dentist or an oral and maxillofacial surgeon.

Dental fractures may be classified as follows:

- Ellis class I (superficial enamel only) – No emergency care is required; follow-up with a dentist is arranged as needed
- Ellis class II (enamel and dentin, with sensitivity to temperature, air, and palpation) – The exposed dentin is covered, preferably with dental cement; the patient is referred to a dentist within 24 hours
- Ellis class III (enamel, dentin, and pulp; a dental emergency) – The fracture is covered with dental cement; patients receive urgent and immediate dental follow-up; topical painkillers increase the risk of infection and thus should not be applied
- Root fractures – Extraction of the coronal segment is required; if no more than one third of the root is involved, a dentist may be able to perform a root canal and salvage the tooth.

Principles of management for dental avulsions include the following:

- An adult tooth that is avulsed should be reimplanted in its socket as soon as possible
- If the tooth cannot be reimplanted, it should be placed in a protective solution; it should never be allowed to dry
- If the tooth has been dry for a significant period, it should be soaked in the appropriate solution (which depends on the length of the dry period)
- Some studies suggest that when a tooth has been out of the mouth for longer than 60 minutes, immediate reimplantation is not required, and a root canal of the tooth should be performed with the tooth outside the mouth before it is reimplanted
- After reimplantation, any other injuries are repaired
- In children with dental avulsions, primary teeth are never reimplanted, because reimplantation of a deciduous tooth can cause harm to the developing permanent tooth.

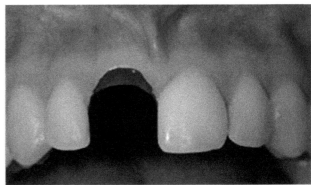

Avulsed tooth

Luxations may be classified as follows:

- Concussion - Mild injury to the periodontal ligament, with some clinical tenderness but no movement of the tooth
- Subluxation - More significant injury to the periodontal ligament, with clinical tenderness and movement of the tooth
- Extrusion - Partial removal of a tooth from its socket
- Lateral luxation - Lateral displacement of a tooth at an angle, with possible fracture of the alveolar bone as well
- Intrusion - Impaction of a tooth into its socket in the fractured alveolar bone

Treatment of luxations includes the following:

- Concussion and subluxation – A soft diet, administration of nonsteroidal anti-inflammatory drugs (NSAIDs), and referral to a dentist; subluxation is a more significant injury and is more often associated with pulpal necrosis
- Extrusion – Restoration of the tooth to its original position; splinting

- Lateral luxation – Repositioning of the tooth, often made more difficult by a fractured alveolar bone; splinting, done by a general practitioner only if the alveolar bone fracture is minimal and done by a dentist or an oral and maxillofacial surgeon if the fracture is more extensive
- Intrusion – Usually, the general practitioner can provide no emergency treatment; referral to a dentist within 24 hours is indicated

Associated injuries to the maxillofacial bones may be classified as follows:
- Le Fort I – Transverse fracture separating the body of the maxilla from the lower portion of the pterygoid plate and nasal septum
- Le Fort II – Pyramidal fracture of the central maxilla and palate; facial tugging moves the nose but not the eyes
- Le Fort III (ie, craniofacial disjunction) – Facial skeleton completely separated from the skull, with the fracture extending through the frontozygomatic suture lines and through the orbit, the base of the nose, and the ethmoid; on physical examination, the entire face shifts with tugging

Cracked teeth

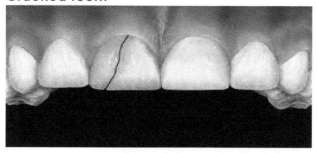

- Are more complicated to treatment plan and treat, and require assessment by a qualified dentist. Attempts should be made to locate missing fragments, and the patient warned about risk of future pain and requirement for future dental work. Sensitive toothpaste, paracetamol and NSAIDs can be recommended for these patient groups to help with pain that is likely to occur on contact with hot/cold food, drinks or other substances.
- In all cases of dental trauma, follow up with a dentist should be advised, as the blood supply to the teeth may be affected, resulting in devitalisation of the tooth pulp.
- This needs to be monitored and treated by a dentist accordingly. It is also useful to advise patients on the use of **0.2% chlorhexidine mouthrinse** as brushing is likely to be very painful.

Ellis I fracture:
- Smooth rough corners with a dental drill or an emery board.

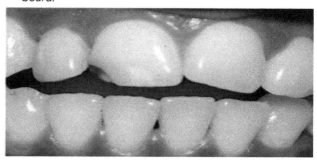

- Treatment of fractures contained solely within the enamel alone requires no urgent care. The tooth can be repaired cosmetically at the convenience of the patient.

Ellis II fracture:

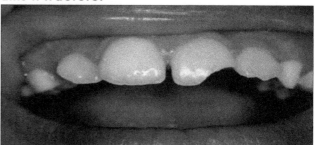

- This type is managed by a bonded resin restoration or by crowning it, and its prognosis is good unless accompanied by a luxation injury.

Ellis III fracture:

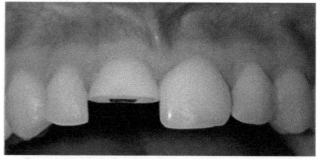

- Cover exposed dentin with a layer of zinc oxide or calcium hydroxide. Bleeding and moisture with this type of fracture usually makes it more difficult for these materials to adhere to the tooth.
- Cover with dental foil and expediently refer the patient to a dentist. Root and dentoalveolar fractures require splinting by a dentist for several weeks.
- Bone wax (Ethicon), which is a combination of beeswax and isopropyl palmitate, is not recommended for open dental fractures because it can cause inflammatory reactions of the surrounding soft tissues (eg, pulp).

III. BLEEDING AND DRY SOCKETS

1. DRY SOCKET

INTRODUCTION

- **A dry socket** is caused by the partial or total loss of a blood clot in the tooth socket after a tooth extraction. Normally, after a tooth is extracted, a blood clot will form as the first step in healing to cover and protect the underlying jawbone.
- If the blood clot is lost or does not form, the bone is exposed and healing is delayed

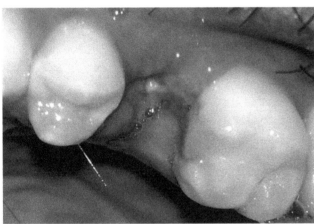
Dry Socket

PRESENTATION

Population:
- More common in women

Risk Factors
- Smoking
- Birth control pills

Most Common Sites of Occurrence
- Distal sites (e.g., third molars)
- More common in the mandible than in the maxilla

Signs
- Occurs 3-5 days following a tooth extraction and can last up to 7 days
- Distress and pain

Symptoms
- Throbbing, radiating pain that is difficult to localize and which may radiate up to the periauricular area.
- Initially, the healing seems to be progressing well with pain diminishing—but then pain increases and seems more severe than at the time of extraction.
- Pain severity:
  - Severe throbbing pain
  - Pain usually lasts anywhere from 24 to 72 h.

DIAGNOSIS

Based on:
- Bone exposure
- Absence of facial swelling or swelling of the lymph nodes
- Pain when the extraction site is irrigated/flushed with fluids

Persistent pain beyond 3 days, exposed bone with an inflammation of the mucosa and evidence of swelling, buccal space and sublingual space might suggest other possible diagnoses.

- Dry sockets usually do not require any special tests, but an x-ray can be useful to rule out tooth fragments being left behind in the socket area.
- OPG long cone periapical radiographs are common views used to do this.

DIFFERENTIAL DIAGNOSIS

- Osteomyelitis or local infection such as subperiosteal abscess
- Osteonecrosis (in medically compromised patients)
- Bisphosphonate- or drug-related osteonecrosis of the jaw
- Myofascial pain

MANAGEMENT

Common Initial Treatment

Alveolar osteitis is not an infection; an antibiotic therapy will not improve the condition.

1. Control the pain with a dressing material (e.g., Alvogyl™ paste, DRESSOL-X™).
   - Irrigate the site with chlorhexidine or saline.
   - Pack the extraction site enough to cover the exposed surgical site with a resorbable or nonresorbable dressing.
   - Instruct the patient to maintain good oral hygiene.
   - If the dressing is nonresorbable, remove it after 2-3 days.
   - If the pain persists, consider repacking the area.
   - Advise the patient to refrain from smoking for at least 6 weeks after the extraction; smoking delays healing and restricts blood supply to the extraction site.
2. Use postoperative analgesics such as NSAIDs (e.g., ibuprofen) or a mixture of narcotic with acetaminophen and codeine (e.g., Tylenol® 3) in case of severe pain.
   - Ibuprofen: for a 70 kg person, 400 mg q.i.d. or q. 4 h.
3. If the pain persists beyond 72 h., take radiographs to rule out the existence of a foreign body at the extraction site, bone destruction, or other possible etiologies.

2. BLEEDING SOCKET

INTRODUCTION

- Low level oozing from a tooth socket in the first 12-24 hours after extraction is normal[144]
  - Reactionary haemorrhage, usually two to three hours post extraction due to wearing off of the vasoconstrictor effect of the local anaesthetic adrenaline
  - Active bleeding beyond this point (infection) requires investigations and treatment (antibiotics)
  - Advise patients (post tooth extraction) to avoid rinsing their mouth, exploring the socket with tongue or fingers.

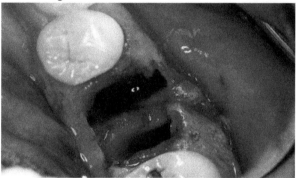

Bleeding Socket

- Most teeth extractions will involve bleeding to some degree, however generally, the application of pressure via a damp gauze will suffice to ensure haemostasis is achieved.
- Bleeding sockets need to be differentiated between a true bleeding socket compared with just some blood-stained saliva. A fresh bleeding socket will be seen oozing, and not just spitting of blood. It is important to investigate potential causes of the bleeding (is the patient clotting normally? is the patient on any anticoagulants?).

INVESTIGATION

- FBC
- Clotting
- INR if appropriate

MANAGEMENT

- Significant active haemorrhage (A, B, C) addressed first
- STOP THE BLEEDing, then IV access, Cross-match etc.
- Application of gauze soaked in tranexamic acid or adrenaline (or adrenaline containing local anaesthetic)

- Application of damp gauze. Use of heamostatic agents such as hemocollagen or surgicel
- Use of resorbable sutures (these are best placed by experienced operators. Beware bleed History (anticoagulated, bleeding/bruising Hx, FHx coagulopathy)
- Beware some meds (e.g. methotrexate, antiplatelet agents) that patient may not associate with bleeding
- Labs as indicated by History / Exam
- Locate the bleeding site - tooth socket, gum or bone (Hx of a difficult extraction)
- Sit patient up, good light, **suction** away and "liver clots" (assoc. with secondary haemorrhage and infection) ±saline syringe to see base of socket.
- Patients with bleeding sockets **should not be encouraged to rinse with water or saline**. This is a common misconception. By doing this, it results in further dislodgement of the blood clot. Any palpable fracture, mobile bony socket or mal-occlusion (fracture)?

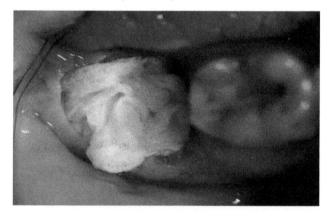

- Beware vomit (irritant blood in stomach)
- Stop bleeding with direct pressure - damp gauze in socket & bite down for 5 minutes
- If bleeding continues, saline wash out the socket, soak new gauze in 10% Tranexamic acid and get patient to bite down for 30 min (alternatively, bite on tea bag as tannin is a procoagulant)
- Refer to Maxillofacial/Haematology- If local measures are unsuccessful
- Bleeding from the soft tissues is usually arrested by placing a horizontal mattress suture across the socket
- Bleeding from the base of the socket, from bone, is usually arrested using a pack such as 'Surgical' or in some instances soaking ribbon gauze in Whitehead's varnish and packing the socket full.

---

[144] *Emed. Post Extraction Dental Haemorrhage [Emed.ie]*

12. Dialysis & Kidney Injury
I. ACUTE KIDNEY INJURY

1. INTRODUCTION:

o The term 'acute kidney injury' (AKI) has replaced 'acute renal failure' to emphasize its potential reversibility in the early stages. Early identification and appropriate management are essential. AKI should be viewed as a spectrum of injury and is characterized by a reduction in kidney function that results in a failure to maintain fluid, electrolyte, and acid–base balance.

o Acute kidney injury (AKI) is a sudden, potentially reversible, kidney dysfunction with partial or complete loss of glomerular filtration resulting in electrolyte and fluid abnormalities as well as retention of nitrogenous waste products. In contrast, Chronic Kidney Disease (CKD) describes loss of kidney function for at least three months. While a decrease in Glomerular Filtration Rate (GFR) is used to categorize CKD, an increase in serum creatinine or decrease in urine output is used to characterize AKI.

o AKI occurs in up to 7% of all patients admitted to hospital, whilst 5-20% of all critically ill patients have an episode of AKI during the course of their illness.

o Approximately 5% of all critically ill patients will at some point require renal replacement therapy (RRT) during their admission. Patients with AKI are also vulnerable to additional harm perioperatively, and care must be taken to reduce long-term risk in this cohort. The international definition of AKI is the presence of one of the following criteria:

   ↓ *Serum creatinine rising by ≥26μmol/L within 48 hours.*
   ↓ *Serum creatinine rising ≥1.5-fold from the reference value, which is known or presumed to have occurred within 1 week.*
   ↓ *Urine output is <0.5mL/kg/h for >6 consecutive hours.*

o The reference serum creatinine should be the lowest creatinine value recorded within 3 months of the event.

RIFLE CLASSIFICATION

o In 2004, the Acute Dialysis Quality Initiative (ADQI) group developed the RIFLE system to standardize the classification of AKI.

o AKI is classified according to the acronym RIFLE, which includes three classes of severity (risk/injury/failure) and two outcome classes (loss and end-stage).

o The three severity classes are based on changes in either serum creatinine or urine output. The two outcome criteria are defined by the duration of loss of kidney function at 4 weeks and 3 months, respectively.

o The RIFLE criteria are summarized in Table below.

	GFR criteria	Urine output criteria
Risk	Increased Creatinine 1.5x or GFR reduction >25%	<0.5mL/kg/h for 6h
Injury	Increased Creatinine 2x or GFR reduction >50%	<0.5mL/kg/h for 12h
Failure	Increased Creatinine 3x or GFR reduction >75%	<0.3mL/kg/h for 24h or anuria for 12 h
Loss	Persistent renal failure for >4 weeks	
ESRF	Persistent renal failure for >3 months	

2. CLASSIFICATION

o Acute kidney injury is classified into three categories (**Prenal, Intrinsic, or Postrenal**) based on the physiologic mechanism that prevents production or excretion of urine.

o A patient may have more than one cause of acute kidney injury simultaneously due to derangements of any of the above four processes.

o Additionally, most patients with previously normal kidneys may not have an elevation in serum markers in the event of an acute injury to one kidney.

• *Prerenal*

   o **Hypovolemia:** commonly due to decreased intake, increased losses, diuretic use, blood loss, third spacing, salt-wasting nephropathy, hypoaldosteronism.

   o **Hypotension:** shock state, heart failure, antihypertensive use, Addison's disease

   o **Renal artery vascular diseases:** renal artery stenosis or fibrosis, thromboembolic events, aortic dissection, aortic aneurysm, NSAID/ARB/ACE inhibitor use, pre-eclampsia, HUS, DIC, traumatic devascularization

   o **Other:** hepatorenal disease, aortic cross-clamping, renal vein thrombosis

• *Intrinsic*

   o **Interstitial diseases:**
      ▪ Infection (pyelonephritis, infected stone, abscesses, emphysematous pyelitis),

- Infiltration (amyloid, myeloma, sarcoid, lymphoma),
- Autoimmune (SLE),
- Drug-induced interstitial nephritis, loss of parenchyma due to polycystic disease
  - o **Glomerular diseases:** post-infectious glomerulonephritis, HSP, SLE, Wegener's, Goodpasture's, membranoproliferative.
  - o **Nephrotoxins:** may result in interstitial and glomerular injury:
    - **Medications**: NSAIDS, Aminoglycosides, Radiocontrast, Amphotericin, Sulfonamides.
    - Heme moieties from hemolysis or rhabdomyolysis,
    - Uric acid, calcium oxalate, amyloid deposits

- *Postrenal acute kidney injury*
  - o **Intraluminal obstruction:** calculi, obstructed catheters, urethral strictures, posterior urethral valves, vesicoureteral reflux, failed ureteral stents
  - o **Extrinsic compression:** BPH, GU/GYN/GI cancers, pregnancy, ascites, expanding hematoma, penile fractures
  - o **Other:** traumatic disruption, neurogenic bladder, spinal cord injury (cauda equina syndrome), anticholinergic and alpha-adrenergic antagonist toxicity, surgical injury.

3. CLUES FOR ACUTE RENAL INJURY
- o **By aetiology:**
  - *Prerenal Acute Kidney Injury* may present with hypotension, tachycardia, shock, peripheral oedema, vomiting, diarrhoea, acute blood loss, flank or back pain, oliguria or anuria.
  - *Intrinsic Acute Renal Injury* may present with flank and back pain, hematuria, proteinuria, urinary casts and sediments, infectious prodrome, and history or presentation of systemic diseases causing microangiopathy and hemolysis like HUS, TTP, scleroderma, and DIC.
  - *Postrenal Acute Kidney Injury* patients present with obstruction to urine flow associated with a history of renal calculi, urinary urge, failure to void, incontinence, mechanical failure of indwelling catheter, pelvic and flank pain, palpable large urinary bladder, CVA tenderness, and hydronephrosis or hydroureter on imaging studies.
- o **By consequence:**
  - Acute kidney injury may present with a variety signs and symptoms consistent with uraemia, electrolyte disturbances, and fluid status.

- These may include third spacing with shortness of breath, pleural and pericardial effusions, interstitial oedema, and ascites.
- **Hyperkalemia** may present with acutely life-threatening arrhythmias and requires emergent diagnosis and management.
- **Uremia** may present with uremic pericarditis, effusion and life-threatening pericardial tamponade requiring emergent diagnosis and management.
- **Acute hypertension** with hypertensive emergency also requires emergent management.

4. ED-FOCUSED WORK-UP
- o **Labs** – Serum chemistry, CK, BUN/Cr ratio, FeNa, Specific gravity, Microscopic analysis, Urine electrolytes
- o **ECG** – evaluate for changes secondary to electrolyte changes
- o **CXR** – volume status, infection
- o **KUB** – displaced ureteral stents, nephrolithiasis
- o **U/S** – hydronephrosis, hydroureter, bladder distention, flow doppler of the kidney
- o **CT** – nephrolithiasis, abdominal/pelvic masses

5. COMPLICATIONS OF AKI
- *Complications of AKI include:*
  - o **Biochemical**: *Metabolic acidosis, Hyperkalaemia, and other Electrolyte disturbances (Na^+, $PO4^{3-}$, Ca^{2+}).*
  - o **Cardiovascular**: *Pulmonary Oedema, Hypertension, Myocardial Depression, Arrhythmias, Pericarditis.*
  - o **Gastrointestinal**: *GI bleeding, Gastric Stasis, Ileus, Anorexia, Vomiting.*
  - o **Haematological**: *Anaemia, Impaired Haemostasis, Platelet Dysfunction.*
  - o **Neurological:** *Lethargy, Memory Impairment, Encephalopathy, Peripheral Neuropathy.*

6. MANAGEMENT OF AKI IN ED
- The main treatment modalities for AKI in the ED are:
  - o Fluid resuscitation and monitoring of volume status.
  - o Prevention of further injury by stopping nephrotoxic drugs.
  - o Urinary catheterization to relieve any urethral or bladder obstruction.
  - o Treatment of complications (e.g. hyperkalaemia, pulmonary oedema).
  - o Treatment of the precipitant (e.g. sepsis, hypovolaemia).

II. ACUTE RHABDOMYOLYSIS

1. DEFINITION

- Rhabdomyolysis is a complex medical condition involving the rapid dissolution of damaged or injured skeletal muscle. This disruption of skeletal muscle integrity leads to the direct release of intracellular muscle components, including myoglobin, creatine kinase (CK), aldolase, and lactate dehydrogenase, as well as electrolytes, into the bloodstream and extracellular space. Rhabdomyolysis ranges from an asymptomatic illness with elevation in the CK level to a life-threatening condition associated with extreme elevations in CK, electrolyte imbalances, acute renal failure (ARF), and disseminated intravascular coagulation. [145]
- The normal range : **30–190 IU/Litre**. So, readings over 200 can be considered as elevated. **Any value above 950 IU/litre** is diagnostic of rhabdomyolysis.

2. CAUSES

- o Change in medication: Statins
- o Drug abuse/Alcoholism /Overexertion
- o Genetic disorders/ Heatstroke/ Crush injury
- UK most causes: **alcohol abuse**, **muscle overexertion**, **muscle compression** and the **use of certain medications and illicit drugs.**

3. CLINICAL MANIFESTATIONS

- **Local features**: Muscle pain, Weakness, Tenderness, Swelling, Bruising
- **Systemic features**: Dark urine (Tea coloured urine), Fever, Malaise, Nausea and vomiting, Agitation, Delirium, Anuria

4. DIAGNOSIS

- The common scenarios that are associated with rhabdomyolysis will be evident from the patient's history or presentation. In immobilisation, **crush injury and illicit drug use** consideration of the diagnosis is obvious.
- Rhabdomyolysis must also be considered when there is history of recent medication changes, especially **statins.**
- Remember that in non-traumatic rhabdomyolysis patients may only demonstrate muscle weakness, tenderness or stiffness.
- Paralysis and severe weakness may suggest very extensive myonecrosis or coexistent potassium disturbances that can occur as renal function is impaired.
- Do not dismiss as dehydration a patient who complains of darker than normal urine; **obtain a myoglobin dipstick.**

- The number of rhabdomyolysis patients who develop some degree of renal failure is **as great as 50%.**

5. INVESTIGATIONS

- **Blood:** CK, U&E, FBC, Ca^{2+} & $PO4^{3-}$, Urate & clotting test
- **Imaging:** MRI, US, CT
- **Urines:** Myoglobinuria

6. ED MANAGEMENT OF RHABDOMYOLYSIS

- **Find and Treat the cause**
- **Rehydration**
  - o Aggressive intravascular fluid rehydration up to **10 litres of fluid.** The sooner this commences the lower the risk of developing renal failure.
  - o Ideally rehydration commences pre-hospitally at the same time as extrication.
- **Find and treat complications**
  - o Rhabdomyolysis can lead to **cardiac arrhythmias** as a consequence of **metabolic acidosis and hyperkalaemia**. These disturbances are as important to correct as the arrhythmia itself.
- There are two treatments which are unproven and are considered here, the administration of sodium bicarbonate and the use of mannitol.
- **Administration of sodium bicarbonate**
  - o NaHCO3 has been long advocated as a treatment for rhabdomyolysis. The theory was alkalinisation of the urine would clear an increasingly acid load delivered to the kidney. There is no evidence to substantiate this. Furthermore, large doses of bicarbonate may worsen the **hypocalcaemia** especially if hypovolaemia is corrected.
  - o It is likely that large volume of crystalloid alone will produce a diuresis sufficient to alkalinise urine.
- **Use of mannitol**
  - o Mannitol has been suggested, and demonstrated in experimental models, to produce a diuresis that protects against renal failure. However robust evidence is lacking from the literature to confirm its efficacy. Mannitol, like furosemide, is a renal vasodilator and osmotic diuretic and both have been used to attempt to initiate diuresis when the patient becomes anuric. Again, there is little evidence and retrospective studies suggest there is no additional benefit over fluid hydration.
  - o The prognosis in rhabdomyolysis is related to coexistent illness and injury but the renal failure is usually reversible.

---

[145] *Huerta-Alardín AL, Varon J, Marik PE. Bench-to-bedside review: Rhabdomyolysis-- an overview for clinicians. Crit Care. 2005 Apr;9(2):158–169.*

III. HEMODIALYSIS & PERITONEAL DIALYSIS

INTRODUCTIONS

The three primary treatment options for patients with end-stage renal disease (ESRD) are:

- *Hemodialysis (HD),*
- *Peritoneal Dialysis (PD), and*
- *Kidney transplantation.*

INDICATIONS FOR RRT

The classical indications for RRT are (**HAFAS**):

- *Hyperkalaemia (K⁺>6.5mmol/L)*
- *Acidosis (pH<7.2)*
- *Fluid overload*
- *Anuria (for >6h) or oliguria (for >12h).*
- *Symptomatic uraemia (encephalopathy, pericarditis, etc.)*

- In addition, RRT can also be used for the **removal of unwanted drugs and other toxins**. Drugs that are removed by RRT include **Lithium, Metformin, Ethylene Glycol, Salicylates, and many antibiotics.**
- *Digoxin, Tricyclics, Phenytoin, Warfarin, and Macrolide and Quinolone antibiotics are not removed.*

COMPLICATIONS OF RRT

Complications of RRT relate to venous access, the extra-corporeal circuit, and the replacement therapy itself:

- *Haemorrhage*
- *Infection (catheter-related bloodstream infection)*
- *Air emboli*
- *Hypothermia*
- *Platelet consumption and coagulation abnormalities*
- *Electrolyte abnormalities*
- *Haemodynamic instability*

CONTINUOUS vs INTERMITTENT RRT

RRT can be performed continuously or intermittently.

The principal difference **is the speed at which water and wastes are removed.**

- **With intermittent techniques** (e.g. intermittent haemodialysis (IntHD)):
  - Patients are connected to a renal replacement circuit **for 3–5h per session**.
  - Typically, patients require 2 - 3 sessions per week but this can vary.
  - Large volumes of fluid and solute can be removed in a short period of time using IntHD.
- **With continuous techniques** (e.g. continuous renal replacement therapy (CRRT)): Patients are connected to the circuit for several days at a time.

HAEMODIALYSIS vs HAEMOFILTRATION

Both haemodialysis and haemofiltration involve blood being removed from the body and pumped in an extracorporeal circuit through a filter (artificial kidney) that is composed of small hollow fibres to maximize the surface area in contact with the blood flowing within them.

Haemofiltration uses hydrostatic pressure in the circuit to drive fluid across the semi-permeable membrane of the fibres, and into bags that are then removed.

This is termed **ultrafiltration** and is similar to what happens at the glomerulus.

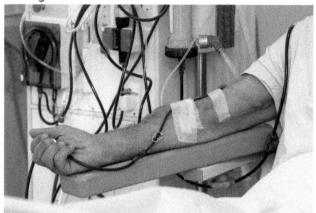

The physical process in ultrafiltration is **convection.**

Large molecules (approximately >50KDa) cannot pass through the membrane, but smaller solutes are pulled through with the fluid (termed solvent drag).

Exogenous fluid is then added to the circuit after the filter to achieve the required fluid balance. Thus, a haemofiltration rate of 1L/h means that 1L of fluid is filtered from the patient's blood and eliminated in the drainage fluid and 1L of replacement fluid is returned to the circuit before it reaches the patient to achieve neutral fluid balance.

The filtration fraction (fraction of 'water' removed from blood) is optimal at about 20–25%.

Haemodialysis also involves a semipermeable membrane but uses a dialysis fluid (**dialysate**) on the other side from the blood. Solutes move across the membrane according to their concentration gradient (Fick's law of diffusion).

The dialysate is a crystalloid solution in which the concentrations of the various solutes have been carefully chosen. The dialysis fluid usually flows in the opposite direction to the blood (counter current) in order to maximize the concentration gradient along the length of the filter.

Both principles can be utilized at the same time in haemo-diafiltration, and this is particularly useful for the clearance of small solutes.

1. HEMODIALYSIS

PRINCIPLES OF HEMODIALYSIS

Hemodialysis, simply stated, consists of the perfusion of blood and a physiologic solution on opposite sides of a semipermeable membrane. Multiple substances, such as water, urea, creatinine, uremic toxins, and drugs, move from the blood into the dialysate, by either passive diffusion or convection as the result of ultrafiltration.

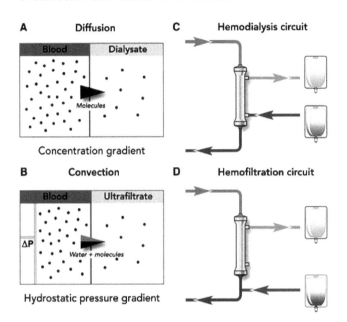

Diffusion is the movement of substances down a concentration gradient, usually for endogenous waste products from the blood to dialysate. The rate of diffusion depends on the difference between the concentration of the solute in blood and dialysate, solute characteristics (i.e., size, water solubility, and charge), the dialyzer membrane composition, and blood and dialysate flow rates. Diffusive transport is rapid for small solutes but slows with increasing molecular size. Other important diffusive solute transport factors include the membrane thickness, porosity, and the steric hindrance between the membrane pores and solute.

Ultrafiltration is the movement of water across the dialyzer membrane as a consequence of hydrostatic or osmotic pressure and is the primary means for removal of excess body water.

Convection occurs when dissolved solutes are "dragged" across a membrane with fluid transport (if the pores in the dialyzer are large enough to allow them to pass). Convection can be maximized by increasing the hydrostatic pressure gradient across the dialysis membrane, or by changing to a dialyzer that is more permeable to water transport.

These two processes of diffusion and convection can be controlled independently; thus, a patient's HD prescription can be individualized to attain the desired degree of solute and fluid removal.

ADVANTAGES

1. Higher solute clearance allows intermittent treatment.
2. Parameters of adequacy of dialysis are better defined and therefore underdialysis can be detected early.
3. Technique failure rate is low.
4. Even though intermittent heparinization is required, hemostasis parameters are better corrected with hemodialysis than with peritoneal dialysis.
5. In-center hemodialysis enables closer monitoring of the patient.

DISADVANTAGES

1. Requires multiple visits each week to the hemodialysis center, which translates into loss of patient independence.
2. Disequilibrium, dialysis-induced hypotension, and muscle cramps are common. May require months before the patient adjusts to hemodialysis.
3. Infections in hemodialysis patients may be related to the choice of membranes, the complement-activating membranes being more deleterious.
4. Vascular access is frequently associated with infection and thrombosis.
5. Decline of residual renal function is more rapid compared with peritoneal dialysis.

HEMODIALYSIS ACCESS

Obtaining and maintaining access to the circulation has been a challenge for long-term use and success of HD. Permanent access to the circulation may be accomplished by several techniques, including the creation of an **AV fistula** or an **AV graft** or by the use of **venous catheters**.

1. AV FISTULA

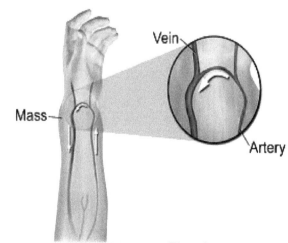

Arteriovenous Fistula

The native AV fistula is created by the anastomosis of a vein and artery (ideally the radial artery and cephalic vein in the forearm).

Advantages:

- Fistulas have the longest survival of all blood-access devices,
- Are associated with the lowest rate of complications such as infection and thrombosis,
- Increased survival and lower hospitalization rates compared with other HD patients,
- AV fistulas is the most cost-effective in terms of placement and long-term maintenance.

Ideally, the most distal site (the wrist) is used to construct the fistula. This fistula is the easiest to create, and in the case of access failure, more proximal sites on the arm are preserved.

Disadvantages:

- Fistulas require 1 to 2 months or more to mature before they can be routinely utilized for dialysis.
- Creation of an AV fistula may be difficult in elderly patients and in patients with peripheral vascular disease (which is particularly common in patients with diabetes).

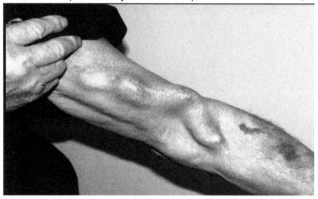

2. ARTERIOVENOUS GRAFT

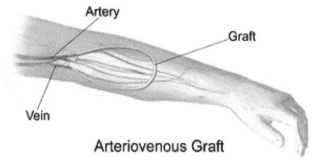

Arteriovenous Graft

The first primary arteriovenous fistula is usually created by the surgical anastomosis of the cephalic vein with the radial artery.

The flow of blood from the higher-pressure arterial system results in hypertrophy of the vein.

The most common AV graft is between the brachial artery and the basilic or cephalic vein. The flow of blood may be diminished in the radial and ulnar arteries since it preferentially flows into the low-pressure graft.

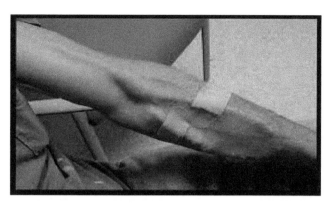

Synthetic AV grafts, usually made of polytetrafluoroethylene, are another option for permanent AV access.

In general, grafts require only 2 to 3 weeks to endothelialize before they can be routinely used.

Disadvantages

- Shorter survival of the grafts,
- Higher rates of infection and thrombosis than do AV fistulas.

3. TUNNELLED OR CENTRAL VENOUS LINES

The least-desirable HD access is via **central venous catheters**, which, unfortunately, are commonly used in chronic HD patients. Venous catheters can be placed in the femoral, subclavian, or internal jugular vein.

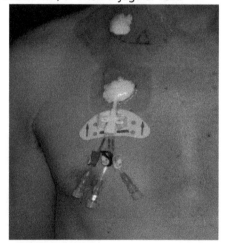

Advantages:

- Can be used immediately.
- Catheters are often used in small children, diabetic patients with severe vascular disease, the morbidly obese, and other patients who have no viable sites for permanent AV access.

Disadvantages:

- Have a short life span and
- Are more prone to infection and thrombosis than either AV grafts or fistulas.
- Some catheters are not able to provide adequate blood flow rates, which can limit the dose of dialysis delivered.

COMPLICATIONS OF HEMODIALYSIS

The most common complications that occur during the HD procedure include:

- Hypotension,
- Cramps,
- Nausea and Vomiting,
- Headache,
- Chest pain,
- Back pain, and
- Fever or chills
- **Vascular access complications (Fistula complications):**
  - Haemorrhage
  - Infection
  - Thrombosis
  - Stenosis
  - Aneurysm

MANAGEMENT OF HD COMPLICATIONS

1. Hemorrhage

- Direct Pressure
- Topical Hemostatic Agents:
  - Gelfoam
  - Thrombin – Recombinant human thrombin (rhThrombin)
  - Reversal of Supra-Therapeutic Anticoagulation – Heparin is commonly used in dialysis centers.
  - Pharmacotherapy – Desmopressin (DDAVP)

2. Infection

The most common infecting organism in the HD population is **Staphylococcus aureus**, followed by **Staphylococcus epidermidis and gram-negative bacteria**.

- Blood cultures
- Intravenous antibiotics:
  - Vancomycin (15mg/kg or 1g IV).
  - Gentamicin (100mg IV initially and after each dialysis treatment) should be given if an infection with gram-negative organisms is suspected.
- Admit
- **Ultrasound** should be utilized to differentiate fistula infection from infected thrombus, local abscess, or infected hematoma which require vascular surgery consultation and oftentimes surgical management.

3. Fistula Stenosis

Stenosis and thrombosis are the most common complications of AV fistulas.

In the ED, Doppler US may be utilized for the assessment of vascular flow. **Vascular surgery should be consulted** for patients presenting to the emergency department with the aforementioned symptomatology, as percutaneous transluminal angioplasty is the treatment of choice.

4. Fistula Thrombosis

AV fistula thrombosis is quickly identified **by examining the fistula site for the absence of a bruit and thrill**.

In the case of thrombosis, **vascular surgery** should be consulted immediately.

5. Fistula Aneurysm or Pseudoaneurysm

Both AV fistula aneurysm and pseudoaneurysms can be identified with the use of Doppler US.

Vascular surgery should be consulted for all detected vessel irregularities for consideration for operative repair.

2. PERITONEAL DIALYSIS

PRINCIPLES OF PERITONEAL DIALYSIS

The three basic components of HD—namely, a blood-filled compartment separated from a dialysate-filled compartment by a semipermeable membrane—are also present in PD.

In PD, the dialysate-filled compartment is the peritoneal cavity, into which dialysate is instilled via a peritoneal catheter that traverses the abdominal wall.

The contiguous peritoneal membrane surrounds the peritoneal cavity.

The cavity, which normally contains about 100 mL of lipid-rich lubricating fluid, can expand to a capacity of several liters. The peritoneal membrane that lines the cavity functions as the semipermeable membrane, across which diffusion and ultrafiltration occur.

The membrane is classically described as a monocellular layer of peritoneal mesothelial cells. However, the dialyzing membrane is also composed of the basement membrane and underlying connective and interstitial tissue.

The peritoneal membrane has a total area that approximates body surface area (approximately 1 to 2 m^2).

Blood vessels supplying and draining the abdominal viscera, musculature, and mesentery constitute the blood-filled compartment.

Unlike HD, the crucial components of peritoneal dialysis are unable to be manipulated to maximize solute and fluid removal.

Because the blood is not in intimate contact with the dialysis membrane as it is in HD, metabolic waste products must travel a considerable distance to the dialysate-filled compartment. In addition, unlike HD, there is no easy method to regulate blood flow to the surface of the peritoneal membrane, nor is there a countercurrent flow of blood and dialysate to increase diffusion and ultrafiltration via changes in hydrostatic pressure.

Similarly, there is no easy means to modify the permeability of peritoneal membrane; most of the control in dialysis dosing during peritoneal dialysis thus involves alterations in dialysate volume, dwell time, and the number of exchanges per day.

For these reasons, PD is a much less efficient process per unit time as compared with HD, and must, therefore, be a virtually continuous procedure to achieve acceptable goals for clearance of metabolic waste products.

ADVANTAGES

1. Hemodynamic stability due to slow ultrafiltration rate.
2. Higher clearance of larger solutes, which may explain good clinical status in spite of lower urea clearance.
3. Better preservation of residual renal function.
4. Convenient intraperitoneal route for administration of drugs such as antibiotics and insulin.
5. Suitable for elderly and very young patients who may not tolerate hemodialysis well.
6. Freedom from the "machine" giving the patient a sense of independence (for continuous ambulatory peritoneal dialysis).
7. Less blood loss and iron deficiency, resulting in easier management of anemia or reduced requirements for erythropoietin and parenteral iron.
8. No systemic heparinization required.
9. Subcutaneous versus intravenous erythropoietin or darbepoetin is usual, which may reduce overall doses and be more physiologic.

DISADVANTAGES

1. Protein and amino acid losses through peritoneum and reduced appetite owing to continuous glucose load and sense of abdominal fullness predispose to malnutrition.
2. Risk of peritonitis.
3. Catheter malfunction, exit site, and tunnel infection.
4. Inadequate ultrafiltration and solute dialysis in patients with a large body size, unless large volumes and frequent exchanges are employed.
5. Patient burnout and high rate of technique failure.
6. Risk of obesity with excessive glucose absorption.
7. Mechanical problems such as hernias, dialysate leaks, hemorrhoids, or back pain more common than with HD.
8. Extensive abdominal surgery may preclude peritoneal dialysis.
9. No convenient access for intravenous iron administration

PERITONEAL DIALYSIS ACCESS

Access to the peritoneal cavity is via the placement of an **indwelling catheter**. Most catheters are manufactured from Silastic, which is soft, flexible, and biocompatible.

A typical adult catheter is 40 to 45 cm long, 20 to 22 cm of which are inside the peritoneal cavity.

Placement of the catheter is such that the distal end lies low in a pelvic gutter.

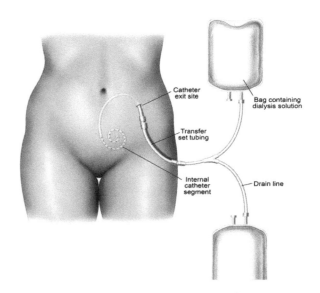

PERITONEAL DIALYSIS PROCEDURES

Several variants of PD are clinically utilized. All variants of PD require the placement of a dialysis solution to dwell in the peritoneal cavity for some period, removing the spent dialysate, and then repeating the process.

The prescribed dose of PD may be altered by changing the number of exchanges per day, by altering the volume of each exchange, or by altering the strength of dextrose in the dialysate for some or all exchanges.

Increasing any one of these variables increases the effective osmotic gradient across the peritoneum, leading to increased ultrafiltration and diffusion (solute removal). If the dwell time is extended, equilibrium may be reached, after which time there will be no further water or solute removal. In fact, after a critical period, reverse water movement may occur.

Continuous ambulatory peritoneal dialysis (CAPD) involves performing the dialysate exchanges manually, whereas automated systems, collectively termed **automated peritoneal dialysis (APD)**, perform the exchanges with a device referred to as a cycler. APD systems are designed for patients who are unable or unwilling to perform the necessary aseptic manipulations, and for those who require more dialysis. APD provides an automated cycler that performs the exchanges. The device is set up in the evening, and the patient attaches the peritoneal catheter to it at bedtime. The machine performs several short-dwell exchanges (usually 1 to 2 hours) during the night. This permits a long cycle-free daytime dwell of up to 12 to 14 hours. Typical APD regimens involve total 24-hour exchanges of approximately 12 L, which include one or more daytime dwells.

This type of regimen is sometimes referred to as APD with a **"wet" day**.

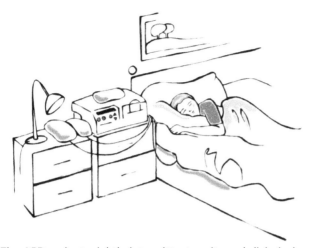

The APD variant, nightly intermittent peritoneal dialysis, has a similar theme, except that the peritoneal cavity tends to be dialysate free during the day. This type of regimen is frequently referred to as APD with a **"dry" day**.

A number of variants exist and depend largely on equipment availability, patient and prescriber preference, and whether the patient retains any residual renal function, which influences the quantity of dialysis prescribed.

In a basic CAPD system, the patient or caregiver is manually responsible for performing the prescribed number of dialysate exchanges. The patient is connected to a bag of prewarmed peritoneal dialysate via the PD catheter by a length of tubing called a transfer set. The most common transfer set used is the **Y transfer set.**

This consists of a Y-shaped piece of tubing that is attached at its stem to the patient's catheter, leaving the remaining two limbs of the Y attached to dialysate bags, one filled with fresh dialysate and the other empty.

The spent dialysate from the previous dwell is drained into the empty bag, and the peritoneum is subsequently refilled from the bag containing fresh dialysate.

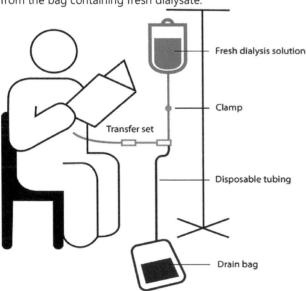

The Y set is then disconnected, and the bag containing the spent fluid and the empty bag that had contained fresh dialysate are detached and discarded. Typically, a patient instills 2 to 3 L of dialysate three times during the day, with each exchange lasting 4 to 6 hours, and then a single dialysate exchange overnight lasting 8 to 12 hours.

At the end of the prescribed dwell period a new Y set is attached and the process is repeated. The process of outflow, aseptic manipulation of the administration set and catheter, and inflow requires a total time of approximately 30 minutes.

COMPLICATIONS OF PERITONEAL DIALYSIS
1. Medical Complications of PD

Cause	Complication	Treatment
Glucose load	Exacerbation of Diabetes Mellitus	Intraperitoneal (IP) insulin
Fluid overload	Exacerbation of CCF Edema Pulmonary congestion	Increase ultrafiltration Diuretics, if the patient has residual renal function
Electrolyte abnormalities	Hypercalcemia Hypocalcemia	Alter dialysate calcium content
PD additives	Chemical peritonitis	Discontinue PD additives
Malnutrition	Albumin loss	Dietary changes
	Loss of amino acids	Parenteral nutrition
	Muscle wasting	Discontinue PD
	Increased adipose tissue	
Unknown	Fibrin formation in dialysate	IP heparin

2. PD PERITONITIS
Peritonitis is a major cause of catheter loss in PD patients.

CLINICAL PRESENTATION AND DIAGNOSIS OF PERITONEAL DIALYSIS–RELATED PERITONITIS

General
- Patients generally present with abdominal pain and cloudy effluent.

Symptoms
- The patient may complain of abdominal tenderness, abdominal pain, fever, nausea and vomiting, and chills.

Signs
- Cloudy dialysate effluent may be observed.
- Temperature may or may not be elevated.

Laboratory Tests
- Dialysate white blood cell count >100/mm^3 (>0.1 × 10^9/L), of which at least 50% are polymorphonuclear neutrophils
- Gram stain of a centrifuged dialysate specimen

Other Diagnostic Tests
- Culture and sensitivity of dialysate should be obtained.

MANAGEMENT OF PD PERITONITIS

- **Intraperitoneal antibiotics** are the first line treatment in patients suspected of having PD peritonitis.
- **Involve the renal team early** as they should be responsible for administering the antibiotics.
- A typical regime would be **intraperitoneal Vancomycin** and **Gentamicin and/or oral Ciprofloxacin.**
- Choice of empiric treatment should be made based on the dialysis center's and the patient's history of infecting organisms and their sensitivities.
- Final choice of therapy should always be guided by culture and sensitivity results.
- Intraperitoneal (IP) administration of antibiotics remains the preferred route over IV therapy.

3. CATHETER-SITE INFECTIONS

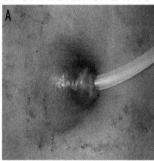
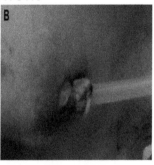

Topical antibiotics and disinfectants appear to be effective agents for the prevention of exit-site infections.

Gram-positive organisms should be treated with oral penicillinase-resistant penicillin or a first-generation cephalosporin such as **cephalexin.**

Rifampin may be added if necessary, in slowly resolving or particularly severe *S. aureus* infections.

Vancomycin should be avoided in routine or empiric treatment of gram-positive catheter-related infections, but it will be necessary for methicillin-resistant *S. aureus*.

Gram-negative organisms should be treated with **oral quinolones**. The effectiveness of oral quinolones may be diminished owing to the chelation drug interactions with divalent and trivalent metal ions, which are commonly taken by dialysis patients. Administration of quinolones should occur at least 2 hours prior to these drugs.

In cases where *Pseudomonas aeruginosa* is the pathogen, a second antipseudomonal drug should be added. **IP ceftazidime** may be considered.

In all cases antibiotics should be continued until the exit site appears normal; 2 to 3 weeks of therapy may be necessary. A patient with a catheter-related infection that progresses to peritonitis will usually require catheter removal.

3. COMMON COMPLICATIONS OF ESRD

MANAGEMENT OF THE SICK DIALYSIS/END-STAGE RENAL DISEASE (ESRD) PATIENT

Case 1
You receive a call from the charge nurse who says you have a new patient in major area. He is here with generalized weakness. The patient is being hooked up to the monitor and the HR is 38. The BP is pending. The patient's family looks concerned due to the low heart rate alarm. Two nurses are looking at you for orders. You ask for atropine as your attending walks into the room.

Case 2
An hour later, your SHO is assigned a patient brought in by EMS complaining of difficulty breathing. The patient is speaking in full sentences but is very tachypneic. You decide to help your SHO and bring in the ultrasound. You notice B-lines, then get a phone call and have to step away from the room. You first relay this information to your SHO, and you both agree it likely represents volume overload from a missed dialysis session. After you are done with your phone call, you hear assistance is required in room 5, and you rush over to see what is happening with the patient.

1. Cardiopulmonary

1.1. Cardiac tamponade
- It is a life-threatening disease that an ED doctor should be mindful of in the patient with hypotension and dyspnea.
- **Assuming the patient's dyspnea is from a missed dialysis session or the natural course of the patient's disease is a common pitfall.**
- One should also be mindful that Beck's triad (hypotension, distended neck veins, muffled heart sounds) is only seen in a minority of cardiac tamponade cases and this applies even more to ESRD patients.
- A quick **bedside ultrasound** can detect a significant pericardial effusion and essentially exclude the diagnosis if normal.
- **A chest x-ray** may also show an enlarging heart size when compared to a previous chest x-ray.
- Electrical alternans on **ECG** would also clue in the ED physician of significant pericardial effusion, however, its absence does not rule out an effusion.
- If this diagnosis is identified, **cardiology or cardiothoracic surgery consultation** should be obtained immediately.
  - If the patient is hypotensive, **IV fluids** should be provided.
  - If the patient is in a peri-arrest state, then the ED physician should perform a **pericardiocentesis**.

1.2. Ischaemic Heart Disease

- Chest pain is also a common complaint, and it is estimated that ischemic heart disease accounts for approximately 50% of deaths in ESRD patients.
- While ESRD patients generally have abnormal ECGs, new ST changes should be acted on immediately.
- Troponin elevation can occur due to reduced renal clearance. However, **previous troponin levels should be compared** and elevated troponin should not be automatically attributed to ESRD.
- If the ESRD patient has acute coronary syndrome, **no dose adjustments are required for aspirin, clopidogrel, heparin, or thrombolytics** if they are being considered. However, if **enoxaparin is to be started, dosage adjustments are required.**

1.3. Hyperkalaemia

- In the setting of cardiac arrest, **hyperkalemia** should be the first of the "Hs and Ts" on the differential.
- This can be treated with **calcium gluconate or calcium chloride** and **sodium bicarbonate**.
- A stat VBG/ABG can confirm hyperkalemia. Otherwise, the patient should be treated as any patient with cardiac arrest without a history of ESRD.
- Common ECG changes of hyperkalemia classically occur in a progressive fashion:
  - Peaked or tall T waves,
  - Shortening QT interval,
  - Lengthening of the PR segment,
  - Followed by widening of the QRS wave that eventually turns into a "sine wave."
- ECG alone should never be used to rule out hyperkalemia. Furthermore, ECG changes do not correlate with the patient's potassium level. Unexplained rhythm abnormalities should be considered as hyperkalemia in the HD patient until proven otherwise.

1.4. Pulmonary Edema

- The most common cause of dyspnea in dialysis patients is **pulmonary edema** or volume overload.
- The patient may have missed dialysis, have uncontrolled high blood pressure, ignored dietary restrictions, or have underlying systolic dysfunction.
- Brain natriuretic peptide (BNP) is **not a reliable serum marker for diagnosing heart failure as it is usually elevated in this population**.
- Inquiring about missed dialysis, dietary indiscretions, and especially any recent weight gains can clue the ED physician that volume overload may be the cause of the patient's dyspnea.
- If IV access is problematic and the patient is normotensive, **sublingual nitroglycerin and non-invasive ventilation** can reduce pre- and afterload.

- Once IV access is obtained, a **nitroglycerin infusion** can be started. Ultimately, these measures only provide symptomatic relief and urgent hemodialysis should be arranged for the patient.
- Vascular access is also a common problem in dialysis patients.
- The hemodialysis access site should not be used except as a last resort in critical situations.
- Blood pressure recording is also contraindicated over the access site.

2. Pharmacology

ESRD patients typically have some degree of anemia due to a **deficiency in erythropoietin** produced by the kidney.

- **If blood transfusion is required, it should occur during dialysis** to correct for the extra volume as well as potassium changes.
- If analgesia is required, NSAIDs agents should be avoided.
- **Opioids** such as morphine and hydromorphone should be started at a dose reduced by approximately 50%.
- Most antibiotics are efficacious and may require dosage adjustment, but **nitrofurantoin should be avoided**.
- If the ESRD patient **requires contrast for radiographic evaluation, the ED physician can order the necessary studies without concern for renal injury**.
- If a decision is made to intubate a HD patient, **succinylcholine should be avoided** if the potassium level is not yet known.
- Succinylcholine causes potassium efflux after binding to skeletal nicotinic receptors, thus causing a rise in potassium.
- While this rise in potassium is usually inconsequential, this rise from succinylcholine can cause **dysrhythmia in patients with hyperkalemia**.
- **Rocuronium** is the RSI paralytic of choice.

3. Infectious Disease

- Patients on dialysis are **immunosuppressed,** making infection a common concern.
- Clinical presentations for common infectious diseases are **not always straightforward**, i.e. patients may only complain of generalised weakness or fatigue and can be afebrile.

3.1. Access site infection

- **Infection of the access site** is a common complication.
- Patients with catheters are at increased risk compared to patients with fistulas.

3.2. Endocarditis

- If a new murmur is detected on your physical exam in the setting of fever, one must consider **endocarditis**.

3.3. Discitis or osteomyelitis
o Patients with back pain without apparent cause raise the possibility of **discitis or osteomyelitis** due to hematogenous spread

3.4. UTI
o **Urinary tract infections** have been diagnosed in dialysis patients who are essentially anuric as well.

- ESRD patients with fever should get a FBC, chest x-ray, and 2 sets of blood cultures prior to antibiotic therapy.
- If there is concern for an infection at the access site, the **catheter should be removed and sent for culture.**
- Patients with suspected infection should be admitted and have **empiric antibiotic therapy covering for both MRSA and gram-negative organisms** started.

3.5. Peritonitis
- For patients with continuous ambulatory peritoneal dialysis (CAPD), **peritonitis** is a common cause of fever.
- Common symptoms include diffuse abdominal pain/tenderness, cloudy dialysate, with nausea and/or vomiting.
- The most common organisms are **Strep and Staph** species. However, one study reported 15-20% **gram-negative organisms** as well as another 15-20% culture negative.
- If one suspects CAPD-associated peritonitis, the dialysate should be sent for **WBC count with differential, gram stain, and culture.**
- Gram stains are usually negative, but still should be performed as it may show the presence of yeast.
- If yeast is detected, antifungal therapy should be initiated and the catheter removed.
- Fungal and mycobacterial species have been isolated in about 1-2% of CAPD-associated peritonitis.
- WBC count greater than **100/uL with > 50% PMNs suggests peritonitis.**
- Begin empiric antibiotic therapy to cover gram positive and gram-negative organisms.
- The preferred route of administration is **intraperitoneal** as it is superior to intravenous administration.

4. Neurology
- Neurologic complaints such as headache, confusion, and altered mental status (AMS) are common.

4.1. Dialysis Disequilibrium Syndrome (DDS)
- The most common cause is **dialysis disequilibrium syndrome (DDS)**, which is thought to occur from removal of blood urea nitrogen and other uremic wastes during HD. This subsequently leads to a decrease in serum osmolality and water to shift into brain tissue, causing **cerebral edema.**

- A clue that DDS is the cause of the patient's headache is if the patient's symptoms started **during or shortly after HD.**
- Treatment is supportive, with the nephrologist making adjustments such as a shorter hemodialysis session.

4.2. Intracranial Hemorrhage
- Other causes of headache and AMS include **intracranial hemorrhage** made more likely by platelet dysfunction.
- **Subdural hematomas** occur 10 times more frequently in HD patients than the general population.
- **Subdural hematomas** can be bilateral and can occur without any focal deficits.

4.3. Strokes
- Strokes are also common in HD patients with 52% of these being hemorrhagic. Therefore, neuroimaging should be considered in all HD patients presenting with headache or AMS.

5. BLEEDING FISTULA, GRAFT& LINES
A 68-year-old man is being conveyed from his own home in a blue light ambulance. He has end-stage renal disease of unknown aetiology and receives haemodialysis 3 times weekly. He had an uneventful dialysis session this morning but since returning home his fistula has started to bleed. The paramedics have applied a bandage and pressure but the bleeding appears to have continued unabated. You have 5 minutes to prepare yourself before the patient arrives.

The following preparatory steps should be taken:
1. Plan to receive the patient in the resuscitation room if at all possible
2. Ensure you have enough pairs of hands - you will need a nurse and a second pair of hands as a minimum
3. This may well get messy - make sure everyone is wearing appropriate PPE (eye and face protection, apron, gloves etc.)
4. Consider giving the renal and vascular team the heads up.

GOLDEN RULES WHEN DEALING WITH GRAFTS AND FISTULA:
- As a general rule, try not to touch a renal patient's access site unless the patient is in extremis - do not take blood from them and do not administer drugs or fluids via them
- Do not use a blood pressure cuff or tourniquet on the same arm as the graft/ fistula - you risk clotting the access
- Always remember that a dialysis patients access site is their lifeline - it is a complete disaster for them to lose their access.

If a patient is **in extremis** and you are considering using their fistula to gain circulatory access, please consider the following:

- Is there really no alternative? (What about ultrasound guided peripheral access or an intraosseous line?)
- Do not use a tourniquet
- Clean the site really, really well
- Avoid puncturing the back wall of the vessel
- Secure the IV catheter in VERY carefully
- Remember you are dealing with a high-pressure system – you will need a pressure bag in order to get fluid into the patient
- Document the presence of a thrill before and after the procedure
- 10-15 minutes of firm pressure will be required on removal of the catheter

The patient arrives and is still bleeding copiously. He is accompanied by 2 stressed looking paramedics.
How do you proceed?

- Get the patient onto a resus bed and whilst the nurses apply monitoring, prepare to examine the fistula,
- Remove the bandage and identify the bleeding point. Press firmly with one finger onto the exact site of bleeding (whilst this sounds obvious, it is often done really poorly. A bandage will likely do nothing to control bleeding and neither will diffusely applied pressure. It really does need to be: one finger, pressing hard at the exact point at where the fistula is spurting).
- A temporising measure (especially if short of hands) may be to **place a gallipot** over the bleeding fistula and secure it firmly with tape.

What are your options now?

- Ensure someone keeps single finger pressure on whilst heads are scratched and specialists consulted
- If the patient has recently dialysed, consider applying **protamine-soaked gauze** to the bleeding fistula
- Consider using a **haemostatic aid** such as Gelfoam if you have it available.
- If the patient has any other bleeding tendency (including anticoagulants and anti-platelet drugs), **speak to the haematologists early**. Remember that all renal patients are likely to bleed like mad – they are anti-coagulated during dialysis, have poorly functioning platelets and an elevated bleeding time secondary to uraemia.

- **Involve a vascular surgeon early** – it may be that the fistula needs to be sutured if usual measures fail
- Applying a tourniquet is an absolute last resort. It will work but will almost certainly result in thrombosis formation and failure of the fistula.

- *It goes without saying that if the patient is shocked, they should be resuscitated in the usual manner.*
- *The ultimate aim is to stop the bleeding without clotting off the fistula. The least invasive way possible of controlling the haemorrhage should be used.*
- *In a dialysis patient, it is no under-statement to say that the patient's access is their lifeline. These access sites should be treated with respect at all times.*
- *There are 3 main categories of access that you may come across (graft, fistula and line) and it is important to be able to tell the difference as they have different properties and susceptibility to problems*

You are informed by the nurse in charge that a patient is being sent in from the local dialysis centre. You are accompanied by a keen medical student who wants to know what general questions you should ask when seeing a haemodialysis patient.

How do you answer them?
Haemodialysis – questions to ask in the history

- What sort of access do they have (fistula/ graft/ tunnelled line) and have they had problems with dialysis access in the past?
- How frequently and for how many hours do they dialyse? Most people (unless on home dialysis) dialyse 3 times a week on set days e.g. Monday, Wednesday, Friday.
- When did they last dialyse? This helps predict what the problem might be e.g. if it is a Monday and they last dialysed on Friday they are much more at risk of fluid overload and hyperkalaemia.
- Take a detailed fluid balance history – what is their dry weight (a clinical estimate of their weight when they are euvolaemic), what is their fluid restriction, how much fluid is normally removed at dialysis and do they still make any urine?
- How has dialysis been going recently?
- Have they had any technical problems or felt unwell on dialysis?
- Are they on the transplant list?

Case Conclusion

Case 1:

Your attending somehow immediately knew the patient was a dialysis patient. She asks for an amp of calcium gluconate and sodium bicarbonate while ordering your RT to get a VBG with stat K. The patient's K+ is 8.2 and you order 10 units of insulin with 2 amps of D50, a salbutamol 5mg neb, and you get the patient's nephrologist on the phone to arrange emergent dialysis. Because the patient will receive dialysis within an hour, you convince the nephrologist to hold off on sodium polystyrene. Prior to the patient leaving the ED, you see the patient's HR is now in the 70s. The patient is dialyzed and eventually leaves the hospital without any neurologic deficits.

Case 2:

The patient's vital signs are BP 84/50, HR 119, RR 30 with O2 sat of 96% on 2L NC. No JVD is apparent, but you decide to perform a bedside ECHO to rule out tamponade. An obvious pericardial effusion with paradoxical septal wall motion is present and your co-resident orders a one-liter bolus and cancels the nitroglycerin order. The patient's BP improves after the IVF and the cardiothoracic surgeon is called in for an emergent pericardial window.

6. HYPOTENSION & DIALYSIS

The paramedics have subsequently phoned through to say the patient is a 46-year-old who has become hypotensive during her dialysis session.

Please give an initial, broad differential diagnosis:

1. *Fluid shifts (removal of too much fluid or fluid removed too quickly)*
2. *Sepsis*
3. *Bleeding*
4. *Cardiac tamponade*
5. *Arrhythmia (due to potassium shifts for example)*
6. *Hypersensitivity reaction – allergic or anaphylactic*
7. *Acute coronary syndrome*
8. *Air embolism*
9. *Dialysis hypotensive syndrome*

The following questions will help you work out a potential aetiology:

- Was the patient unwell beforehand? (any symptoms suggestive of infection or tamponade)
- At what point during dialysis did the patient become hypotensive? (e.g. at the beginning of dialysis, hyperkalaemia is more likely, e.g. at the end of dialysis, hypotension due to fluid shifts is more likely)
- Does the patient have any symptoms of infection? (fever, malaise, systemic upset or focal symptoms of infection)
- Is there any evidence of bleeding? (obvious bleeding site, signs of shock)

- Are they any symptoms or signs of an allergic reaction? (rash, wheeze, breathlessness)
- Are there symptoms or signs suggestive of an air embolism? (e.g. chest pain, breathlessness, hypoxia, tachycardia if the embolus travels to the heart or lungs. Syncope or seizures if the embolus travels to the brain)
- Are there any symptoms indicative of a cardiac cause – ACS, Arrhythmia, Tamponade? (chest pain, palpitations, breathlessness)
- Investigation will clearly be guided by the history and examination findings. Specific tests helpful in particular contexts are discussed further below

THINGS YOU SHOULD DEFINITELY DO:

↓ *Search for a source of infection (e.g. CXR)*
↓ *Culture the patient*
↓ *Administer broad spectrum antibiotics as soon as possible (aiming for < 1 hour as per national sepsis guidelines)*

THINGS YOU PROBABLY SHOULDN'T DO:

- Immediately remove the tunnelled line
- Catheterise the patient
- Give the patient a stat one litre fluid bolus
- Insert a central line

- **Sepsis** is the second most common cause of death in ESRD patients (**cardiac causes** are the commonest).
- Mortality is higher in ESRD patients compared with the general population.
- Generally, it should be treated as per national sepsis guidance with prompt administration of antibiotics.
- Patients should be cultured prior to receiving antibiotics and a lactate measured (although the lactate may have been removed if they have dialysed recently).
- Patients with ESRD pass little or no urine and there is therefore little point in catheterising.
- Cautious administration of crystalloids in 250ml aliquots is sensible followed by reassessment after each bolus.
- **Antibiotics** can generally be given as per local guidance but may need to be dose adjusted for the renal function.
- Involve a renal physician or microbiologist if unsure. Remember that nephrotoxic antibiotics can't make things worse if the patient has no preserved renal function but care should be taken if the patient has any preserved renal function.

- Any residual renal function is very important to a haemodialysis patient (as it may mean that their daily fluid restriction can be slightly less severe) so **nephrotoxic medications** should still be avoided in dialysis patients who report that they still pass urine in less critical circumstances.
- If the patient is very unwell then a risk/benefit assessment may suggest nephrotoxic antibiotics are indicated even if there is a degree of preserved renal function.
- Dialysis patients require careful assessment of their **fluid balance** – however a central line is rarely required to guide fluid resuscitation.
- Every effort should be made to preserve future potential access sites and putting in a central line is a potential risk to this. If a line or graft infection is suspected, every effort should still be made to preserve the access site. The only exception would be a patient who is critically ill – access removal should be considered but would be a decision to be made jointly with the renal and critical care teams.
- *Do not be frightened to give septic patients with ESRF fluids – just be aware of the difficulties and the need for frequent assessment.*
- *Dialyses can remove lactate which may be misleading in the context of sepsis*

POTENTIAL CAUSES OF HYPOTENSION IN A PATIENT HAVING HAEMODIALYSIS:

1. Bleeding
Renal patients have a multitude of reasons to bleed. A bleeding access site will be obvious but they can also bleed into hidden spaces such as intracranially and intra-abdominally. Of note they also have an increased tendency to thromboembolism.

2. Cardiac tamponade
This may be due to bleeding or secondary to uraemia. In any hypotensive patient with ESRD consider an early ultrasound unless there is an obvious alternative cause. Treatment in the compromised patient revolves around optimising right ventricular filling with fluids and pericardiocentesis.
Emergency dialysis is the treatment of choice in uraemic tamponade.

3. Arrhythmia
Electrolyte shifts during dialysis may lead to arrhythmias (**particularly hyperkalaemia**).
A high potassium may also activate an ICCD if the patient has one as the ECG changes may be misinterpreted as VT.

Get an ECG early. It is also useful to know what the patients' potassium usually runs at to see how worried you need to be!

4. Hypersensitivity reaction
This may occur as a reaction against components of the dialysis membrane or to foreign substances in the extra-corporeal circuit.
Standard allergy/ anaphylactic management applies.

5. Acute Coronary Syndrome
Dramatic fluid shifts during haemodialysis inevitably place additional stress on the heart and it is not uncommon to precipitate symptoms of cardiac ischaemia especially as many renal patients have co-existent coronary artery disease. 50% of all deaths in ESRD patients are cardiac in origin.

6. Air embolism
This occurs when air is inadvertently let into the system during dialysis. Symptoms and signs are dependent upon where the embolus goes.
For example, an embolus in the heart or lungs may lead to chest pain and breathlessness. The patient may be hypoxic, tachycardic and hypotensive.
If the embolus travels to the brain the patient may experience seizures, syncope, headache or other neurological symptoms such as ataxia. All of these symptoms may be explained by alternative causes so a high index of suspicion is required. The biggest clue is that the symptoms are temporally related to dialysis. As ED physicians we are unlikely to be there at the exact time of onset.
However, patients are increasingly being dialysed at off-site satellite units and the patients may therefore arrive in the ED shortly afterwards. Management is uncertain but the following are recommended in addition to the usual A, B, C approach.
Put the patient into the **left lateral decubitus position** to try and prevent further propagation of the air through the right side of the heart and into the pulmonary arteries. **Try and suck** any remaining air out of the catheter (hopefully this will have been done by the dialysis team already). If the patient is in cardiac arrest, **chest compressions** may help to break up the embolus. It is worth considering a longer period of resuscitation. As a last-ditch effort, a **thoracotomy** could be considered in order to try and suck air out of the right ventricle

7. Dialysis hypotension Syndrome
Multifactorial and poorly understood.
Not a diagnosis an ED Doctor needs to worry about.

13. Diarrhoea

I. ACUTE BLOODY DIARRHOEA

INTRODUCTION

- Acute bloody diarrhea should be considered a medical emergency. Its causes are frequently serious or actionable or both and are usually identified. However, acute bloody diarrhea as a stand-alone clinical presentation has received little scholarly attention in the past several decades.
- Although the range of possible causes of acute bloody diarrhea is broad, infectious considerations are paramount and should always be prioritized in the evaluation of such patients.[146]

CAUSES OF ACUTE BLOODY DIARRHEA

- **Infectious**
  - Bacteria: Campylobacter jejuni, Salmonella, E coli O157:H7 & selected STEC, V. parahaemolyticus, Shigella, Yersinia, Aeromonas, C difficile
  - Viruses: Cytomegalovirus
  - Parasites: Entamoeba histolytica, Schistosomiasis
- **Ischemic colitis**
- **Inflammatory bowel disease**
- **Diverticulitis**
- **Anatomic gastrointestinal bleeding**
  - Gastric ulcer
  - Angiodysplasia
  - Hemorrhoids
- **Colon cancer**
- **Radiation**
- **Medications**
  - Nonsteroidal anti-inflammatory drugs
  - 5-Flucytosine
  - Chemotherapy
- **Systemic disorders**
  - Amyloidosis
  - Vasculitides
  - Blood dyscrasias (multiple myeloma)
- **Rare causes**
  - Meckel's diverticulum
  - Typhlitis (neutropenic colitis)
  - Intussusception
  - Stercoral ulceration

---

[146] Lori R. Holtz, Marguerite A. Neill, Phillip I. Tarr. *Acute Bloody Diarrhea: A Medical Emergency for Patients of All Ages* [online]

PRACTICAL APPROACHES

- Patients with severe illness who are immunocompromised and have coagulopathy or brisk bleeding are likely to have an anatomic disorder and warrant **hospital admission** for close monitoring.
- Patients admitted to hospital should be placed on contact precautions until it is clear that they are not infected with an enteric pathogen.
- **Stools with pus or mucus and blood** should be sent for bacterial culture; adult stool samples should be handled with the same considerations as those of children.
- **Tests for faecal ova and parasites** should be performed if bacterial cultures and C difficile toxin assays are negative and if the patient has lived or visited areas where amoebiasis or schistosomiasis is endemic.
- In patients known to have IBD, **microbiologic analyses** should be performed if they have flares of unusual severity or do not respond to their usual treatment, because enteric infections can complicate this chronic condition. These patients almost invariably undergo an **abdominal CT scan**, which includes administration of oral contrast that might make subsequent stool specimens difficult to analyse by microscopic or microbiologic evaluation. Plain films have limited usefulness in the evaluation of bloody stools in adults.
- CT scans, to be most helpful, should be performed with oral as well as intravenous contrast; if profound ileus is present, patients can be rescanned a few hours later.
- Although CT scans do not establish a specific cause, they contribute information that can be used to fully assess adults with bloody diarrhoea, such as anatomic localization and extent of bowel involvement (diverticulitis or bowel-wall thickening), complications such as perforation (free air) or pneumatosis coli, and occasionally, vascular thrombosis. A colonoscopic biopsy can detect infections that are unexpected (e.g., schistosomiasis) or that cannot be diagnosed with other tests (e.g., cytomegalovirus colitis); both are treatable entities. In addition, the biopsy can differentiate acute self-limited (probably infectious) colitis from IBD. However, the diagnostic yield from a biopsy should be considered against the risk of perforation; a biopsy can often be deferred for several days to diminish this risk.

II. PSEUDOMEMBRANOUS COLITIS (C. DIFFICILE)

- Clostridium difficile colitis results from a disturbance of the normal bacterial flora of the colon, colonization by C difficile, and the release of toxins that cause mucosal inflammation and damage.
- Antibiotic therapy is the key factor that alters the colonic flora. C difficile infection (CDI) occurs primarily in hospitalized patients.

SIGNS AND SYMPTOMS

- Symptoms of C difficile colitis often include the following:
  - Mild to moderate watery diarrhea, rarely bloody
  - Cramping abdominal pain
  - Anorexia
  - Malaise
- **Physical examination may reveal the following:**
  - Fever: Especially in more severe cases
  - Dehydration
  - Lower abdominal tenderness
  - Rebound tenderness: Raises the possibility of colonic perforation and peritonitis

DIAGNOSIS

- The diagnosis of C difficile colitis should be suspected in any patient with diarrhea who has received antibiotics within the previous 3 months, has been recently hospitalized, and/or has an occurrence of diarrhea within 48 hours or more after hospitalization.[147]
- In addition, C difficile can be a cause of diarrhea in community dwellers without previous hospitalization or antibiotic exposure.

LABORATORY STUDIES

- **FBC:** Leukocytosis may be present (the levels can be very high in severe infection)
- **U&Es:** Dehydration, anasarca, and electrolyte imbalance may accompany severe disease
- **Albumin levels:** Hypoalbuminemia may accompany severe disease
- **Serum lactate level:** Lactate levels are generally elevated (≥5 mmol/L) in severe disease
- **Stool examination:** Stool may be positive for blood in severe colitis, but grossly bloody stools are unusual; fecal leukocytes are present in about half of cases

---

[147] McDonald LC, Coignard B, Dubberke E, Song X, Horan T, Kutty PK. Recommendations for surveillance of Clostridium difficile-associated disease. Infect Control Hosp Epidemiol. 2007 Feb. 28(2):140-5.

IMAGING STUDIES AND PROCEDURES

- **CT Scan Abdomen** is the imaging modality of choice for C difficile colitis when pseudomembranous colitis, complications of CDI, or other intra-abdominal pathology is suspected.
- **PFA:** In patients with sepsis due to suspected megacolon, abdominal radiography may be performed instead of CT scanning to establish the presence of megacolon in a timely manner.
- **Endoscopy**: is less sensitive for diagnosing C difficile than are stool assays. Endoscopy may demonstrate the presence of raised, yellowish white, 2- to 10-mm plaques overlying an erythematous and edematous mucosa.

MANAGEMENT

- Patient with a diagnosis of CDI should have any **precipitating antibiotics discontinued**. If it is not possible to discontinue the precipitating antibiotics immediately then an alternative antibiotic regimen should be considered.
- **All suspected cases must be isolated**
- Treatment for CDI varies according to its severity.
- Interventions include the following:
  - **Asymptomatic carriers:** No treatment is necessary
  - **Mild, antibiotic-associated diarrhea without fever, abdominal pain, or leukocytosis:** Cessation of antibiotic(s) may be the only treatment necessary
  - **Mild to moderate diarrhea or colitis:** oral metronidazole (500 mg PO TDS 10/7) is recommended as the initial treatment or vancomycin PO X 10/7
  - **Severe or complicated disease:** suitable antibiotic regimens include vancomycin (125 mg 4 times daily for 10 days; may be increased to 500 mg 4 times daily) or fidaxomicin (200 mg twice daily for 10 days).
  - **Additional management measures:**
    - Discontinuing unnecessary antimicrobial therapy,
    - Adequate replacement of fluids and electrolytes,
    - Avoiding antimotility medications, and
    - Reviewing the use of proton pump inhibitors.
- Relapse occurs in 20-27% of patients. Once a patient has 1 relapse, the risk for a second relapse is 45%.
- Relapses should be treated as follows:
  - **First relapse:** The choice of antibiotic should be based on the severity of C difficile diarrhea/colitis
  - **Subsequent relapses:** For every relapse after the first, vancomycin or fidaxomicin with or without probiotics is recommended.

III. HEMOLYTIC UREMIC SYNDROME

OVERVIEW

- Hemolytic uremic syndrome (HUS) is a clinical syndrome characterized by the triad of thrombotic microangiopathy, thrombocytopenia, and acute kidney injury. Hemolytic uremic syndrome represents a heterogeneous group of disorders with variable etiologies that result in differences in presentation, management and outcome. [148]
- HUS is the most common cause of acute kidney injury in children and is increasingly recognized in adults.
- Thrombotic thrombocytopenic purpura (TTP), childhood HUS, and adult HUS have different causes and demographics but share many common features, especially in adults, which include similar pathologic changes such as microangiopathic hemolytic anemia, thrombocytopenia, and neurologic or renal abnormalities[149].
- HUS can be broken down into two classifications:
  1. Diarrhea (typical) vs. no-diarrhea (atypical) and
  2. Primary vs. secondary.
- Primary refers to defects in the complement activation system, while secondary includes infection (E. coli, S. pneumonia, and HIV), drug toxicity, autoimmune disorders, and several other etiologies.
- Most cases of HUS in pediatric patients are secondary (non-complement mediated) and occur after a prodrome of diarrhea (typical).

ETIOLOGY

- HUS occurs most commonly during the summer in children under 3 years.
- The most common cause of HUS in pediatric patients is **Shiga-toxin producing *Escherichia coli* (STEC),** which accounts for 90% of cases in pediatric patients.
- The most common serotype leading to HUS is **Enterohemorrhagic *E. coli* (EHEC) O157:H7,** which produces Shiga toxin 1 and 2. While exposure to STEC results in 38-61% of patients developing hemorrhagic colitis, only 6-9% of patients infected with STEC experience HUS[150].
- The second most common cause of HUS in children is infection with **Streptococcus pneumoniae.**

CLINICAL PRESENTATIONS

History

- History findings may include the following:
  - Prodromal gastroenteritis – Fever, bloody diarrhea for 2-7 days before the onset of renal failure
  - Irritability, lethargy
  - Seizures
  - Acute renal failure, Anuria

Physical Examination

- Physical findings may include the following:
  - Hypertension
  - Edema, fluid overload
  - Pallor, often severe

DIFFERENTIAL DIAGNOSES

- Disseminated Intravascular Coagulation
- Malignant Hypertension
- Pediatric Antiphospholipid Antibody Syndrome
- Preeclampsia
- Thrombotic Thrombocytopenic Purpura (TTP)

LABORATORY

- Microangiopathic hemolytic anemia
- Thrombocytopenia
- Acute renal damage

MANAGEMENT

- There is no specific therapy. Priority should be given to supportive treatment.

Supportive treatment:

- Adjustment of fluid and electrolyte balance,
- control of blood pressure and regulation of dialysis
- **Hypertension:** Calcium channel blockers; nifedipin at a dose of 0.25 mg/ kg or amlodipin at a dose of 0.1 mg/kg can be intitated.
- **Dialysis:** Symptomatic uremia
- **Anemia**: Erythrocyte transfusion is recommended in patients with a hemoglobin level of <6 g/dL.
- **Thrombocytopenia:** Platelet transfusion is recommended only for patients with life threatening bleeding or in the preperation period of surgery.
- **Plasma treatment:** There is no sufficient evidence indicating that administration of this treatment. Plasma exchange may be useful in patients with neurological involvement.
- **Eculizumab:** Eculizumab is a monoclonal C5 antibody which inhibits complement activation and used in treatment of complement-related HUS.

---

[148] Canpolat N. Hemolytic uremic syndrome. Turk Pediatri Ars. 2015;50(2):73-82. Published 2015 Jun 1. doi:10.5152/tpa.2015.2297

[149] Malvinder S Parmar. Hemolytic-Uremic Syndrome. [Medscape online]

[150] Brit Long. Hemolytic Uremic Syndrome (HUS): Pearls and Pitfalls [emdocs online]

14. Dizziness & Vertigo

INTRODUCTION

- **Vertigo** and **dizziness**, are **symptoms** rather than a disease. They do differ subtly with dizziness a potential symptom of someone suffering from vertigo.
- People often use the word "**dizziness**" when they are talking about a variety of **symptoms**, including[151]:
  - **Vertigo:** a feeling of spinning or whirling when you are not actually moving. **Pathological vertigo** is usefully divided into two types; **central and peripheral**.
  - **Unsteadiness**: a sense of imbalance or staggering when standing or walking.
  - **Lightheadedness** or feeling as if you are **about to faint** (presyncope). This may mean there is a heart problem or low blood pressure.
  - **Dizziness** caused by breathing too rapidly (hyperventilation) or anxiety.
- **Central vertigo** results from dysfunction of the central connections of the vestibular apparatus including the vestibular nuclei **in the brainstem** and their connections, especially to the cerebellum.

DIFFERENTIAL DIAGNOSIS OF VERTIGO

PERIPHERAL
- Benign Paroxysmal Positional Vertigo (BPPV)
- Labyrinthitis (viral or post-infectious)
- Meniere's disease
- CN VIII tumour
- Perilymphatic fistula
- Drug-induced (e.g., aminoglycosides)

CENTRAL
- Vertebrobasilar ischemic stroke (cerebellar, brainstem)
- Vertebrobasilar haemorrhagic stroke (cerebellar, brainstem)
- Demyelinating (Multiple Sclerosis)
- Tumour – of the cerebellar-pontine angle, brainstem or cerebellum.
- Migraine (vertebrobasilar)
- Partial seizure
- Infection (abscess)
- Neurodegenerative disease involving brainstem and/or cerebellum
- Drug induced (e.g., anticonvulsants)

- The vestibular nerve (CN VIII) is usually considered part of the peripheral vestibular system (essentially being a peripheral nerve). However, in the case of an acoustic neuroma of CN VIII, if the neuroma is large, it can compress the **cerebellopontine angle** and result in central vertigo as well.
- **Peripheral vertigo** generally refers to vertigo which arises from dysfunction of the vestibular apparatus **in the inner ear** or its connecting vestibular nerve (CN VIII).

PROVOKING FACTORS FOR DIFFERENT CAUSES OF VERTIGO

PROVOKING FACTOR	SUGGESTED DIAGNOSIS
Changes in head position	Acute labyrinthitis; benign positional paroxysmal vertigo; cerebellopontine angle tumor; multiple sclerosis; perilymphatic fistula
Spontaneous episodes (i.e., no consistent provoking factors)	Acute vestibular neuronitis; cerebrovascular disease (stroke or transient ischemic attack); Ménière's disease; migraine; multiple sclerosis
Recent upper respiratory viral illness	Acute vestibular neuronitis
Stress	Psychiatric or psychological causes; migraine
Immunosuppression (e.g., immunosuppressive medications, advanced age, stress)	Herpes zoster oticus
Changes in ear pressure, head trauma, excessive straining, loud noises	Perilymphatic fistula

CLINICAL ASSESSMENT

History

- History alone reveals the diagnosis in roughly three out of four patients complaining of dizziness, although the proportion in patients specifically complaining of vertigo is unknown. When collecting a patient's history, the physician first must determine whether the patient truly has vertigo versus another type of dizziness.
- This can be done by asking, "When you have dizzy spells, do you feel light-headed or do you see the world spin around you?"

---

[151] J. Miller, S.Armfield. *Vertigo & Dizziness.* [Online]

- An affirmative answer to the latter part of this question has been shown to accurately detect patients with true vertigo

TYPICAL DURATION OF SYMPTOMS FOR DIFFERENT CAUSES OF VERTIGO

DURATION OF EPISODE	SUGGESTED DIAGNOSIS
A few seconds	Peripheral cause: unilateral loss of vestibular function; late stages of acute vestibular neuronitis; late stages of Ménière's disease
Several seconds to a few minutes	Benign paroxysmal positional vertigo; perilymphatic fistula
Several minutes to one hour	Posterior transient ischemic attack; perilymphatic fistula
Hours	Ménière's disease; perilymphatic fistula from trauma or surgery; migraine; acoustic neuroma
Days	Early acute vestibular neuronitis*; stroke; migraine; multiple sclerosis
Weeks	Psychogenic (constant vertigo lasting weeks without improvement)

Physical Examination
- Physicians should pay particular attention to physical findings of the neurologic, head and neck, and cardiovascular systems.

1. NEUROLOGIC EXAMINATION
- The cranial nerves should be examined for signs of palsies, sensorineural hearing loss, and nystagmus. Vertical nystagmus is 80 percent sensitive for vestibular nuclear or cerebellar vermis lesions
- Spontaneous horizontal nystagmus with or without rotatory nystagmus is consistent with acute vestibular neuronitis.
- Patients with peripheral vertigo have impaired balance but are still able to walk, whereas patients with central vertigo have more severe instability and often cannot walk or even stand without falling.
- The Dix-Hallpike maneuver[152] may be the most helpful test to perform on patients with vertigo. It has a positive predictive value of 83 percent and a negative predictive value of 52 percent for the diagnosis of BPPV[153].

- After the initial test, the intensity of induced symptoms typically wanes with repeated maneuvers in peripheral vertigo but does so less often in central vertigo.
- The combination of a positive Dix-Hallpike maneuver and a history of vertigo or vomiting suggests a peripheral vestibular disorder.
- If the maneuver provokes purely vertical (usually downbeat) or torsional nystagmus without a latent period of at least a few seconds, and does not wane with repeated maneuvers, this suggests a central cause for vertigo such as a posterior fossa tumor or hemorrhage[154]

2. HEAD AND NECK EXAMINATION
- The tympanic membranes should be examined for vesicles (i.e., herpes zoster oticus [Ramsay Hunt syndrome]) or cholesteatoma.
- **Hennebert's sign** (i.e., vertigo or nystagmus caused by pushing on the tragus and external auditory meatus of the affected side) indicates the presence of a perilymphatic fistula.
- Pneumatic otoscopy may cause similar findings. The Valsalva maneuver (i.e., forced exhalation with nose plugged and mouth closed to increase pressure against the eustachian tube and inner ear) may cause vertigo in patients with perilymphatic fistulaeor anterior semicircular canal dehiscence[155]; its clinical diagnostic value, however, is limited.

3. CARDIOVASCULAR EXAMINATION
- Orthostatic changes in systolic blood pressure (e.g., a drop of 20 mm Hg or more) and pulse (e.g., increase of 10 beats per minute) in patients with vertigo upon standing may identify problems with dehydration or autonomic dysfunction. Carotid sinus stimulation should not be performed; it has been shown to be not useful diagnostically[156] and potentially is dangerous.

INVESTIGATION STRATEGIES
- Laboratory tests such as electrolytes, glucose, blood counts, and thyroid function tests identify the etiology of vertigo in fewer than 1 percent of patients with dizziness.
- They may be appropriate when patients with vertigo exhibit signs or symptoms that suggest the presence of other causative conditions.
- Audiometry helps establish the diagnosis of Ménière's disease[157].

152 Derebery MJ. The diagnosis and treatment of dizziness. Med Clin North Am. 1999;83:163–77.

153 Hoffman RM, Einstadter D, Kroenke K. Evaluating dizziness. Am J Med. 1999;107:468–78.

154 Buttner U, Helmchen C, Brandt T. Diagnostic criteria for central versus peripheral positioning nystagmus and vertigo: a review. Acta Otolaryngol. 1999;119:1–5.

155 Buttner U, Helmchen C, Brandt T. Diagnostic criteria for central versus peripheral positioning nystagmus and vertigo: a review. Acta Otolaryngol. 1999;119:1–5.

156 Herr RD, Zun L, Mathews JJ. A directed approach to the dizzy patient. Ann Emerg Med. 1989;18:664–72.

157 Ronald H. Labuguen. Initial Evaluation of Vertigo [Online]

Radiologic Studies
- Physicians should consider neuroimaging studies in patients with vertigo who have neurologic signs and symptoms, risk factors for cerebrovascular disease, or progressive unilateral hearing loss

NYSTAGMUS
- Spontaneous nystagmus, when present, may indicate whether vertigo has a central or peripheral origin.

	PERIPHERAL VERTIGO	CENTRAL VERTIGO
Effect of fixation	Decreases with fixation	Persists with fixation
Fatigability	Fatigues	Does not fatigue
Direction	Usually horizontal, never vertical	Any direction
Direction on movement	One direction only	Direction of nystagmus may change with direction of gaze
Duration	Resolves within 48 hours	Persists beyond 48 hours

ASSOCIATED SYMPTOMS FOR DIFFERENT CAUSES OF VERTIGO

SYMPTOM	SUGGESTED DIAGNOSIS
Aural fullness	Acoustic neuroma; Ménière's disease
Ear or mastoid pain	Acoustic neuroma; acute middle ear disease (e.g., otitis media, herpes zoster oticus)
Facial weakness	Acoustic neuroma; herpes zoster oticus
Focal neurologic findings	Cerebellopontine angle tumor; cerebrovascular disease; multiple sclerosis (especially findings not explained by single neurologic lesion)
Headache	Acoustic neuroma; migraine
Hearing loss	Ménière's disease; perilymphatic fistula; acoustic neuroma; cholesteatoma; otosclerosis; transient ischemic attack or stroke involving anterior inferior cerebellar artery; herpes zoster oticus
Imbalance	Acute vestibular neuronitis (usually moderate); cerebellopontine angle tumor (usually severe)
Nystagmus	Peripheral or central vertigo
Phonophobia, photophobia	Migraine
Tinnitus	Acute labyrinthitis; acoustic neuroma; Ménière's disease

CAUSES OF VERTIGO ASSOCIATED WITH HEARING LOSS

DIAGNOSIS	CHARACTERISTICS OF HEARING LOSS
Acoustic neuroma	Progressive, unilateral, sensorineural
Cholesteatoma	Progressive, unilateral, conductive
Herpes zoster oticus (i.e., Ramsay Hunt syndrome)	Subacute to acute onset, unilateral
Ménière's disease	Sensorineural, initially fluctuating, initially affecting lower frequencies; later in course: progressive, affecting higher frequencies
Otosclerosis	Progressive, conductive
Perilymphatic fistula	Progressive, unilateral
Transient ischemic attack or stroke involving anterior inferior cerebellar artery or internal auditory artery	Sudden onset, unilateral

MANAGEMENT OF VERTIGO IN THE ED
- Do not expect to be able to make a definitive diagnosis in every patient with vertigo, concentrate on making a distinction between central and peripheral vertigo.
- Vestibular suppressants: **Diazepam 2mg, Lorazepam 0.1mg**
- Anticholinergics: **Hyoscine**
- Antihistamines with anticholinergic (and antiemetic) properties: **Cyclizine**.
- Antiemetics: **Prochlorperazine** and **Metoclopramide** are also commonly used but may be associated with **acute dystonic reactions**.
- **Mobilisation:** Patients prescribed a vestibular suppressant should be encouraged to mobilise and to use their medication for the minimum time possible.
- **Vestibular Neuritis**
  - In addition to vestibular suppressant / antiemetic treatment, one study has shown that **steroids** may have a beneficial effect on the short- and long-term recovery of vestibular function although symptoms were not assessed.

I. WEBER'S AND RINNE'S TESTS

- The Weber and Rinne tests are more than just a way to evaluate the Vestibulocochlear nerve (cranial nerve VIII).
- They are screening tests to determine the presence of hearing loss. They are performed using tuning forks at the frequencies of 512- and 1024-Hz.
- Tuning forks with these different frequencies are utilized so that both low (512-Hz) and high (1024-Hz) frequency hearing loss may be revealed.
- *The Weber test is able to test for and distinguish between* **conductive hearing loss (CHL) and sensorineural hearing loss (SNHL)**, *while the Rinne test* **assesses for the presence of CHL only.**

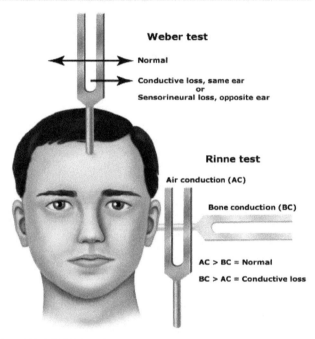

1. THE WEBER TEST

- The Weber test is a test of lateralisation and establishes where a tone is perceived[158]. It is executed by hitting the tuning fork and then holding it in the middle of the patient's forehead. If the patient is unable to hear the tuning fork in this position, it can also be placed on the nasal bone or in the middle of the front two teeth.
- The patient is then asked to determine where the sound is heard the best. A normal result is when the sound is the same in both ears.
  - **If the sound is louder in one ear**, *it is indicative of conductive hearing loss (CHL) in that ear or sensorineural hearing loss (SNHL) in the opposite ear.*
  - **If the sound is quieter in one ear**, *it is indicative of SNHL in that ear or CHL in the opposite ear.*

- At first glance, the results of the Weber test seem opposite to what you would normally think.
- However, the key to understanding it is realizing that the tuning fork is measuring how well the sound conducts through the bone (termed bone conduction), and the patient reports how well this sound is heard.
- Additionally, outside sound is still being conducted through the air (termed air conduction) to the patient's ear (if no CHL is present). The bone conduction is a measure of SNHL, while the air conduction is a measure of CHL.
  - If bone conduction is intact on both sides (therefore no SNHL), the patient will report a louder sound in the ear with CHL. This is because the ear with the CHL is only receiving input from the bone conduction and no air conduction, and the sound is perceived as louder in that ear.
  - If air conduction is intact on both sides (therefore no CHL), the patient will report a quieter sound in the ear with the SNHL. This is because the ear with the SNHL is not receiving input from the bone conduction, and the sound is perceived as louder in the normal ear.

2. THE RINNE TEST

- This test is a comparison of loudness of perceived air conduction to bone conduction in one ear at a time[159]. It is executed by hitting the tuning fork and then holding it on the patient's mastoid process.
- After the patient states the sound can no longer be heard, the tuning fork is then moved to just outside the external auditory meatus.
  - *If the sound is able to be heard again, it is a normal result. This is termed a positive test because the air conduction (AC) is greater than the bone conduction (BC).* **AC> BC=Normal**
  - *A negative test is when the sound cannot be heard again, and the BC > AC. If there is no air conduction, then CHL must be present.* **BC> AC=CHL**

II. DIX-HALLPIKE MANEUVER

1. INDICATIONS

- The Dix-Hallpike maneuver, also termed the "head-hanging positioning maneuver," is helpful in confirming the clinical suspicion of benign paroxysmal positional vertigo (BPPV). This maneuver provokes abnormal nystagmus, which is a characteristic feature of BPPV.

---

158 *British Society of Audiology. Rinne and Weber tuning fork tests. September 2016* [Online]

159 *British Society of Audiology. Rinne and Weber tuning fork tests. September 2016* [Online]

2. CONTRAINDICATIONS

- Severe cervical spine disease.
- Unstable spinal injury.
- High-grade carotid stenosis.
- Unstable heart disease.
- Elderly patients may not tolerate this maneuver.
- There is no need to perform this test in the presence of nystagmus at rest.

3. COMPLICATIONS

- Vertigo
- Nausea

5. PROCEDURE

- This test is performed by rapidly moving the patient from a sitting position to the supine position with the head turned 45° to the right. After waiting approximately 20-30 seconds, the patient is returned to the sitting position. If no nystagmus is observed, the procedure is then repeated on the left side[160].
- The ear that is down when the greatest symptoms of nystagmus are produced is the affected ear, which can be treated using canalith-repositioning maneuvers.
- To prevent nausea and vomiting when these symptoms are not tolerable for the patient, premedicate him with an antiemetic such as metoclopramide (Reglan), 10 mg IV, or ondansetron (Zofran), 4 mg IV.

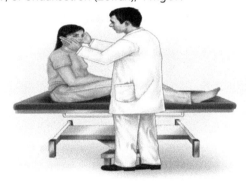

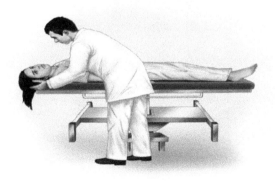

III. EPLEY MANEUVER

- Particle Repositioning or Canalith Repositioning Procedure. During the Dix-Hallpike test, the particles move in the canal and trigger a burst of upbeat-torsional nystagmus.
- The Epley maneuver is now widely used as a first-line treatment of vertical (posterior or anterior) canal BPPV[161]. The Epley maneuver causes resolution of positional nystagmus. This maneuver is effective in about 80 % of patients with benign paroxysmal positional vertigo (BPPV).

1. INDICATIONS

- Performed to alleviate the symptoms of posterior canal BPPV

2. CONTRAINDICATIONS

- Back or spine injuries or other problems
- Presence of detached retina

3. COMPLICATIONS

- When performing this maneuver, caution is advised should neurological symptoms occur.
- Occasionally such symptoms are caused by **compression of the vertebral arteries**; if it persists for a long period of time, a **stroke** can occur.

4. PROCEDURE

- With the patient seated, the patient's head is rotated 45 degrees toward the affected ear.
- The patient is then tilted backward to a head-hanging position, with the head kept in the 45-degree rotation.
- The patient is held in this position (same as the Dix-Hallpike position with the affected ear down) until the nystagmus and vertigo abate (at least 20 seconds, but most clinicians recommend 4 minutes in each position). The head is then turned 90 degrees toward the unaffected ear and kept in this position for another 3 to 4 minutes. With the head remaining turned, the patient is then rolled onto the side of the unaffected ear.
- This may again provoke nystagmus and vertigo, but the patient should again remain in this position for 3 to 4 minutes.
- Finally, the patient is moved to the seated position, and the head is tilted down 30 degrees, allowing the canalith to fall into the utricle.
- This position is also held for an additional 3 to 4 minutes

---

[160]https://www.medscape.com/answers/884261-46057/how-is-the-dix-hallpike-maneuver-performed-and-which-findings-indicate-benign-paroxysmal-positional-vertigo-bppv

[161] Hilton MP, Pinder DK. The Epley (canalith repositioning) manoeuvre for benign paroxysmal positional vertigo. Cochrane Database Syst Rev. 2014 Dec 8. 12:CD003162. [Medline].

15. Environmental Emergencies

I. DROWNING

INTRODUCTION

- Drowning remains a significant worldwide public health concern, ranking as the third leading cause of unintentional injury death and accounting for 7% of all injury-related deaths.
- It is a major cause of disability and death, particularly in children. At least one third of survivors sustain moderate-to-severe neurologic sequelae[162].

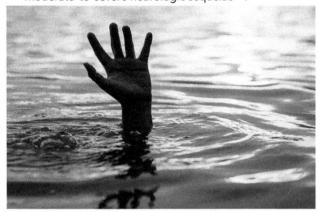

- Drowning is defined as "the process of experiencing respiratory impairment from submersion/immersion in a liquid" by the World Health Organization.
- Drowning begins with respiratory impairment due to submersion (victim's airway under the surface of the water) or immersion (water splashes over the victim's face). Although no longer recommended, the classifications of "near drowning" and "drowning" are still commonly used in literature and among laypersons.
- **Near drowning** refers to respiratory impairment from submersion/immersion without mortality.
- **Drowning** refers to mortality from water submersion/immersion. The preferred terms to use now are **"drowning without morbidity," "drowning with morbidity"** and **"drowning with death."**
- Drowning is most common among toddlers and teenage boys. It typically occurs in home swimming pools, bathtubs or buckets. Males are 4 times more likely to drown than females and black children have a 1.3 times higher rate of drowning than children in other ethnic groups.

- Alcohol use is common among older drowning victims.
- Pre-existing conditions including seizures and pre-existing cardiac disease also increase risk of drowning. Trauma may coexist as a result of diving or falls.

INITIAL ACTIONS AND PRIMARY SURVEY

- The initial approach to a patient with suspected drowning is similar to the approach to any other critically ill patient.
- Initial efforts should focus on resuscitation, including evaluation and treatment of airway, breathing and circulation. Because respiratory arrest is the most common cause of cardiac arrest in drowning victims, the traditional A-B-C approach should be used for drowning victims. Resuscitation with rescue breaths may begin in the water if responders are properly trained.
- Chest compressions should not be attempted in the water as they will not be effective.
- Mechanism of injury should also be considered to determine whether spinal immobilization and further trauma evaluation is indicated.
- Drowning victims are at high risk for hypothermia and should be treated for hypothermia if indicated.

PRESENTATION

- The history from the patient, witnesses or EMS are vital in diagnosing drowning. When the event was not witnessed it is important to remember to evaluate for trauma and other medical conditions.
- The clinical presentation varies from asymptomatic to benign conditions like a mild cough to more serious conditions including respiratory failure with cardiac arrest, depending on various factors: the reason for submersion, time of submersion, temperature of the water, and amount of water aspirated.
- Healthy patients who have been rescued from drowning and have no respiratory symptoms, clear lungs and normal mental status may not need any further care. These patients should receive explicit directions about when to return as some respiratory symptoms may be delayed up to 24 hours.
- Symptomatic patients can present with symptoms such as respiratory distress, tachypnea, hypoxia, coughing, or foaming from the mouth or nose. Auscultation of the lungs may reveal rhonchi or rales.

[162] Szpilman D, Sempsrott J, Webber J, Hawkins SC, Barcala-Furelos R, Schmidt A, et al. 'Dry drowning' and other myths. Cleve Clin J Med. 2018 Jul. 85 (7):529-535.

- Vomiting is also common. Hypothermia may be present.
- Traumatic injuries, especially from falls or diving may also be present.
- Drowning begins when the patient's airway is occluded by a liquid medium. When a person can no longer keep their airway clear of water, the typical response is to hold one's breath. At some point the respiratory drive becomes too high and water is aspirated, causing coughing.
- Laryngospasm can occur, but usually is overcome by brain hypoxia.
- Water aspiration continues until respiratory arrest occurs. Cardiac arrest ensues, typically after a period of tachycardia followed by bradycardia.
- The initial rhythm in the arrest is PEA followed by asystole.
- About half of drowning resuscitations begin with bystander CPR. Patients requiring CPR will often present with CPR still in progress or in the peri-resuscitation stages.
- Drowning should be considered in any unconscious patient found submerged in water; however, it is critical to evaluate for trauma and medical conditions that could have led to drowning.

DIAGNOSTIC TESTING

- Diagnostic testing will vary based on the severity of illness. Vital signs and most importantly SpO2 should be obtained on all patients with suspected drowning.
- **An ABG** should be obtained in mechanically ventilated patients. Core temperature should be measured to assess for hypothermia.
- **Chest radiography** should be obtained to evaluate for aspiration. Even in patients with mild symptoms, this can be important for use as a baseline.
- **Cardiac monitoring and/or ECG** should also be obtained. This is especially important if the patient may have had a medical etiology for drowning.
- A trauma work up, especially **c-spine imaging**, should be obtained in any patient with a mechanism or exam concerning for trauma and in any obtunded patient for whom the cause of drowning is unknown.
- In the teenage and young adult population diving injuries commonly occur with drowning.

MANAGEMENT

- Initial treatment should focus on correcting any airway and breathing difficulties with a goal of correcting hypoxemia and acidosis.
- **Supplemental oxygen** can be used for patients with mild symptoms. Patients with persistent hypoxia may require a trial of **CPAP or even intubation**.

- Patients with hypoxia and altered mental status will require endotracheal intubation.
- The treatment of pulmonary injury due to drowning is similar to the treatment of ARDS and applicable protocols should be utilized. Once a patient has been intubated, weaning should not occur for at least 24 hours as local pulmonary injury is unlikely to resolve in shorter timeframes.
- **Hypothermia** is common in submersion patients. Depending on the degree of hypothermia, passive or active rewarming may be needed. Hypothermia has been shown to be neuroprotective in patients with prolonged time prior to ROSC.
- **There is no role for antibiotics** in the initial treatment of drowning, but close monitoring for infection is indicated as bacterial pneumonia does occur from aspiration of water or vomit. This typically appears after 3-4 days, once pulmonary edema resolves.
- CNS infections have also been reported. In either situation, there is no evidence that empiric prophylactic treatment with antibiotics is efficacious. If pneumonia develops, antibiotic therapy can be tailored by using samples obtained from bronchial alveolar lavage.
- The degree of hypoxia and amount of supplemental oxygen required will determine whether patients should be further observed in a general bed, telemetry bed or ICU.

PEARLS AND PITFALLS

- Always consider the mechanism of injury and evaluate for trauma.
- Even on warm days, hypothermia is a real threat.
- Remember to evaluate for underlying medical causes including seizures, dysrhythmias, or cardiac etiologies.
- Respiratory symptoms may be delayed. If asymptomatic patients are discharged, ensure they have appropriate return precautions and the ability to access care.

References

- Cushing, T, Hawkins, S, et al. "Submersion Injuries and Drowning". Wilderness Medicine. 2012; 1494-1513.
- David Szpilman, M.D., Joost J.L.M. Bierens, M.D., Ph.D., Anthony J. Handley, M.D., and
- James P. Orlowski, M.D. "Drowning" N Engl J Med 2012; 366:2102-2110
- van Beeck EF, Branche CM, Szpilman D, Modell JH, Bierens JJLM. A new definition of drowning: towards documentation and prevention of a global public health problem. Bull World Health Organ 2005;83:853-856

II. HEAT RELATED ILLNESS

INTRODUCTION

- Heat-related illness is classically taught to represent a spectrum of hyperthermic disease ranging from heat cramps, heat syncope, heat exhaustion, and – in extreme cases – heat stroke.
- Symptoms present when the body is exposed to heat with inability to properly cool core body temperature.
- Normal core temperature ranges between 36-38° Celsius. Below 35° C, radiation represents 60% of heat dissipation with an additional 30% from evaporation; above 35° C, this native process becomes overwhelmed and insufficient to maintain adequately cooled core body temperature. Subsequently, thermoregulatory failure occurs and the body is unable to release heat quickly, leading to elevated core temperatures.

TYPES OF HEAT ILLNESS

- Heat-related illness may be classified as exertional or non-exertional (classic).
  - **Exertional type** is related to the endogenous heat production of physical activity and generally occurs in young, healthy individuals.
  - **Non-exertional type** tends to be environmentally related and occurs insidiously in children and the elderly.
- Classic heat-related illness occurs during periods of high environmental heat stress, and physical exertion is not required. In non-exertional heat illness, the increase in core temperature is generally slow, occurring over hours to days. Subsequently, these individuals are likely to develop volume or electrolyte disturbances.
- Exertional heat injuries tend to occur in young, physically fit individuals performing under conditions of high heat, including sports, recreational physical activity, firefighting, and military training.

INCIDENCE AND RISK FACTORS

- Because reporting of heat-related illness is not mandatory, the incidence is likely underestimated. A heat wave is defined as >3 consecutive days of sustained temperatures > 32.2° C.
- **Non-environmental risk factors include:**
  - Heavy clothing or equipment,
  - Children younger than 4 years of age,
  - Adults older than age 65,
  - Obesity,
  - Underlying medical conditions such as diabetes, heart, and pulmonary disease.
  - Mental illness

  - Drugs (diuretics, blockers, alcohol, stimulants, phenothiazines, anticholinergics)
  - Young individuals participating in strenuous activity during warm weather increases their risk of heat-related illness.
- **Environmental risk factors include:**
  - Warm temperatures and humidity,
  - Medical care,
  - Cooling centers,
  - Occupational (miners, fire fighters, military recruits)
  - Lack of air conditioning (lower socioeconomic groups)

TREATMENT

- The best treatment for heat-related illnesses is public education and prevention. Air-conditioning is the No. 1 protective factor against developing heat-related illness and death.[163] During a heat wave, public facilities with air conditioning should be made available.
- In mass participation events, several measures can be taken by organizers and medical staff to reduce the risk of developing heat-related illness.
- Care should be taken to avoid scheduling during hot and humid months, and events should be held during the cooler hours of the day. If possible, athletes should prepare with heat acclimatization; a process of increasing activity duration and intensity during the preceding 10-14 days.

HEAT EDEMA

- It is a self-limited process defined as dependent pretibial edema of the lower extremities and/or hands during the first few days of exposure to increased temperature.
- Although it usually resolves within days of onset, patients may be symptomatic for up to 6 weeks.
- No specific treatment is necessary; elevation and compression stockings may accelerate recovery and aid in symptomatic relief. Diuretics are not indicated and may precipitate more severe heat-related illness.

PRICKLY HEAT

- Known as **miliaria rubra** or **heat rash**, is a pruritic, maculopapular, erythematous rash due to inflammation, dilation, and rupture of the sweat glands, producing small vesicles that presents over clothed areas of the body.

---

163 Davis RE, Knappenberger PC, Novicoff WM, Michaels PJ. Decadal changes in heat-related human mortality in the eastern United States. Climate Research. 2002;22(2):175–184.

- Patients generally complain of itching, which responds well to antihistamines. Wearing light, loose-fitting clothing will reduce likelihood of developing heat rash. Talc and baby powder do not help; chlorhexidine lotion may provide relief.

HEAT CRAMPS

- They are painful, involuntary muscle contractions, typically of the calves, occurring in sweating individuals with inadequate volume replacement or who are hydrating with hypotonic fluids.
- Cramps may occur during exercise or commonly during a rest period following physical activity.
- Although self-limited, patients may present to the emergency department due to persistent myalgias.
- Cramping is usually isolated to a specific muscle group and rarely leads to the development of rhabdomyolysis.

ELECTROLYTE DISTURBANCES

- include hyponatremia and hypochloremia.
- Primary treatment is with oral isotonic fluid replacement and rest in a cool environment. Oral hydration with 0.1% saline solution or with commercially available electrolyte drinks are adequate for most patients. Patients with severe symptoms may require IV rehydration.
- Prevention is directed at maintaining sufficient hydration with either water and salt tablets or commercial electrolyte drink.

HEAT TETANY

- It is caused by hyperventilation and subsequent respiratory alkalosis, presenting as paresthesias of the extremities, perioral area, and carpopedal spasm.
- It is often confused with heat cramps; however, it is a separate clinical entity typically not accompanied by muscle cramps.
- Treatment is directed at moving the patient to a cooler area and reducing their respiratory rate.

HEAT SYNCOPE

- It is due to a combination of volume depletion, peripheral vasodilation, and decreased vasomotor tone resulting in postural hypotension.
- Evaluation includes workup of other causes of syncope including cardiac, metabolic, and neurologic etiologies, and treatment is directed at rehydration, rest, and removing the patient from the area of heat exposure.
- Hospitalization is often unnecessary.

HEAT EXHAUSTION

- is the result of both hypovolemia and hyponatremia. Hypovolemia occurs in individuals in warm environments with inadequate water replacement; hyponatremia occurs when individuals replace fluid losses with water or other hypotonic fluids.

- **Symptoms** include headache, nausea and vomiting, malaise, dizziness, muscle cramps, and other clinical indicators of hypovolemia. Notably, patients do not have altered mentation. Patients are tachycardic and may have positional hypotension, temperature is elevated but typically below 40° C.
- **Laboratory evaluation** reflects hemoconcentration; patients may have hypotonic or isotonic hypovolemia.
- **Treatment** is directed at fluid replacement, electrolyte correction, removal from warm environment and rest. These patients may require active cooling, especially if not responding to the first 30-60 minutes of therapy.

HEAT STROKE

- A true Medical Emergency, Heat stroke, whether classical or exertional, is the most serious presentation of heat-related illness. Mortality rates range from 30-80% and is universally fatal if left untreated.
- The diagnosis is generally clinical and defined by **encephalopathy and hyperthermia > 40° C,** although temperature less than 40° C should not be exclusive criteria for treatment. **The presence of mental status changes in a hot and/or humid environment should be considered heat stroke until proven otherwise.**
- **Anhidrosis** is not diagnostically reliable.
- **Ataxia** is an early symptom due to sensitivity of the cerebellum; patients may also have irritability, confusion, behavior changes, combativeness, hallucinations, decorticate and decerebrate posturing, hemiplegia, and coma.
- **Seizures** are common. Neurologic injury is a function of duration of exposure and maximum temperature.
- The patient may be tachycardic, tachypneic, and/or hypotensive.

DIFFERENTIAL DIAGNOSIS
Differential diagnosis in suspected heat stroke:

- Polypharmacy
- Toxic ingestions
- Meningitis, Sepsis, Malaria, Thyphoid
- Status epilepticus
- Neuroleptic malignant syndrome,
- Malignant hyperpyrexia
- Serotonin syndrome,
- Anticholinergic toxicity
- Salicylate toxicity
- Thyroid storm,
- Phaeochromocytoma
- Intracerebral haemorrhage
- Alcohol withdrawal, Cocaine, Amphetamine

INVESTIGATION

- It is important for the provider to consider other causes of altered mentation and to assess for end organ damage. Diagnostic studies include Full blood count, metabolic panel, blood gas, creatine phosphokinase, myoglobin, coagulation panel, urinalysis. An ECG and chest radiograph should be obtained.
- **Lumbar puncture** and **head CT** should be considered.

Haematological and Biochemical abnormalities of heatstroke:

Test	Findings	Explanation
Acid/base balance	Metabolic acidosis +/- respiratory compensation, elevated lactate	Poor peripheral perfusion
Electrolytes	Hyper/hyponatraemia, Hyper/hypokalaemia	Water and electrolyte loss
Renal function	Elevated creatinine and urea	Reduced renal perfusion, Myoglobinuria in rhabdomyolysis
Liver function	Elevated ALT and AST	Centrilobular hepatocyte necrosis
Muscle function	Elevated creatine kinase, Hyperkalaemia and hypocalcaemia	Rhabdomyolysis
FBC and coagulation	Neutrophilia, thrombocytopenia, prolonged clotting times, hypofibrinogenaemia	Disseminated Intravascular Coagulation

HEAT STROKE MANAGEMENT

- Initial treatment of exertional heat stroke is directed at removing the patient from the offending environment and immediate cooling with cold-water immersion, as it has been shown to be the fastest cooling modality.[164]

COOLING TECHNIQUES

- If cold water immersion is not available, cold water dousing and wet ice towel rotation may be used, but these have not been found to be as efficient.
- The length of time that core body temperature is elevated has been linked with increased morbidity and mortality, with practitioners aiming to lower body temperature below 39° C within 30 minutes to decrease these risks.[165]

- Because external thermometry is unreliable, accurate temperature measurement with a core temperature is essential; regardless, cold-water immersion should be initiated as soon as the diagnosis is suspected.
- Rapid cooling should be discontinued once temperature reaches 39° C to avoid rebound hypothermia.
- Heat stroke is a medical emergency and patient should be transported to hospital for further evaluation.

ED APPROACH

- In the ED, treatment is directed at addressing the ABCs of airway, breathing, and circulation, along with volume resuscitation and continued active cooling of the patient.
- Simple adjuncts to cooling such as the use of **cooled peripheral intravenous fluids** and **placing of icepacks in the groin and axillae** are often used. Care must be taken with ice packs as prolonged skin contact may cause tissue damage.
- **Cold fluid peritoneal and gastric lavage** and **cardiopulmonary bypass** have also been described, but are not usually necessary. The aim of cooling is not to achieve rapid normothermia, this would result in **overshoot hypothermia**.
- *The target core temperature when cooling should be 38.5°C.*
- **Antipyretics and dantrolene** are not indicated for temperature reduction.
- Intravenous fluid resuscitation should be isotonic fluids with a target urine output of **2-3 mL/kg/hr.**

EARLY COMPLICATIONS

- ARDS,
- Metabolic acidosis,
- Respiratory alkalosis,
- Electrolyte imbalance,
- Hypoglycemia,
- Increased cpk,
- Rhabdomyolysis,
- Leukocytosis,
- Coagulation disorder,
- Hepatic dysfunction.

LATE COMPLICATIONS

- Acute renal failure,
- Pulmonary edema,
- Stroke and
- Hepatic failure.

All patients presenting with heat stroke require admission to the hospital.

---

[164] Hadad E, Rav-Acha M, Heled Y, Epstein Y, Moran DS. Heat Stroke: a review of cooling methods. Sports Med. 2004;34(8): 501-511.

[165] Costrini A. Emergency treatment of exertional heatstroke and comparison of whole body cooling techniques. Med Sci Sports Exerc. 1990;22(1):15-18.

III. FROSTBITE

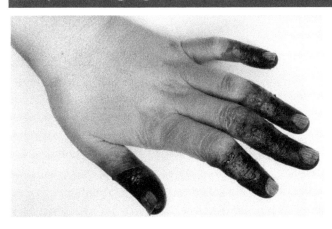

DEFINITION

- Frostbite, the most common type of freezing injury, is defined as the freezing and crystalizing of fluids in the interstitial and cellular spaces as a consequence of prolonged exposure to freezing temperatures.

RISK FACTORS

- **Environmental factors:**
  - Alcohol abuse
  - Inadequate shelter
  - Inadequate or constrictive clothing
  - Winter season
  - Wind chill factor
  - High altitude
  - Prolonged exposure to cold
  - Homelessness,
  - Altered mental status,
- **Medical factors:**
  - Thyroid disease
  - Stroke
  - Diabetes.
  - Arthritis
  - Malnutrition,
  - Infection,
  - Peripheral vascular disease

CLINICAL ASSESSMENT

History

- Frostbite is a completely preventable injury that can occur with or without hypothermia.
- Below –10°C, any tissue that feels numb for more than a few minutes may become frostbitten.
- Progressive symptoms of frostbitten areas are as follows:
  - Coldness
  - Stinging, burning, and throbbing
    - Numbness followed by complete loss of sensation (This history of anesthesia suggests a frostbite injury.)
    - Loss of fine muscle dexterity (ie, clumsiness of fingers)
    - Loss of large muscle dexterity (ie, difficulty ambulating)
    - Severe joint pain
- Numbness over the affected area is the initial symptom of frostbite. After rewarming, severe throbbing and hyperemia begin and may last for weeks. Many patients complain of paresthesias. Long-term symptoms include cold sensitivity, sensory loss, and hyperhidrosis.

PHYSICAL EXAMINATION

- The initial appearance of frostbite does not accurately predict the eventual extent and depth of tissue damage.
- **Signs and symptoms** vary according to severity of the frostbite injury. The hands, feet, ears, and nose are the most commonly affected.
- **Physical examination** in patients with superficial frostbite reveals the presence of soft, palpable skin. If a thumbprint can be left in the skin, the patient usually has more viable underlying tissue. Individuals with deeper frostbite effects present with skin that is hard to the touch.
- Other signs may include the following:
  - Excessive sweating
  - Joint pain
  - Pallor or blue discoloration
  - Hyperemia
  - Skin necrosis
  - Gangrene

DIAGNOSIS

- The diagnosis of frostbite is a clinical one, although imaging may help to assess severity.
- **Routine x-ray** at presentation and again at 4-10 weeks post injury may demonstrate specific abnormalities, such as osteomyelitis.
- The imaging of choice in frostbite assessment is **scintigraphy.**
- **Tc-99m (Technetium 99)** pertechnetate scintigraphy is sensitive and specific for tissue injury. In addition, scintigraphy is useful in assessing the response of damaged tissue to therapy.

MANAGEMENT OF FROSTBITE

Pre-hospital Care

- As a general principle, always address the ABCs and treat any life-threatening conditions (eg, hypothermia) first.
- Correct any systemic hypothermia to a core temperature of 34°C before treating the frostbite.
- Remove the patient from cold.
- Replace wet and constrictive clothing with dry loose clothing. Remove jewelry from the affected area.
- Dress the extremity in a manner that minimizes mechanical trauma.
- Rewarm the frostbitten area if no danger of refreezing is present. However, rewarming should be avoided if it cannot be maintained (freeze-thaw-freeze cycle).
- Walking on frozen frostbitten areas and risking tissue chipping and fracture is considered better than thawing and refreezing. Reports from Canada show that forced-air rewarming with portable units can be used effectively to warm victims of hypothermia and frostbite in the field and during transport to a regional medical center. [166]
- Ibuprofen 400mg orally **prior to re-warming may improve** tissue salvage. Do not rub frostbitten areas in an attempt to rewarm them; this can cause further tissue damage.

Emergency Department

- Rapid rewarming is the single most effective therapy for frostbite.[167] On admission, rapidly rewarm the affected area in circulating water (ie, a whirlpool bath) at a temperature of **40-42°C** by thermometer measurement.
- Warming is continued for 15-30 minutes or until thawing is, by clinical assessment, complete (ie, when the distal area of the extremity is flushed, soft, and pliable). The addition of an antiseptic solution such as povidone-iodine or chlorhexidine to the bath may be beneficial. Avoid inadvertent slow rewarming or overheating. Encourage active gentle motion of the frostbitten area during the rewarming. Constantly monitor water temperature.
- Thawing takes about 20-40 minutes for superficial injuries and as long as 1 hour for deep injuries.

- The most common error in this stage of treatment is premature termination of the rewarming process because of reperfusion pain.
- Reperfusion is intensely painful and **parenteral analgesia is often required**.
- Partial thawing and refreezing generate more damage than does prolonged freezing alone, through the release of multiple inflammatory mediators. In patients who experience a refreezing injury of thawed areas, rewarming should be delayed until it can be maintained.
- Clear blisters should be debrided and aloe vera applied the affected area every 6 hours.
- Haemorrhagic blisters should be left infect but aloe vera should again be used topically.
- The injured extremities should be kept elevated to minimize oedema formation.
- Sterile dressings should be applied and involved areas handled gently. Persistent cyanosis in the extremities after a complete thaw may reflect increased fascial compartment pressure.
- Because of the cold-induced anaesthesia, this and other occult soft tissue injuries are often not appreciated by the patient or physician.
- **Tetanus prophylaxis** should be considered
- **Antibiotics** are not routinely needed unless there are signs of infection.
- **Referral to a physiotherapist** at an early stage.
- It may be a 4-6-week period before the extent of the injury is known and surgical debridement should not be considered before then.

DISPOSITION

- The patient should be there are any features suggestive of deep frostbite.
- Superficial frostbite can generally be discharged from the ED with follow up at 24-48 hours and instructions to return if they experience worsening or new symptoms.

PREVENTION

- The best management of frostbite is, of course, prevention.
- Preventative measures that may be effective include minimising direct skin exposure, avoiding tight boots or multiple sock layers in large boots, keeping the head, neck and face covered, wearing mittens instead of gloves, staying hydrated, having an adequate caloric intake and avoiding direct skin-metal or skin-fluid contact.

[166] *Ducharme MB, Giesbrecht GG, Frim J, Kenny GP, Johnston CE, Goheen MS, et al. Forced-air rewarming in -20 degrees C simulated field conditions. Ann N Y Acad Sci. 1997 Mar 15. 813:676-81.*

[167] *Britt LD, Dascombe WH, Rodriguez A. New horizons in management of hypothermia and frostbite injury. Surg Clin North Am. 1991 Apr. 71(2):345-70.*

IV. INDUSTRIAL CHEMICAL INCIDENT

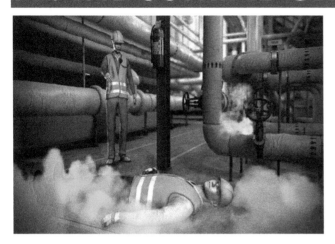

INTRODUCTION

- A **chemical disaster** is the unintentional release of one or more hazardous substances which could harm human health and the environment.
- **Chemical hazards** are systems where chemical accidents could occur under certain circumstances. Such events include fires, explosions, leakages or release of toxic or hazardous materials that can cause people illness, injury, or disability.
- While chemical accidents may occur whenever toxic materials are stored, transported or used, the most severe are industrial accidents, involving major chemical manufacturing and storage facilities.
- The most dangerous chemical accident in recorded in history was the 1984 Bhopal gas tragedy in India, in which more than 3,000 people had died after a highly toxic vapour, (methyl isocyanate), was released at a Union Carbide Pesticides factory.
- **Hazchem** (UK Hazard Identification System) is a UK system for managing chemicals and information.

CAUSES OF CHEMICAL ACCIDENTS[168]

1. Equipment failure
- Inappropriate equipment includes **chemical storage** (for example, using non-flammable storage units to store flammable chemicals), mishandling of **containment barriers** or spill kits, and malfunctioning valves.
- The use of pressure relief systems in place of fully functioning valves are adequate to relive the pressure flow and therefore will results in a chemical accident.

2. Inadequate safety review/analysis
- A key issue in many workplaces is the total lack or absence of a solid **chemical safety risk assessment process**. Particularly in large scale workplace **chemical accidents**, investigations afterwards almost always tend to discover flaws in the chemical review and analysis procedures. Failure to regularly assess chemical safety and storage procedures meant that workplaces were more vulnerable to chemical hazards.

3. Operator error
- Chemical accidents are likely to happen if an uniformed or untrained member of personnel is handling or encounters chemicals in the workplace. This can lead to a host of chemical safety risks not only to the operator themselves but to the entire workplace. Operator errors usually occur due to a lack of understanding or training when it comes to safely handling hazardous chemicals.
- **Only allowing authorised personnel to handle chemicals or enter chemical storage areas.**

4. Warnings ignored
- Many large scale chemical accidents come as a result of ignoring warning signs such as smaller chemical incidents, spills or injuries.
- Minor chemical spills are merely cleaned up so that operations can continue without the source of the spill or leak being fully investigated or remedied, which can lead to an even larger scale chemical spill in the future.
- Minor **chemical combustions** are not properly investigated and therefore root causes such as improper chemical storage are not identified until after a major chemical explosion.

PREVENTING CHEMICAL ACCIDENTS IN THE WORKPLACE
- The high level of chemical incidents in U.K. workplaces every year emphasis a real need for training and knowledge of chemical safety and chemical storage best practices.
- Understanding the top four causes of chemical accidents can help you to identify high risk areas in your facility and appropriate safety practices to mitigate these risks.

CLINICAL ASSESSMENT
History
- What exposed to?
- How much in terms of volume and concentration?
- What route?
- Any protective measures taken?
- Any treatment given?

---

[168] *Safety storage systems, Top 4 Causes of Chemical Accidents in the Workplace [Online]*

HOW CHEMICALS ENTER THE BODY[169]

- **Inhalation**: Breathing in contaminated air is the most common way that workplace chemicals enter the body
- **Skin contact**: Some chemicals, by direct or indirect contact, can damage the skin or pass through the skin into the bloodstream
- **Ingestion**: Workplace chemicals may be swallowed accidentally if food or hands are contaminated
- **Injection**: Can occur when a sharp object (e.g. needle) punctures the skin and injects a chemical directly into the bloodstream
- **The eyes** may also be a route of entry. Only very small quantities of chemicals in the workplace enter through the mouth or the eyes.
- Regardless of the way the chemical gets into the body, once it is in it can be distributed to anywhere in the body by the bloodstream. In this way, the chemicals can attack and harm organs that are far away from the original point of entry
- **Acute effects** are those that show up immediately after a chemical exposure occurs. A good example of an acute effect is the spillage of acid on the skin – a chemical burn will occur immediately.
- **Chronic effects** are those that occur after a significant amount of time passes and usually are the result of multiple exposures over a period of time. **Cancer** is a typical example of a chronic effect because cancers caused by chemical exposures often do not show up until twenty or more years after the initial exposure.
- Some common examples of the effects of hazardous chemicals include:
  - Skin irritation, dermatitis or skin cancer from frequent contact with oils.
  - Injuries to hands and eyes from contact with corrosive liquids.
  - Asthma resulting from sensitisation to isocyanates in paints and adhesives.
  - Long-term disability from lung diseases following exposure to dusty environments (e.g. exposure to respirable crystalline silicate).
  - Death or injury from exposure to toxic fumes (e.g. carbon monoxide).
  - Cancer causing death many years after first exposure to carcinogens at work (e.g. asbestos).
- Chemicals vary widely in how toxic (poisonous) they are.
- Exposure to small amounts of highly toxic chemicals can be a greater danger than exposure to large amounts of less toxic chemicals person is unique.
- While there are many similarities in response to chemical

exposures, responses may vary dramatically among individuals. For example, males and females can react differently and special concern is afforded to pregnant employees. Some individuals are allergic or hypersensitive to certain chemicals.

- Exposure is a function of the concentration of poison that the patient is exposed to, and time. Exact symptoms will depend on the toxidrome of the chemical.
- One-time exposures that are of short duration are of less concern than multiple exposures of longer duration, all other factors being equal. Thus, when there has been a chemical exposure, it is important to know its duration and frequency.

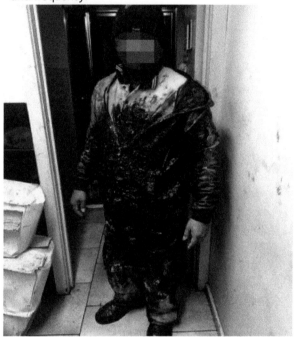

ANTIDOTES OF CERTAIN TOXIDROMES

Poison	Toxidrome	Antidote
Methaemoglobin	Normal pupil size, cyanosis despite good oxygenation, decreased respiratory rate	**Methylene Blue**
Hydrofluoric acid	Rapid onset severe pain and erythema	**Calcium Gluconate**
Carboxy-Haemoglobin	Normal pupils size, Pink or cyanosed skin, Decreased conscious level and respiratory rate	**Oxygen**
Hydrogen Sulphide	Mydriasis, cyanosis, Increased respiratory rate	**Sodium Nitrite**

---

[169] *Workplace Health Toolkit to Assist Small Businesses, Chemicals [Online]*

MANAGEMENT
General principles of care of contamination[170]
Contamination has three phases:

- **Primary** is from the incident and can only be minimised before the event (by safety measures, Personal Protective Equipment (PPE), handling plans etc).
- **Secondary** comes from contaminated people leaving the scene and taking the chemical with them, and may occur from the exhalation of patients with certain poisonings, such as cyanide.
- **Tertiary** results to the environment, including air and water-borne spread.

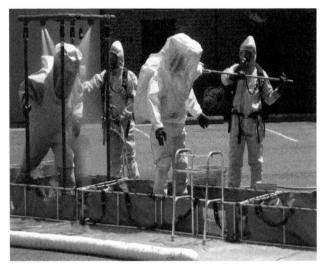

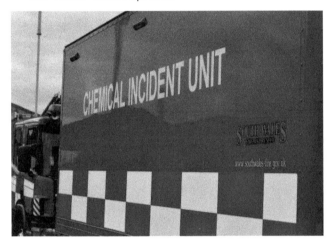

- Following an overt release of hazardous materials, decontamination may be needed to reduce the risk of harm to the patient, to others, or to the wider environment.
- Casualties should ideally be decontaminated at the scene, but it should be expected that contaminated casualties may also self-present to emergency department.
- The first indication of a CBRN incident may be the arrival of contaminated or symptomatic patients at your emergency department or urgent care centre.
- Prompt decontamination after chemical exposure is needed if caustic or irritating injuries are present, or organophosphate (nerve agent) poisoning is suspected.
- Remove all contaminated clothes (to be treated as hazardous waste)

- Decontamination is NOT NEEDED if the chemical agent released is a gas.
- In a radiation incident, treat and stabilise life-threatening injury before decontamination Be alert to the unusual, the unexpected, and the unexplained – and if in doubt, seek expert advice.
- Decontamination methods to be preferred are: •
  o Disrobing
  o Improvised dry decontamination
  o Improvised wet decontamination
- Standard Fire and Rescue Service frontline decontamination systems should only normally be used for planned and structured decontamination.
- NHS secondary care decontamination facilities should be used to manage any casualties self-presenting at hospitals or where contaminated casualties have been transported directly to hospital and the nature of the contaminant may pose a risk to the secondary care environment if decontamination is not performed before admitting.
- Other people in the waiting room may also be contaminated, and the department may become unusable.
- All waste should be bagged for disposal.

---

[170] *Public health England, Chemical, biological, radiological and nuclear incidents: clinical management and health protection [Online]*

V. ACUTE RADIATION SYNDROME

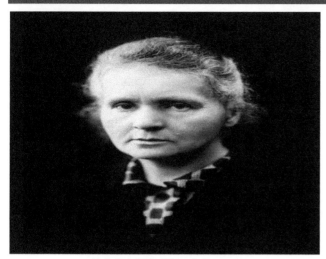

Marie Curie 1920 - Wikimedia Commons

INTRODUCTION

- Since the time nuclear energy has been harnessed and was put to use in industry, medicine, scientific research, military and numerous other fields, undesirable radiation incidents or accidents of variable scales have time and again overshadowed the benefits reaped from it by the mankind.[171]
- Human exposure to nuclear radiations due to accidents, sabotage and terrorism are a reality and leave in their wake perplexing challenges to competent but relatively unprepared healthcare providers.
- The primary principles and objectives of response to nuclear/radiological emergencies includes mitigation of accidents at the site of occurrence and of individual health hazards, rendering primary first aid and imparting injury treatment, reduction of chances of delayed outcomes in the general population, protection of environment and addressing to their psychological impact.
- On the basis of severity of the nuclear/radiological events and their effects, necessary response should be mobilized without any delay through a trained and equipped team.[172]

---

[171] *Coeytaux K., Bey E., Christensen D., Glassman E.S., Murdock B., Doucet C. Reported radiation overexposure accidents worldwide, 1980– 2013: a systematic review. Carpenter DO, ed. PLOS ONE. 2015;10(3):e0118709.*

[172] *National Disaster Management Authority (IN); February; New Delhi: 2009. National Disaster Management Guidelines—Management of Nuclear and Radiological Emergencies. 170 pp. http://nidm.gov.in/pdf/guidelines/new/managementofnuclearradiologic alemergencies.pdf.*

- Each radiation accident may lead to an acute emergency. Assessment for ionizing radiation exposure and the extent to which the patient is afflicted with radiation induced damage is to be done immediately.
- This is important to arrive at the provisional diagnosis, and to decide the requirement of hospitalization, type of hospital facility and super-specialty care imperative in the case.
- The following primary aspects are required to be deliberated for patient care in accidents due to radiation:
  (a)Assessment of damage and its extent
  (b)Choosing the type of healthcare facility
  (c)Providing suitable medical care
  (d)Prognosis assessment

CLINICAL MANIFESTATION OF ACUTE RADIATION SYNDROME

- Prodromal signs and symptoms develop within 1-72 hrs of an individual exposed to a dose of 10-20 Gy or more, which include fever, loss of appetite, nausea and vomiting, loose motions, fluid and electrolyte derangement.
- These may gradually lead to hypotension, loss of consciousness, damage to other organ systems and finally result in death within a few days.
- A severe and rapid prodromal phase predicts a poor clinical prognosis.
- It is difficult to ascertain the prognosis from prodromal response if the exposure is less than 2-10 Gy.
- Subsequent to the prodromal phase occurs the illness targeting various organ systems.
- The critically important organ systems primarily affected in Acute Radiation Syndrome are hematopoietic, cutaneous, gastrointestinal and the neurovascular.

NEUROVASCULAR SYNDROME

- Focal transient aberration of the nervous system results from low dose exposure to radiation.
- Impairment of capillary circulation, acute inflammation, interstitial edema, petechial hemorrhages and meningitis are some of the transient changes.

- EEGs may show paroxysmal spike and wave discharges and CT scans head and MRIs may show the presence of edema.[173]

CUTANEOUS SYNDROME

- Moist desquamation and erythema of the skin may occur within 1-2 days after early exposure, however the complete manifestations may take years. Such lesions can present simultaneously in various parts of the body, subject to the extent of exposure. The commonly seen signs and symptoms are pruritus, blisters, and bullae, ulceration of skin, subcutaneous tissue, muscle or bone. Blister and bullae associated with or without necrosis generally appear 1-3 weeks after exposure of more than 3 Gy.
- It is imperative to grade the severity of involvement of various systems at the earliest after exposure to significant radiation for planning future management strategies.

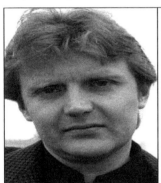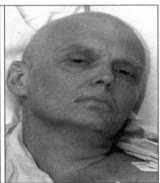

Image source CBS news

GASTROINTESTINAL SYNDROME

- Doses between 05 and 12 Gy may lead to mild gastrointestinal symptoms like mild diarrhea, abdominal pain and electrolyte imbalance. However, the recovery is almost certain.
- Extensive damage to the gastrointestinal tract may lead to ulceration and necrosis of the bowel and severe complications like stenosis, ileus, and perforation.

HAEMATOPOIETIC SYNDROME

- Clinical manifestations of Haematopoietic Syndrome (HS) may be seen primarily in patients having significant radiation exposure (more than 2 Gy) due to radiation induced damage of the haematopoietic tissue of the bone marrow.

- Significant radiation exposure leads to aplasia or hypoplasia which may lead to peripheral blood cytopenias.
- Mild cytopenias without significant bone marrow damage are induced at lower doses of less than 2 Gy radiations, while complete myeloablation without any chance of autologous recovery results from very high dose of more than 10 Gy.
- The severity of hematotoxicity can be graded from degree 1 to degree 4 based on the polymorphonuclear leucocytosis level, lymphocytic, platelet count, and the associated blood loss or infectio.
- The management depends on severity of involvement of hematological toxicity.

STAGES OF ACUTE RADIATION SYNDROME

The four stages of ARS are[174]:

- **Prodromal stage (N-V-D stage):** The classic symptoms for this stage are nausea, vomiting, as well as anorexia and possibly diarrhea (depending on dose), which occur from minutes to days following exposure. The symptoms may last (episodically) for minutes up to several days.
- **Latent stage:** In this stage, the patient looks and feels generally healthy for a few hours or even up to a few weeks.
- **Manifest illness stage:** In this stage the symptoms depend on the specific syndrome (see Table 1) and last from hours up to several months.
- **Recovery or death:** Most patients who do not recover will die within several months of exposure. The recovery process lasts from several weeks up to two years.

LABORATORY EVALUATION

- Take **FBC at 12h then 4 hourly**.
- Lymphocyte counts decrease depending on the absorbed dose to the body and consequent severity of radiation sickness.
- A fall in absolute lymphocyte count is a practical and reliable approach for early assessment based on the radiation exposure dose.
- Three main elements which are essential for assessment of prognosis and selection of treatment are:
  o Time required for onset of vomiting,
  o Depletion of lymphocytes and its kinetics, and
  o Chromosomal changes.

[173] Gorin N.C., Fliedner T.M., Gourmelon P. Consensus conference on European preparedness for haematological and other medical management of mass radiation accidents. Ann Hematol. 2006;85:671–679.

[174] Centers for Disease Control and Prevention. Acute Radiation Syndrome: A Fact Sheet for Clinicians [Online]

TRIAGE

- Majority of casualties may not require immediate medical attention and the "well and worried" might form a large number.
- The concerned department shall be made responsible for limiting further damage, decontamination, protection of general public, and disposal of radioactive material. In addition to a hematologist, a trauma specialist, burns specialist, neurologist and dermatologist may be made available.
- Detailed clinical assessment should be done at the earliest on receiving the patient. Health care institutions should develop protocols which are in tandem with the local resources and health care teams. Bigger incidents warrant a national response system to be in place.

EMERGENCY MEDICAL TEAMS: ROLE AND RESPONSIBILITY

- Subsequent to triage, victims of radiation exposure should be immediately moved to the nearest appropriate health care facility where a preliminary evaluation and treatment can be started. Overlapping roles of various specialists will be instrumental in management of each patient. A well-structured and coordinated care by various specialties supported by good nursing care for inpatients, especially those admitted in ICU will be the bedrock for successful outcomes.
- To overcome the detrimental effects on the psychology of the patients and their relatives, the role of Psychiatrists and Social workers cannot be negated.[175]
- Based on the signs and symptoms severity each patient is given a "response category".

SUPPORTIVE THERAPY

- **Personnel safety**: recommendations are that:
  - At **0.1mGy/hr:** personnel can enter and do lifesaving/ time critical/ treatments,
  - At exposures **> 0.1Gy/hr exposure** is life threatening so personnel should not proceed.
- The following are the indispensable components of the support therapy:
  - Dose estimation
  - Psychological support
  - Fluid and electrolyte estimation

- If a patient has had a complete body dose of more than 2-3 Gy, reverse isolation, antacids and H2 blockers are given. If severe Granulocytopenia is observed, reverse barrier nursing, prophylactic antimicrobials should be given.
- Blood component products are introduced if patient has severe bone marrow damage.[176]

SPECIFIC THERAPEUTIC APPROACHES

- Colony Stimulating Factor (CSF).
- Haematopoetic CSFs like Granulocyte Colony Stimulating Factor (G-CSF), Pegylated Granulocyte Colony Stimulating Factor (PEG-G-CSF or Pegfilgrastim), Recombinant Granylocyte Macrophage Colony Stimulating Factor (GM-CSF), Erythropoietin (EPO), Thrombopoietin analogs and Thrombopoietin receptor agonists like Eltrombopag are available.
- CSFs facilitate neutrophil recovery in radiation induced bone-marrow suppression as they promote multiplication and differentiation of granulocyte progenitors for generation of neutrophils. Newer modalities being evaluated are novel cytokine therapies like interleukin-7 and keratinocyte growth factor. Allogenic haematopoietic stem cell transplant (HSCT)
- For patients with severe bone marrow aplasia HSCT is lifesaving, however the approach is complicated by concomitant burns and traumatic injuries. Generally, the approach should be that a sample for HLA typing is taken initially, followed by a potential donor search, however transplant is undertaken not before the minimal observation period of 14-21 days is elapsed. HSCT is undertaken only after considering the factors like irradiation source, patient specific issues, any additional injuries and previous diseases.

CONCLUSION

- Nuclear and radiation accidents are a reality in the present world. Multi organ system pathology is generally the outcome of radiation exposure.
- The management of victims of these accidents is challenging and needs to be undertaken with meticulous assessment of the various factors.
- Awareness of these medical challenges is the need of the hour and a structured organizational approach will deliver desirable outcomes.

---

175 Fliedner T.M., Friesecke I., Beyrer K., British Institute of Radiology, editors. Medical Management of Radiation Accident—Manual on the Acute Radiation Syndrome (METREPOL European Commission concerted action) British Institute of Radiology; Oxford: 2001. pp. 1–66. compendium p. C1–C21.

176 Fliedner T.M., Friesecke I., Beyrer K., British Institute of Radiology, editors. Medical Management of Radiation Accident—Manual on the Acute Radiation Syndrome (METREPOL European Commission concerted action) British Institute of Radiology; Oxford: 2001. pp. 1–66. compendium p. C1–C21.

VI. BITES & ENVENOMATIONS IN UK

1. SNAKE BITE

- There are many snakes that are not poisonous. However, when a person is bitten by a venomous snake this will often result in a medical emergency.
- UK poisons centres are consulted about an average of 100 human and a dozen veterinary cases each year. In about 70% of patients, envenoming is negligible or purely local, causing pain, swelling, and inflammation of the bitten digit.
- Only 14 fatalities have been reported since 1876[177], the last in a 5 year old child in 1975, but adder bites should not be underestimated. On rare occasions, envenoming can be life threatening, especially in children, and many adults experience prolonged discomfort and disability after the bite. The toxins released through the poison glands of a snake will often subdue or kill the victim, and there are some bites that can actually begin to break down the victim's tissue.
- The affects can be fatal within a very short space of time.
- A child would need immediate attention due to their small size and the ability of the poison to work its way around the body quickly.
- If an antidote for the venom is readily available then it can be suitably treated, but if there is not one available then the results can be fatal. Snakes known to be poisonous include the rattlesnake, cobra and coral snake.
- Three species of snake are native to the mainland UK:
  o *Vipera berus* (adder or viper)
  o *Natrix natrix* (grass snake)
  o *Coronella austriaca* (smooth snake)
- *In the UK, **adders** (pictured below) are the only venomous snakes found in the wild.*
- *People also keep foreign (exotic) venomous snakes, sometimes illegally.*

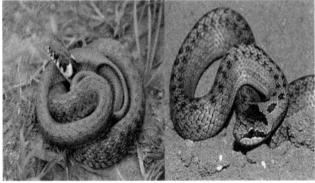
Vipera berus

---
[177] *Reid HA. Adder bites in Britain. BMJ 1976; 2: 15*

- It occurs throughout mainland Britain (it is the only snake in Scotland) and on some of the islands off western Scotland but not in the Channel Isles, Isle of Man, Ireland, Outer Hebrides, Orkneys and Shetland.
- It can be identified by its grey/brown body and distinctive dark zigzag pattern along its back. Bites are rare in the winter when the snake hibernates.
- *Snake bites, particularly those that occur in the UK, usually aren't serious and are only very rarely deadly*
- Some *V. berus* bites cause no envenoming but systemic features occur in about 30% of cases. Most bites occur on the hands or feet.

CLINICAL FEATURES
1. NON-VENOMOUS BITES:
Local *V. berus* envenoming:

- A sensation of tingling and local swelling that spreads proximally occur up to 30 minutes after the bite.
- Pain, tenderness, erythema, swelling, and regional lymph node enlargement ensue within hours, together with reddish lymphatic lines and bruising.
- Depending on severity the whole limb may become swollen and bruised with involvement of the trunk, and in children the whole body, within 24 hours.
- Massive extravasation into the bitten limb may occur, requiring volume resuscitation. Necrosis and intra-compartmental syndromes are extremely rare.

Systemic *V. berus* envenoming:
This is less common than local envenoming in the UK.
- **Acute anaphylaxis-like**: nausea, vomiting, abdominal pain, transient, recurrent or persistent hypotension, urticaria, angio-oedema, and bronchospasm - and last for up to 48 hours.
- **Bleeding diathesis**: *Bleeding is made worse by administration of heparin, which should not be given.*
- **Acute renal failure** especially in children.
- **Increased capillary permeability** causes angio-oedema (causing airway occlusion), pulmonary oedema, and cerebral oedema.
- **Coma and convulsions**
- **Cardiac effects:** tachy or brady-dysrhythmias, heart block, global ECG changes suggesting ischaemia and myocardial infarction precipitated by hypotension.

- **GI effects:** gastric dilatation, ileus, and acute pancreatitis.
- **Deaths** have occurred 6-60 hours after the bite.
- Patients may **develop complications** such as hypotension 12-24 hours after the bite.

INVESTIGATIONS

- Neutrophil leucocytosis is common.
- Initial haemo-concentration and later anaemia result from extravasation into the bitten limb and perhaps haemolysis. Concentrations of serum creatine kinase, transaminases, urea, and creatinine may be raised, and bicarbonate may be reduced.
- Thrombocytopenia and mild coagulopathy—reflected by prolonged prothrombin time (international normalised ratio), activated partial thromboplastin time, hypofibrinogenaemia, and raised fibrin degradation products or D-dimer—is sometimes detected.
- Consumption coagulopathy and incoagulable blood (20 minute whole blood clotting test) are uncommon.[178]
- Electrocardiographic changes include tachyarrhythmias, bradyarrhythmias, atrial fibrillation, flattening or inversion of T waves, ST elevation or depression, second degree heart block, and frank myocardial infarction.[179]

EMERGENCY DEPARTMENT MANAGEMENT

- Any interference with the bite site should be avoided.
- Do not cut into or suck from the site, or apply tourniquets, ligatures, or compression bandages

FIRST AID

- Initial management is to reassure, give paracetamol to control pain, and immobilise the whole patient (especially the bitten limb with a splint or sling) during urgent transport to hospital.
- Early anaphylactoid symptoms can be treated with an oral or parenteral H_1 blocker or adrenaline (epinephrine) (Epi-Pen), depending on severity. Any interference with the wound should be avoided.
- Tourniquets, ligatures, and compression bandages should not be used.

HOSPITAL TREATMENT

- In hospital, rapid clinical assessment of the degree of envenoming and resuscitation may be needed, followed by careful monitoring of the blood pressure and evolution of envenoming over at least 24 hours.
- The most important decision is whether antivenom should be given.

ANTIVENOM

- This specific antidote prevents mortality and reduces hospital stay and morbidity,[180] but it is underused in the UK. Zagreb antivenom has been provided to NHS hospitals since 1969.
- Other effective antivenoms are Protherics ViperaTAb and Sanofi-Pasteur Viperfav. Zagreb antivenom has also proved safe and effective in *V berus* envenomed dogs. Indications for antivenom are:
  - Hypotension with or without signs of shock
  - Other signs of systemic envenoming (see above), electrocardiographic abnormalities, peripheral neutrophil leucocytosis, elevated serum creatine kinase, or metabolic acidosis
  - Local swelling that is either extensive (involving more than half the bitten limb within 48 hours of the bite) or rapidly spreading (beyond the wrist after bites on the hand or beyond the ankle after bites on the foot within about four hours of the bite).
- Two ampoules of Zagreb antivenom are given (exactly the same dose for infants and children) by slow intravenous injection or infusion; 0.1% adrenaline (plus intravenous antihistamine and hydrocortisone) should be drawn up in case of early anaphylactoid antivenom reactions, which complicate about 10% of treatments with Zagreb antivenom.
- These reactions are not predicted by intradermal hypersensitivity tests. Their frequency may be reduced by giving prophylactic subcutaneous adrenaline (adult dose 0.25 mg of 0.1%)[181] but is not affected by H_1 blockers.
- If no clinical improvement has occurred after one hour, the initial dose of two ampoules of antivenom can be repeated. Late serum sickness reactions can be treated with oral H_1 blockers or corticosteroids.

OTHER MANAGEMENT

- Intravenous fluids or blood transfusion may be needed to correct hypovolaemia and anaemia from massive extravasation into the tissues.
- The bitten limb should be nursed in the most comfortable position, but excessive elevation should be avoided. Contractures (such as result in equinus deformity) from prolonged bed rest must be prevented by splinting, and rehabilitation physiotherapy should be started as early as possible.

[178] Karlson-Stiber C, Persson H. Antivenom treatment in Vipera berus envenoming—report of 30 cases. J Intern Med 1994; 235: 57

[179] Persson H, Irestedt B. A study of 136 cases of adder bite treated in Swedish hospitals during one year. Acta Med Scand 1981; 210: 4339.

[180] Theakston RDG, Reid HA. Effectiveness of Zagreb antivenom against envenoming by the adder, Vipera erus. Lancet 1976; ii: 1215.

[181] Premawardhena AP,de Silva CE, Fonseka MM,Gunatilake SB, de Silva HJ. Low dose subcutaneous adrenaline to prevent acute adverse reactions to antivenom serum in people bitten by snakes: randomised, placebo-controlled trial. BMJ 1999; 318: 10413.

VII. HIGH ALTITUDE EMERGENCIES

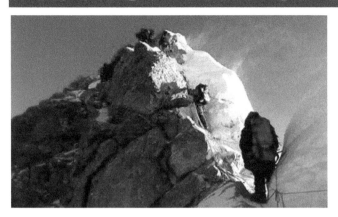

INTRODUCTION

- Preventive measures, along with prompt recognition and treatment of altitude-related illness, are essential to improving outcomes and preventing life-threatening sequelae. Patients participating in occupational and sports-related activities requiring ascent to high elevations are at risk of developing a range of high-altitude illnesses. Prompt recognition and treatment are paramount to improving outcomes and preventing life-threatening sequelae. High-elevation locations are the setting of many recreational activities for outdoor enthusiasts. As such, illnesses associated with high altitude may be encountered by those summiting peaks, traveling by air, or working in flight medicine or as part of an emergency rescue team.
- The altitude syndromes discussed in this review are acute mountain sickness (**AMS**), high-altitude cerebral edema (**HACE**), and high-altitude pulmonary edema (**HAPE**).
- While these conditions do not represent all altitude-related illnesses, they are the primary pathological processes for which ED physicians should be familiar when working with high-altitude populations.

PHYSIOLOGICAL RESPONSE TO ALTITUDE

- The normal acclimatization response to high elevation involves an increase in alveolar ventilation, referred to as **hypoxic ventilatory response (HVR)**.
- The HVR is initiated by the carotid body, which acts as a peripheral chemosensor.
- **Over the first 2 weeks at elevation,** an increased sensitivity to hypoxia leads to a **rise in ventilation**. This precipitates an increase in alveolar oxygen pressure and arterial oxygen concentration, and a **decrease in arterial carbon dioxide**.
- **Cardiac output increases,** ventilation perfusion-matching is improved, and pulmonary arterial pressure rises.

- **Respiratory alkalosis** develops secondary to this hyperventilation; as a compensatory response, increased **excretion of bicarbonate** by the kidneys occurs, leading to a normalization of pH, which peaks at about 7 days.
- These physiological changes result in **hyperventilation**, increased **urinary output**, periodic nighttime breathing, and dyspnea on exertion.
- **Periodic nighttime breathing** is characterized by periods of hyperpnea followed by apnea during sleep.
- The duration of apnea is commonly 3 to 10 seconds, but may last up to 15 seconds. These symptoms may be considered normal at elevations above 2500 meters.

THE LAKE LOUISE CRITERIA

- The following definitions on the diagnosis of altitude illness were adopted at the 1991 International Hypoxia Symposium, held at Lake Louise in Alberta, Canada[182].

AMS	In the setting of a recent gain in altitude, the presence of **headache** and at least one of the following symptoms: ○ GIT (Anorexia, Nausea or Vomiting) ○ Fatigue or Weakness ○ Dizziness or Lightheadedness ○ Difficulty Sleeping
HACE	Can be considered **"end stage"** or **severe AMS**. In the setting of a recent gain in altitude, either: ○ The presence of a change in mental status and/or ataxia in a person with AMS ○ Or, the presence of both mental status changes and ataxia in a person without AMS
HAPE	In the setting of a recent gain in altitude, the presence of the following: • **Symptoms: at least two of:** ○ Dyspnea at rest ○ Cough ○ Weakness or decreased exercise performance ○ Chest tightness or congestion • **Signs: at least two of:** ○ Crackles or wheezing in at least one lung field ○ Central cyanosis ○ Tachypnea/ Tachycardia

[182] Roach RC, Bärtch P, Hackett PH, Oelz O, and the Lake Louise AMS Scoring Consensus Committee. The Lake Louise Acute Mountain Sickness Scoring System. In: Hypoxia and Molecular Medicine. Proceedings of the 8th International Hypoxia Symposium. Burlington, VT: Queen City Printers; 1993:272-274.

1. ACUTE MOUNTAIN SICKNESS

- Acute mountain sickness (AMS) comprises a constellation of symptoms caused by the atmospheric changes at elevations above approximately 2,500 m.
- It is the most common form of high-altitude illness, affecting 25% of travelers at moderate altitude and 50% to 85% above 4,000 m.[183]

SYMPTOMS

- The onset of symptoms (eg, headache, anorexia, nausea, vomiting, weakness) may occur at 2,000 m in the setting of rapid ascent—most commonly at 6 to 12 hours, but onset can range from 1 hour to 2 days after ascent. If symptoms begin after 3 days, other diagnoses should be considered.
- Symptoms of AMS are generally worse after the first night of sleep at elevation. On physical examination, vital signs are usually normal, though **postural hypotension and tachycardia** are possible.
- Oxygen saturation may be markedly decreased after rapid ascent, and chest auscultation may reveal **rales in 20%** of patients[184]. **Peripheral and facial edema** may also be present. Funduscopic examination may show venous tortuosity and dilation, and **retinal hemorrhage** is common in ascents over 4,800 m.

  ↓ *High altitude retinal hemorrhages are more common at altitudes above 5000m. They are usually asymptomatic and typically resolve over a few weeks. They may be found in HAPE and HACE, as well as the otherwise well person.*
  ↓ *Central scotomata can occur if the macula is involved.*

DIFFERENTIAL DIAGNOSIS

The differential diagnosis for AMS is broad and includes hypothermia, dehydration, exhaustion, subarachnoid hemorrhage, intracranial mass, carbon monoxide poisoning, alcohol hangover, intoxication, central nervous system infection and migraine.

Risk factors for developing AMS are:

- *A previous history of altitude illness,*
- *Rapid ascent, and*
- *Lack of previous acclimatization.*
- ↓ *Interestingly, physical fitness does not protect a person from developing AMS.*

MECHANISM OF AMS

- The true mechanism of AMS is uncertain, but it is clear that a fall in barometric pressure results in hypobaric hypoxia.

- This is thought to lead to an increased blood volume in the brain and increased cerebral blood flow, possibly precipitating an enlarged brain. A mechanism related to vasogenic edema has been proposed due to patients' clinical improvement with dexamethasone therapy[185].
- Acute mountain sickness does appear to be related to overall fluid balance, as an increase in reninangiotensin, aldosterone, and antidiuretic hormone has been observed in patients with the condition.
- Elevation of these hormones is contrary to the appropriate physiological response of diuresis.

TREATMENT

- Treatment of AMS **begins with descent from elevation as soon as possible.** Descent should be at least 500 m from the aggravating elevation. Patients should remain at least 1 to 2 days at this lower elevation before attempting reascent. If descent is not feasible, any further ascent should be delayed until symptoms have resolved.
- **Dexamethasone** The initial dose is **8 mg followed by 4 mg QID.**
- **Acetazolamide** 250 **mg BD.**
- **Ibuprofen** 600 **mg tds** reduces the severity of AMS.
- **Oxygen 1 to 2 L/min via nasal cannula for 12-24 hrs**
- **A portable hyperbaric oxygen (HBO) bag** (eg, a Gamow bag) can be used to create an effective altitude of approximately 1,500 to 2,000 m inside the bag. The patient is placed completely within the bag, the zipper is sealed shut, and the bag is inflated with a foot pump. Treatment in such a chamber can be provided in 1-hour increments and repeated as needed. However, if descent is possible, use of the HBO chamber should not prevent or delay descent.

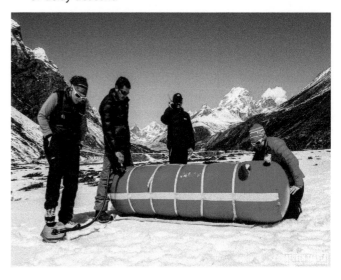

[183] Eide RP 3rd, Asplund CA. Altitude illness: update on prevention and treatment. Curr Sports Med Rep. 2012;11(3):124-130.

[184] Milzman DP, Damergis JA, Napoli AM. Rapid ascent changes in vitals at altitude. Ann Emerg Med. 2008;51(4):536.

[185] Hackett PH, Roach RC. Medical therapy of mountain illness. Ann Emerg Med. 1987;16(9):980-986.

Disclaimer: Information and images included in these notes originate from multiples sources such as academic journals, textbooks, published articles, Emergency Medicine websites and Blogs etc. The Editor and the Publisher have gone to every effort to seek permission from and acknowledge the sources of clinical guidelines and images which appear in this compilation that is public on the internet. Nevertheless, should there be any cases where Copyright holders have not been identified or suitably acknowledged, the author welcome advice from such Copyright holders and will endeavor to amend the text accordingly on future prints

PREVENTION OF AMS

Strategies to prevent AMS are similar to those used to treat the condition. These include gradual ascent and prophylactic drug therapy.

- **Gradual ascent** is the primary strategy to prevent AMS.
- At altitudes above 3,000m, each subsequent night should not be spent at an elevation 300 m higher than the previous night.
- **Acetazolamide 125 mg bd,** and should be started the day before ascent.
- **Dexamethasone 2 mg qid or 4 mg bd**. However, unlike acetazolamide, which acts to facilitate acclimatization, dexamethasone only prevents symptoms. Thus, cessation of the drug can result in rebound AMS symptoms, and prolonged use can result in adrenal suppression. *Therefore, it should not be used for more than 10 days.*
- **Ibuprofen 600 mg tds** can be initiated the day prior to ascent, and has been shown to decrease the incidence of AMS[186].

2. HIGH-ALTITUDE CEREBRAL EDEMA

- High-altitude cerebral edema (HACE), a condition that can be considered on a continuum with AMS, is hallmarked by progressive neurological symptoms.
- It is defined by either the presence of a change in mental status and/or ataxia in a person with AMS, or the presence of both mental status changes and ataxia in a person without AMS. Clinical signs are truncal ataxia, hallucinations, confusion, vomiting, decreased activity, mild fever, upper motor neuronal signs, stupor, or coma. Development of HACE usually requires at least 2 days of altitudes above 4000 m[187].

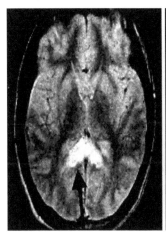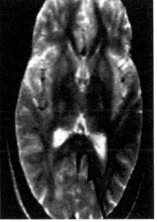

TREATMENT

- Current recommendations for treating HACE are similar to treatment strategies for AMS.
- **Descent:** A therapeutic priority, descent may prove challenging as the patient may be ataxic, have altered mental status, and have difficulty facilitating his or her own descent.
- **Airway Management:** If the patient has significantly altered mental status, appropriate airway management must be initiated.
- **Oxygen:** A portable HBO bag can be used to simulate descent until evacuation is possible.
- Supplemental oxygen should be applied immediately.
- **Dexamethasone:** In treating HACE, dexamethasone may be administered at a loading dose of **8 mg, followed by 4 mg every 6 hours**[188].

3. HIGH ALTITUDE PULMONARY EDEMA

- The most common cause of death from altitude illness is HAPE[189], a form of noncardiogenic pulmonary edema.
- This condition generally occurs at elevations above 3,000 m. Symptoms begin 2 to 5 days after ascent and progress in a typical pattern. A patient will initially experience a **nonproductive cough** and **dyspnea at rest.**
- The dyspnea worsens, and the cough becomes productive of pink, frothy sputum. Without medical intervention, lethargy, coma, and death may follow.
- Symptoms of HAPE generally worsen following a night of sleep at elevation. Physical examination reveals crackles, tachycardia, tachypnea, and hypoxia.

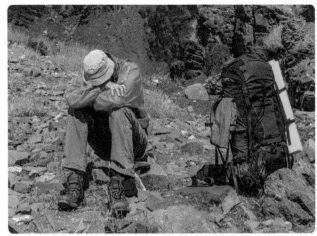

Image source| News medical

[186] Lipman GS, Kanaan NC, Holck PS, Constance BB, Gertsch JH; PAINS Group. Ibuprofen prevents altitude illness: a randomized controlled trial for prevention of altitude illness with nonsteroidal anti-inflammatories. Ann Emerg Med. 2012;59(6): 484-490.

[187] Bärtsch P, Swenson ER. Clinical practice: Acute high-altitude illnesses. N Engl J Med. 2013;368(24):2294-2302.

[188] Eide RP 3rd, Asplund CA. Altitude illness: update on prevention and treatment. Curr Sports Med Rep. 2012;11(3):124-130.

[189] Gallagher SA1, Hackett PH. High-altitude illness. Emerg Med Clin North Am. 2004;22(2):329-355.

Diagnosis requires at least two of the following signs:
- Crackles or wheezing in at least one lung field
- Central cyanosis
- Tachypnea
- Tachycardia.

In addition to the above signs, **at least two of the following symptoms must also be present:**
- Dyspnea at rest
- Cough
- Weakness or decreased exercise performance
- Chest tightness
- Congestion.

- **Chest X-ray** typically reveals patchy opacities at varying locations. There are often infiltrates in the right middle lobe.
- **Ultrasound** has been used to facilitate the diagnosis of HAPE in the field.
- **The "comet-tail" sign** is a term used to describe echogenic patterns in the lung as a result of increased lymphatic flow. This sign, if seen in the clinical setting of HAPE, may aid in the diagnosis and monitoring of treatment efficacy[190].

TREATMENT OF HAPE
- **Descent and warming** of the patient as soon as possible,
- **Oxygen: 4 to 6 L/min**; if the patient improves clinically and can maintain oxygen saturations greater than 90%, oxygen may be decreased with a goal to maintain saturation above 90%.
- **Nifedipine: 20 to 30 mg** of the sustained release form **every 12 hours.**
- **Salmeterol/Albuterol and expiratory positive airway pressure:** The oral inhalers salmeterol or albuterol may be used for bronchodilation; however, there is little evidence to support their effectiveness in HAPE. Ventilation with expiratory positive airway pressure can be employed if available.

PREVENTION
- For patients with a predisposition to HAPE, preventive measures should be considered prior to ascent. As with all forms of altitude illness, gradual ascent is the most effective prevention method available.
- **Phosphodiesterase Inhibitors:** Phosphodiesterase inhibitors act via pulmonary vasodilation to prevent HAPE in some patients.

- **Tadalafil at a dose of 10 mg BD or 20 mg OD** has been shown to reduce the incidence of HAPE or **Sildenafil 50 mg TDS** may be used.
- **Acetazolamide and β-agonists:** Although both acetazolamide and β-agonists such as albuterol have been theorized to aid in preventing HAPE, this has not been proven[191].

RECOMMENDED DOSAGES FOR MEDICATIONS USED IN THE PREVENTION & TREATMENT OF ALTITUDE ILLNESS

Medication	Indication	Route	Dosage
Acetazolamide	AMS, HACE prevention	Oral	125mg BD Paeds: 2.5mg/kg 12hly
	AMS treatment	Oral	250mg BD Paeds: 2.5mg/kg 12 hly
Dexamethasone	AMS, HACE prevention	Oral	2mg 6hly or 4mg 12hly Paeds: should not be used for prophylaxis
	AMS, HACE treatment	Oral, IV, IM	AMS: 4 mg 6hly HACE: 8 mg once then 4 mg 6hly Paeds: 0.15mg/kg/dose 6hly
Nifedipine	HAPE prevention	Oral	30mg SR version 12hly or 20mg SR version 8hly
	HAPE treatment	Oral	30mg SR version 12hly or 20mg SR version 8hly
Tadanafil Sildenafil Salmeterol	HAPE prevention	Oral	10mg BD
	HAPE prevention	Oral	50mg 8hly
	HAPE prevention	Inhaled	125µg BD

190 Fagenholz PJ, Gutman JA, Murray AF, Noble VE, Thomas SH, Harris NS. Chest ultrasonography for the diagnosis and monitoring of high-altitude pulmonary edema. Chest. 2007;131(4): 1013-1018.

191 Schoene RB. Illnesses at high altitude. Chest. 2008;134(2):402-416.

VIII. DECOMPRESSION ILLNESS

INTRODUCTION
- Decompression illness (DCI) encompasses two diseases, **Decompression Sickness (DCS)** and **Arterial Gas Embolism (AGE)**.
- DCS is thought to result from bubbles growing in tissue and causing local damage, while AGE results from bubbles entering the lung circulation, traveling through the arteries and causing tissue damage at a distance by blocking blood flow at the small vessel level.

RISK FACTORS
- Scuba divers,
- Aviators,
- Astronauts and
- Compressed-air workers.

1. DECOMPRESSION SICKNESS
- Decompression sickness **(the bends or caisson disease)** is the result of inadequate decompression following exposure to increased pressure.
- In some cases, the disease is mild and not an immediate threat. In other cases, serious injury does occur; when this happens, the quicker treatment begins, the better the chance for a full recovery.
- During a dive, the body tissues absorb nitrogen from the breathing gas in proportion to the surrounding pressure.
- As long as the diver remains at pressure, the gas presents no problem. If the pressure is reduced too quickly, however, the nitrogen comes out of solution and forms bubbles in the tissues and bloodstream.
- A variety of classification systems have been established for DCS. One common approach is to describe cases as Type 1 or Type 2.

Type 1 DCS
- Type 1 DCS is usually characterized by musculoskeletal pain and mild cutaneous, or skin, symptoms.
- Common Type 1 skin manifestations include itching and mild rashes (as distinct from a clear mottled or marbled and sometimes raised discoloration of the skin – a condition that is known as **cutis marmorata** that may presage the development of the more serious symptoms of Type 2 DCS). Less common but still associated with Type 1 DCS is obstruction of the lymphatic system, which can result in swelling and localized pain in the tissues surrounding the lymph nodes – such as in the armpits, groin or behind the ears.
- The symptoms of Type 1 DCS can build in intensity.

- For example, pain may originate as a mild ache in the vicinity of a joint or muscle and then increase in magnitude. However, the pain associated with DCS does not typically increase upon movement of the affected joint, although holding the limb in one position rather than another may reduce discomfort.
- Such pain can ultimately be quite severe.

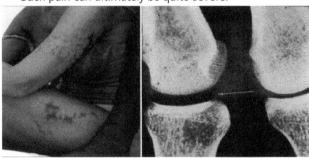

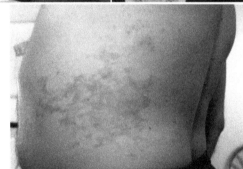

Skin mottling like this is characteristic of cutis marmorata, a condition that can warn of likely development of more serious Type 2 symptoms.

Type 2 DCS
Type 2 symptoms are considered more serious. They typically fall into three categories: **neurological, inner ear and cardiopulmonary**.
- **Neurological symptoms** may include numbness; paresthesia, or an altered sensation, such as tingling; muscle weakness; an impaired gait, or difficulty walking; problems with physical coordination or bladder control; paralysis; or a change in mental status, such as confusion or lack of alertness.
- **Inner-ear symptoms** may include ringing in the ears, known as "tinnitus"; hearing loss; vertigo or dizziness; nausea; vomiting; and impaired balance.
- **Cardiopulmonary symptoms**, known commonly as "**the chokes,**" include a dry cough; chest pain behind the sternum, or breastbone; and "dyspnea."
- **The respiratory complaints,** which are typically due to high bubble loads in the lungs, can compromise the lungs' ability to function – threatening the affected diver's health, and even life, if treatment is not sought promptly.

2. ARTERIAL GAS EMBOLISM

- If a diver surfaces without exhaling, air trapped in the lungs expands with ascent and may rupture lung tissue - called **pulmonary barotrauma** - which releases gas bubbles into the arterial circulation. This distributes them to body tissues in proportion to the blood flow. Since the brain receives the highest proportion of blood flow, it is the main target organ where bubbles may interrupt circulation if they become lodged in small arteries.

- This is arterial gas embolism, or AGE, considered the more serious form of DCI. In some cases, the diver may have made a panicked ascent, or he may have held his breath during ascent. However, AGE can occur even if ascent appeared completely normal, and pulmonary disease such as obstructive lung disease may increase the risk of AGE. The most dramatic presentation of air embolism is the diver who surfaces unconscious and remains so, or the diver who loses consciousness within 10 minutes of surfacing. In these cases, a true medical emergency exists, and rapid evacuation to a treatment facility is paramount.

- On the other hand, air embolism may cause fewer spectacular symptoms of neurological dysfunction, such as sensations of tingling or numbness, a sensation of weakness without obvious paralysis, or complaints of difficulty in thinking without obvious confusion in individuals who are awake and easily aroused. In these cases, there is time for a more thorough evaluation by a diving medical specialist to rule out other causes of symptoms.

SYMPTOMS OF AGE
- Dizziness
- Visual blurring
- Areas of decreased sensation
- Chest pain
- Disorientation

SIGNS OF AGE
- Bloody froth from mouth or nose
- Paralysis or weakness
- Convulsions
- Unconsciousness
- Cessation of breathing
- Death

PREVENTION OF AGE
- Always relax and breathe normally during ascent.
- Lung conditions such as asthma, infections, cysts, tumors, scar tissue from surgery or obstructive lung disease may predispose a diver to air embolism.

COMPLICATIONS
- Residual paralysis,
- Myocardial necrosis.

EMERGENCY DEPARTMENT CARE
The treatment for DCI is **recompression.**

- **Administer 100% oxygen** to wash nitrogen out of the lungs and set up an increased diffusion gradient to increase nitrogen offloading from the body.

- **Do not put the patient into the Trendelenburg position.** Placing the patient in a head-down posture used to be considered a standard treatment of diving injuries to prevent cerebral gas embolization. This practice should be abandoned. The process actually increases intracranial pressure and exacerbates injury to the blood-brain barrier. It also wastes time and complicates movement of the patient.

- **Perform intubation and aggressive resuscitation** including advanced cardiac and trauma life support.

- If **tension pneumothorax:** perform needle decompression followed by chest tube thoracostomy, if indicated.

- **If pneumoperitoneum** from ruptured viscus: perform Emergent needle decompression of the peritoneum is the corrective procedure.

- **Administer intravenous fluids** for rehydration until urinary output is **1-2 mL/kg/h**. Rehydration improves circulation and perfusion.

- **Aspirin** is commonly considered and given in diving accidents for antiplatelet activity if the patient is not bleeding. However, there are no current data to support this practice. The nitrogen bubbles interact with platelets, leading to adhesion and activation, which is thought to contribute to micro venous obstruction and resultant ischemia in DCS. However, no studies or trials of the effect or benefit of aspirin on this process have been conducted. Giving aspirin could increase bleeding, especially in severe DCS.

- Treat the patient for nausea, vomiting, pain, and headache.

- **Contact the closest hyperbaric facility** to arrange transfer and try to keep all diving gear with the diver.

- The diving gear may provide clues as to why the diver had trouble (eg, faulty air regulator, hose leak, carbon monoxide contamination of the compressed air).

- Patients with type I or mild type II DCS can dramatically improve and have complete symptom resolution. This improvement should not dissuade the practitioner from **HBO referral or transfer**, as relapses have occurred with worse outcomes.

16. Endocrine Emergencies
I. ADRENAL INSUFFICIENCY

INTRODUCTION

- **Adrenal crisis** and **severe acute adrenocortical insufficiency** are often elusive diagnoses that may result in severe morbidity and mortality when undiagnosed or ineffectively treated.
- Although it is thought by experts that more than 50 steroids are produced within the adrenal cortex, **cortisol** and **aldosterone** are by far the most abundant and physiologically active. Do not confuse acute **adrenal crisis** with **Addison disease**.
- **Adrenal crisis** is a life-threatening condition that requires emergency medical treatment.
- The patient or a family member or friend should immediately give an emergency injection of a glucocorticoid at the first signs of adrenal crisis.
- **Addison disease** described a syndrome of long-term adrenal insufficiency that develops over months to years, with weakness, fatigue, anorexia, weight loss, and hyperpigmentation as the primary symptoms.
- In contrast, an acute adrenal crisis can manifest with vomiting, abdominal pain, and hypovolemic shock. Usually caused by concurrent illness, surgery, failure to take medications
- **In primary adrenocortical insufficiency**, glucocorticoid and mineralocorticoid properties are lost; however, in **secondary adrenocortical insufficiency** (i.e., secondary to disease or suppression of the hypothalamic-pituitary axis), mineralocorticoid function is preserved.
- As suggested by its occurrence in both causes of adrenal insufficiency, both mineralocorticoid and glucocorticoid deficiency can participate in the development of adrenal crisis.
- The physiologic basis for this is the ability of aldosterone or synthetic mineralocorticoid to promote sodium retention as well as to enhance vasoconstrictor responses of the vasculature[192].

PATHOPHYSIOLOGY

- **Adrenal medullae** normally secrete **80% epinephrine** and **20% norepinephrine**. Sympathetic stimulation results in secretion.

- The adrenal cortex produces cortisol, aldosterone, and androgens.

PHYSIOLOGIC EFFECTS OF ALDOSTERONE

- Aldosterone is produced by multiple hydroxylations of deoxycorticosterone and is normally 60% protein bound.
- The renin-angiotensin system stimulates aldosterone release.
- Increased potassium stimulates aldosterone production, and decreased potassium inhibits production.
- Chronic adrenocorticotropic hormone (ACTH) deficiency may inhibit production.
- **Excess aldosterone** results in sodium retention, hypokalemia, and alkalosis.
- **Aldosterone deficiency** results in sodium loss, hyperkalemia, and acidosis.
- Hyperkalemia stimulates aldosterone release to improve potassium excretion.
- Aldosterone is the first-line defense against hyperkalemia.

1. PRIMARY ADRENAL INSUFFICIENCY

- Primary adrenal insufficiency, which can be acute or chronic, may be caused by the anatomic destruction of the gland.
- This destruction can have various causes, including tuberculosis or fungal infection, other diseases infiltrating the adrenal glands, and hemorrhage. However, the most frequent cause is **idiopathic atrophy**, which is probably autoimmune in origin.
- Primary adrenal insufficiency also may be caused by metabolic failure (eg, insufficient hormone production).
- This failure may be a result of congenital adrenal hyperplasia (CAH), enzyme inhibitors (eg, metyrapone), or cytotoxic agents (eg, mitotane).
- Primary adrenocortical insufficiency is rare and occurs at any age. The male:female ratio is 1:1.

---

192 Feldman RD, Gros R. Vascular effects of aldosterone: sorting out the receptors and the ligands. Clin Exp Pharmacol Physiol 2013; 40:916.

2. SECONDARY ADRENAL INSUFFICIENCY

- Secondary adrenal insufficiency may be caused by **hypopituitarism** due to hypothalamic-pituitary disease or may result from suppression of the hypothalamic-pituitary axis by exogenous steroids or endogenous steroids (i.e., tumor).
- Secondary adrenocortical insufficiency is relatively common. Extensive therapeutic use of steroids has greatly contributed to increased incidence.

CAUSES

CAUSES OF ADRENAL INSUFFICIENCY
Primary causes
• Idiopathic/Autoimmune
• Infective: TB, AIDS, Fungal infection.
• Haemorrhage: anticoagulant therapy, Waterhouse-Friderichsen syndrome (haemorrhage into the adrenal gland secondary to fulminant meningococcal septicaemia).
• Infiltration : carcinoma, lymphoma, sarcoidosis, amyloidosis.
• Drugs: ketoconazole, Etomidate
Secondary causes
• Abrupt withdrawal of long-term steroids
• Trauma to infundibular stalk
• Necrosis (Sheehan's syndrome)
• Neoplasms and granulomatous disease of pituitary
• Radiation to pituitary

3. ADRENAL CRISIS

HISTORY

The following are important elements in the history of patients with adrenal crisis or adrenal insufficiency:
- Weakness, Pigmentation of skin, Weight loss
- Abdominal pain, Salt craving, Diarrhea
- Constipation, Syncope, Vitiligo

PHYSICAL

- Patients with **mineralocorticoid insufficiency** may show signs of sodium and volume depletion (eg, orthostatic hypotension, tachycardia). Evidence of hyperpigmentation is observed, particularly in areas exposed to the sun or areas subject to friction or pressure.

INVESTIGATION

- U&E, Serum Cortisol & Plasma ACTH
- Infective Screen and ECG
- **Adrenocortical deficiency results in:**
  - Hyponatraemia.
  - Hyperkalaemia.
  - Hypoglycaemia.
  - Elevated urea and creatinine.
  - Metabolic acidosis.
  - Raised Ca2+ (primary only)
  - Eosinophilia
  - *Serum cortisol and plasma ACTH levels should be sent, but should not delay treatment with hydrocortisone.*

- **Interpretation of the cortisol and ACTH results:**
  - Low serum cortisol (<200nmol/L): indicates adrenal insufficiency.
  - A raised ACTH in this context suggests primary adrenal insufficiency and a low ACTH suggests secondary.
  - High serum cortisol (>550nmol/L): excludes adrenal insufficiency.
  - Intermediate serum cortisol (200-550 nmol/L): requires further investigation with a Synacthen (tetracosactrin) test.

DIFFERENTIAL DIAGNOSES

- Acute Hypoglycemia
- Acute Hypopituitarism
- Anorexia Nervosa
- Appendicitis
- Cholecystitis and Biliary Colic
- Urinary Tract Infection (UTI) and Cystitis
- Hypercalcemia, Hyperkalemia, Hyponatremia
- Hypothyroidism and Myxedema Coma
- Metabolic Acidosis

4. MANAGEMENT

- Obtain a blood glucose, since hypoglycaemia is a danger in adrenal crisis.
- Hydrocortisone 100-200 mg IV as soon as the diagnosis is suspected can be lifesaving and is the mainstay of treatment.
- Take an ECG to look for signs of hyperkalaemia.
- ABG to assess the severity of shock (metabolic acidosis).
- A septic screen: inflammatory markers and blood cultures, midstream urine collection, and CXR.
- IV resuscitation and rehydration should also be instituted, but remember that the hypotension will not respond to fluids until the glucocorticoid deficiency has been treated with IV steroid.
- Treat any underlying infection; (broad-spectrum antibiotic such as intravenous cefuroxime 1.5 g).
- As TB is a possible cause of the adrenal crisis, an ultrasound of the adrenals would be inappropriate further investigation once the patient is stable.
- Admit to HDU or ITU.

II. PHEOCHROMOCYTOMA

INTRODUCTION

o Catecholamine-secreting tumors that arise from chromaffin cells of the adrenal medulla and the sympathetic ganglia are referred to as "pheochromocytomas" and "catecholamine-secreting paragangliomas" ("extraadrenal pheochromocytomas"), respectively.

o Because the tumors have similar clinical presentations and are treated with similar approaches, many clinicians use the term "pheochromocytoma" to refer to both adrenal pheochromocytomas and catecholamine-secreting paragangliomas.

CLINICAL ASSESSMENT

o Pheochromocytoma is usually suggested by the history in a symptomatic patient, discovery of an incidental adrenal mass, or the family history in a patient with familial disease.

o In one report of 107 patients, the average age at diagnosis was 47 years, and the average tumor size was 4.9 cm[193].

o **Classic triad** – The classic triad of symptoms in patients with a pheochromocytoma consists of episodic headache, sweating, and tachycardia[194].

o Approximately one-half have paroxysmal hypertension; most of the rest have either primary hypertension (formerly called "essential" hypertension) or normal blood pressure. Most patients with pheochromocytoma do **not** have the three classic symptoms, and patients with primary hypertension may have paroxysmal symptom[195].

o Hypertension is frequently associated with profound **tachycardia, pallor and a feeling of anxiety or impending doom**. The diagnosis should be considered in any patient presenting with acute hypertension or with a hypertensive crisis but be aware that hypertension can be episodic or absent and consider the diagnosis if there is a syndrome of appropriate clinical features compatible with the diagnosis.

o Precipitants can include abdominal compression, anaesthesia, opiates, dopamine antagonists, cold medications, radiographic contrast media, catecholamine reuptake inhibitors and childbirth.

---

[193] Guerrero MA, Schreinemakers JM, Vriens MR, et al. Clinical spectrum of pheochromocytoma. J Am Coll Surg 2009; 209:727.

[194] Bravo EL. Pheochromocytoma: new concepts and future trends. Kidney Int 1991; 40:544.

[195] Young WF Jr, Maddox DE. Spells: in search of a cause. Mayo Clin Proc 1995; 70:757.

DIFFERENTIAL DIAGNOSIS

• **Endocrine:** Hyperthyroidism, Hypoglycaemia, Menopausal syndrome

• **Cardiovascular:** Heart failure, Arrythmias and IHD

• **Neurological:** Migraine, Stroke, Postural orthostatic tachycardia syndrome

• **Miscellaneous:** Essential hypertension, Alcohol withdrawal, Pre-eclampsia, Porphyria, Panic Disorder or Anxiety, Drug treatment, Illegal Drug Use

INVESTIGATION STRATEGIES

• ECG, Capillary Blood Glucose and FBC.

• **CT scan** of the abdomen & **MRI**: Sensitivity 93-100%

• Specific investigation for pheochromocytoma is not usually instigated in the ED; appropriate subsequent tests include assay of plasma and urine metanephrines, catecholamines and urine vanillylmandelic acid (VMA).

• The most sensitive test is **Plasma Metanephrine Assay** (99% sensitivity with a specificity of 89%).

MANAGEMENT OF PHEOCHROMOCYTOMA

• Definitive treatment is by **surgical resection of the tumour**, normally using a laparoscopic approach.

• Prior to surgery the acute crisis is treated medically to control the effects of excess catecholamines. This is normally achieved by **alpha adrenoceptor blockade:**

PHENOXYBENZAMINE

o It is advocated as it blocks adrenoceptors irreversibly and therefore its effect cannot be overcome by increasing catecholamine concentrations.

o **Phenoxybenzamine IV 10-40 mg over one hour.**

o It acts within one hour and its effects last for up to four days. It can be given orally in a dose of **10-60 mg/day in divided doses.**

o **Side effects include** hypotension, dizziness, sedation, dry mouth, paralytic ileus and impotence.

PHENTOLAMINE

• **5-10 mg:** used in the diagnosis and perioperative management of pheochromocytoma. It causes vasodilatation, but also has positive inotropic and chronotropic effects. It exerts its effect predominantly by competitive alpha adrenoceptor blockade.

• **Side effects** include orthostatic hypotension, dizziness, abdominal discomfort and diarrhoea.

• Cardiovascular collapse has occurred following treatment of pheochromocytoma.

• Beta adrenoceptor blockade can be instituted to control tachycardia, but this should only be done after adequate alpha blockade, otherwise unopposed alpha activity can lead to worsening hypertension

III. THYROID EMERGENCIES

1. HYPERTHYROIDISM IN THE ED

INTRODUCTION

- **Hyperthyroidism** occurs when an excess of thyroid hormones (thyrotoxicosis) is produced by an overactive thyroid gland.
- **Thyroid storm** is a rare, life-threatening condition characterized by severe clinical manifestations of thyrotoxicosis[196].
- **Graves' disease**, which is caused by thyroid stimulating hormone (TSH) receptor stimulating autoantibodies, is responsible for most cases, and nodular thyroid disease accounts for most of the rest.

CLINICAL FEATURES

- **Symptoms**
  - Dyspnoea, palpitations.
  - Hyperactivity, emotional lability, insomnia, irritability, nervousness, anxiety.
  - Exercise intolerance, fatigue, muscle weakness.
  - Frequent bowel movements, diarrhoea.
  - Heat intolerance, increased sweating.
  - Increased appetite with weight loss or gain.

- **Signs**
  - Agitation.
  - Sinus tachycardia, atrial fibrillation, heart failure, resting tachycardia, dependent oedema.
  - Thyroid enlargement.
  - Tremor.
  - Warm, moist skin; palmar erythema.

THYROID STORM PRECIPITANTS

- **Medical**
  - Infection/sepsis
  - Cerebral vascular accident
  - Myocardial infarction
  - Congestive heart failure
  - Pulmonary embolism
  - Visceral infarction
- **Trauma**
  - Thyroid surgery
  - Nonthyroid surgery
  - Blunt and penetrating trauma to the thyroid gland
  - Vigorous palpation of the thyroid gland
  - Burns

- **Endocrine**
  - Hypoglycemia
  - Diabetic ketoacidosis
  - Hyperosmolar nonketotic coma
- **Drug-Related**
  - Iodine-131 therapy
  - Premature withdrawal of antithyroid therapy
  - Ingestion of thyroid hormone
  - Amiodarone therapy
  - Iodine ingestion
  - Anaesthesia induction
  - Miscellaneous drugs (chemotherapy, pseudoephedrine, organophosphates, aspirin)
- **Pregnancy-Related**
  - Hyperemesis gravidarum
  - Parturition and the immediate postpartum period

- The diagnosis of hyperthyroidism is based upon thyroid function tests. In patients in whom there is a clinical suspicion of hyperthyroidism, the best initial test is serum TSH. If the value is normal, the patient is very unlikely to have primary hyperthyroidism. Many laboratories have instituted algorithms in which serum free T4 and T3 are automatically measured if a low serum TSH value is obtained[197].

- If hyperthyroidism is suspected, the TSH level should be checked. If it is below the reference range, measurement of free thyroxine (FT4) and free triiodothyronine (FT3) is recommended. A normal TSH level effectively excludes primary thyroid disease. Typically, hyperthyroidism causes a low TSH and raised FT4 and FT3 levels.

DRUGS USED IN THE MANAGEMENT OF THYROID STORM

- **Beta-blockers**
  - Provides relief of adrenergic symptoms, b-adrenergic blockade and decreases t3-t4 conversion.
  - Propanolol 0.5-1.0 mg iv repeat every 15 min to desired effect.
    - Propanolol 60–80 mg PO
    - Metoprolol 50 mg PO
- If Beta blocker contraindicated -calcium channel blocker - diltiazem for relief of adrenergic symptoms
- **Corticosteroids**
  - Inhibits T4 to T3 conversion, treats relative adrenal insufficiency.

[196] Sarlis NJ, Gourgiotis L. Thyroid emergencies. Rev Endocr Metab Disord 2003; 4:129.

[197] Davey RX, Clarke MI, Webster AR. Thyroid function testing based on assay of thyroid-stimulating hormone: assessing an algorithm's reliability. Med J Aust 1996; 164:329.

- Hydrocortisone 200mg IV ,
- Dexamethasone 4mg IV
- **Thionamide therapy**
  - Inhibits thyroid hormone synthesis
    - Carbimazole – inhibits thyroid hormone production
    - Propylthiouracil- impairing T4 to T3 conversion.
- **Inorganic Iodine**
  - Blocks the release of thyroid hormone
  - Potassium Iodide
  - Lugols Iodine solution
  - Sodium iodide
  - If allergic to iodine lithium carbonate
- **Lorazepam or diazepam**
  - Anxiolytics, decreases central sympathetic outflow.

COMPLICATIONS
- Graves' ophthalmopathy.
- Thyroid storm (thyrotoxic crisis).
- Atrial fibrillation.
- Congestive cardiac failure.
- Osteoporosis.
- Increased risk of miscarriage, eclampsia, premature labour, low birthweight, and neonatal thyrotoxicosis in untreated pregnant women.

IMMEDIATE TREATMENT/ DISPOSITION
- For patients with clinical features of thyroid storm or with severe thyrotoxicosis who do not fully meet the criteria for thyroid storm (ie, impending storm), we begin immediate treatment with a beta blocker (**propranolol** in a dose to achieve adequate control of heart rate, typically 60 to 80 mg orally every four to six hours, with appropriate adjustment for heart rate and blood pressure) and either **propylthiouracil** (PTU) 200 mg every four hours or **methimazole** (20 mg orally every four to six hours)[198].
- Admission to hospital if the person has severe symptoms and signs of hyperthyroidism.
- Referring all other individuals with overt hyperthyroidism for specialist management.
- Secondary care treatments options include carbimazole or propylthiouracil, total or near-total thyroidectomy, and radioiodine treatment.
- Interim treatment with a beta-blocker to provide relief of adrenergic symptoms (if present).
- All pregnant women with hyperthyroidism should be urgently referred for specialist management.

[198] Douglas S Ross. Thyroid storm. [Uptodate Online]

2. MYXEDEMA COMA
DESCRIPTION
- Myxedema coma is an uncommon presentation of **severe hypothyroidism** that is potentially fatal.
- Myxedema coma is defined as severe hypothyroidism leading to decreased mental status, hypothermia, and other symptoms related to slowing of function in multiple organs.
- It is a medical emergency with a high mortality rate. Fortunately, it is now a rare presentation of hypothyroidism, likely due to earlier diagnosis as a result of the widespread availability of thyroid-stimulating hormone (TSH) assays.

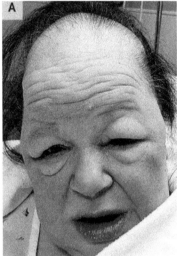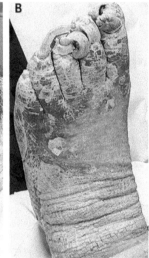

INCIDENCE
- Demographics of patients who develop myxedema coma are those of hypothyroidism in general, with older women being most often affected[199].
- Myxedema coma can occur as the culmination of severe, longstanding hypothyroidism or be precipitated by an acute event in a poorly controlled hypothyroid patient, such as infection, myocardial infarction, cold exposure, surgery, or the administration of sedative drugs, especially opioids.
- It can occur in patients who have any of the usual causes of hypothyroidism, particularly chronic autoimmune thyroiditis, because its insidious course may lead the diagnosis to be overlooked, compared with postsurgical or postablative hypothyroidism .
- Myxedema coma can occur in patients with central hypothyroidism, or lithium-induced hypothyroidism, and there are a dozen case reports of myxedema coma in patients taking amiodarone[200].

[199] Ono Y, Ono S, Yasunaga H, et al. Clinical characteristics and outcomes of myxedema coma: Analysis of a national inpatient database in Japan. J Epidemiol 2017; 27:117.

[200] Hawatmeh A, Thawabi M, Abuarqoub A, Shamoon F. Amiodarone induced myxedema coma: Two case reports and literature review. Heart Lung 2018; 47:429.

CLINICAL MANIFESTATION

o Myxedema coma can be precipitated by several factors.
o **Infections,** especially pneumonia, are perhaps the most common precipitating factor. Even occult bacterial infections have been implicated and, as such, infections should be thoroughly evaluated for as a potential etiologic factor.
o Cardiac events (myocardial infarction, congestive heart failure), cerebral infarction, trauma, haemorrhage, hypothermia, hypoglycemia, and respiratory depression secondary to anesthetics or sedatives have also been implicated. Clinical findings in myxedema coma are similar to those encountered with hypothyroidism, but they are typically seen in greater magnitude. In short, it is a state of profound decreased metabolic activity.
o Cardinal features include:
  ▪ ***Impaired thermoregulation*** *(hypothermia),*
  ▪ ***Hypotension,***
  ▪ ***Bradycardia,***
  ▪ ***Mental status depression.***
o Mental status depression is a common clinical feature and may progress to stupor, obtundation, or frank coma.
o The hypometabolic state and mental status depression may result in centrally mediated hypoventilation and hypercapnic respiratory failure.
o Concomitant endocrinopathies are commonly encountered, most notably **adrenal insufficiency**, which may contribute to the electrolyte, thermoregulatory, and cardiovascular derangements commonly seen.
o **Hyponatremia** resulting from an increased release of antidiuretic hormone and **hypoglycemia** caused by decreased gluconeogenesis, infection, or adrenal insufficiency are common features.

DIAGNOSIS

o Myxedema is characterized by generalized skin and soft tissue swelling, periorbital edema, ptosis, macroglossia, and the presence of cool, dry skin.
o Unlike thyroid storm, most patients with myxedema coma have a prior diagnosis of hypothyroidism.
o Although it is necessary to confirm the diagnosis, thyroid function testing can be confusing. The diagnosis is suspected clinically and confirmed with TFT.
o Treatment should not be delayed for laboratory confirmation
o ***Hypothyroidism*** *is diagnosed in individuals with elevated TSH levels and low levels of free T4 and T3.*
o ***In myxedema coma, T3 and T4 levels may be profoundly diminished or even undetectable.***
o The degree of TFT abnormalities does not distinguish hypothyroidism from myxedema coma.

o Rather, the distinction is based on clinical findings.
o Abnormal TFT can be seen in other acute illnesses and does not necessarily reflect myxedema coma or even hypothyroidism. It is important for the clinician to be able to differentiate hypothyroidism from **euthyroid sick syndrome**, in which patients **have a reduction in both TSH and thyroid hormone levels.**
o Given the common association with adrenal insufficiency, a **cosyntropin stimulation test** should be considered, especially in those with hemodynamic instability.

EMERGENCY TREATMENT

o The treatment of myxedema coma involves **rapid replacement of thyroid hormone, treatment of the precipitating cause, and general supportive measures.** A stated, despite a prompt diagnosis and initiation of treatment, mortality from myxedema coma can still exceed 30%.
o **Thyroid hormone replacement**: High-dose intravenous **thyroxine** is given as a bolus of **300-500 mcg**, followed by **50-100 mcg daily** depending on the patient's age, weight, and risk of complications. This method provides a more rapid recovery of symptoms but carries the potential for unwanted cardiac events resulting from the rapid replacement of thyroxine. In the low-dose method, **thyroxine 25 mcg** is given **daily for 1 week** followed by a gradually increased dose until the patient is able to resume normal thyroxine orally.
o Alternatively, **5 mcg of triiodothyronine** can be given **twice daily** during the loading period.
o IV triiodothyronine can be used as well and may provide a more rapid resolution of symptoms and improved mental status, although high levels of triiodothyronine have been correlated with increased mortality.
o **Triiodothyronine is given as an initial bolus dose of 10-20 mcg, followed by 10 mcg every 4 to 24 hours, with taper to 10 mcg every 6 hours.**
o Regardless of the replacement method used, all patients should be continuously monitored for hypertension and cardiac ischemia, which portend the greatest risk of death among patients with myxedema coma.
o Treatment should also be directed at identifying and reversing the underlying cause.

SUPPORTIVE CARE

o **Ventilatory support,** passive external rewarming, and correction of underlying electrolyte abnormalities are commonly required.
o **Glucose and steroid replacement** should also be considered until recovery.
o Given the strong association with infectious causes, **antimicrobial therapy** should be considered.

IV. PITUITARY DISEASE

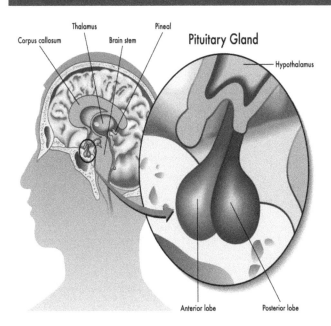

Pituitary Gland

Thalamus
Pineal
Corpus callosum
Brain stem
Hypothalamus
Anterior lobe
Posterior lobe

INTRODUCTION

- The pituitary is an endocrine gland located in the sella turcica in the skull base.
- Superior to it is the hypothalamus and the optic chiasm, laterally is the cavernous sinus through which run the III, IV, V, and VI cranial nerves.
- The pituitary is divided into anterior and posterior parts.
- The anterior pituitary produces and secretes hormones; it is regulated by hypothalamic hormones and negative feedback from target organs.
- The posterior pituitary is mainly a neuronal extension of the hypothalamus and secretes hormones made in the hypothalamus.
- Hormones secreted by the anterior and posterior pituitary:

Anterior pituitary

- Adrenocorticotropic hormone (ACTH)
- Growth hormone (GH)
- Follicle-stimulating hormone (FSH)
- Luteinizing hormone (LH)
- Thyroid-stimulating hormone (TSH)
- Prolactin (PRL)

Posterior pituitary

- Anti-diuretic hormone (ADH)
- Oxytocin

1. PITUITARY APOPLEXY

- Sudden hemorrhage into the pituitary gland is called pituitary apoplexy. Hemorrhage often occurs into a pituitary adenoma. In one report, the prevalence of pituitary apoplexy among patients with nonfunctioning pituitary macroadenomas was 8 percent[201].
- An existing pituitary adenoma is usually present.
- The anterior pituitary gland has an unusual vascular supply being perfused by a portal venous system, making it an area prone to infarction.

PREDISPOSING FACTORS

o Head trauma,
o Anticoagulation,
o Pituitary radiotherapy,
o Endocrine stimulation tests,
o Drugs, e.g. oestrogens, bromocriptine.

- **Sheehan's syndrome**: during pregnancy the pituitary hypertrophies, however the blood supply from the low-pressure portal venous system remains unchanged. If major haemorrhage or hypotension occurs during the peripartum period the anterior pituitary may infarct.
- The posterior pituitary is usually spared due to its direct arterial blood supply.

✦ *Sheehan's syndrome, also known as postpartum pituitary gland infarction, is hypopituitarism (decreased functioning of the pituitary gland), caused by ischemic necrosis due to blood loss and hypovolemic shock during and after childbirth.*

CLINICAL FEATURES

o The sudden enlargement of the pituitary mass, due to acute hemorrhage, results in a range of acute clinical findings[202]:
o Severe headache,
o Nausea & vomiting,
o Photophobia
o Loss of consciousness,
o Meningism,
o Visual field defect—bitemporal hemianopia.
- **Cranial nerve palsies:**

---

[201] Vargas G, Gonzalez B, Guinto G, et al. Pituitary apoplexy in nonfunctioning pituitary macroadenomas: a case-control study. Endocr Pract 2014; 20:1274.

[202] Capatina C, Inder W, Karavitaki N, Wass JA. Management of endocrine disease: pituitary tumour apoplexy. Eur J Endocrinol 2015; 172:R179.

- o CN III (unilateral dilated pupil, ptosis, and a globe deviated inferiorly and laterally),
  - o CN IV (inability to look down and in, resulting in vertical diplopia),
  - o CN V (facial pain or sensory loss),
  - o CN VI (unable to abduct eye, resulting in horizontal diplopia).
- Patients may have a history suggestive of pre-existing endocrine dysfunction (e.g. amenorrhoea, hypogonadism, decreased libido, obesity, lethargy, constipation, etc.).

INVESTIGATIONS
- o CT or MRI head.
- o Blood should be taken to measure pituitary hormones (ACTH, TSH, FSH, LH, and prolactin) and the effects these hormones have on target organs (oestradiol—women, testosterone— men, T4, T3, cortisol).
- o Electrolytes and glucose should be monitored.

MANAGEMENT
- o Supportive therapy (ABCDE),
- o **Hydrocortisone** 100 mg IV 6-hourly'
- o Urgent neurosurgical opinion.

2. CUSHING'S SYNDROME

- **Cushing's syndrome** is a debilitating endocrine disorder characterized by excessive cortisol levels in the blood which may be the result of a tumor of the pituitary gland, adrenal glands (located above the kidneys) or from tumors or cancer arising elsewhere in the body (ectopic ACTH producing tumors). The cause of Cushing's Syndrome is a pituitary adenoma in over 70% of adults and in approximately 60-70% of children and adolescents. Most pituitary ACTH-secreting adenomas are small in size (microadenomas).
- **Cushing's disease** refers specifically to excessive ACTH secretion by a pituitary tumor (also called pituitary adenoma). Overall, Cushing's Disease is relatively rare, affecting 10 to 15 of every million people each year, and most commonly affects adults aged 20 to 50 years. Women account for over 70% of cases.

SYMPTOMS AND SIGNS:
- o Change in body habitus: weight gain in face (moon face), above the collar bone (supraclavicular) and on back of neck (buffalo hump)
- o Skin changes with easy bruising, purplish stretch marks (stria) and red cheeks (plethora)
- o Excess hair growth (hirsutism) on face, neck, chest, abdomen, and thighs
- o Generalized weakness and fatigue, Loss of muscle

- o Menstrual disorders in women (amenorrhea)
- o Decreased fertility and/or sex drive (libido)
- o Hypertension, Diabetes mellitus
- o Depression with wide mood swings

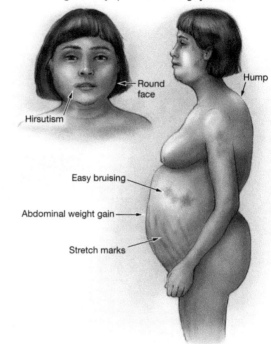

Signs and symptoms of Cushing syndrome

DIAGNOSIS
- o Comparison of old and recent photographs will often demonstrate the marked changes in facial appearance and body habitus of patients who develop Cushing's syndrome or Cushing's disease. However, the diagnosis of Cushing's disease is often long delayed and can be difficult to make. An endocrinologist should always supervise the evaluation for Cushing's disease.

- o **Hormonal Diagnosis:**
  - ▪ The first step in diagnosing Cushing's disease is to confirm the presence of **excessive cortisol secretion** (Cushing's syndrome).
  - ▪ This diagnosis is most easily made by performing a low-dose **dexamethasone suppression test** or a **24-Hour urine collection** to quantitate cortisol levels.
  - ▪ The low-dose dexamethasone suppression test involves taking a small dose of dexamethasone (1mg) at 11 pm and having blood drawn for cortisol the following morning at 8 am.
  - ▪ Once the diagnosis of Cushing's syndrome is established, the source of the excess cortisol needs to be determined: either from an adrenal gland tumor, an ectopic ACTH-producing tumor or a pituitary ACTH-producing adenoma.

- A high dose dexamethasone test, ACTH levels, metyrapone test, and/or sometimes a CRH test are used for this determination.
- In some individuals with depression, alcohol abuse, anorexia nervosa or high oestrogen levels, cortisol levels may be chronically elevated.
- These patients with "**pseudo-Cushing's**" may be difficult to distinguish from those with true Cushing's disease. Additional hormonal tests are often needed to clarify the diagnosis in these individuals.

o **PETROSAL SINUS SAMPLING:**
  - Petrosal Sinus Sampling is an angiographic and endocrinological test used to distinguish between ectopic ACTH production or pituitary ACTH production (Cushing's disease).
  - It is also used to help determine on which side of the pituitary gland an adenoma is located in patients with normal MRIs of the pituitary but with hormonal studies strongly suggesting Cushing's disease.
  - Petrosal sinus sampling should never be performed before the diagnosis of Cushing's syndrome is established.

o **Imaging:**
  - If laboratory tests suggest a pituitary adenoma as the cause of Cushing's, then a pituitary MRI is performed to confirm the diagnosis.
  - In approximately 70% of cases an adenoma can be seen.
  - A CT scan will detect only about 50% of adenomas.
  - CT scans of the adrenal glands are very useful for determining the presence or absence of an adrenal tumor causing Cushing's syndrome.

TREATMENT

o Cushing's syndrome does not require acute treatment in the ED. However, patients with Cushing's syndrome are more prone to fractures, infections, and poor wound healing, so may present with complications that require treatment.

o If the cause of Cushing's syndrome is exogenous steroids, these may be gradually tapered off and eventually stopped, if possible.

o Definitive treatment for Cushing's disease is **selective removal of the pituitary adenoma**.

o If the source cannot be located, **bilateral adrenalectomy** may be required.

3. DIABETES INSIPIDUS

- Diabetes insipidus (DI) is due to impaired water resorption by the kidney because of reduced secretion of ADH from the posterior pituitary (cranial DI) or impaired response of the kidney to ADH (nephrogenic DI).

- Central diabetes insipidus (CDI) is characterized by decreased release of antidiuretic hormone (ADH, also called arginine vasopressin or AVP), resulting in a variable degree of polyuria. Lack of ADH can be caused by disorders that act at one or more of the sites involved in ADH secretion: the hypothalamic osmoreceptors; the supraoptic or paraventricular nuclei; or the superior portion of the supraopticohypophyseal tract[203].

CAUSES OF DIABETES INSIPIDUS

CRANIAL DI	NEPHROGENIC DI
• Head injury	• Low potassium
• Hypophysectomy	• High calcium
• Meningitis	• Drugs (e.g. lithium)
• Pituitary tumour	• Pyelonephritis
• Metastases	• Hydronephrosis
• Craniopharyngioma	• Polycystic kidney disease
• Vascular lesion	• Inherited
• Idiopathic (50%)	

CLINICAL FEATURES

o Polyuria.
o Polydipsia.
o Dilute urine.
o Dehydration.

INVESTIGATION

o Plasma osmolality–high.
o Urine osmolality–low.
o Serum sodium–high.
o Check serum potassium and calcium as potential causes.
o CT head if a cranial cause suspected.
o Measure pituitary function (TSH, ACTH, LH, FSH, and Prolactin).

EMERGENCY TREATMENT

o Cranial DI–**desmopressin 1mcg intranasally.**
o Nephrogenic DI–**treat the cause.**
o Rehydrate–match input to fluid losses and aim to gradually reduce the serum sodium.

---

[203] *Rose BD, Post TW. Clinical Physiology of Acid-Base and Electrolyte Disorders, 5th ed, McGraw-Hill, New York 2001. p.751.*

V. HYPOGLYCAEMIA

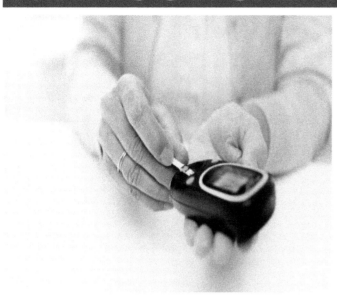

*A 55-year-old female with a previous medical history of hypertension, hyperlipidemia, and diabetes, presents to the emergency department with slurred speech and dysarthria. As you enter the room, an anxious family member hands you a list detailing the following medications: lisinopril, clopidogrel, and glimepiride. VS: HR 110, RR 14, BP 132/88, T 37.3°C. Accucheck: **2.6 mmol/l.***

INTRODUCTION

- Hypoglycaemia is a lower than normal level of blood glucose. It can be defined as "mild" if the episode is self-treated and "severe" if assistance by a third party is required (DCCT, 1993).
- For the purposes of people with diabetes who are hospital inpatients, any blood glucose less than 4.0mmol/L should be treated[204].
- This condition typically arises from abnormalities in the mechanisms involved in glucose homeostasis.
- The most common cause of hypoglycemia in patients with diabetes is injecting a shot of insulin and skipping a meal or overdosing insulin[205].
- Severe hypoglycaemia is less common in people with insulin treated type 2 diabetes mellitus (T2DM) but still represents a significant clinical problem.
- Patients with insulin treated T2DM are more likely to require hospital admission for severe hypoglycaemia than those with T1DM (30% versus 10% of episodes)

(Donnelly et al., 2005).

RISK FACTORS OF HYPOGLYCEMIA

Medical issues
- Strict glycaemic control
- Previous history of severe hypoglycaemia
- Long duration of type 1 diabetes
- Duration of insulin therapy in type 2 diabetes
- Lipohypertrophy at injection sites
- Impaired awareness of hypoglycaemia
- Severe hepatic dysfunction
- Impaired renal function (including those patients requiring renal replacement therapy)
- Sepsis
- Inadequate treatment of previous hypoglycaemia
- Terminal illness
- Cognitive dysfunction/dementia

Lifestyle Issues
- Increased exercise (relative to usual)
- Irregular lifestyle
- Alcohol
- Increasing age
- Early pregnancy
- Breast feeding
- No or inadequate blood glucose monitoring

Reduced Carbohydrate intake/absorption
- Food malabsorption e.g.gastroenteritis, coeliac disease
- Bariatric surgery involving bowel resection

SIGNS & SYMPTOMS OF HYPOGLYCEMIA

- Glycemic thresholds for hypoglycemic symptoms in diabetic patients are difficult to define.
- Patients who have recently experienced a severe hypoglycemic event may not become symptomatic until blood glucose levels are dangerously low.
- On the contrary, patients with poorly controlled blood glucose levels may experience symptoms of hypoglycemia when glucose levels are within normal limits[206].
- The diabetic patient should be questioned regarding symptoms experienced, recent HgbA1C levels, average blood glucose levels, most recent medication injection/ingestion, and recent food intake.

---

204 *Joint British Diabetes Societies, The Hospital Management of Hypoglycaemia in Adults with Diabetes Mellitus 3rd edition [Online]*

205 *Mathew P, Thoppil D. Hypoglycemia. 2018 Jan.*

206 *Dagogo-Jack S, Craft S, Cryer P. Hypoglycemia-associated autonomic failure in insulin-dependent diabetes mellitus. Recent antecedent hypoglycemia reduces autonomic responses to, symptoms of, and defense against subsequent hypoglycemia. J Clin Invest 1993;91:819–828.*

- Signs and symptoms of hypoglycemia in non-diabetic patients are relatively easier to predict.
- **Autonomic symptoms:** nervousness, anxiety, tremulousness, sweating, palpitations, shaking, dizziness, hunger
- **Neuroglycopenic symptoms:** confusion, weakness, drowsiness, speech difficulty, incoordination, odd behavior
- **In severe cases:** hypoglycemia may result in seizure, coma, or death.

SOMOGYI EFFECT

- The Somogyi phenomenon (also known as post-hypoglycemic hyperglycemia, chronic Somogyi rebound) describes a rebound high blood glucose level in response to low blood glucose[207].
- The counter-regulatory hormones cause transient insulin resistance. This results in post hypoglycaemic hyperglycaemia known as the Somogyi effect. The duration of the effect is different for each of the main hormones:
  - Glucagon <2 h
  - Epinephrine 4-6 h
  - Cortisol and Growth hormone up to 12 h

- The Dawn Effect (or Dawn Phenomenon) is a morning rise in blood sugar which occurs as a response to waning levels of insulin and a surge in growth hormones[207]

DRIVING AND DVLA

- **Patient with Impaired awareness of hypoglycaemia –'hypoglycaemia unawareness'** must not drive and must notify the DVLA.
- It is the doctor's duty to inform the patient of this and to explain their responsibility to notify the DVLA.
- If there are episodes of severe hypoglycaemia from any cause other than diabetes treatment driving must stop while the liability to episodes remains.
- Examples include hypoglycaemia post-bariatric surgery or in association with eating disorders, and the restriction applies for both car and motorcycle, and bus and lorry drivers.

TREATING THE HYPOGLYCEMIC ADULT PATIENT
(Glucose <4.0 mM for adult patients)

1. **If conscious and able to drink:**
- 100 mls Lucozade or 150 mls normal Coke / 7UP / fruit juice
- Repeat after 5 minutes if glucose < 3.5 mM.
- If next meal is more than an hour away, 1 slice of brown bread recommended.

2. **If unconscious or unable to drink:**
- Establish IV access.
- **Give 20 mls of 20% dextrose IV push** using 3 way tap connected to a syringe for ease of administration and check glucometer after 1 minute.
- If glucometer <4.5 mM, repeat IV push again after 1 minute
- Repeat same every minute until glucometer > 4.5 mM
- The patient should not require more than 100mls of 20% dextrose to reverse hypoglycaemia.
- If the hypoglycaemia is secondary to sulphonylurea therapy, consider IV infusion of 20% dextrose for 24 hours starting at 50mls per hour and checking glucometer hourly.
- If IV access not available, inject **glucagon (Glucogen) 1mg intramuscularly.** This will not work if patient is in fasting state.
- 500mls bags of 20% dextrose are now available on the wards and ED.
- **The use of 50% dextrose is discouraged as it can lead to thrombophlebitis and extravasation will lead to skin necrosis.**

---

[207] *Somogyi Phenomenon – Rebound Hyperglycemia, Diabetes UK*

VI. HYPERGLYCEMIC HYPEROSMOLAR SYNDROME

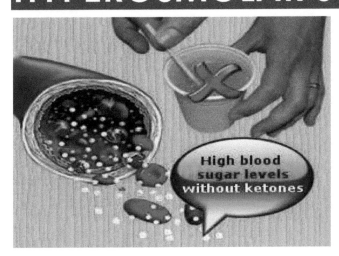

DEFINITION

- An acute decompensated state in which patients manifest a change in mental status in the setting of hyperglycemia, hyperosmolarity and severe volume depletion.
- Altered mental status can present as focal neurologic defects or global encephalopathy.
- In HHS, there is little or no ketoacid accumulation, the serum glucose concentration frequently exceeds 1000 mg/dL (56 mmol/L), the plasma osmolality (Posm) may reach 380 mOsmol/kg, and neurologic abnormalities are frequently present (including coma in 25 to 50 percent of cases)[208]

PATHOPHYSIOLOGY

- Decreased activity of insulin leads to increased serum glucose via gluconeogenesis, glycogenolysis and decreased cellular glucose uptake
- Resultant hyperglycemia leads to fluid shift from intracellular to extracellular space
- Increased circulating glucose spills into urine resulting in osmotic diuresis
- Decreased circulating volume leads to reduction in glomerular filtration rate (GFR) and hypotonic urine
- Hypotonic diuresis produces dehydration and creates cycle of hyperglycemia, hypernatremia and increased osmolarity

---

[208] Kitabchi AE, Umpierrez GE, Fisher JN, et al. Thirty years of personal experience in hyperglycemic crises: diabetic ketoacidosis and hyperglycemic hyperosmolar state. J Clin Endocrinol Metab 2008; 93:1541.

CAUSES

- Non-compliance with medications and/or diet
- Inadequate access to fluids to counteract losses
- Common acute conditions exacerbating chronic diabetes: infection (i.e. sepsis), myocardial ischemia/infarction, pulmonary embolism, trauma, burns, GI hemorrhage etc.

CLINICAL MANIFESTATIONS

- The development of HHS is typically prolonged in comparison to DKA.
- **History**
  - Polydipsia, polyuria, polyphagia
  - Weakness
  - Weight loss
  - Nausea/Vomiting
  - Confusion
  - 20% without a known history of DM II
  - Chronic renal insufficiency a common comorbid condition

- **Physical Examination**
  - Hypotension
  - Tachycardia
  - Dehydration (dry mucous membranes, delayed capillary refill)
  - Neurologic Manifestations
    - Decreased level of consciousness
    - Seizures
    - Focal neurologic findings
    - Stroke-like syndromes

DIAGNOSTIC TESTING

- *Hyperglycaemia (Glucose > 30 mmol/l)*
- *Total osmolality > 340mOsm/kg*
- *Serum bicarbonate >15mmol/l*
- *Urinary ketones < 1+ plus*

- **Renal Function**
  - Elevated Urea:Cr ratio common indicating pre-renal causes
  - Acute Kidney Injury (AKI) from hypoperfusion will often co-exist
- **Electrolyte disturbances**
  - **Profound hypokalemia** secondary to osmotic diuresis

- **Hyponatremia** often results from hyperglycemia and will correct without directed management on sodium
- **Phosphate and Magnesium** levels commonly low

Basics: ABCs, IV, Cardiac Monitor and 12-lead EKG

- Establish at least 2 large-bore (16-18 gauge) peripheral IVs as patients may require multiple medications
- Carefully consider underlying cause of decompensation and HHS

INITIAL MANAGEMENT

- **Intravenous fluids**
  - **Role**
    - Replenish intravascular depletion resulting from osmotic diuresis
    - Correct increased serum osmolarity
    - Correct decreased GFR

  - **Initial Fluid Dose**
    - Patients with HHS frequently have concomitant comorbid conditions like CHF and chronic renal insufficiency
    - May not tolerate large volumes of fluid well
    - Consider smaller boluses (10 ml/kg) with repeat cardiac and lung assessment

  - **0.9% NaCl (Normal Saline)**
    - Most commonly employed fluid
    - Problems:
    - NS is far from "normal"
    - Large volume infusions (> 2-3 liters) can cause hyperchloremic metabolic acidosis (unclear impact on patient)

  - **Hartmann's solution**
    - Closer to physiologic solution
    - Does not cause hyperchloremic metabolic acidosis
  - Other options: balanced solutions (i.e. Plasma-Lyte)

- **Insulin therapy**
  - Patients with HHS will typically have adequate basal insulin levels and additional insulin may not be necessary.

- **Electrolyte Disorder Correction**
  - **Potassium**
    - Aggressive repletion frequently necessary
    - Patients hundreds of mEq depleted
    - Supplementation (see hypokalemia post)

- **Oral:** KCl 40 mEq every hour (if patient safe for oral route)
- **Intravenous:** KCl 10-40 mEq in each liter of fluid (caution: infusion of > 10 mEq potassium/hour will cause burning in peripheral vein)

- **Sodium**
  - Typically, dilutional hyponatremia
  - Will correct without specific treatment

- **Magnesium**
  - **HypoK = HypoMg** (Boyd 1984)
  - Both electrolytes lost during osmotic diuresis
  - Cannot replete intracellular potassium without magnesium
  - Serum magnesium level may not correlate with total body stores
  - Dose: **1-2 gm MgSO₄**

- **Phosphorous**
  - If PO_4 < 1.0 mEq, consider repletion with KPO_4

TAKE HOME POINTS

- HHS is defined by hyperglycemia and hyperosmolarity due to volume depletion with resultant altered mental status
- Profound hypokalemia is common as a result of osmotic diuresis. Replete aggressively
- Hypokalemia = hypomagnesemia. Replete both of these electrolytes simultaneously
- Fluid repletion is the key point in management but careful repletion is vital as patients may not tolerate aggressive administration
- All patients should have an exhaustive investigation of the cause of their decompensation. Look for signs of infection, ischemia, trauma etc.

Osmolality

2 x Na⁺ + Urea + Glucose

Usually > 350 mOsm/kg

VII. DIABETIC KETOACIDOSIS IN ADULT

1. INTRODUCTION

- **BMJ[209] defines DKA as:**
  o *Hyperglycaemia (>14 mM).*
  o *Metabolic acidosis (pH<7.35 and bicarbonate <15 mM).*
  o *High anion gap.*
  o *Ketonaemia/heavy (3+) ketonuria.*

2. KEY POINTS IN DIAGNOSIS OF DKA[219]

- There are no specific physical symptoms or signs
- Rule out DKA and other causes of metabolic acidosis before making a diagnosis of hysterical hyperventilation
- Check capillary blood glucose early but always follow this with a formal venous blood glucose level
- Test urine for ketones
- Arterial blood is **NOT** needed as routine
- Blood potassium levels should be measured hourly (hyperkalaemic and hypokalaemic cardiac arrest are common causes of death in patients with DK)
- Venous blood glucose should be measured hourly during insulin infusion
- A chart should be started to continuously record vital signs, urine output, and the results of all tests.

3. CLINICAL ASSESSMENT

- No specific clinical signs that confirm or refute the diagnosis of DKA.
- Nausea, vomiting, or abdominal pain may predominate.
- Polyuria, polydipsia, and weakness are usually present
- The diagnosis is comparatively straight forward where there is a clear history that the patient has diabetes but can cause serious diagnostic difficulty where the patient is unconscious or DKA is the first presentation of diabetes (a past history of diabetes mellitus will be absent in 1 in 10 patients).
- The possibility of DKA (or other metabolic acidosis) should be considered whenever assessing a patient who presents with "hyperventilation" and it is always essential to measure the blood glucose early in the resuscitation of any unconscious patient.
- If the patient is already being treated with insulin, there may be a history of reduced or omitted insulin. Chest pain may be described if DKA complicates acute myocardial infarction, although silent infarction may occur.
- On examination the patient has an increased depth and rate of respiration.

- The mouth, tongue and lips are dry. The majority of doctors can smell ketones on the patient's breath but this is an unreliable sign. There may be other signs of volume depletion. Signs of infection (for example, lobar pneumonia) should be sought; absence of fever does not exclude infection.

4. INVESTIGATIONS

- A capillary glucose measurement
- Defining DKA as serum glucose >250 mg/dl (>14 mM), metabolic acidosis with corrected pH<7.30 or serum bicarbonate <15 mM and ketonaemia, the sensitivity of urine ketone dip test for ketonaemia in patients with DKA is 97% (95% CI 92% to 99%)
- The absence of ketonuria makes the diagnosis of DKA unlikely. It is possible that clinical staff in the study were using negative urine dip stick test to rule out DKA; the study would therefore overestimate its sensitivity. Few laboratories offer an urgent ketone level; an estimate of the severity of ketonaemia can be made from the anion gap (available immediately on some "blood gas analysers"); an anion gap >20 mM is abnormal.

5. DKA MANAGEMENT

- Get experienced help
- Obtain good venous access and send off blood samples
- Consider nasogastric tube if patient not alert
- Consider urinary catheter if haemodynamically unstable
- 0.9% saline 500 ml/h for four hours then 250 ml/h until euvolaemic is an effective fluid regime (unless the patient is shocked at presentation)
- Insulin, by continuous intravenous infusion at 0.1 unit/kg/h. The fall in [glucose] should not exceed 5 mM/h.
- Start potassium supplementation *after* insulin treatment once [K$^+$] is below the upper limit of the reference range.
- The administration of bicarbonate does **NOT** increase biochemical or clinical recovery.

6. DKA COMPLICATIONS

- **Hypokalaemia and hyperkalaemia:** potassium should not be prescribed with the initial litre of fluid or if the serum potassium level remains above 5.5 mmol/l since severe dehydration may cause acute pre-renal failure
- **Hypoglycaemia:** with the correction of ketoacidosis, blood glucose levels will fall very rapidly
- **Cerebral oedema:** usually occurs within a few hours of initiation of treatment
- **Pulmonary oedema:** rare complication of DKA

---

209 Hardern RD, Quinn ND. Emergency management of diabetic ketoacidosis in adults. Emergency Medicine Journal 2003;**20**:210-213.

7. MANAGEMENT OF DKA IN THE ED

ED

Adult Diabetic Keto-Acidosis

Initial management to be completed within 1 hour of arrival.	**Establish Diagnosis** Known Diabetes or High Blood Glucose or BM: 11 or Higher + Ketones: Urinalysis 2+ ketones or more Acidosis: Blood gas (Venous or arterial) pH 7.30 or lower or Bicarbonate 15 or lower or BE worse than -10	All patients with BM 11 or more must have a urinalysis DKA may be the 1st presentation of Diabetes

MOVE TO RESUS

Pitfalls:
Euglycaemia DKA
Non-Ketotic DKA

Inform **ED Middle Grade** or **Consultant**
Inform **Medical & O&G Registrar** immediately if patient is pregnant
Contact Medical Registrar ± ITU middle grade to assist at any time

Investigations and Monitoring:

FBC, U&E, Blood Glucose (Before treatment)
Blood Cultures
Consider urinary catheter
Urine culture

Attach cardiac & Sats monitoring
Obtain IV access (minimum 18G cannula)
ECG
CXR only if indicated

If Systolic BP <90mmHg:
Consider stat dose 500mls 0.9% Saline
Call for senior help
Caution: Young adults 18-24 yrs, pregnancy, elderly, heart failure (Refer to Trust policy.)

Treatment:

1. Fluids

BM <14: Give 10% Glucose and 0.9% saline
    1L 10% Glucose over 8 hours (125mL/Hr)
    1L 0.9% Saline as per Saline regime
Run through 2 separates lines at the same time
If Hypoglycaemia occurs, INCREASE rate of Glucose infusion to permit insulin administration.
	BM 14 or more: Give 0.9% saline
	    1L over 1 hour
	    1L over 2 hours
	    1L over 2 hours
	    1L over 4 hours
	    1L over 4 hours
		Continue 0.9% Saline infusion until volume replete
		Add KCl as per guideline below, EXCEPT 1ST BAG

2. INSULIN (Whatever BM)
No stat dose
Start fixed rate INSULIN infusion of 50Units ACTRAPID in 50mL 0.9% Saline (1 U/ml) solution
Run at 0.1U/Kg/hr (May need to estimate weight)
Aim: Fall in Blood Glucose by 3 mmol/hr or rise in HCO3 by 3 mmol/hr
Consider increasing rate of insulin infusion by 1 U/hr to achieve this.

3. POTASSIUM: Do not add K$^+$ to first bag of fluid
Await results before adding K+ to IV Fluids
Replace at rate no greater than 20mmols/hr via peripheral line
    K$^+$>5.5: NIL
    K$^+$3.5 -5.5: ADD 40mmol in 1L 0.9% Saline
    K$^+$<3.5: may require additional KCL (seek expert help)

4. BM
Check hourly
When BM<14, patient needs to have 10% Glucose (1L over 8hrs) as well as 0.9% saline
Avoid hypoglycaemia whilst on insulin infusion. Prescribe appropriately on drug chart

Recheck Blood gas, U&E, Blood Glucose, CK within 2 hours

17. E.N.T. Emergencies

I. ACUTE SORE THROAT

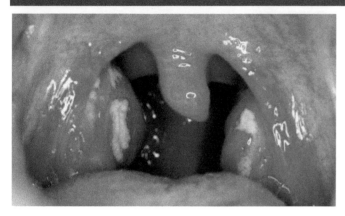

1. INTRODUCTION
- **Common Causes:**
  - Tonsillitis
  - Pharyngitis
  - Peritonsillar Abscess (quinsy)
  - Infectious mononucleosis

- **Less common and/or dangerous causes of a sore throat include:**
  - Epiglottis
  - Scarlet fever/ Diphtheria
  - Bacterial Tracheitis
  - Ludwig's Angina
  - Retropharyngeal abscess
  - Angioedema or anaphylaxis
  - Lemierre's syndrome due to *Fusobacterium necrophorum*
  - Painful cervical lymphadenopathy
  - Trauma, e.g. foreign body or caustic ingestion

2. CAUSATIVE AGENTS
- The most important bacterial cause of a throat infection is group A β-hemolytic streptococcus (GABHS), which is responsible for about one-third of sore throats in children aged 5 to 15 years[210].
- In adults and in younger children, only 10% of sore throats are caused by GABHS.
- Carriers of GABHS do not need treatment.
  - Viruses are responsible for 85% to 95% of adult sore throats.
  - Viruses cause 70% of sore throats in children aged 5 to 16.

- Viruses cause 95% of sore throats in children younger than 5 years.
- The most common bacterial cause of sore throat is GABHS.
- At least 30% of GABHS cultured in primary care are due to carriers who are not sick and are at very low risk of infecting other people.

- **OTHER LESS COMMON BACTERIAL CAUSES OF PHARYNGITIS/ TONSILITIS INCLUDE:**
  - *Group C and G strep*
  - *Fusobacterium necrophorum*
  - *Neisseria gonorrhoea*
  - *Corynebacterium diphtheriae*
  - *Mycoplasma pneumoniae and several chlamydial species*

3. COMPLICATIONS
- Complications of GABHS infection are categorised into suppurative and non-suppurative:
  - **Suppurative complications[211]:**
    - Tonsillopharyngeal cellulitis or abscess
    - Otitis media
    - Sinusitis
    - Necrotizing fasciitis
    - Streptococcal bacteremia

  - **Non-suppurative complications:**
    - Acute rheumatic fever (ARF)
    - Poststreptococcal reactive arthritis (PSRA)
    - Scarlet fever
    - Streptococcal toxic shock syndrome
    - Acute glomerulonephritis
    - Pediatric autoimmune neuropsychiatric disorder associated with group A streptococci (PANDAS)

4. RED FLAG SYMPTOMS
  - Inability to swallow
  - Drooling of saliva
  - Significant systemic upset
  - Severe pain
  - Stridor (airway obstruction)
  - Severe neck stiffness
  - Patient holding a tripod position

---

[210] Worrall G. J. (2007). Acute sore throat. *Canadian family physician Medecin de famille canadien*, 53(11), 1961–1962.

[211] *Michael E Pichichero, Complications of streptococcal tonsillopharyngitis [Uptodate Online]*

5. RISK STRATIFICATION
CENTOR CLASSIFICATION[212]

MODIFIED CENTOR OR McISAAC SCORE

History of fever or T⁰ > 38∘C	+1
Absence of cough	+1
Tender anterior cervical lymphadenopathy	+1
Tonsillar swelling or exudates	+1
Age 3-15 yrs	+1
Age 15 to < 45yrs	0
Age ≥45 years	-1

POINTS	SUGGESTED MANAGEMENT
-1 or 0	No culture or antibiotic
1	No culture or antibiotic
2	Culture all treat those with +ve culture
3	Culture all treat those with +ve culture
4 or 5	Treat with antibiotic

6. INVESTIGATIONS

- **Throat swabs** - in general, throat swabs are of little value in the management of sore throat as up to 20% of patients carry strep. pyogenes as a commensal; there are no criteria for distinguishing between carriage and infection
- Full Blood Count and Monospot may be helpful if glandular fever or blood dyscrasia is suspected

7. INDICATIONS FOR ANTIBIOTHERAPY

- Antibiotics are unnecessary for most patients with sore throat as it is a self-limiting condition, which resolves by one week in 85% of people, whether it is due to streptococcal infection or not[213],
- Serious complications are rare
- The centor criteria may be useful to predict patients who are at higher risk of group a beta-haemolytic streptococcus (GABHS) and complications, who may benefit from antibiotics:
  - Tonsillar exudate
  - Tender anterior cervical lymph nodes
  - Absence of cough
  - History of fever
- In patients with tonsillitis who are unwell, and have three out of four of these criteria, the risk of quinsy is 1:60 compared with 1:400 in those who are not unwell

- if antibiotics are clinically indicated, **phenoxymethylpenicillin** is an appropriate first choice (adult dose: 500mg two to four times a day for 10 days)
- In penicillin allergic patients, **Erythromycin or Clarithromycin** should be used.
- Patients given antibiotics are more likely to reattend if they have another similar infection
- A delayed prescription, for use after three days if symptoms are not starting to resolve or are getting significantly worse, may be more appropriate for some patients
- Offer advice and reassurance, and recommend analgesics for symptom relief in all patients
- As most patients with a sore throat do not see a doctor it is worth asking why they came.

8. SPECIFIC MANAGEMENT
1. TONSILLOPHARYNGITIS

- **Current recommendation:** No initial antibiotics are given and the patient is advised to return to their GP if their symptoms are not settling after a few days.
- Antibiotic treatment has been shown to reduce symptom severity and hasten the rate of recovery in patients with streptococcal pharyngitis[214].
- However, even without antibiotic therapy, symptoms typically resolve in about three to five days for most patients[215], making the prevention of complications a key goal of care.

2. SCARLET FEVER

- Scarlet fever is a GABHS exotoxin-mediated illness which occurs far more commonly in children.
- Other than **standard antibiotic treatment** for GABHS, consideration must also be made of **hydration status and intravenous fluid rehydration** may be required.

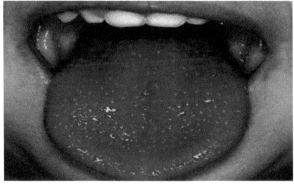

[212] *Nice Guideline NG84, Sore throat (acute): antimicrobial prescribing guideline [Nice NG84]*

[213] *MeReC Bulletin 2006;17(3):12-14.*

[214] *Spinks A, Glasziou PP, Del Mar CB. Antibiotics for sore throat. Cochrane Database Syst Rev 2013; :CD000023.*

[215] *BRINK WR, RAMMELKAMP CH Jr, DENNY FW, WANNAMAKER LW. Effect in penicillin and aureomycin on the natural course of streptococcal tonsillitis and pharyngitis. Am J Med 1951; 10:300.*

3. PERITONSILLAR ABSCESS

SYMPTOMS

o Fever
o Dysphagia
o Otalgia
o Odynophagia
o Progressively worsening sore throat, often localized to one side

PHYSICAL EXAMINATION

o Erythematous, swollen tonsil
o Contralateral uvular deviation
o Trismus
o Oedema of palatine tonsils
o Purulent exudate on tonsils
o Drooling
o Muffled, **"hot potato" voice**
o Cervical lymphadenopathy

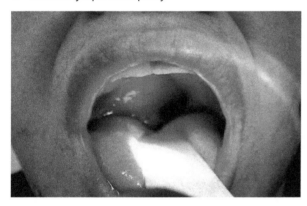

- Uncomplicated peritonsillar abscess may be managed in the ED although it is common practice for patients to be referred to an ear, nose and throat (ENT) specialist due to a lack of familiarity with treatment techniques.
- Both **needle aspiration and incision and drainage techniques** may be used employed and have been found to be equally effective. The clinician must be aware of the potential complications of both the problem e.g. **Lemierre's syndrome** (extension of infection involving the jugular vein) and its management e.g. **accidental puncture of the carotid artery.**

4. EPIGLOTTITIS

o Since the advent of Hib vaccination, this is now more commonly an infection affecting adults.
o The main complication of airway obstruction may be predicted by the presence of specific clinical features:
  ▪ *Stridor*
  ▪ *Muffled voice*
  ▪ *Rapid clinical course*
  ▪ *History of diabetes*

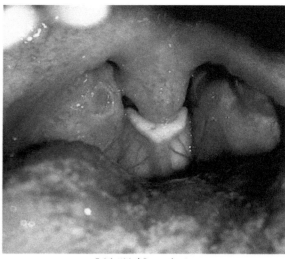

Epiglottitis | Researchgate

o **Routine intubation was unnecessary** as over 90% of patients recovered with a conservative watchful approach.
o Antibiotics – **IV Ceftriaxone 2g BD X 7days and Metronidazole** are recommended to cover the spectrum of organisms responsible.

5. RETROPHARYNGEAL ABSCESS

- Although very uncommon, a combination of *sore throat, fever, neck stiffness and stridor* should alert the clinician to consider this diagnosis. Swelling or oedema of the posterior pharynx should prompt a consideration of advanced airway care and an urgent ENT opinion.
- Mortality rates are high when complications such as airway obstruction and mediastinitis arise.

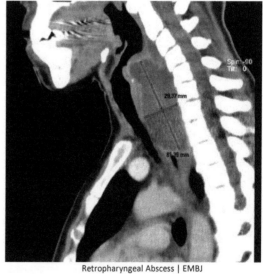

Retropharyngeal Abscess | EMBJ

- Signs suggestive of potential airway obstruction are: **stridor, altered voice, inability to swallow saliva, tripod position >>> call ENT and Anaesthetist immediately.**

II. POST TONSILLECTOMY HAEMORRHAGE

BACKGROUND

- Post tonsillectomy bleeding is an uncommon, but potentially devastating event. The main difficulties arise from airway obstruction and hypovolaemic shock
- The risk is reduced if on antibiotics, adequate oral intake and adequate analgesia.
- Postoperative hemorrhage following tonsillectomy can be classified as:
  - **Primary (most common)** – within 24 hours and rarely dealt with in ED
  - **Secondary** – from 24 hours to 14 days post operation, most commonly 6-10 days
- The incidence is variable, depending in part upon how hemorrhage is defined and measured. Primary hemorrhage typically ranges from 0.2 to 2.2 percent and secondary hemorrhage between 0.1 and 3 percent[216].

ASSESSMENT

- Management of bleed occurs concurrently with history and examination.
- Bleeding is often occult in children as they swallow blood rather than spit it out.
- The amount of blood loss is usually more than you estimate. Children can tolerate blood loss up to a certain point then will decompensate.

HISTORY

- Timing of operation
- Analgesia given (especially if ibuprofen or aspirin has been given)
- Past history, especially of bleeding disorders
- Intercurrent illnesses, especially URTI or other febrile illnesses.
- Estimated amount of blood observed to be lost

EXAMINATION

- Calm manner and reassuring tone (for parents and child)
- Heart rate, respiratory rate, blood pressure, capillary refill, pallor, fever
  - If prolonged central capillary refill or low BP, then major blood loss has already occurred
  - Watch pulse changes closely – beware of an increasing tachycardia
- Look at the back of the throat (within limits of patient cooperation) for signs of active bleeding and/or clot.

ED MANAGEMENT

- Postoperative hemorrhages usually stop spontaneously, but they sometimes require a return to the operating room for hemorrhage control. They seldom require blood transfusion. In rare cases, they can be life threatening[217]. In addition, postoperative hemorrhage can cause difficulty in securing the airway by intubation, leading to an anoxic injury[218].
- Contact the ENT registrar +/- anaesthetics as soon as condition is recognised. For patients being transferred, ETA should be determined and ENT made aware of time they are needed. Transferred patients may need a medical escort from the transferring hospital.

Initial management

- Manage patient in **resuscitation bay** or appropriate high acuity area
- **Early intravenous access**: a large cannula if possible
- **IO access** if no IV access can be obtained
- Obtain bloods for:
  - **FBC** – baseline Hb and platelets (this may not be representative of blood loss)
  - **Coagulation profile and von Willebrand's screen** (for unrecognised coagulopathy)
  - **Group and Hold +/- crossmatch** (depending on severity of symptoms/signs)
- **IV fluids**: 10-20mL/kg boluses of 0.9% saline to correct physiologic parameters
- If unstable, **give packed cells** (O neg/group specific)
- **Apply co-phenylcaine spray** to the oropharynx or adrenaline 1:10 000
- Administer **intravenous tranexamic acid**
- **DDAVP** may also be given on advice of ENT or senior ED doctor
- Keep **Nil Per Mouth**
- **Allow to sit upright**, leaning forward if necessary (to help keep blood out of airway)
- **Intubation** in an emergency is extremely difficult and should be done by the most experienced airway doctor available in the hospital
- All post tonsillectomy bleeding will need admission for observation or operating theatre.

[216] De Luca Canto G, Pachêco-Pereira C, Aydinoz S, et al. Adenotonsillectomy Complications: A Meta-analysis. Pediatrics 2015; 136:702.

[217] Windfuhr JP, Schloendorff G, Sesterhenn AM, et al. A devastating outcome after adenoidectomy and tonsillectomy: ideas for improved prevention and management. Otolaryngol Head Neck Surg 2009; 140:191.

[218] Subramanyam R, Varughese A, Willging JP, Sadhasivam S. Future of pediatric tonsillectomy and perioperative outcomes. Int J Pediatr Otorhinolaryngol 2013; 77:194.

III. EPISTAXIS

INTRODUCTION

- Epistaxis is defined as acute hemorrhage from the nostril, nasal cavity, or nasopharynx.
- It is a frequent emergency department (ED) complaint and often causes significant anxiety in patients and clinicians. However, the vast majority of patients who present to the ED with epistaxis (likely more than 90%) may be successfully treated by an emergency physician[219].
- Emergency physicians have a 90% success rate at treating epistaxis in emergency department, and only have to refer 10% to ENT for further assessment and management

CAUSES OF EPISTAXIS

Local trauma:	Coagulopathies
• Nose picking • Facial trauma • Foreign bodies • Nasal or sinus infections • Nasal septum deviation	• Von Willebrand disease, • Haemophilia A& B • Splenomegaly • Thrombocytopenia • Platelet disorders • Liver disease • Renal failure • Chronic alcohol abuse • AIDS
Environmental	**Iatrogenic**
• Dry cold conditions (presentations increase during winter) • Prolonged inhalation of dry air (Oxygen)	• Nasogastric tube insertion • Nasotracheal intubation
Vascular Abnormalities	**Medicinal**
• Sclerotic vessels • Hereditary haemorrhagic telangiectasia • Arteriovenous malformation • Neoplasm, Aneurysms • Septal perforation • Septal deviation • Endometriosis	• **Anticoagulants:** Aspirin, NOACs, warfarin, platelet inhibitors • Topical corticosteroids and antihistamines • Solvent inhalation (huffing) • Snorting cocaine

1. HYPERTENSION:

- The association between epistaxis and hypertension has long been disputed. Several population-based studies have failed to show an association between hypertension and nasal bleeding[220].

- These studies, however, address the question "Is epistaxis more common in patients with hypertension?"
- Karras, et al. looked at an ED population with elevated blood pressures on presentation and questioned the patients regarding recent blood pressure associated symptoms, including epistaxis[221].
- They found no correlation between elevated ED blood pressures and recent epistaxis. Both the population-based studies and the ED-based study by Karras are subjected to significant recall bias.

2. ANATOMY & PHYSIOLOGY OF EPISTAXIS

- The blood supply of the nose is rich and complex with branches arising from both the internal and external carotid arteries with multiple anastomoses. 90% of epistaxis occurs in the anterior nasal septum, from **Littles area** which contains the **Kiesselbach plexus of vessels (LEGS Vessels).** The other 10% occur posteriorly, along the nasal septum or lateral nasal wall.
- The external carotid artery supplies the nose via the facial and internal maxillary branches. The superior labial branch of the facial artery supplies the anterior nasal floor and nasal septum. The internal maxillary artery divides into multiple branches in the pterygomaxillary fossa.
- The blood supply of the nasal septum is from the **internal carotid** through the **anterior and posterior Ethmoidal arteries,** and from **external carotid** through the **Greater palatine, Sphenopalatine and superior Labial arteries.**

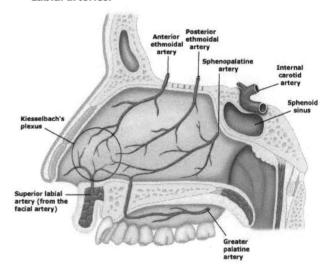

219 Van Wyk FC, Massey S, Worley G, Brady S. Do all epistaxis patients with a nasal pack need admission? A retrospective study of 116 patients managed in accident and emergency according to a peer reviewed protocol. J Laryngol Otol. 2007 Mar. 121(3):222-7.

220 Beran M, Petrusno B. Occurrence of epistaxis in habitual nose-bleeders and analysis of some etiological factors. ORL J Otorhinolaryngol Relat Spec 1986;48:297-303.

221 Karras DJ, Ufberg JW, Harrigan RA, et al. Lack of relationship between hypertension-associated symptoms and blood pressure in hypertensive ED patients. Am J Emerg Med 2005;23:106-110.

3. ASSESSMENT OF THE PATIENT PRESENTING WITH EPISTAXIS:

- **History:**
  - Obtain the following:
    - Laterality, duration, frequency, Severity, estimated blood loss
    - Any contributing or inciting factors
    - Family history or bleeding disorder, Past medical history
    - Current medications
- **Physical Examination:**
  - Application of a vasoconstrictor before the examination may reduce hemorrhage and help to pinpoint the precise bleeding site.
  - Topical application of a local anesthetic reduces pain associated with the examination and nasal packing.
  - Gently insert a nasal speculum and spread the naris vertically. This permits visualization of most anterior bleeding sources. Approximately 90% of nosebleeds can be visualized in the anterior portion of the nasal cavity. Blood dripping from the posterior nasopharynx confirms a nasal source.
  - A posterior bleeding source is suggested by failure to visualize an anterior source, by hemorrhage from both nares, and by visualization of blood draining in the posterior pharynx.

4. INVESTIGATIONS

- **FBC, U&E, LFT** (renal failure = U&E, chronic alcohol abuse = LFTs)
- **INR:** Patients taking warfarin
- **Coagulation**: only of benefit in patients with a known coagulopathy or chronic liver disease, and should not be routine in patients presenting with epistaxis.
- Radiological investigations have little role in the management of epistaxis,
- **CT scan** is indicated if neoplasm suspected, and would generally be arranged post consultation with your ENT specialist.

5. MANAGEMENT OF EPISTAXIS IN ED

FIRST AID MEASURES TO STEM NASAL BLEEDING:

- **Lean the patient forwards in an upright position**; Encourage the patient to **spit out** any blood passing into the throat
- **Firmly pinch the soft part of the nose** compressing the nostrils for at least 10 minutes. If unable to comply then an alternative technique is to **ask a relative** or **staff member** or apply **swimmers nose clip.**
- **Use of ice:** to the neck or forehead; sucking on an ice cube or applying an ice pack ice directly to the nose may help

- **Equipment and Personal Protection**
  - Gloves, mask and visor
  - Essential items for managing epistaxis: light source, Suction apparatus
  - A combination anaesthetic and vasoconstrictor agent: lidocaine with phenylephrine.
  - Nasal speculum
- **Nasal Cautery**: silver nitrate application stick or equipment for electrocautery
  - ⤷ *__Do not cauterize both side of the nasal septum__: There is a risk of septal perforation due to decreased vascular supply from the perichondrium*

- **Topical Treatment**
  - In children, it is normally the case that adequate first aid measures will stop bleeding.
  - Children with recurrent nose bleeds and nasal crusting should be treated with **topical nasal antiseptic (Naseptin) cream applied twice daily for 4 weeks.**
  - In the presence of a visible vessel on the septum, cauterisation with silver nitrate is recommended.
  - *Topical antiseptic cream is as effective as silver nitrate cautery in preventing further nosebleeds in children with recurrent epistaxis.*

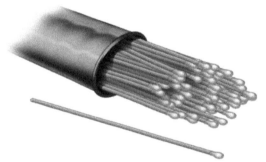

- **Nasal Packing**: ribbon gauze packs
  - ⤷ *Insertion of Foley catheters to stop uncontrolled posterior bleeding is a technique of last resort when immediate specialist help is unavailable.*

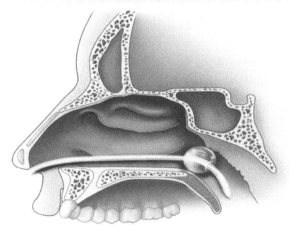

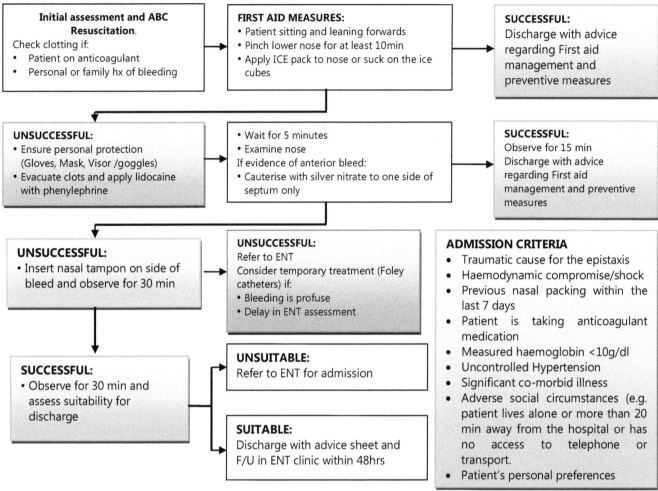

Initial assessment and ABC Resuscitation.
Check clotting if:
• Patient on anticoagulant
• Personal or family hx of bleeding

FIRST AID MEASURES:
• Patient sitting and leaning forwards
• Pinch lower nose for at least 10min
• Apply ICE pack to nose or suck on the ice cubes

SUCCESSFUL:
Discharge with advice regarding First aid management and preventive measures

UNSUCCESSFUL:
• Ensure personal protection (Gloves, Mask, Visor /goggles)
• Evacuate clots and apply lidocaine with phenylephrine

• Wait for 5 minutes
• Examine nose
If evidence of anterior bleed:
• Cauterise with silver nitrate to one side of septum only

SUCCESSFUL:
Observe for 15 min
Discharge with advice regarding First aid management and preventive measures

UNSUCCESSFUL:
• Insert nasal tampon on side of bleed and observe for 30 min

UNSUCCESSFUL:
Refer to ENT
Consider temporary treatment (Foley catheters) if:
• Bleeding is profuse
• Delay in ENT assessment

ADMISSION CRITERIA
• Traumatic cause for the epistaxis
• Haemodynamic compromise/shock
• Previous nasal packing within the last 7 days
• Patient is taking anticoagulant medication
• Measured haemoglobin <10g/dl
• Uncontrolled Hypertension
• Significant co-morbid illness
• Adverse social circumstances (e.g. patient lives alone or more than 20 min away from the hospital or has no access to telephone or transport.
• Patient's personal preferences

SUCCESSFUL:
• Observe for 30 min and assess suitability for discharge

UNSUITABLE:
Refer to ENT for admission

SUITABLE:
Discharge with advice sheet and F/U in ENT clinic within 48hrs

7. PROGNOSIS & FOLLOW UP STRATEGIES

• No follow-up is necessary for patients in whom the epistaxis has either stopped spontaneously or by 1st aid measures or cautery alone.
• However, it is important to provide advice to prevent recurrence of the nosebleed and first aid measures for future episodes.

8. ADVICE TO PREVENT RECURRENCE OF EPISTAXIS

o **Avoidance of:**
  ▪ Blowing the nose for one week.
  ▪ Sneezing through the nose: keep the mouth open.
  ▪ Hot and spicy drinks and food, including alcohol for two days.
  ▪ Heavy lifting, straining or bending over.
  ▪ Vigorous activities for one week.
  ▪ Picking the nose.
• For those patients who have an anterior nasal pack, it should be left in place for **24-48 hours** and follow-up arranged with the ENT department for its removal and further assessment.

⊥ Routine antibiotic cover is unnecessary for patients with an anterior pack in place for less than 48 hours.

SEPTAL HAEMATOMA

• Blood has collected in the cavity between the **cartilage and the supporting perichondrium**.
• This is typically caused by a shearing force stripping the perichondrium away from the underlying cartilage.
• Septal haematomas should be **drained** by needle aspiration to avoid complications occurring.
• Following drainage, the nose should be **firmly packed** to avoid re-accumulation of the haematoma and **broad-spectrum antibiotics** should be given.
• Left untreated septal haematomas are associated with the following complications:
  o *Septal abscess formation*
  o *Cartilage necrosis*
  o *Collapse of nasal bridge ('saddle nose')*
• Following treatment, the patient should be **followed up in the ENT clinic in one week**.

IV. OTITIS

1. ACUTE OTITIS MEDIA

1. DEFINITION
- Acute otitis media is the presence of a middle ear effusion accompanied by rapid onset of one of otalgia, otorrhoea, irritability in an infant or toddler, or fever.
- Acute otitis media (AOM) is a common problem in early childhood with 2/3 of children experiencing at least one episode by age 3, and 90% have at least one episode by school entry.
- Peak age prevalence is **6-18 months**

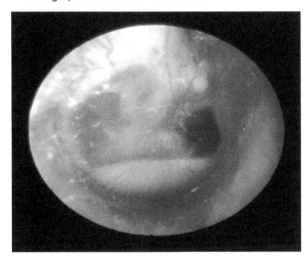

2. AETIOLOGY
- In children: **Streptococcus pneumoniae** and **Haemophilus influenzae**, with **Moraxella catarrhalis**[222].
- Globally: **S. pneumoniae** and **H. influenzae** combined caused 50 to 60 percent of pediatric AOM cases, while M. catarrhalis was responsible for 3 to 14 %[223].
- **Group A streptococcus** and **Staphylococcus aureus** are less frequent causes of AOM in general pediatric populations, although S. aureus may be a significant pathogen in adults based upon limited studies.
- Viral (25%)

3. INDICATIONS TO ADMINISTER ANTIBIOTICS FOR AOM
- Children under 2 years with bilateral infection
- Presence of purulent discharge from ear
- If systemically unwell (e.g. fever and vomiting)
- Recurrent infections

[222] Pichichero ME. Otitis media. Pediatr Clin North Am 2013; 60:391.

[223] Ngo CC, Massa HM, Thornton RB, Cripps AW. Predominant Bacteria Detected from the Middle Ear Fluid of Children Experiencing Otitis Media: A Systematic Review. PLoS One 2016; 11:e0150949.

- **Amoxicillin** is the recommended first-line antibiotic for AOM, where antibiotics are indicated.
- **Five days** treatment at the following doses is sufficient for uncomplicated ear infections in children.
- The doses are as follows:
  - **Neonate (7-28 days):** 30mg/kg TDS
  - **1 month-1 yr:** 125mg TDS
  - **1-5 years:** 250mg TDS
  - **5-18 years:** 500mg TDS
- If the patient is penicillin allergic then **Erythromycin** (or suitable macrolide antibiotic alternative) should be prescribed for **5 days**. The doses are as follows:
  - **<2 years:** 125mg QDS
  - **2-8 years:** 250mg QDS
  - **8-18 years:** 250-500mg QDS

4. POTENTIAL COMPLICATIONS OF AOM
- *Chronic secretory otitis media*
- *Conductive hearing loss*
- *Tympanic membrane perforation*
- *Acute mastoiditis*
- *Meningitis*
- *Facial nerve palsy*
- *Brain and Dural abscesses*
- *Endocarditis*

2. OTITIS EXTERNA
- It is infection and inflammation of the ear canal.
- Common symptoms include pain, itching and discharge from the ear. Otoscopy will reveal erythema of the ear canal with pus and debris present. Various conditions can predispose to otitis externa including skin conditions, such as psoriasis and eczema. It is also more prevalent in people that have regular exposure to water in the ear canal, such as swimmers (**Swimmer's ear**).

- **RISK FACTORS**
  - Swimming
  - Congenital narrowing of the ear canal
  - Foreign object in the ear canal e.g. cotton bud or hearing aid
  - Trauma to the ear canal e.g. overly vigorous cleaning
  - Skin conditions e.g. eczema or psoriasis
- **The commonest causative organisms are:**
  - *Pseudomonas aeruginosa* (50%)
  - *Staphylococcus aureus* (23%)
  - Gram negative bacteria e.g. *E. coli* (12%)
  - *Aspergillus* and *Candida* species (12%)

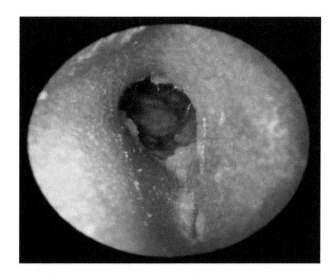

ED MANAGEMENT OF OTITIS EXTERNA

- **Cleaning the ear canal** – Cleaning out the external canal (aural toilet) is the first step in treatment. The removal of cerumen, desquamated skin, and purulent material from the ear canal greatly facilitates healing and enhances penetration of ear drops into the site of inflammation[224].
- Keep the ear dry and advise against inserting anything into the ear.
- Simple analgesia.
- Topical ear drops e.g. combined corticosteroid and antibiotic.
- An aminoglycoside is contraindicated if the tympanic membrane is perforated.
- A referral to the on-call ENT team would be warranted if any of the following are present:
  o *Concurrent skin infection e.g. erysipelas or cellulitis*
  o *Presence of necrotizing otitis externa (osteomyelitis)*
  o *Failure to respond to first line treatment*
  o *Aural toilet required*
  o *History of chronic ear condition*

3. MALIGNANT OR NECROTISING OTITIS EXTERNA

- Malignant (necrotizing) external otitis (also termed malignant otitis externa) is an invasive infection of the external auditory canal and skull base, which typically occurs in elderly patients with diabetes mellitus.
- Increasing reports of malignant external otitis in patients infected with the human immunodeficiency virus (HIV) implicate a compromised immune system as a predisposing factor in this disease.

- **Pseudomonas aeruginosa** is nearly always the responsible organism. The widespread use of oral and topical fluoroquinolones for the treatment of otitis may make the isolation of *P. aeruginosa* more difficult and has contributed to the emergence of *P. aeruginosa* resistant to ciprofloxacin[225].
- Otitis externa with severe pain, out of proportion to the otoscopic findings, discharge, headaches and CN findings are all suggestive of malignant or necrotising otitis externa.
- Elderly diabetic patients are overwhelmingly the population at risk for malignant external otitis. More than 90 percent of adults with this disease were found to have some form of glucose intolerance in one review[226].
- There is progression of infection from the EAM to the auditory canal, temporal bone and base of skull.
- There is less local blood flood and the earwax in these groups is less acidic and has fewer lysosomes.
- Cranial nerve involvement/palsy is due to both direct neurotoxic effect and the swelling and inflammation causing compression.
- The first nerve to be involved is the facial nerve at the stylomastoid foramen and with progression the IX,X and XI as the jugular foramen is involved.
- Imaging modalities include computed tomographic (CT) scanning Head, technetium Tc 99m medronate methylene diphosphonate bone scanning, and gallium citrate Ga 67 scintigraphy.
- With progression of the infection there is risk of meningitis, brain abscesses, dural sinus thrombosis and this reflects the mortality of near 80% if there is cranial nerve involvement.

MANAGEMENT

- Treatment of necrotizing external otitis includes correction of immunosuppression (when possible), local treatment of the auditory canal, long-term systemic antibiotic therapy and, in selected patients, surgery.
- Meticulous cleaning and debridement plus topical application of antimicrobial agents (antibiotics and others)
- IV Antibiotics
- ENT referral

[224] Kaushik V, Malik T, Saeed SR. Interventions for acute otitis externa. Cochrane Database Syst Rev 2010; :CD004740.

[225] Bernstein JM, Holland NJ, Porter GC, Maw AR. Resistance of Pseudomonas to ciprofloxacin: implications for the treatment of malignant otitis externa. J Laryngol Otol 2007; 121:118.

[226] Rubin Grandis J, Branstetter BF 4th, Yu VL. The changing face of malignant (necrotising) external otitis: clinical, radiological, and anatomic correlations. Lancet Infect Dis 2004; 4:34.

4. MASTOIDITIS

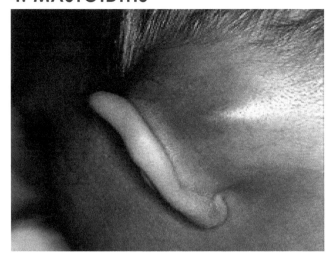

- Mastoiditis is an infection of the mastoid process of the temporal bone.
- A purist's definition of mastoiditis includes all inflammatory processes of the mastoid air cells of the temporal bone.
- As the mastoid is contiguous to and an extension of the middle ear cleft, virtually every child or adult with acute otitis media (AOM) or chronic middle ear inflammatory disease has mastoiditis.
- In most cases, the symptomatology of the middle ear predominates (eg, fever, pain, conductive hearing loss), and the disease within the mastoid is not considered a separate entity[227].
- It is fortunately an uncommon complication of acute otitis media but can lead to intracranial infection.
- **Clinical features** that help identify mastoiditis:
  o Erythema, swelling, and tenderness over the mastoid process.
  o Displacement of the pinna forwards and outwards.
  o Narrowing of the external auditory canal.
  o Failure of treatment in acute otitis media.
- **Workup** includes the following:
  o Fu blood count (FBC)
  o Audiometry
  o Tympanocentesis/myringotomy
  o Computed tomography (CT) scanning - CT scanning of the temporal bone is the standard for evaluation of mastoiditis, with published sensitivities ranging from 87-100%

ED MANAGEMENT OF MASTOIDITIS
- Intravenous broad-spectrum antibiotics.
- Urgent ENT referral.

[227] Minovi A, Dazert S. Diseases of the middle ear in childhood. GMS Curr Top Otorhinolaryngol Head Neck Surg. 2014. 13:Doc11.

5. CHOLESTEATOMA

- Cholesteatoma is an erosive disorder of the middle ear and mastoid, which can lead to life-threatening intracranial infection.
- It can be caused by a tear or retraction of the tympanic membrane.
- It can be congenital (present from birth), but it more commonly occurs as a complication of chronic ear infections[228].

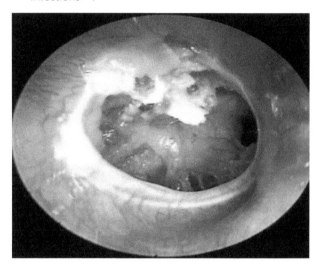

SIGNS AND SYMPTOMS
- Painless otorrhea, either unremitting or frequently recurrent.
- Conductive hearing loss
- Dizziness: Relatively uncommon
- Drainage and granulation tissue in the ear canal and middle ear: Unresponsive to antimicrobial therapy.
- Occasionally, cholesteatoma initially presents with symptoms of CNS complications, including the following[229]:
  o Sigmoid sinus thrombosis
  o Hearing loss in one ear
  o Dizziness (vertigo)
  o Facial Paralysis
  o Persistent ear drainage
  o Epidural abscess
  o Meningitis
- Patient should be referred urgently to ENT for a CT scan and surgical removal of the lesion.

[228] Cholesteatoma. MedlinePlus. May 25, 2016; http://www.nlm.nih.gov/medlineplus/ency/article/001050.htm.

[229] Cholesteatoma. American Academy of Otolaryngology-Head And Neck Surgery. http://www.entnet.org/content/cholesteatoma. Accessed 4/28/2017.

V. EAR INJURIES

1. TYMPANIC PERFORATION

- Traumatic tympanic perforation may be caused by barotrauma, direct penetrating injury (e.g. cotton bud), or following a base of skull fracture.
- The patient experiences pain, reduced hearing, and sometimes a bloody discharge.
- Most perforations will heal spontaneously and the patient should be advised to **keep the ear clean and dry**. They should not put anything into the auditory canal.
- **GP follow-up** should be arranged to ensure adequate healing.

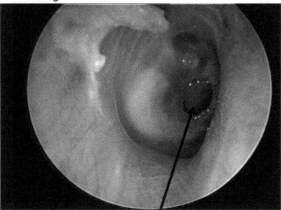

2. AURICULAR HAEMATOMA ('CAULIFLOWER EAR')

- Blunt trauma to the external ear can result in a haematoma forming under the perichondrium.
- This separates the cartilage, which is avascular, from the perichondrium, which supplies it, resulting in **necrosis.**
- The haematoma should be aspirated acutely and a firm dressing applied over the ear and around the head.
- **ENT follow-up** should be arranged.

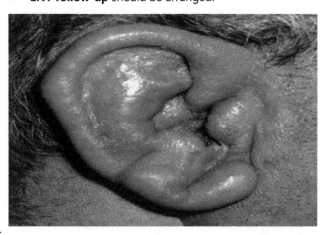

PANCOAST TUMOUR

- It is a tumour that occurs at the apex of the lung, most are non-small cell cancers.
- **The growing tumour can cause compression of a number of nearby structures including:**
  - *Recurrent laryngeal nerve (causing hoarseness)*
  - *The sympathetic ganglion (causing Horner's syndrome)*
  - *Phrenic nerve*
  - *Brachiocephalic vein*
  - *Subclavian artery*
  - *Superior vena cava*
- Approximately 5-15% of lung cancer patients develop hoarseness as a consequence of recurrent laryngeal nerve compression and the left side is most commonly affected.
- **Horner's syndrome** is a combination of symptoms that arises when the sympathetic ganglion is damaged.
- The following clinical **features classically** occur on the same side as the lesion:
  - **M**iosis
  - **A**nhidrosis
  - **P**tosis
  - **E**nophthlamos

Pancoast tumor

Phrenic nerve — Sympathetic trunk
Vagus nerve —
C8 —
T1 —
Brachial plexus
Rib 1
Rib 2
Rib 3
Subclavian artery & vein   Pancoast tumor   Recurrent layrngeal nerve

18. Fever in the ED
I. THE RETURNING TRAVELLER

1. FEVER IN THE RETURNING TRAVELLER
INTRODUCTION

- International travel to tropical destinations is increasingly popular. The majority of these trips are for tourism, with the second largest group being UK residents visiting friends and relatives who live overseas.
- It is estimated that around 10% of travellers will seek medical attention while abroad or after they have returned home.
- In addition, migration into the UK has increased in recent years, and these individuals may present with fever or other health problems soon after arrival in the UK from a tropical country.
- The list of potential infectious causes of fever in a returning traveller from the topics is long.
- However, for all of these patients the attending clinician should consider the following infections early on in their assessment[230]:
  - Malaria
  - Enteric fever (typhoid and paratyphoid)
  - Dengue
  - HIV seroconversion
  - Rickettsial infection
- Some of these diagnoses may be disregarded if there has been no exposure, e.g. no travel to a malarious region, but this list at least serves as a reminder of some of the more important and common infections imported into the UK.
- The annual number of cases of imported malaria in the UK is approximately 1,500, with those visiting friends and relatives overseas accounting for more than 70% of these cases.
- There are between five and ten deaths each year, and in many cases of death there has been a delay in the diagnosis. It must also be remembered that many causes of fever in returning travellers are not specifically 'tropical infections'.
- These might include urinary tract infections, pneumonia, or viral infections like influenza, EBV, or cytomegalovirus.

---

230 *DJ Bell, Fever in the returning traveller [Available online]*

HISTORY

- A detailed and structured history is the key to the diagnosis, appropriate investigation, and the initiation of prompt effective therapy. The following points should be considered:
  - **Countries visited or transited through.**
    - Information resources on infections common in different geographical locations and current disease outbreaks are listed in the further reading list.
  - **Dates of travel and illness onset.**
    - Most tropical infections will cause symptoms within one month of leaving the tropics, though malaria may present many months later. The dates of travel are also particularly important for **Viral Haemorrhagic Fever** (VHF) risk assessment.
  - **Pre-travel vaccinations and malaria prophylaxis taken,** though one must be aware that none of these measures guarantee protection.
  - **Type of travel.**
    - Clearly the range of exposures to different infections will be different for a healthcare worker who has been working in rural Africa and a tourist returning from a safari.
  - **Activities while abroad.**
    - Table below lists risk factors or activities for exposure to specific infections.
  - **VHF risk assessment.**
    - This group of viruses, including **Lassa fever, Crimean-Congo haemorrhagic fever, Marburg and Ebola**, pose a potential risk to healthcare workers because they can be transmitted person-to-person in body fluids. Because of the serious nature of these infections, most UK hospitals have policies for the risk assessment of travellers who present unwell within 21 days of leaving countries where these infections are found.
    - High-risk patients require strict isolation and close liaison with infection diseases and microbiology specialists. These infections are very rare in the UK and specialist isolation facilities are available in Newcastle and London.

- ○ **The patient's immune status.**
  - HIV-infected travellers are at increased risk of certain travel-related infections and opportunistic infections, including malaria, visceral leishmaniasis, gastrointestinal infection (bacterial and parasitic), and invasive fungal infections.

EXAMINATION

- The examination should pay particular attention to look for hepatomegaly, splenomegaly, lymphadenopathy, rash, eschars (dark crusted bites), urticaria, jaundice, haemorrhage (e.g. conjunctival), and features meningism. Clinical features that may be associated with particular tropical infections:

Physical signs	Possible infection
Jaundice	• Viral Hepatitis, Malaria, • Leptospirosis
Maculopapular rash	• Dengue, HIV, Syphilis, • Typhus, Chikungunya
Eschar	• Typhus
Urticarial rash	• Acute Schistosomiasis (Katayama Fever), • Strongyloides
Bloody diarrhoea	• Shigella, Salmonella, • Amoebiasis
Hepatomegaly	• Enteric Fever, Leptospirosis, • Viral hepatitis
Splenomegaly	• Malaria, Visceral leishmaniasis

INVESTIGATIONS

Initial investigations recommended for febrile travellers are:

- FBC, LFT, U&E
- At least three malaria blood films or rapid diagnostic tests (RDTs) **over two days**
- Blood cultures
- HIV test
- Urine and stool culture and microscopy
- Serology ± PCR for Dengue and other arbovirus infections, Rickettsia, Q fever, Brucella
- CXR and ultrasound of liver and spleen

A large Dutch study of febrile returned travellers noted that:

- ❖ **Malaria** was predicted by splenomegaly, thrombocytopenia (platelet count < 150 x10⁹/ml)
- ❖ **Dengue** by rash, thrombocytopaenia, and leukopaenia (leucocyte count < 4 x10⁹/ml)
- ❖ **Acute schistosomiasis** by eosinophil count ≥ 0.5 x 10⁹/ml
- ❖ **Enteric fever** by splenomegaly and elevated liver transaminases.

1. MALARIA

- All patients with fever who have travelled to a malarious region within the past year must be investigated for malaria. Malaria parasites may be in the blood at very low concentrations, especially in patients who have taken prophylaxis, and the parasites may not be visible in the peripheral blood at different stages of their life cycle.
- It is, therefore, advisable to take **three malaria blood tests over 2–3 days** in order to rule out malaria with confidence. Malaria can be diagnosed by microscopy of a blood film, or using a rapid diagnostic antigen test.

COMPLICATED FALCIPARUM MALARIA

- ○ **CNS:** *Impaired consciousness or seizures*
- ○ **Respiratory:** *Pulmonary oedema or ARDS*
- ○ **GIT:** *Jaundice*
- ○ **Renal:** *Renal impairment*
- ○ **Metabolic:** *Acidosis (pH < 7.3), Hypoglycaemia (<2.2 mmol/l)*
- ○ **CVS:** *Shock (BP < 90/60 mmHg)*
- ○ **Hematologic abnormalities**: *Spontaneous bleeding/DIC, Anaemia (Hb <8 g/dL) and*
- ○ **Renal**: *Haemoglobinuria (without G6PD deficiency/ **Black water fever**)*
- Anaemia in the setting of malaria occurs as a result of the following factors:
  - ○ *Haemolysis of parasitized red cells*
  - ○ *Increased splenic sequestration and clearance of erythrocytes with diminished deformability*
  - ○ *Shortened erythrocyte survival*
  - ○ *Cytokine suppression of haematopoiesis*
  - ○ *Repeated infections and ineffective treatments*

ENTERIC FEVER

- **Blood cultures** should be taken on all patients prior to antibiotics, preferably several sets. These are important for the diagnosis of enteric fever, but also for other bacteraemic illnesses.

HIV & OTHERS

- In the very early days of an HIV infection, the **HIV combined antibody and antigen test** that is used in UK hospitals may be negative. If clinical suspicion is high, this should be repeated after a few days.
- **Antibody tests** are available at UK reference laboratories for many imported infections including rickettsial infections, Q fever, leptospirosis, Brucella and arbovirus infections (dengue, chikungunya).

VHF

- If there is a high suspicion of VHF infection, blood sampling should be limited to avoid risks to healthcare workers (consult local guidelines).

PARASITES

- **A raised eosinophil count** (>0.45 x10^9 /L) is reported in up to 10% of returning travellers and may indicate a tropical parasite infection. The most commonly identified parasites are **intestinal helminths, schistosomes, strongyloides, and filarial infections.**
- These can be diagnosed **serologically**, or by identification of their eggs in stool, urine or sputum samples.
- Investigations performed in early infection may be negative and should be repeated after several months.
- If the eosinophilia persists and no parasitic cause is found, non-infective causes including haematological malignancy and vasculitis should be sought.

MANAGEMENT

- Treatment of many of these infections will require specialist input from infectious diseases physicians and microbiologists.
- Drug-resistant malaria is widespread and up-to-date treatment guidelines or advice should be followed.
- **For malaria** (see Malaria section below), the British Infection Society treatment guidelines are available.
  Patients with confirmed non-falciparum malaria may be treated as outpatients, but all those with falciparum or cases where the malaria species is uncertain should be admitted for treatment. Severe malaria may develop within hours, even in migrants to the UK from malaria endemic countries.
- Where there is a strong suspicion of **enteric fever,** antibiotic treatment should be started without delay.
  - Asian origin: **oral azithromycin** or IV **ceftriaxone**
  - African origin: **ciprofloxacin**.
- **Rickettsial infections** responds to **doxycycline**.
- **Dengue**: judicious fluid replacement and supportive care.
- Travel-related infections **MUST BE NOTIFIED TO PUBLIC HEALTH SERVICES** so that epidemiological data can be collected and where necessary infection prevention and control measures initiated.
- Finally, we have a duty to our patients to educate them so that they take all available measures to prevent ill health on future travel.
- This should include advice on vaccine preventable infections, safe sex, food and drink hygiene, malaria prophylaxis and the importance of compliance and insect bite avoidance.

2. TRAVELLERS' DIARRHOEA (TD)
COMMON PATHOGENS TD

Bacterial – commonest
Escherichia coli- enterotoxic or enteroinvasive – haemorrhagic
Shigella
Campylobacter
Salmonella
Others such as Vibrio, Yersinia

Viral
Rotavirus - children
Noroviruses - cruise ships
Astrovirus

Parasitic
Giardia lambia
Entamoeba histolytica
Strongyloidis stercoralis

- **Travellers' Diarrhoea** (TD) can affect up to 80 percent of international travellers each year (Source: World Health Organization,). It is caused by any one of a number of organisms that can be ingested through the consumption of contaminated food or water.
- Developing countries present the highest risk of TD.
- TD starts suddenly and in addition to diarrhoea may include fever, vomiting, stomach cramps and fatigue.
- Most cases of TD last only a few days and are not life threatening, though some cases may last up to a month.
- Normally, the only treatment that is needed is **fluid replacement**. Special rehydration packs can be bought before leaving home, but any clear fluid will do; non-caffeinated fluids are recommended.
- In severe cases, especially if fever and/or bloody diarrhoea are present, **antibiotics may be required.**
- The Centers for Disease Control do not recommend using antibiotics to prevent TD. Unwarranted use of antibiotics may cause infection with resistant organisms.
- Furthermore, antibiotics do not protect against viruses or parasites that can cause TD.
- If TD does occur and the symptoms are moderate to severe (for example, accompanied by bloody stool, cramping or vomiting), the use of antibiotics is recommended. **Ciprofloxacin** is the medication of choice, at a dose of 500 mg twice daily for three days.
- There is disagreement about the use of anti-diarrhoea medicine such as **Imodium®.** These drugs may increase the time the infecting organism stays in the body, thus increasing the risk of serious complications.
- Anti-diarrhoea drugs should be used only in very severe cases, and never in people with fever or bloody diarrhoea. If TD symptoms continue despite medication, rule out a parasitic infection.

II. BACTERIAL MENINGITIS

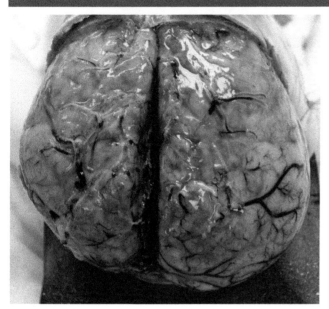

1. OVERVIEW

- Bacterial meningitis is defined as infection of the arachnoid mater, subarachnoid space, and the cerebrospinal fluid (CSF). Approximately 1.2 million cases of bacterial meningitis occur annually worldwide[231].
- Poor outcomes caused by bacterial meningitis often stem from delays in diagnosis and treatment.
- Initial evaluation of patients with bacterial meningitis usually occurs in ED.
- Therefore, it is critically important for ED physicians to diagnose accurately and treat promptly patients with bacterial meningitis to achieve optimal patient outcomes.

2. RISK FACTORS

- CSF leak (e.g. base of skull fracture)
- Head and neck surgery or prostheses (e.g. cochlear implants, VP shunt, ICP monitor, EVD, craniectomy)
- Extremes of age (e.g. Pneumococcus and listeria)
- Head and neck infections (e.g. Sinusitis, mastoiditis, otitis media)
- Comorbidities (e.g. Liver and renal failure)
- Immunosuppression (e.g. Functional asplenia, splenectomy, hypogammaglobulinemia, complement deficiency, steroids, diabetes mellitus)
- Malnutrition/ Low socioeconomic status and overcrowding/ Exposure to epidemic.

---

[231] Scheld WM, Koedel U, Nathan B, Pfister HW. Pathophysiology of bacterial meningitis: mechanism(s) of neuronal injury. J Infect Dis 2002; 186 Suppl 2:S225.

3. ETIOLOGY

COMMUNITY-ACQUIRED MENINGITIS

- *Streptococcus pneumoniae* (pneumococcus) is the most common pathogen since routine immunization of infants with Haemophilus type b conjugate vaccine began.
- However, the decrease in incidence of *H. influenzae* meningitis is seen only in vaccinated infants and children; *H. influenzae* remains among the common culprits in adult patients. Along with pneumococcus and *H. influenzae*, **Neisseria meningitides (meningococcus)**, *Listeria monocytogenes*, and **Group B streptococci** account for nearly all of community-acquired cases in patients up to age 60.
- **Meningococcus** primarily affects younger adults and is associated with individuals living in crowded spaces, such as dormitories and military barracks.
- **Listeria** burdens persons at the extremes of age, pregnant women, and immunocompromised patients.

NOSOCOMIAL MENINGITIS

- *Gram-negative bacilli*, especially from the Enterobacteriaceae family,
- *Staphylococcus aureus,*
- *Coagulase-negative staphylococci.*

Major risks for nosocomial meningitis include **neurosurgery or head trauma** within the previous month, **indwelling medical devices, and CSF leak.**

4. CLINICAL FEATURES

- **History**
  - The classic symptoms of meningitis are **fever, stiff neck, and headache**. Headaches associated with meningitis are typically nonpulsatile, nonfocal, and severe.
  - **Altered mental status** in a patient with fever, even in the absence of headache or stiff neck, should still prompt concern for meningitis.
  - **Rash (petechial, purpuric, or even maculopapular)** in the setting of headache and stiff neck is an alarming sign of meningococcal or pneumococcal disease.

- **Examination**
  - Physical exam manoeuvres traditionally have been used to evaluate neck stiffness by eliciting meningeal irritation: **Kernig and Brudzinski signs.**

- Together, these manoeuvres have reportedly low sensitivity (5%) but high specificity (95%).
- Because of their low sensitivity and false positives among the elderly, the Kernig and Brudzinski signs have limited clinical utility.

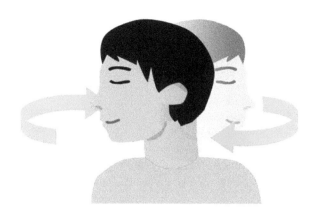

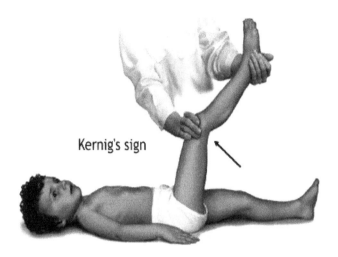

Kernig's sign

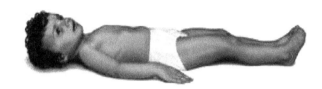

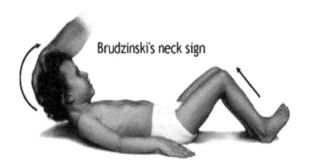

Brudzinski's neck sign

THE JOLT ACCENTUATION TEST

o It is an excellent manoeuvre to help rule out meningitis in a low-risk, nontoxic patient with headache and fever.
o The patient rotates his or her head horizontally at a frequency of two rotations per second; **a positive test is the exacerbation of an existing headache.**
o The jolt accentuation test has a sensitivity of 97% and specificity of 60% for the presence of CSF pleocytosis.
o *Therefore, a negative test essentially can exclude meningitis in patients with fever and headache, and a positive result aids in the decision to proceed with lumbar puncture (LP).*

5. INVESTIGATION

o **LP**: Ideally prior to antibiotics
o **CT Head** first if:
  - *Altered mental Status*
  - *Focal neurologic signs*
  - *Papilloedema*
  - *Immunocompromised*
  - *Seizure within the previous week*
o **Routine blood tests**, **Blood cultures**, **Enterovirus** and **HSV PCR**
o **Bacterial PCR** (Pneumococcus, Meningococcus), Cryptococcal antigen an India Ink
o Neurosyphilis/ Mycobacterium culture or PCR
o Immunocompromised + Gram positive rods = Listeria

Common CSF Findings in Meningitis				
Index	Normal	Bacterial	Viral	Fungal
WBC/mcL	<5	>1,000	<1,000	<1,000
Differential	<15% Neutrophils	>80% Neutrophils	<15% Neutrophils	<15% neutrophils
Glucose (mg/dL)	45-65	reduced	normal	reduced
CSF: blood glucose	0.6	reduced	normal	reduced
Protein (mg/dL)	20-45	>250	50-250	>250
Opening pressure (cm/H20)	<20	Normal to high	Normal to high	Normal to high

6. ED MANAGEMENT OF MENINGITIS

- Antibiotics are essential to the treatment of bacterial meningitis.
- The initial choice should be governed by the patient's age and allergies, as well as resistance patterns of pathogens.
- *Vancomycin plus a third-generation cephalosporin are the mainstays of treatment in most cases of community-acquired bacterial meningitis.*

- In patients who are older than 50 years, immunocompromised, or alcoholics, ampicillin should be added for Listerial infection.
- Coverage for Pseudomonas should be added in nosocomial cases.
- In addition to antibiotics, **steroids should be given in virtually all suspected cases of bacterial meningitis.**
- Intravenous **Dexamethasone (0.15 mg/kg)** is given just prior to or concomitantly with antibiotic administration, and continued **every 6 hours for the next 4 days.**
- Steroids have been shown **to reduce overall mortality** and **neurological sequelae from meningitis**, probably by attenuating the intense inflammatory response in the CNS.
- While this is particularly true for pneumococcus, steroids should be continued regardless of the culprit bacterial pathogen.

EMPIRIC TREATMENT

- Antibiotics within 30 min of initial assessment
- Dexamethasone 0.15mg/kg Q6 hourly with or before the first dose of antibiotics
- Ceftriaxone (immunocompetent) or vancomycin + ciprofloxacin
- Ceftriaxone + benzylpencillin (immunocompromised to cover Listeria)
- Add vancomycin if staph seen on gram stain or at risk (e.g. indigenous, permanent lines, recent hospitalisation, known to be colonised)

DIRECTED TREATMENT

- **Neisseria meningitidis** - Benzylpenicillin or Ceftriaxone or Ciprofloxacin
- **Streptococcus pneumonia**
  - MIC* <0.125mg/L to Penicillin -> Benzylpenicillin,
  - MIC* = 0.125mg/L to Penicillin -> Ceftriaxone + Vancomycin or Rifampicin or Moxifloxacin
  *MIC: Minimum Inhibitory Concentration

- **Haemophilus influenzae** - Ceftriaxone or Cefotaxime or Amoxicillin or Ciprofloxacin
- **Listeria monocytogenes** - Penicillin or Amoxicillin or Co-Trimoxazole
- **Streptococcus agalactiae** – Benzylpenicillin
- **Cryptococcus neoformans or gattii** - Amphotericin B + Flucytosine then go to Fluconazole once CSF clear.

COMPLICATIONS
Intracranial:
- Abscess,
- Cerebritis,
- Deafness,
- Cognitive impairment,
- Hydrocephalus

Extracranial:
- Septic shock,
- Adrenal insufficiency from infarction (Waterhouse Friderichsen syndrome),
- ARF,
- Purpura fulminans,
- Necrotising vasculitis -> skin necrosis and digital gangrene.

PUBLIC HEALTH CONSIDERATIONS
- **Neisseria meningitidis**
  - Requires droplet precautions
  - Post-exposure prophylaxis needed for close contacts if <24h treatment with appropriate antibiotics
    - **Ciprofloxacin 500 mg** (child younger than 5 years: 30 mg/kg up to 125 mg; child 5 to 12 years: 250 mg) orally, as a single dose, OR
    - **Ceftriaxone 250 mg** (child 1 month or older: 125 mg) IM, as a single dose (preferred option for pregnant women), OR
    - **Rifampicin 600 mg** (neonate: 5 mg/kg; child: 10 mg/kg up to 600 mg) orally, 12-hourly for 2 days.

III. URINARY TRACT INFECTION

1. DEFINITIONS
o Emergency physicians encounter urinary tract infections (UTIs) in a wide spectrum of disease severity and patient populations.
o The challenges of managing UTIs in an emergency department include limited history, lack of follow-up, and lack of culture and susceptibility results.
o Most patients do not require an extensive diagnostic evaluation and can be safely managed as outpatients with oral antibiotics.

- **Pyelonephritis**
  o Acute pyelonephritis is a bacterial infection of the renal parenchyma that can be organ- and/or life-threatening and that often leads to renal scarring.
  o The bacteria in these cases have usually ascended from the lower urinary tract, but may also reach the kidney via the bloodstream. Timely diagnosis and management of acute pyelonephritis has a significant impact on patient outcomes[232].

- **Cystitis**
  o Cystitis describes a broad range of diseases with diverse etiology and pathologic mechanisms but with similar clinical presentations. it refers to the inflammatory response of the bladder to infection[233].
  o The leading symptoms are dysuria, frequency, urgency, and, occasionally, suprapubic pain. However, these symptoms are nonspecific and may also be associated with infection of the lower genitourinary tract (urethra, vagina) or with noninfectious conditions such as bladder carcinoma, urethral diverticulum, and calculi.

- **Acute prostatitis**
  o Prostatitis is an infection or inflammation of the prostate gland that presents as several syndromes with varying clinical features. The term prostatitis is defined as microscopic inflammation of the tissue of the prostate gland and is a diagnosis that spans a broad range of clinical conditions.

- **Uncomplicated UTIs**
  o Occurs in patients who have a normal, unobstructed genitourinary tract, who have no history of recent instrumentation, and whose symptoms are confined to the lower urinary tract.
  o Uncomplicated UTIs are most common in young, sexually active women.

- **Complicated UTIs**
  o Occur in certain patient populations. These include UTIs in the elderly (>65), men, in the presence of structural or functional abnormality such as obstruction and neurogenic bladder. They also include the presence of renal stones or foreign body (catheter), pregnancy, recent instrumentation or presence of comorbidity (diabetes, malignant disease).

- **Etiologies**
  o **Escherichia coli** remains the predominant uropathogen (80%) isolated in acute community-acquired uncomplicated infections,
  o **Staphylococcus saprophyticus** (10% to 15%).
  o **Klebsiella, Enterobacter, and Proteus species, and enterococci** infrequently (5-10%) cause uncomplicated cystitis and pyelonephritis.
  o The pathogens traditionally associated with UTI are changing many of their features, particularly because of antimicrobial resistance.
  o The etiology of UTI is also affected by underlying host factors that complicate UTI, such as age, diabetes, spinal cord injury, or catheterization.
  o Consequently, complicated UTI has a more diverse etiology than uncomplicated UTI, and organisms that rarely cause disease in healthy patients can cause significant disease in hosts with anatomic, metabolic, or immunologic underlying disease[234].

2. CLINICAL ASSESSMENT OF COMPLICATED UTIS
- **Cystitis**
  o Cystitis commonly presents with one or more of dysuria, urinary frequency, haematuria, urgency and suprapubic discomfort, especially in the young adult woman.
- **Pyelonephritis**
  o The classic presentation in patients with acute pyelonephritis is as follows:
    - **Fever** - This is not always present, but when it is, it is not unusual for the temperature > 39.4°C
    - **Costovertebral angle pain** - Pain may be mild, moderate, or severe; flank or costovertebral angle tenderness is most commonly unilateral over the involved kidney, although bilateral discomfort may be present

232 Belyayeva M, Jeong JM. Acute Pyelonephritis. 2019 Jan.

233 Reka G Szigeti, Pathology of Cystitis [Medscape]

234 Allan Ronald, The etiology of urinary tract infection: traditional and emerging pathogens [Online]

- **Nausea and/or vomiting** - These vary in frequency and intensity, from absent to severe; anorexia is common in patients with acute pyelonephritis
    o **Gross hematuria** (hemorrhagic cystitis), unusual in males with pyelonephritis, occurs in 30-40% of females, most often young women, with the disorder.
    o Symptoms usually develop over hours or over the course of a day but may not occur at the same time.
    o If the patient is male, elderly, or a child or has had symptoms for more than 7 days, the infection should be considered complicated until proven otherwise.
    o The classic manifestations of acute pyelonephritis observed in adults are often absent in children, particularly neonates and infants. In children aged 2 years or younger, the most common signs and symptoms of urinary tract infection (UTI) are as follows:
        - Failure to thrive
        - Feeding difficulty
        - Fever
        - Vomiting
    o Elderly patients may present with typical manifestations of pyelonephritis, or they may experience the following:
        - Fever
        - Mental status change
        - Decompensation in another organ system
        - Generalized deterioration
    o **Pyelonephritis** will most often require a **7-10-day course of antibiotics**. It also always requires a **renal ultrasound** to be performed. This may be acutely on admission or as part of discharge follow up.
- **Acute bacterial prostatitis**
    o Typically presents as an acute onset of fever, chills, malaise, dysuria, and perineal or rectal pain.
    o One study cited that over 96% of patients present with a triad of pain, prostate enlargement, and failure to void and 92% present with fever[235].
    o It may also present as dysuria, urinary frequency, urinary urgency, and, occasionally, urinary retention.

3. INVESTIGATIONS

o Urine dipstick, Urine microscopy and culture
o Imaging: mainly ultrasound, but occasionally CT in certain complicated UTIs.

- **Imaging**
    o It may reveal complications of urinary tract infection such as **renal calculi**, **hydronephrosis and renal abscess.**
    o Severely unwell patients, those who fail to resolve and those in which diagnostic uncertainty exists, require urgent imaging.
    o **CT** will detect any renal calculi, hydronephrosis and abscess, yet is most usually saved for renal colic or diagnostic uncertainty.

4. MANAGEMENT OF UTIs IN THE ED

1. ACUTE CYSTITIS

A. ACUTE UNCOMPLICATED CYSTITIS
o In young female, non-pregnant patients in areas with low E. coli resistance, **trimethoprim** is still a reliable empiric treatment.
o **Nitrofurantoin** must not be used if pyelonephritis is suspected, as it has poor efficacy in the upper urinary tract.

B. ACUTE COMPLICATED CYSTITIS
o **Ciprofloxacin or cephalexin** may be used.
o Avoid Trimethoprim.

2. ACUTE PYELONEPHRITIS

A. ACUTE UNCOMPLICATED PYELONEPHRITIS
o **Ciprofloxacin** is the initial treatment of choice for uncomplicated pyelonephritis.
o If intravenous treatment is required, a **single dose of gentamicin** followed by ciprofloxacin is a reasonable approach.
o The IV dose can be given in the ED allowing the patient to be discharged on oral antibiotics.
o *Uncomplicated pyelonephritis in a well patient can usually managed as an out-patient initially.*

B. ACUTE COMPLICATED PYELONEPHRITIS
o **Admit**
o **IV Ciprofloxacin, Piperacillin-Tazobactam** or **IMI/Meropenem.**
o **Gentamicin** may be useful.

3. UTI IN PREGNANCY
o UTIs in pregnancy are complicated.
o **Cystitis**: Use **Nitrofurantoin, Cephalexin** or **Amoxicillin.**
o **In pyelonephritis,**
    - **Ceftriaxone** may be used, but in later pregnancy there is a risk of kernicterus.
    - **Piperacillin-tazobactam** may also be used.

---

235 *Tibor Fulo, Acute Pyelonephritis [Medscape]*

19. Fits /Seizure
I. FIRST TIME SEIZURE IN THE ED

DEFINITION

Excessive, abnormal cortical neuronal activity resulting in a variety of physical symptoms.

- **Provoked seizure:** An acute symptomatic seizure that occurs at the time of or within 7 days of an acute neurologic, systemic, metabolic, or toxic insult.
- **Unprovoked seizure:** A seizure occurring in the absence of acute precipitating factors and includes remote symptomatic seizures, as well as seizures that are not established to have a cause.

SEIZURE CLASSIFICATION

Questions that can help guide your ED management decisions

- *Is the patient back to his baseline neurological status?*
  - Get collateral information for accurate answer
- *Is this a first-time seizure?*
  - Be aware that 50% of "first time seizures" have had prior events
  - Consider Syncope!
- *Is the seizure provoked or unprovoked?*

Seizure classification

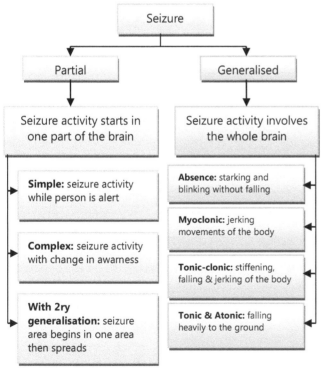

DIFFERENTIAL DIAGNOSIS

Medications	Vital Signs	CNS Abnormalities
Bupropion	Hypoxia	TBI
Camphor	Hyperthermia	SAH
Clozapine	Hypertensive	CVA
Cyclosporine	Emergency	Traumatic ICH
Fluoroquinolones	Hypoglycemia	Space Occupying
Imipenem	Hyperglycemia	Lesion (i.e. Tumor)
Isoniazid		
Lead		
Lidocaine Lithium		
Metronidazole		
Theophylline		
TCAs		

Withdrawal Syndromes	Infectious	Metabolic
Alcohol	Meningitis	Hepatic
AEDs	Encephalitis	Encephalopathy
Benzodiazepines	CNS Abscess	Hypocalcemia
Baclofen		Hypercalcemia
		Hyponatremia
		Uremia

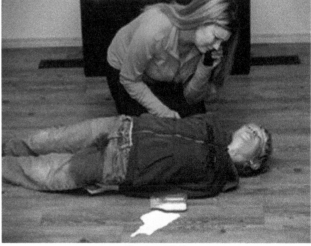

Courtesy JEMS

ED WORKUP OF 1ST TIME SEIZURE

1. Non-Contrast Head CT (CT Brain)

- Unprovoked, back at baseline: CT not indicated
- Provoked or unprovoked, NOT at baseline: Obtain CT
  - CT abnormal in up to 80% of patients with focal neurological deficit after seizure (Harden 2007)

- **Provoked and back at baseline**[236]:
  - No definitive recommendations
  - CT unlikely to have high-yield
  - If provoking factor addressed and patient can reliably follow up, may consider outpatient imaging

2. Electroencephalogram (EEG)

- Provoked or unprovoked, **NOT at baseline = Emergent EEG**
  - Concern for status (nonconvulsive) epilepticus
  - Mortality rates estimated to be as high as 40%
- If patient returns to baseline, EEG can be deferred to outpatient.

3. ELECTROCARDIOGRAM

- **Always obtain an ECG in first time seizure patients**
- **The challenge:** Significant overlap in presentation with syncope often having myoclonic or tonic jerks (12-75%) due to cerebral hypoperfusion.
- **The importance:** Misdiagnosing syncope as seizure can lead to application of incorrect treatment and, thus mortality and morbidity
- **Can't miss ECG findings:**
  - *Wolff-Parkinson-White syndrome*
  - *Prolonged QT interval (especially in younger patients)*
  - *Brugada syndrome: RBBB pattern with STE in V1-V3*
  - *Hypertrophic cardiomyopathy*
  - *Arrhythmogenic RV dysplasia: Negative T waves in V1-V3 with or without epsilon waves*
  - *Bi/tri fascicular blocks or undetermined intraventricular conduction abnormalities*
  - *High degree AV blocks*

4. Lumbar Puncture

- Indicated if there's a concern for a CNS infection (i.e. meningitis, encephalitis)
- Lower threshold to LP if patient is immunocompromised (increased rate of CNS toxoplasmosis, CNS abscess etc)
- Provoked or unprovoked
  - At baseline: No LP
  - NOT at baseline: Obtain LP

5. Starting Anti-Epileptic Drugs (AEDs)

- Current best literature does not uniformly recommend starting AEDs after a first time seizure.
- Early treatment does not seem to provide protection from future seizures.

KEY LEARNING POINTS:

- It is critical to determine if the event was a seizure or syncope. Look for a post-ictal period and get an ECG in all patients
- Review the differential for seizure in all patients, particularly those with a 1st time seizure.
- Consider vital sign abnormalities, toxic/metabolic, CNS and infectious causes
- In 1st time seizures, always carefully consider whether the seizure was provoked or unprovoked and whether the patient is back at his baseline as this can drastically effect management.
- There is no specific testing that is required in all patients with a 1st time seizure.
- Testing is based on your history and physical examination

References

1. *Bergfeldt, L. Differential diagnosis of cardiogenic syncope and seizure disorder. Heart 2003; 89(3): 353-358. PMID: 1767616*
2. *Harden CL et al. Reassessment: neuroimaging in the emergency patient presenting with seizure (an evidence-based review): report of the Therapeutics and Technology Assessment Subcommittee of the American Academy of Neurology. Neurology 2007; 69 (18): 1772-1780. PMID 17967993*
3. *Huff JS et al. Clinical policy: critical issues in the evaluation and management of adult patients presenting to the emergency department with seizures. Ann Emerg Med 2014; 63 (4): 437-447.e415. PMID 24655445*
4. *Knake S, et al. Status epilepticus: a critical review. Epilepsy Behav 2009; 15 (1): 10-14. PMID 19236943*
5. *McMullan J et al. Seizure disorders, in Marx JA, Hockberger RS, Walls RM, et al (eds): Rosen's Emergency Medicine: Concepts and Clinical Practice, ed 8. St. Louis, Mosby, Inc., 2010, (Ch) 102: p 1375-1385.*
6. *Raskin NH et al. Neurologic Disorders in Renal Failure. NEJM 1976; 294 (3): 143-148. PMID 1105188*
7. *Tardy B et al. Adult first generalized seizure: etiology, biological tests, EEG, CT scan, in an ED. Am J Emerg Med 1995; 13 (1): 1-5. PMID: 7832926*

---

[236] *Adapted from RICH WHITE, MD (CORE EM) https://coreem.net/core/1st-time-seizure*

II. STATUS EPILEPTICUS

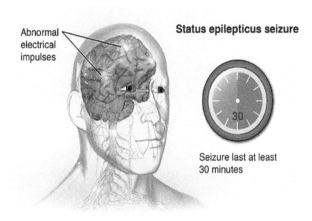

Abnormal electrical impulses

Status epilepticus seizure

30

Seizure last at least 30 minutes

1. DEFINITIONS

- Status epilepticus (SE) is a medical emergency associated with significant morbidity and mortality. SE is defined as a continuous seizure lasting more than 30 min, or two or more seizures without full recovery of consciousness between any of them.
- Based on recent understanding of the pathophysiology, it is now considered that any seizure that lasts more than 5 min probably needs to be treated as SE.
- There is a growing body of support for the definition to refer to seizures that persist for greater than 5 minutes without intervention. Status epilepticus (SE) is a common medical emergency associated with high morbidity, if not mortality. Mortality from SE varies from 3–50% in different studies. In elderly patients, refractory status epilepticus (RSE) may lead to death in over 76% cases[237].
- **Impending Status Epilepticus** has been advocated to describe continuous or intermittent seizures that persist **beyond 5 minutes** without neurological recovery.
- **Established SE** refers to clinical or electrographic seizures that persist for **30 minutes** or longer without full neurological recovery in between.
- **Refractory SE:** About 9-31% of patients with SE may fail to respond to standard treatment. This subgroup of RSE has greater morbidity and mortality. RSE is defined as continuous or repetitive seizures lasting longer than 60 min despite treatment with a benzodiazepine (lorazepam) and another standard anticonvulsant (usually phenytoin/fosphenytoin) in adequate loading dose[238].

- **Malignant SE** is a severe variant of RSE, in which the seizure fails to respond to aggressive treatment with even anesthetic agents. It typically occurs in young patients (18–50 years) in the setting of encephalitis.
- SE may be subdivided into convulsive and non-convulsive forms.

2. MANAGEMENT OF S.E. IN THE ED (See algorithm)[239]

- **Pre-hospital**
  - **ABC**: attention to airway, breathing and circulation, with the application of high flow oxygen where available.
  - **Blood glucose** should be checked and intravenous dextrose used to treat hypoglycaemia as indicated.
  - **Benzodiazepines**: **Diazepam** (rectal) or **Midazolam** (buccal or intranasal) may be used for this purpose.
- **On arrival in the ED**
  - Check **ABC**
  - Administer high-flow oxygen
  - Measure **blood glucose** and do **Pregnancy test**
  - **Drug regime**
    - **IV access**: Lorazepam **0.1 mg/kg IV**
    - **No IV access**: Diazepam **0.5 mg/kg PR**
- **10min later; continued seizure:**
  - **Drug regime**
    - **IV access**: Lorazepam **0.1 mg/kg IV**
    - **No IV access**: Paraldehyde **0.4 ml/kg (in same volume of olive oil) PR**
- **20min later; continued seizure:**
  - Request senior help, if not already present
  - Consider intraosseous access, consider IV cutdown if IV access not already established
  - **Drug regime**
    - Phenytoin **20 mg/kg IV** OR Phenobarbitone **20 mg/kg IV**
    - And Paraldehyde **0.4 ml/kg** (in same volume of olive oil) PR if not already given.
- **40 min later; continued seizure:**
  - Rapid sequence intubation
  - Transfer to intensive therapy unit (ITU)
  - **Drug regime:** Thiopental **4 mg/kg**

---

237 Logroscino G, Hesdorffer DC, Cascino GD, Annegers JF, Bagiella E, Hauser WA. Long-term mortality after a first episode of status epilepticus. Neurology. 2002;58:537–41.

238 Shorvon S. Status epilepticus: Its clinical features and treatment in children and adults. Cambridge, England: Cambridge University Press; 1994. p. 201e.

239 APLS 6th Manual.

STATUS EPILEPTICUS- APLS ALGORITHM

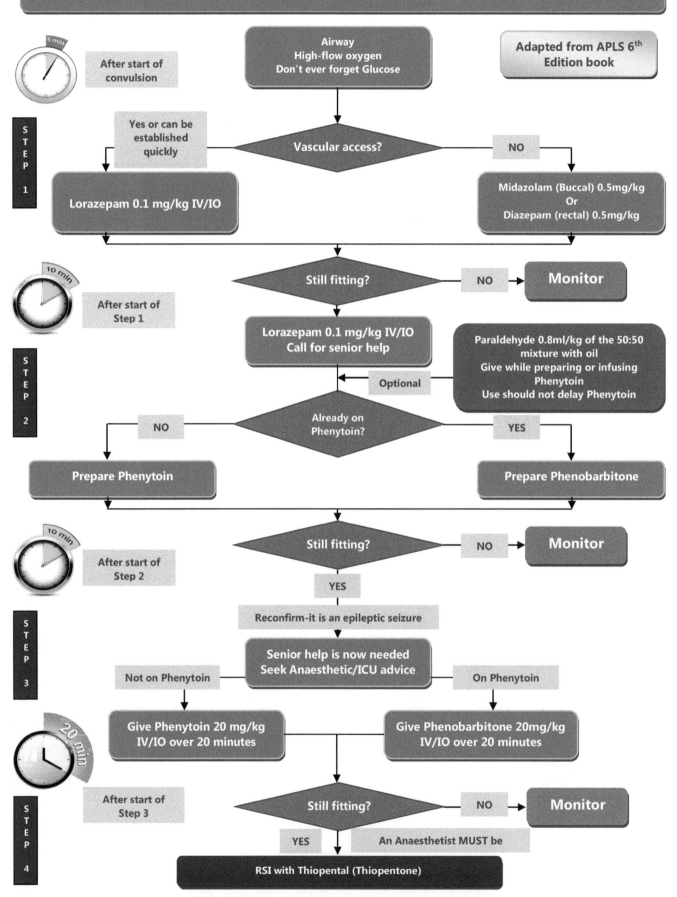

III. NON EPILEPTIC ATTACK DISORDER (NEAD)

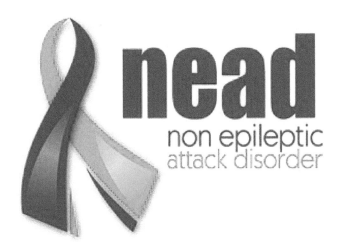

INTRODUCTION

- 'NEAD' stands for Non Epileptic Attack Disorder. Other names include Psychogenic Non Epileptic Seizures (PNES) which is mainly used in the USA, functional seizures and dissociative seizures.
- NEAD are paroxysmal episodes that resemble and are often misdiagnosed as epileptic seizures; however, NEAD are psychological (i.e., emotional, stress-related) in origin.
- Men, women and children of all ages can develop functional seizures. These seizures look like epileptic seizures but are not caused by electrical activity in the brain. Associated symptoms may include fatigue, cognitive difficulties, memory loss, confusion on coming round from the seizure and temporary paralysis of parts of the body. Functional seizures can also co-exist with Epilepsy and other functional neurological symptoms.
- The differential diagnosis of suspected seizures is long but over 90% of self-limiting episodes of unprovoked transient loss of consciousness (TLOC) are caused by epileptic seizures, vasovagal syncope and NEAD[240].

- As with Epilepsy, the seizures differ from person to person and can range from staring blankly (dissociation), to blackouts, to falling to the ground with various parts of the body, or the whole body, twitching and jerking. People are generally aware (but not always) of what is occurring but are unable to respond[241].

CAUSES OF NEAD
- It is currently believed that functional seizures are triggered by the brain's response to overwhelming stress, which can be from emotional or physical (e.g. pain) triggers, but there may be other causes.
- For some people symptoms may proceed a specific traumatic incident (such as abuse, accident or death of a loved one), and for others, an accumulation of stress over time. Many people are confused by the diagnosis as they don't feel particularly stressed.

PHYSICAL EXAMINATION
- **Physical and neurologic findings** are usually normal, but the examination can also uncover suggestive features. For example, overly dramatic behaviors, give-way weakness, and a weak voice or stuttering can be useful predictors.
- **Psychological features** suggestive of psychogenic episodes include anxiety, depression, inappropriate affect or lack of concern (*la belle indifference*), multiple and vague somatic complaints suggestive of somatization disorder, and abnormal interaction with family members.

DIAGNOSTIC
- As already stated, getting a diagnosis may take quite some time. People may initially be diagnosed with epilepsy and be put on anti-epileptic medication. It may be that when these medications don't work, the patient will be referred for further tests.
- Laboratory studies are useful only in excluding metabolic or toxic causes of seizures (e.g., hyponatremia, hypoglycemia, drugs).
- **Prolactin and creatine kinase (CK)** levels rise after generalized tonic-clonic seizures and not after other types of episodes.

[240]Shorvon S, Cook M, Guerrini R, et al.Malmgren K, Reuber M, Appleton R. Differential diagnosis of epilepsy. In: Shorvon S, Cook M, Guerrini R, et al., eds. Oxford textbook of epilepsy and epileptic seizures. Oxford: Oxford University Press, 2013:81–94.

[241] FND Action, Non Epileptic Attack Disorder (NEAD) [FNDaction Online]

- However, sensitivity is too low to be of any practical value (i.e., lack of elevation does not exclude epileptic seizures).
- Although imaging findings are normal in psychogenic nonepileptic seizures (NEAD), images should be obtained to exclude organic pathology.
- Incidental abnormalities are occasionally seen on imaging. However, they should not confound the diagnosis if results of EEG video monitoring firmly establish NEAD.
- If the diagnosis is still uncertain, the patient may be referred for a **video telemetry test**.
- The patient will be taken into hospital for a number of days, usually three to five, and will be connected to an EEG machine. They will be videoed constantly during their stay and will be closely monitored by medical staff.
- They may be required to go without sleep, be subjected to flashing lights or asked to hyperventilate in an effort to safely provoke an attack.

HOW PEOPLE ARE AFFECTED

- The potential impact of NEAD on the person and those close to them cannot be overstated. Many are afraid to go out in case they have a seizure and become increasingly isolated. Depending on the type of seizure, people can also be physically harmed.
- All aspects of life can be affected with many losing their jobs, often because employers are unwilling to make reasonable adjustments as required by law.
- NEAD sufferers are unable to drive for certain periods of time and may be wary of using public transport.
- Relationships can suffer with family members having to step in to the carer's role. Lack of knowledge amongst health professionals, especially those in emergency care, leads to people being accused of faking, drug abuse or attention seeking.
- Correct diagnosis can take up to five years, with many being treated unnecessarily for epilepsy with attendant risks.
- People may become increasingly incapacitated and no longer able to care for themselves, needing help with normal day-to-day activities such as washing and getting dressed.
- Anxiety and depression are common co-morbidities.

TREATMENT

- The currently accepted medical treatment is specialist **Cognitive Behavioural Therapy (CBT)** although this does not work for everyone and there are very long waiting lists. Other treatments such as **Eye Movement Desensitization and Reprocessing (EMDR)**, for those with traumatic triggers, are being investigated.
- There are currently no approved medications for NEAD.
- Some people may be prescribed anti-anxiety medication or antidepressants if appropriate.
- People may benefit from trying self-care techniques such as grounding/distraction when they feel a seizure coming on, however some may not have any warning.
- If people also present with other functional neurological symptoms, a collaborative care approach should be considered.
- The main obstacle to effective treatment is effective delivery of the diagnosis. The physician delivering the diagnosis must be compassionate, remembering that most patients are not faking, but also firm and confident to avoid the use of ambiguous and confusing terms.
- Most patients with psychogenic symptoms have previously received a diagnosis of organic disease (e.g., epilepsy); therefore, patients' reactions typically include disbelief and denial, as well as anger and hostility. For example, they may ask "Are you accusing me of faking?" or "Are you saying that I am crazy?"
- Patients who accept their diagnosis and follow through with therapy are more likely to experience a successful outcome; therefore, patient education is crucial.

20. Headache

I. PRIMARY & SECONDARY HEADACHES

- Headache is the most common neurological problem presented to general practitioners and to neurologists.
- Headache accounts for 4% of primary care consultations and up to 30% of neurology appointments[242].
- Headache disorders are classified as primary or secondary:
  o The most common **primary headache** disorders are tension-type headache, migraine and cluster headache.
  o **Secondary headaches** are attributed to underlying disorders and include headache associated with giant cell arteritis, raised intracranial pressure and medication overuse..

1. CLINICAL ASSESSMENT

- Most patients will be discharged, and many require no investigation beyond a focussed clinical history and examination.

Clinical history

- The clinical history is the single most important assessment tool when determining the cause of a headache.
- Red flags suggest headache secondary to intracranial pathology (usually serious) and warrant further investigation. The 2008 SIGN Guideline gives the following list of red flag features on history and examination:
  o Worsening headache with fever
  o Sudden-onset headache reaching maximum intensity within 5 minutes
  o New-onset neurological deficit
  o New-onset cognitive dysfunction
  o Change in personality
  o Impaired level of consciousness
  o Recent (typically within the past 3 months) head trauma
  o Headache triggered by cough, valsalva (trying to breathe out with nose and mouth blocked) or sneeze
  o Headache triggered by exercise
  o Orthostatic headache (headache that changes with posture)

  o Symptoms suggestive of giant cell arteritis
  o Symptoms and signs of acute narrow angle glaucoma
  o A substantial change in the characteristics of their headache. **[2012**
  o New onset headache in a patient with a history of human immunodeficiency virus (hiv) infection.
  o New onset headache in a patient with a history of cancer.
- *The presence of any 'red flag' feature mandates further investigation of a patient presenting with headache.*

- **Examination**
  o The most important features of the clinical examination are:
    - Cognitive state,
    - Vital signs
    - Neck movement,
    - Pupils – symmetry and fundi
    - Motor function – Pronator drift
    - Gait
- If any of these are abnormal, further investigation is required. Approximately 10% of patients will have signs or symptoms of headache due to a secondary cause.

2. INVESTIGATIONS

- The most important investigation is the **neurological examination itself**.
- Most patients with a normal neurological examination and a 'non-thunderclap' headache will require no further investigation.
- In about 10% of ED headache patients, the history and/or the examination will suggest the possibility of a secondary cause. Such patients will need to undergo a **Brain Computerised Tomography (CT) scan.**
- CT scanning is indicated on first presentation to exclude subarachnoid haemorrhage (SAH)/structural lesion.
- **A CT scan** is **not** indicated in patients with symptoms of a tension-type headache**,** cluster headache and trigeminal neuralgia.

---

242 *NICE clinical guideline: Headaches [NICE CG150]*

HEADACHE TYPES

HEADACHE TYPES	CHARACTERISTICS
Primary headaches	• Migraine. • Tension-type headache. • Cluster headache. • Miscellaneous: Benign Cough Headache, Benign Exertional Headache, Headache associated with Sexual Activity.
Secondary headaches	• Head injury (including post-traumatic headache). • Vascular disorders (e.g. subarachnoid haemorrhage (SAH), stroke, intracranial haematoma, cavernous sinus thrombosis, hypertension, unruptured arteriovenous malformation, temporal arteritis). • Non-vascular disorders (e.g. idiopathic intracranial hypertension, intracranial tumour, post-lumbar puncture). • Headaches associated with substances or their withdrawal (including analgesia, caffeine, nitrates, alcohol, and carbon monoxide). • Infections (e.g. Encephalitis, Meningitis, Sinusitis). • Metabolic (e.g. Hypoxia, Hypercapnia, Hypoglycaemia). • Craniofacial disorders (e.g. pathology of skull, neck, eyes, nose, ears, sinuses, mouth, and temporomandibular joints causing pain; this includes headache secondary to glaucoma). • Headache attributed to psychiatric disorders. • Cranial neuralgias (e.g. trigeminal neuralgia).

CLUSTER HEADACHES
- Unilateral; Pain is in and around one Eye
- Severe temporal headache, Ipsilateral rhinorrhoea
- Ipsilateral eye tearing and redness of the eye

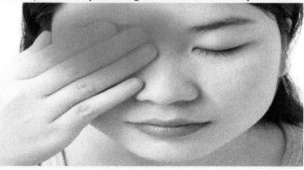

TENSION HEADACHES
- Bilateral Pain is like hand/Band squeezing the head
- Associated with stress in life
- Occurs 3-4 times a week, mostly at the end of the day

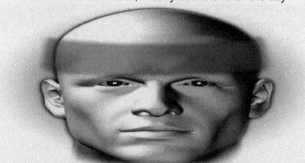

MIGRAINE HEADACHES
- Pain is **POUND**ing: **P**ulsatile, **O**nset 4-72hrs, **U**nilateral, **N**ausea & Vomiting, **D**isabling
- Associated with aura, Lasts 2-3 hours

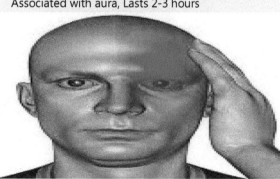

SINUS HEADACHES
- Pain behind the forehead and/or cheekbones
- Fever,
- Headache and nasal discharge

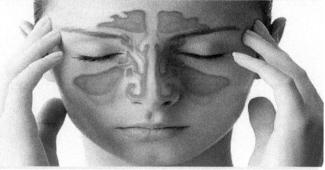

TYPES	CLINICAL FEATURES	MANAGEMENT

PRIMARY HEADACHES

Migraine	**The best predictors for migraine** can be summarised as follows:
	o **POUND**ing: **P**ulsating, Duration of 4-72 h**O**urs, **U**nilateral, **N**ausea, **D**isabling
	o Builds up over minutes to hours.
	o Variable duration but may last up to 72h.
	o May be preceded by an aura (15-33% of patients).
	o Moderate to severe in intensity.
	o Often disabling.
	o Associated with nausea and vomiting.
	o Exacerbated by light (photophobia), sound (phonophobia), and physical activity.
	o Episodic (patient may have a history of previous migraines).
	o Sensitivity to light between attacks.
	o Positive family history of migraine.
		o **Analgesics**
		o **Anti-emetics:** Metoclopramide and Domperidone
		o **Non-specific Therapies**
		  ▪ Chlorpromazine 25-50 mg IM
		  ▪ Prochlorperazine 10mg IV/IM
		o **Specific Therapies:**
		  ▪ The triptans: **Sumatriptan 6 mg sub-cut**
		  ▪ **Ergotamine tartrate 1-2 mg** if migraine does not respond to triptans.
		
		Prevention:
		o Biofeedback;
		o Propranolol, Timolol
		o Divalproex sodium
		o Calcium Blockers and NSAIDs

Tension- type headache	o Pain is typically bilateral. o Pressing or tightening ('band-like') in quality. o Non-throbbing pain o Mild to moderate intensity. o No nausea or vomiting. o Not aggravated by physical activity. o May have pericranial tenderness. o May have sensitivity to light or noise.	o Rest; Aspirin; Paracetamol; o Ibuprofen; Naproxen sodium; o Combinations of analgesics with caffeine; o Ice packs; Muscle relaxants; o Antidepressants, o **Prevention:** Avoidance of stress; use of biofeedback; relaxation techniques; or antidepressant medication.
Cluster headache	o Severe unilateral headache. o Excruciating pain in the vicinity of the eye; tearing of the eye; nose congestion; and flushing of the face. o Pain frequently develops during sleep and may last for several hours. o Attacks occur every day for weeks, or even months, and then disappear for up to a year. o 80% of cluster patients are male, most between the ages of 20 and 50. o **Precipitating Factors:** Alcoholic beverages; excessive smoking	o **High flow O$_2$ therapy**: 10 L/minute for 15 minutes is usually effective. o **Sumatriptan,** 6 mg, sub-cut o **Ergotamine** o Intranasal application of local anaesthetic agent o **Prevention:** Use of steroids; ergotamine; calcium channel blockers; and lithium
Exertional Headaches **Headache associated with sexual activity (coital cephalgia)**	o Explosive headache indistinguishable from a SAH. o Related to sexual activity usually at or near orgasm. o Classically the headache is severe and throbbing. o The first-time a patient experiences coital cephalgia a subarachnoid haemorrhage should be actively excluded.	o Treated with **Aspirin, Indomethacin, Propranolol.** o Extensive testing is necessary to determine the cause. o Surgery is occasionally indicated to correct the organic disease. o **Prevention:** Alternative forms of exercise; avoid jarring exercises

SECONDARY HEADACHES

Subarachnoid haemorrhage (SAH)	o Sudden-onset, 'worst-ever' headache. o Maximum intensity usually reached in less than 1 min. o Usually occipital and may be described like a blow to the back of the head. o May be associated with vomiting, neck pain, and photophobia. o The patient may present with a transient loss of consciousness or fits. o The patient may be drowsy and/or confused. o May have a history of a 'warning headache' days to weeks earlier. o Fundoscopy may show subhyaloid retinal haemorrhage (haemorrhage near the optic nerve head). o May have focal neurological deficits depending on the location of the aneurysm (e.g. IIIrd nerve palsy with posterior communicating artery aneurysms).
Meningitis	o Generalized headache in an unwell/drowsy patient. o May have neck stiffness and photophobia. o May be pyrexial. o May have a rash (meningococcal).
Space-occupying lesion (raised ICP)	o Headache exacerbated by lying down and Valsalva manoeuvres (e.g. coughing, straining, laughing, bending forwards). o Headache may wake the patient from sleep. o Visual obscurations (transient changes in vision) with change in posture or Valsalva suggest raised intracranial pressure. o Seizures, Cognitive change or focal neurological signs and Papilloedema.
Temporal arteritis	o Patient age >50 years. o Diffuse, throbbing headache. o **Scalp tenderness, jaw claudication, and tender temporal artery with reduced pulsation.** o **Visual disturbance.** o A normal ESR makes the diagnosis unlikely. **Management:** *Carbamazepine, Phenytoin, Valproate, Lamotrigine and Gabapentin* o Approximately 30% of patients do not respond to drug therapy, and these patients may need **surgical intervention**.
Acute angle closure glaucoma	o Unilateral headache. o Eye pain. o Mid-dilated, red eye. o Halos around lights. o Reduced visual acuity.
CO2 Poisoning	o Headache that improves on leaving the environment. o Nausea and vomiting. o Dizziness, Muscle weakness and Blurred vision.

- **COMMON CAUSES OF THUNDERCLAP HEADACHES**
  - o *SAH*
  - o *Benign Exertional Headache*
  - o *Cervical Arterial Dissection*
  - o *Cerebral Venous Thrombosis*
  - o *Pituitary Apoplexia*
  - o *Ischaemic Stroke*
  - o *Hypertensive Crisis*
  - o *Spontaneous Intracranial Hypotension*
  - o *Benign Orgasmic Headache*

II. NON-TRAUMATIC SAH

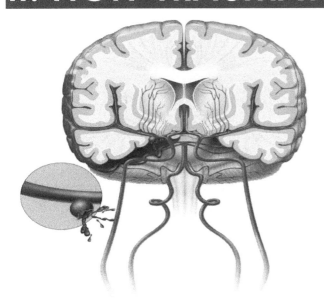

INTRODUCTION
- The term subarachnoid hemorrhage (SAH) refers to extravasation of blood into the subarachnoid space between the pial and arachnoid membranes (see the image below). It occurs in various clinical contexts, the most common being head trauma. However, the familiar use of the term SAH refers to nontraumatic (or spontaneous) hemorrhage, which usually occurs in the setting of a ruptured cerebral aneurysm or arteriovenous malformation (AVM)[243].

AETIOLOGY[244]
- Berry aneurysm (80%)
- AVM
- Polycystic kidney disease
- SLE · Moyamoya disease
- Syndromes: Marfan, Ehlers-Danlos, Osler- Weber-Rendu, Klippel-Trenaunay-Weber
- Metastatic tumours eg atrial myxoma, choriocarcinoma (very rare)
- Vasculitis (very rare)
- Fungal / bacterial infections (very rare)

SIGNS AND SYMPTOMS
- Classically presents with what's known as a 'thunderclap' headache.
- Signs and symptoms of SAH range from subtle prodromal events to the classic presentation.
- The most common premonitory symptoms are as follows:

- o Headache (48%)
- o Dizziness (10%)
- o Orbital pain (7%)
- o Diplopia (4%)
- o Visual loss (4%)

- **Signs present before SAH include the following**:
- o Sensory or motor disturbance (6%)
- o Seizures (4%)
- o Ptosis (3%)
- o Bruits (3%)
- o Dysphasia (2%)

- As to how short in duration a headache can be and still be a SAH, no-one knows, however an arbitrary time of **1 hour** has been suggested.
- Prodromal signs and symptoms usually are the result of sentinel leaks, mass effect of aneurysm expansion, emboli, or some combination thereof.

- **The classic presentation can include the following:**
- o Sudden onset of severe headache (the classic feature)
- o Accompanying nausea or vomiting
- o Symptoms of meningeal irritation
- o Photophobia and visual changes
- o Focal neurologic deficits
- o Sudden loss of consciousness at the ictus
- o Seizures during the acute phase

- **OTHER FEATURES:**
- o Vomiting is **not** predictive.
- o Seizure at onset is.
- o 2/3rds have a reduced level of consciousness.
- o Neck stiffness may develop – but usually only after several hours and is due to an inflammatory reaction to the blood in the subarachnoid space, and it may not develop at all if there's only a small amount of blood.
- o **3rd nerve palsy due to an aneurysm in the posterior communicating artery.**
- o 1 in 7 will have intraocular haemorrhages.
- o **Ischaemic changes (of any type) on ECG** are common
  - Possibly due to a catecholamine surge or a change in autonomic vascular tone.
- o 3% will have a cardiac arrest
  - Aggressive resuscitation is essential as they appear to have a high rate of ROSC and half of the survivors will regain independent living.

---

243 Tibor Becske, Subarachnoid Hemorrhage [Medscape Online]

244 Barts Health Acute Care Guideline Group, Subarachnoid Haemorrhage [RCEM Website]

RISK FACTORS FOR ANEURYSM RUPTURE[245]
- *Smoking and alcohol*
- *Age 20 – 65 most common*
- *Hypertension (BP > 160/100 high risk)*
- *Coagulopathy does not cause rupture, but is associated with a poor outcome*

2. PERIMESENCEHALIC HAEMORRHAGE
- o Haemorrhage restricted to the cisterns about the brainstem and suprasellar cistern and a negative cerebral angiogram.
- o Has a much better prognosis than standard SAH with a much lower rate of rebleeding or vasospasm.
- o 1 out of 29 patients rebled and died in one retrospective study.
- o Has a presumed venous aetiology but some neurosurgeons are sceptical of this as an entity and advocate a repeat of the angiogram.

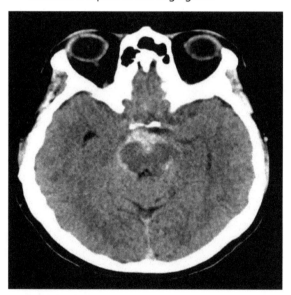

INVESTIGATIONS
- • The **most widely accepted approach** to the investigation of thunderclap headaches is a combination of CT, followed by a lumbar puncture (LP) 12 hours after onset of headache if the CT is negative.

1. CT Scan
- o Modality of choice; The distribution of blood on the initial CT Head scan can be helpful in distinguishing aneurismal SAH from perimesencephalic haemorrhage.
- o However, non-contrast CT brain appearances are not unique and **CT angiography (CTA)** is required in these patients to exclude a ruptured vertebrobasilar aneurysm.

2. CT ANGIOGRAPHY AND ANGIOGRAPHY
- • All patients with CT-proven SAH should undergo **CTA or formal Angiography** to identify the aneurysm responsible or confirm the absence of such in cases of perimesencephalic haemorrhage.
- • A negative CT alone is not yet enough evidence to exclude SAH.

3. LUMBAR PUNCTURE
- o Since CT does not have 100% sensitivity, the concern is that a SAH may be missed despite a normal scan.
- o Traditional teaching and expert opinion still mandate a lumbar puncture (LP) and cerebrospinal fluid (CSF) analysis for **xanthochromia** in every patient with a negative or non-diagnostic CT head scan as evidenced by national guidelines in the United Kingdom (UK) and the United States (US).

- ☩ Patients in whom the diagnosis of SAH is considered but in whom the CT is normal must subsequently undergo an **LP at least 12 hrs after the onset of symptoms.**

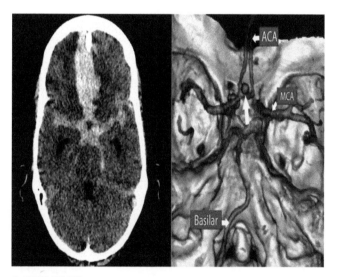

4. MRI SCAN
- o Appears comparable to CT in acute phase.
- o Small studies hint it may even be better.
- o May help localise 'CT negative, LP positive' patients.
- o May pick up pathologies not detected by CT
  - ▪ E.g.: Cerebral venous sinus thrombosis (CVT), Parenchymal lesions.

---

[245] *Barts Health Acute Care Guideline Group, Subarachnoid Haemorrhage [RCEM Website]*

ED MANAGEMENT OF SAH
Acute severe headache suggestive of SAH:
- Insert iv cannula and take blood for FBC, clotting, VBG, ECG. Assess GCS

- **CT brain To be completed within 1 hour of request:**
  - **CT normal completed within 6 hours of onset: SAH Unlikely**
    - Discuss with senior
    - Risk of SAH less than 1%
    - **Risks of LP[246]:**
      - Low pressure headache up to 10%
      - Risk of local infection and epidural haematoma less than 1%
      - If good history discuss with neurosurgery (highest risk age 30 – 65)
    - Discharge with clinical advice

  - **CT normal completed more than 6 hours from onset: SAH Possible**
    - Refer Medical
    - LP is HIGH RISK if GCS < 15:
      - discuss with consultant
      - LP to be carried out minimum 12 hours post onset of symptoms (may remain positive up to 1 week later)
      - The sample must reach lab as soon as possible
      - The last CSF sample should be protected from the light and transported quickly to the laboratory for analysis (by spectrophotometry in the UK) for xanthochromia.
      - Paired serum bilirubin needed
    - **LP positive Or non-diagnostic:**
      - Refer Neurosurgeons
      - Discuss non-diagnositic LP and clinical suspicion
      - Consider further imaging with MRI / MRA / CT angio
    - **LP negative:** High clinical suspicion? (good history, appropriate age, no history of chronic headaches)
      - Refer Neurosurgeons
      - Discuss non-diagnositic LP and clinical suspicion
      - Consider further imaging with MRI / MRA / CT angio
    - **LP negative:** no suspicion
      - Discharge with clinical advice

  - **CT shows SAH** (if shows alternate diagnosis, exit pathway and manage as appropriate): **SAH Confirmed**
    - Discuss with Neurosurgery
    - Consider need for intubation
    - Maintenance 0.9% saline iv
    - BP control – aim for sBP < 180 mmHg but > 120 mmHg
    - CAUTION if chronic HT or low GCS, Prescribe either: Metoprolol 2.5 mg iv, slow boluses (max 10 mg) or GTN infusion 1 to 10 mL per hour (50 mg in 50 mL 0.9% saline) (20 to 200 mcg per min)
    - Arrange critical transfer

- Patients with acute severe headache <2 weeks from the index episode should get non-contrast CTB.
- If CTB normal:
  - LP should be performed at least 12 hours from the start of the headache.
  - If both CT and LP are negative within two weeks, then SAH can be excluded.
- Patients presenting >2 weeks from the index headache or in whom results of either CT or LP have been unobtainable or dubious should be discussed with a neurosurgical team.

COMPLICATIONS OF SAH
- Rebleeding
- Hydrocephalus
- Cerebral vasospasm
- SIADH, resulting in hyponatraemia.
- Neurological deficits from cerebral ischaemia
- Neurogenic pulmonary oedema
- Aspiration pneumonia
- Myocardial ischaemia or infarction due to excessive catecholamine release
- Left ventricular dysfunction due to excessive catecholamine release
- Death.

PROGNOSIS

HUNT – HESS SCALE		Survival
1	Asymptomatic / mild headache	70%
2	Moderate / severe headache; neck stiffness +/or cranial nerve palsy	60%
3	Altered mental status +/- mild focal neurological deficits	50%
4	Reduced GCS +/or hemiplegia	20%
5	Coma or decerebrate posturing	10%

III. TRIGEMINAL NEURALGIA (TN)

INTRODUCTION

- Trigeminal neuralgia is characterized by facial pain often accompanied by a brief facial spasm or tic.
- Pain distribution is unilateral and follows the sensory distribution of cranial nerve V, typically radiating to the maxillary (V2) or mandibular (V3) area.
- At times, both distributions are affected.
- Physical examination will usually eliminate alternative diagnoses. Signs of dysfunction of other cranial nerves or other neurologic abnormality exclude the diagnosis of classic trigeminal neuralgia and suggest that pain may be secondary to a structural lesion.
- In symptomatic trigeminal neuralgia, the pain syndrome is secondary to tumor, multiple sclerosis, or other structural abnormalities[247].

HISTORY

- History is the most important factor in the diagnosis of typical or classical trigeminal neuralgia (TN).
- Symptomatic trigeminal neuralgia secondary to intracranial processes may have a different history.

Nature of pain

- Pain is brief and paroxysmal, but it may occur in volleys of multiple attacks.
- Pain is stabbing or shocklike and is typically severe.

Distribution of pain

- One or more branches of the trigeminal nerve (usually maxillary or mandibular in unilateral distribution) are involved.
- Pain is unilateral in classical trigeminal neuralgia.
- Bilateral pain suggests symptomatic trigeminal neuralgia.

Duration of pain

- It is typically from a few seconds to 1-2 minutes.
- Pain may occur several times a day; patients typically experience no pain between episodes.

Trigger points

- Various triggers may commonly precipitate a pain attack.
- Light touch or vibration is the most provocative.
- Activities such as shaving, face washing, or chewing often trigger an episode.
- Stimuli as mild as a light breeze may provoke pain in some patients.
- Pain provokes brief muscle spasm of the facial muscles, thus producing the tic.

PHYSICAL

Physical examination findings should show no abnormality unless there is a prior or concomitant neurologic process. A normal neurologic examination is part of the definition of typical or classic trigeminal neuralgia (TN).

Perform a careful examination of the cranial nerves, including the corneal reflex.

- Be alert to the presence of any abnormality on physical examination. Abnormality suggests that the pain syndrome is secondary to another process.
- Trigeminal sensory deficits suggest symptomatic trigeminal neuralgia.
- Remember that patients report pain following stimulation of a trigger point; thus, some patients may limit their examination for fear of stimulating these points.

CAUSES

- Idiopathic: in about 85% of cases
- Abnormal vascular course of the superior cerebellar
- Small arteries or veins compressing the facial nerve.
- Aneurysms,
- tumors,
- Chronic meningeal inflammation
- Multiple sclerosis may be the precipitant.

IMAGING STUDIES

- Patients with characteristic history and normal neurologic examination may be treated without further workup.
- Some physicians recommend **elective MRI** for all patients to exclude an uncommon mass lesion or aberrant vessel compressing the nerve roots.

EMERGENCY DEPARTMENT CARE

- Care in the ED is generally limited to correct identification of trigeminal neuralgia (TN), consideration of alternative diagnosis, pain relief, and coordination of follow-up care.
- **Carbamazepine** is regarded by most as the medical treatment of choice
- Other anticonvulsants including **phenytoin, oxcarbazepine, clonazepam, lamotrigine, valproic acid, and gabapentin** are reportedly beneficial in some patients.
- Coordinate therapy for refractory pain of trigeminal neuralgia with the primary care physician or consultants.

---

[247] *Cruccu G, Gronseth G, Alksne J, et al. AAN-EFNS guidelines on trigeminal neuralgia management. Eur J Neurol. 2008 Oct. 15(10):1013-28.*

IV. IDIOPATHIC INTRACRANIAL HYPERTENSION

INTRODUCTION

- Benign Intracranial Hypertension or Idiopathic intracranial hypertension (IIH) is a disorder of unknown etiology that predominantly affects **obese women of childbearing age**.
- Although IIH, pseudotumor cerebri, and benign intracranial hypertension (BIH) are synonymous terms in the literature, IIH is the preferred term.
- The primary problem is chronically **elevated intracranial pressure (ICP),** and the most important neurologic manifestation is, which may lead to secondary progressive optic atrophy, **visual loss, and possible blindness**.

RISK FACTORS

- Exposure to or withdrawal from certain exogenous substances (eg, drugs)
- Systemic diseases (eg, infectious etiologies)
- Disruption of cerebral venous flow (eg, venous sinus thrombosis, dural fistula)
- Certain endocrine or metabolic disorders

COMMON CAUSES

- Vitamin A excess
- Anabolic steroids
- Obesity
- Oral contraception

SIGNS AND SYMPTOMS

- Symptoms in BIH are non-specific and are those of increased intracranial pressure.
- Headaches, nausea/vomiting, and visual disturbances are the most common presenting symptoms[248]. Other Symptoms of increased ICP may include the following:
  - Diplopia (typically horizontal due to nonlocalizing sixth nerve palsy but rarely vertical)
  - Pulsatile tinnitus
  - Radicular pain (typically in the arms, uncommon)
- Rarely, patients presenting with increased ICP with related optic nerve edema may be asymptomatic.
- Visual symptoms of papilledema may include the following:
  - Transient visual obscurations, often predominantly or uniformly orthostatic
  - Progressive loss of peripheral vision in one or both eyes (nerve fiber layer defects, enlargement of the blind spot)
  - Sudden visual loss (eg, fulminant IIH)
  - Blurring and distortion (i.e., metamorphopsia) of central vision due to macular edema or optic neuropathy
- Nonspecific symptoms of IIH may include dizziness, nausea, vomiting, photopsias, and retrobulbar pain.
- The most significant physical finding is **bilateral disc edema secondary to the increased ICP**. Rarely, in more pronounced cases, macular involvement with subsequent edema and diminished central vision may be present.
- By definition, the neurological examination is normal apart from papilloedema or a sixth nerve palsy. **Sixth nerve palsy** is the most common neurological abnormality reported in 9-48% of children with BIH[249].

DIAGNOSIS

- FBC, U&Es, Bicarbonate, Coagulation profile
- Combined **MRI/MRV of the brain with gadolinium is the preferred study.**
- **CT Scan of the Brain** to rule out an intracranial lesion can be performed if a MRI is not immediately available.
- **Lumbar Puncture.**

DIAGNOSTIC CRITERIA

Dandy criteria:

- Increased opening csf pressure
- Focal CN V1 pathology
- Normal CSF
- Normal to small slit ventricles on Ct Scan

MANAGEMENT

The goal is to preserve optic nerve function while managing increased ICP. Pharmacologic therapy may include:

- **Acetazolamide** (the most effective agent for lowering ICP) and furosemide or, rarely, other diuretics
- **Primary headache prophylaxis** (eg, amitriptyline, propranolol, other commonly prescribed migraine prophylaxis agents, or topiramate)
- **Corticosteroids** (for lowering ICP in IIH of inflammatory etiology or for supplementing acetazolamide)
- If visual function deteriorates while on maximal medical therapy, surgical interventions should be strongly considered.

COMPLICATIONS

The only severe and permanent complication of IIH is **progressive blindness** from postpapilledema optic atrophy.

---

[248] Babikan P, Corbett J, Bell W (1994) Idiopathic intracranial hypertension in children: the Iowa experience. J Child Neurol **9**:144–149.

[249] Babikan P, Corbett J, Bell W (1994) Idiopathic intracranial hypertension in children: the Iowa experience. J Child Neurol **9**:144–149.

21. Haematemesis & Melaena
I. UPPER GASTROINTESTINAL HAEMORRHAGE

INTRODUCTION

- Patients with acute upper gastrointestinal (GI) bleeding commonly present with hematemesis (vomiting of blood or coffee-ground-like material) and/or melena (black, tarry stools).
- The initial evaluation of patients with acute upper GI bleeding involves an assessment of hemodynamic stability and resuscitation if necessary.
- Diagnostic studies (usually endoscopy) follow, with the goal of both diagnosis, and when possible, treatment of the specific disorder.

CLINICAL ASSESSMENT
HISTORY

- Patients should be asked about symptoms as part of the assessment of the severity of the bleed and as a part of the evaluation for potential bleeding sources.
- Symptoms that suggest the bleeding is severe include orthostatic dizziness, confusion, angina, severe palpitations, and cold/clammy extremities.
- Specific causes of upper GI bleeding may be suggested by the patient's symptoms[250]:
  - **Peptic ulcer:** Upper abdominal pain
  - **Esophageal ulcer:** Odynophagia, gastroesophageal reflux, dysphagia
  - **Mallory-Weiss tear:** Emesis, retching, or coughing prior to hematemesis
  - **Variceal hemorrhage or portal hypertensive gastropathy:** Jaundice, abdominal distention (ascites)
  - **Malignancy:** Dysphagia, early satiety, involuntary weight loss, cachexia

PHYSICAL EXAMINATION

- The physical examination is a key component of the assessment of hemodynamic stability.
- Signs of hypovolemia include[251]:
  - Mild to moderate hypovolemia (less than 15 percent of blood volume lost): Resting tachycardia.
  - Blood volume loss of at least 15 percent: Orthostatic hypotension (a decrease in the systolic blood pressure of more than 20 mmHg and/or an increase in heart rate of 20 beats per minute when moving from recumbency to standing).
  - Blood volume loss of at least 40 percent: Supine hypotension.
- **Examination of the stool color** may provide a clue to the location of the bleeding, but it is not a reliable indicator.
- In a series of 80 patients with severe hematochezia (red or maroon blood in the stool), 74 percent had a colonic lesion, 11 percent had an upper GI lesion, 9 percent had a presumed small bowel source, and no site was identified in 6 percent[252].
- **Nasogastric lavage** may be carried out if there is doubt as to whether a bleed originates from the upper GI tract.

If there is any evidence of haemodynamic instability then involve senior ED physician.

- High concentration oxygen delivered via a variable deliver mask with reservoir bag
- Two large bores peripheral intravenous cannulae
- Bloods (see investigations)
- Intravenous fluids crystalloid (colloids if known liver disease) administer 1-2 litres immediately and reassess
- If not improving administer red cells (O-neg if necessary)
- Gastric tube and aspirate stomach widely used in US not in UK.
- Urinary catheter and measure urine volumes
- Urgent referral to senior GI specialist and Critical Care.

---

[250] Cappell MS, Friedel D. Initial management of acute upper gastrointestinal bleeding: from initial evaluation up to gastrointestinal endoscopy. Med Clin North Am 2008; 92:491.

[251] Cappell MS, Friedel D. Initial management of acute upper gastrointestinal bleeding: from initial evaluation up to gastrointestinal endoscopy. Med Clin North Am 2008; 92:491.

[252] Jensen DM, Machicado GA. Diagnosis and treatment of severe hematochezia. The role of urgent colonoscopy after purge. Gastroenterology 1988; 95:1569.

1. VARICEAL BLEEDS

- Variceal bleeding is a gastrointestinal emergency that is one of the major causes of death in patients with cirrhosis. The outcome for patients with variceal bleeding depends on achieving hemostasis and avoiding complications related to bleeding or underlying chronic liver disease.
- A variceal bleed is suggested by evidence of decompensated liver disease such as **jaundice, ascites or encephalopathy**.
- A rise in portal pressure (portal hypertension) occurs when there is resistance to outflow from the portal vein. Varices develop in order to decompress the hypertensive portal vein and return blood to the systemic circulation.
- The formation and progression of varices are discussed separately.
- All patients should be referred for urgent endoscopy and admitted to a critical care area.

RISK ASSESSMENT TOOL
A. ROCKALL SCORE

- The most widely used system is the Rockall score which was developed from an audit of patients presenting with acute gastrointestinal bleeding to several English regions.
- This score is based upon age, the presence of shock, medical co-morbidity and a range of endoscopic findings.
- The Rockall score was developed to define the risk of death, but has also been use for other end-points including re-bleeding and duration of admission[253].
- The score consists of three clinical parameters (**age**, presence of **shock** and **co-morbidity**) and two parameters that rely on endoscopic findings (**blood** and **diagnosis**). The maximum **pre-endoscopy Rockall score is 7** and **post-endoscopy 11.**
- A Rockall score of 3 before endoscopy approximates with a 10% mortality rate and a score of 6 a 50% mortality rate.
- The main disadvantage of the Rockall score is that it requires findings at endoscopy to calculate all the components of the score. However, the modified pre-endoscopy score is widely used in the UK.

Variable	0	1	2	3
Age	<60	60-79	>80	
Shock	none BP>100 P<100	tachycardia BP>100 P>100	hypotension BP<100	
Co-morbidity	None		Cardiac failure or IHD	Renal failure, liver failure or disseminated malignancy
Endoscopy	No blood or dark spot only		Blood in upper GI tract, adherent clot or spurting vessel	
Diagnosis	Mallory-Weiss tear	All other diagnoses	GI tract malignancy	

ROCKALL SCORE ASSOCIATED MORTALITY

Score	Mortality %
0	0.2
1	2.4
2	5.6
3	11
4	24.6
5	39.6
6	48.9
7	50

B. BLATCHFORD SCORE

- The Blatchford score was developed from an audit of patients presenting with acute upper gastrointestinal bleeding in the west of Scotland[253]
- It aspires to define the need for intervention (particularly urgent endoscopy) and is based upon simple clinical observations, haemoglobin and blood urea concentrations and, whilst it is a little more cumbersome to use than the Rockall score, it has the advantage that it can be calculated at an early stage after hospital admission, and does not require the results of endoscopy.

- ❖ *Both the Blatchford and Rockall scores are useful tools in identifying high risk upper GI bleeds.*
- ❖ *Rockall scores are more widely used in the UK.*

---

253 *National Clinical Guideline Centre (UK). Acute Upper Gastrointestinal Bleeding: Management. London: Royal College of Physicians (UK); 2012 Jun. (NICE Clinical Guidelines, No. 141.) 5, Risk Assessment (risk scoring)* [*Available Online*]

Risk marker	Score
Blood urea (mmol/L)	2
>6.5 <8.0	3
>8.0 <10.0	4
>10.0 <25.0	6
>25.0	
Haemoglobin (g/L) for men	1
>120 <130	3
>100 <120	6
<100	
Haemoglobin (g/L) for women	1
>100 <120	6
<100	
Systolic blood pressure (mmHg)	1
100-109	2
90-99	3
<90	
Other markers	1
Pulse >100	1
Melaena	2
Syncope	2
Hepatic disease	2
Cardiac failure	

RISK IS CATEGORISED IN THE FOLLOWING WAY:

- **Very low risk:** no objective evidence of GI bleed consider discharge
- **Low risk:** admit to MAU or observation unit for next day or out-patient endoscopy
- **Moderate risk:** admit to appropriate inpatient specialty (local protocols) for urgent endoscopy
- **High risk:** (Rockall Score (pre-endoscopy) =>3): haemodynamic instability, known varices resuscitate, admit to critical care area for emergency endoscopy.

INVESTIGATIONS

Upper GI haemorrhage is largely a clinical diagnosis is largely based on the patient's history.

- ECG,
- ABG,
- FBC, U&ES, LFT
- Coagulation screen
- Cross Match RBC
- PR and FOB
- CXR

MEDICAL THERAPY

- The 2008 Scottish Intercollegiate Guidelines Network (SIGN) guideline on the management of acute upper and lower GI bleeding recommends that an initial (pre-endoscopic) Rockall score be calculated for all patients presenting with an acute UGIB[254].
- In patients with an initial Rockall score >0, endoscopy is recommended for a full assessment of bleeding risk.

1. MANAGEMENT OF NON-VARICEAL BLEEDS

PPI

- The relative efficacy of proton-pump inhibitors (PPIs) may be due to their superior ability to maintain a gastric pH at a level above 6.0, thereby protecting an ulcer clot from fibrinolysis[255].
- Current guidelines recommend a regimen of an intravenous (IV) PPI 40-mg are widely used.
- *There is little evidence to support the administration of IV PPIs pre-endoscopy although it is reasonable to give them to patients who are medium or high risk after risk assessment*
- Theoretically, they reduce bleeding by increasing the pH of the acid environment leading to clot stability.
- They have been shown post-endoscopy to reduce the re-bleeding rate and need for surgery but have no effect on overall mortality.
- A pragmatic approach is to give high dose PPIs to high risk patients with upper GI bleeds, particularly when a delay to endoscopy is envisaged.
- Patients without haemodynamic instability or vomiting can be given high dose oral PPIs.

SOMATOSTATINS

- Occasionally in severe acute non-variceal upper GI haemorrhage, Infusions such as **Octreotide infusions** can be used occasionally.
- Preferably if a delay to endoscopy is likely.

ANTIFIBRINOLYTIC THERAPY

- There is little evidence to support the administration of **Tranexamic Acid** to patients with upper GI haemorrhage.

---

[254] *Scottish Intercollegiate Guidelines Network (SIGN). Management of acute upper and lower gastrointestinal bleeding. A national clinical guideline. Edinburgh (Scotland): Scottish Intercollegiate Guidelines Network (SIGN); 2008 Sep. (SIGN publication; no. 105):*

[255] *Lau JY, Leung WK, Wu JC, et al. Omeprazole before endoscopy in patients with gastrointestinal bleeding. N Engl J Med. 2007 Apr 19. 356(16):1631-40.*

2. MANAGEMENT OF VARICEAL BLEEDS
SOMATOSTATINS AND VASOPRESSINS

- The use of intravenous vasopressors such as terlipressin, **somatostatin and octreotide** for acute variceal haemorrhage have been shown, in a meta-analysis of 30 RCTs, to reduce 7-day all-cause mortality and give lower transfusion requirement[256].
- **Terlipressin** is a synthetic analogue of vasopressin and it causes systemic vasoconstriction and reduces portal blood flow, portal-systemic collateral blood flow and hence variceal pressure.
- **Somatostatins** cause a relaxation of vascular smooth muscle and reduce portal venous pressure.
- In a meta-analysis of seven RCTs, terlipressin was shown to improve survival (RR = 0.66, 95%CI 0.49-0.88) and reduce the failure to control bleeding (RR = 0.66, 95%CI 0.55-0.93)[257].
- It is therefore current practice that, as soon as a variceal bleed is suspected, a vasoactive drug be commenced. In the UK, we use **terlipressin 2 mg qds for 24–72 hours** or until satisfactory haemostasis has been achieved.
- In fact, once haemostasis has been achieved with endoscopic band ligation, 24 hours of terlipressin is as effective as 72 hours[258].

ANTIBIOTICS

- The current guidelines recommend routine antibiotics in all cases of acute variceal haemorrhage regardless of Child-Pugh class and regardless of whether there is a confirmed infection or suspected focus of infection.
- In patients with known liver disease and upper GI haemorrhage intravenous broad-spectrum antibiotics, such as **Ceftriaxone**, have been shown to reduce mortality by 27% and the incidence of infection by 60%.

VITAMIN K

- There is no evidence of efficacy for the administration of Vitamin K in patients with liver disease who have an upper GI haemorrhage.

NON-MEDICAL THERAPY
ENDOSCOPY

- An upper GI endoscopy should be performed as soon as possible after the patient has been stabilized and adequately resuscitated..
- It can be helpful to give a prokinetic about an hour before the endoscopy (e.g. metoclopramide or erythromycin) in order to help clear the stomach of blood and clots, as long as there are no contraindications such as QT prolongation[259].
- **Mallory Weiss tears** normally stop without endoscopic intervention.
- Stable patients can be admitted to a medical ward or observation unit for next-day endoscopy.

BALLOON TAMPONADE

- Balloon tamponade using, for example, a **Sengstaken-Blakemore Tube** (SBT) in patients with massive variceal haemorrhage or refractory bleeding can be a very effective holding measure or bridge to more definitive therapy.
- A SBT should only be left in place for a maximum of 24-48 hours.
- It can stem the acute bleed in about 90% of patients; however, 50% re-bleed when the gastric balloon is deflated[260].
- In addition, it is associated with severe complications such as ulceration, and oesophageal and tracheal rupture.
- An RSI should be performed and the patient should be intubated to prevent aspiration.
- In general, try not to keep in for more than 24 hours and deflate the balloon for a short time every 6 hours.

COMPLICATIONS

- Oesophageal necrosis and perforation from inflation of oesophageal balloon
- Aspiration if airway not secured first
- Mucosal ulceration from pressure
- Proximal migration of tube causing airway obstruction

[256] Wells M,Chande N, Adams P et al. Meta-analysis: vasoactive medications for the management of acute variceal bleeds. Aliment Pharmacol Ther 2012; 35:1267–78.

[257] Ioannou G, Doust J, Rockey DC. Terlipressin for acute esophageal variceal hemorrhage. Cochrane Database Syst Rev 2003; 1:CD002147.

[258] Azam Z, Hamid S, Jafri W et al. Short course adjuvant terlipressin in acute variceal bleeding: a randomized double blind dummy controlled trial. J Hepatol 2012; 56:819–24.

[259] de Francis R, Baveno VI faculty. Expanding consensus in portal hypertension: report of the Baveno VI consensus workshop: Stratifying risk and individualising care for portal hypertension. J Hepatol 2015; 63:743–52.

[260] Teres J, Cecilia A, Bordas JM et al. Esophageal tamponade for bleeding varices: controlled trial between the Sengstaken-Blakemore tube and the Linton-Nachlas tube. Gastroenterology 1978; 75:566–9.

22. Jaundice

INTRODUCTION

- Jaundice (icterus) is the result of accumulation of bilirubin in the bloodstream and subsequent deposition in the skin, sclera, and mucous membranes.
- The normal range for total bilirubin is 3.4 to 20.0 micromol/L (0.2 to 1.2 mg/dL).
- Jaundice may not be clinically evident until serum levels >51 micromol/L (3 mg/dL).
- With a focused history and physical examination, an accurate diagnosis is possible in approximately 85% of patients[261].

PATHOPHYSIOLOGY[262]

Unconjugated (indirect) hyperbilirubinemia:

- Unconjugated bilirubin is the direct breakdown product of heme, is water insoluble, and is measured as indirect bilirubin:
  - **Hemolytic:**
    - Excessive production of unconjugated bilirubinE
    - Anything that causes increased rate of red cell breakdown (haemolysis) will lead to jaundice due to increased haem metabolism and saturation of enzymes.
      - Malaria
      - Sickle cell anaemia
      - Spherocytosis, G6PD deficiency
  - **Hepatic:**
    - Decreased hepatobiliary excretion of bilirubin by:
      - Defective uptake (drugs, Crigler–Najjar syndrome)
      - Defective conjugation (Gilbert syndrome drugs)
      - Defective excretion of bilirubin by the liver cell (drugs, Dubin–Johnson syndrome)

Conjugated (direct) hyperbilirubinemia:

- Conjugated bilirubin is water soluble and measured as direct bilirubin.
- In conjugated hyperbilirubinemia, bilirubin is returned to the bloodstream after conjugation in the liver instead of draining into the bile ducts[262].

- **Hepatocellular dysfunction:**
  - Hepatitis
  - Cirrhosis
  - Tumor invasion
  - Toxic injury
- **Intrahepatic (nonobstructive) cholestasis**
- **Extra(Post)hepatic (obstructive) cholestasis**
  - Obstructive causes are due to inability to excrete bile
  - Conjugated bilirubin is excreted into biliary and cystic ducts as part of bile. In the small intestine, it is converted by enzymes to urobilinogen.
  - Urobilinogen can be further converted to stercobilinogen and passes out with faeces or reabsorbed by intestinal cells and transported in blood to the kidneys where it is oxidised to urobilin and passed out with urine.
  - **Stercobilin and urobilin** are responsible for colouration of faeces and urine respectively.
  - **Post-hepatic causes of jaundice include**
    - Choledocholithiasis (common bile duct gallstones)
    - Pancreatic cancer of the pancreatic head
    - Biliary tract strictures
    - Biliary atresia
    - Primary biliary cholangitis
    - Cholestasis of pregnancy
    - Acute Pancreatitis
    - Chronic Pancreatitis
    - Pancreatic pseudocysts
    - Mirizzi's syndrome
    - Parasites ("liver flukes" of Opisthorchiidae and Fasciolidae)

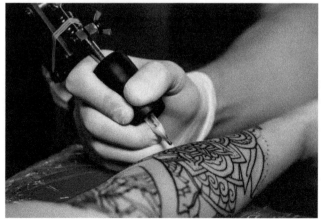

Image source CNBC

---

[261] Greenberger NJ. History taking and physical examination for the patient with liver disease. In: Schiff ER, Sorrell MF, Maddrey WC, eds. Schiff's diseases of the liver. 9th ed. Philadelphia, PA: Lippincott, Williams & Wilkins; 2003:3-5.

[262] 5-Minute Emergency Consult, jaundice [Online]

RISK FACTORS

- Alcohol use disorder
- Using illicit drugs
- Hepatotoxic medications
- Exposure to hepatitis A , hepatitis B , or hepatitis C
- Exposure to certain industrial chemicals
- Transfusion of blood products
- Foreign Travel history
- Tattoos or body piercing
- Needle stick injury

CLINICAL ASSESSMENT

- The history should focus on questioning about:
  - **Colour of urine and stool**,
  - **Weight loss**
  - **Family history of jaundice**

History

- Life-threatening conditions with jaundice include cholangitis, hemolysis (massive), hepatic failure, acute fatty liver of pregnancy, acetaminophen overdose[263].
- Accurate history and exam are essential components of patient evaluation, as history and exam display an 86% sensitivity for determining intrahepatic versus extrahepatic disease.
- Patients may complain of nausea/vomiting, malaise, pruritis, weight changes, edema, and/or ascites.
- Ask about pain, fever, prior surgeries, time of onset, medications, herbal medications, alcohol/drug use, HIV history, travel, work, and family history.

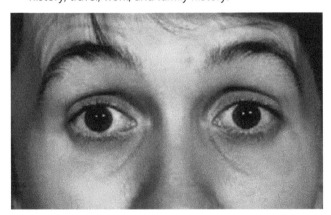

Exam

- Exam must include vital signs (fever/hypotension – cholangitis), mental status, neurologic exam, presence of asterixis, lungs (crackles, pleural effusions), CV (evidence of heart failure), presence of ascites, abdominal tenderness (Murphy's sign), hepatosplenomegaly, and skin.

---

[263] Brit Long, jaundice in Adults [emDOCS Online]

LABORATORY ASSESSMENT

- Obtain direct and indirect bilirubin.
  - Unconjugated bilirubin is reported as indirect bilirubin, and conjugated as direct bilirubin.
  - These are not exactly equivalent, as indirect bilirubin underestimates the actual unconjugated form, while direct bilirubin tends to overestimate the conjugated form[263].
- Other labs include FBC, LFT, ALP, albumin, GGT, coagulation panel, acetaminophen, lipase, albumin, and urinalysis.
  - Elevation of ALP and GGT together suggest hepatobiliary disease.
  - Elevation of liver function enzymes relative to ALP and GGT suggest intrahepatic etiology. Elevation of ALP and bilirubin relative to liver function suggest intrahepatic or extrahepatic disease.
- FBC is warranted to assess for abnormal WBC, Hgb/Hct, thrombocytopenia, and reticulocyte index.
- The liver is responsible for production of clotting factors, and PT/INR will elevate with significant hepatic dysfunction.
- Albumin serves as a marker of liver synthetic function.
- Lactate is warranted in toxic appearing patients; however, lactate is cleared through the liver.
- Acetaminophen level is warranted to assess for overdose.
- If hemolysis is a concern, obtain LDH, haptoglobin, peripheral smear, Coombs test.
- Hepatitis panel may be needed based on history and exam (Hep A/B/C, CMV, EBV, HSV, VZV).

IMAGING

- **US:** Warranted to assess gallbladder and biliary system.
  - Evaluate common bile duct (CBD), as > 5 mm in patients < 50 years suggests obstruction..
- **CT:** Sensitivity 80% and specificity 99% for CBD stones.
  - CT allows for evaluation of other abdominal organs, as well for the presence of a mass and staging of any tumors. CT can evaluate liver parenchyma, vasculature, and mass.
- **HIDA:** Useful in detection of cholelithiasis or cholecystitis if US is negative but clinical concern is present. However, it cannot diagnose complications of cholecystitis or evaluate for hepatic dysfunction.
- **ERCP:** Can visualizes the biliary tree and pancreatic ducts. Superior to CT & US for extrahepatic dysfunction and provides therapeutic options during the procedure.
- **MRCP:** Most sensitive noninvasive method for detecting biliary stones. Can be an alternative to ERCP in certain conditions (ductal tumor, periductal compression, choledocholithiasis).

MANAGEMENT
Dependent on underlying condition[263]

- Resuscitate if patient is critically ill with IV fluids and antibiotics.
- Fluid resuscitate if in shock or hypotensive.
- Provide antiemetics and analgesics.

HEMOLYSIS
- Transfusion for those with low Hbg/Hct and symptoms due to anemia. HUS/TTP = plasma exchange and corticosteroids.

EXTRAHEPATIC OBSTRUCTION
- If cholangitis is present, provide antibiotics and consult gastroenterology team.
- For other conditions such as gallstone/stricture, Refer Surgery.
- For those with malignant mass, discuss with GI and surgery.

HEPATOCELLULAR INJURY
- Encephalopathy: Grade encephalopathy and treat based on this grade (lactulose, rifaximin)
- Coagulopathy: FFP for active bleeding. If not bleeding, no FFP is required. PCC should be considered for severe bleeding. Platelets may be needed for those with levels < 20,000/mm^3.
- Antibiotics: Provide broad-spectrum antibiotics if toxic.
- Fluid resuscitate if in shock or hypotensive.

PARACETAMOL OVERDOSE
- Use Matthew-Rumack nomogram.
- If over toxic level/line, provide NAC (oral or IV).
- May require charcoal (< 1-2 hours from ingestion) and/or dialysis.

CHOLANGITIS
- It is a serious and often life-threatening infection of the biliary tree[263].
- It is typically caused by ascending infection from the gastrointestinal tract into the biliary tree in the setting of biliary stasis, such as in the case of an obstruction from a gallstone, stricture, or mass.
- More rarely, cholangitis can be seen in patients without an obstruction who develop biliary stasis secondary to total parenteral nutrition.
- Organisms commonly implicated in cholangitis include *E. coli* and **enterococcus and bacteroides species**. **Charcot's triad** of **fever, jaundice,** and **right upper quadrant abdominal pain** is classically seen with cholangitis.

- In more severe disease, **Reynolds' pentad** may be seen, with the **addition of altered mental status and shock** to the triad of symptoms named above.
- ED management of cholangitis includes prompt initiation of antibiotics and hemodynamic stabilization through fluid and vasopressor administration, as necessary.
- Surgical and gastrointestinal consultation are also important as emergent biliary decompression through ERCP or cholecystostomy placement may be necessary.

PREGNANCY
- Jaundice can occur due to the previously mentioned conditions and several others such as hyperemesis gravidarum, intrahepatic cholestasis[263] of pregnancy (3rd trimester, pruritis, cholestatic lab findings), infection (Hep E, HSV), acute fatty liver of pregnancy (3rd trimester, microvesicular fat in hepatocytes, N/V, RUQ pain, presents similar to HELLP).

POST LIVER TRANSPLANT
- Discuss with transplant physician. Jaundice can be due to mechanical obstruction, infection, graft malfunction, rejection, drug toxicity, hepatic artery thrombosis.

23. Joint Swelling-Atraumatic

I. GOUT & PSEUDOGOUT

- Gout and pseudogout are the 2 most common crystal-induced arthropathies. Gout is caused by monosodium urate monohydrate crystals; pseudogout is caused by calcium pyrophosphate crystals and is more accurately termed calcium pyrophosphate disease.
- Crystal deposition can be asymptomatic, but gout and calcium pyrophosphate disease (CPPD) can develop into debilitating illnesses marked by recurrent episodes of pain and joint inflammation that result from the formation of crystals within the joint space and deposition of crystals in soft tissue[264].
- The age range is usually 40-70 years and risk factors include **excess alcohol consumption, male sex, obesity, renal impairment and drugs** (low-dose aspirin and diuretics).

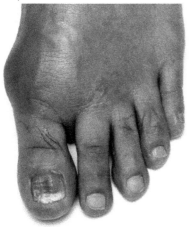

- **A raised serum urate level** is neither specific nor sensitive enough to assist in the diagnosis, since it is often normal in acute episodes of gout.
- Other blood tests (FBC and CRP) that are often performed in the ED in attempts to differentiate the causes of acute monoarthropathy are equally lacking in sensitivity and specificity.
- *The diagnosis of crystal arthropathy is confirmed by the presence of birefringent crystals viewed on polarized light microscopy.*
- **Treatment options** in the acute phase include intra-articular steroid injection, non-steroidal anti-inflammatory drugs (NSAIDs) or colchicine.

II. REACTIVE ARTHRITIS

- Reactive arthritis (ReA), formerly termed Reiter syndrome, is an autoimmune condition that develops in response to an infection[265].
- It has been associated with gastrointestinal (GI) infections with Shigella, Salmonella, Campylobacter, and other organisms, as well as with genitourinary (GU) infections (especially with Chlamydia trachomatis).
- This usually develops 2-4 weeks after a genitourinary (Chlamydia) or gastrointestinal (Shigella, Salmonella or Campylobacter) infection, although approximately 10% of cases do not have a preceding symptomatic infection.
- Only a minority of patients will have the classical triad (conjunctivitis, urethritis and arthritis) described by Reiter. The age range is typically 2-40 years.
- Onset is usually acute and can resemble septic arthritis, but will often affect more than one joint. Elevated white cell count (WCC) and CRP are common, and joint aspiration will be needed to exclude septic arthritis.
- The disease is self-limiting in 3-12 months, but will require management with NSAIDs or steroids (either systemic or intra-articular).

III. SEPTIC ARTHRITIS

- Septic arthritis, also known as infectious arthritis, may represent a direct invasion of joint space by various microorganisms, most commonly caused by bacteria. However, viruses, mycobacteria, and fungi have been implicated.
- Reactive arthritis is a sterile inflammatory process that may result from an extra-articular infectious process.

1. RISK FACTORS INCLUDE:
- ○ *Immunosuppression*
- ○ *Extremes of age*
- ○ *Diabetes*
- ○ *Chronic arthritides (especially rheumatoid arthritis)*
- ○ *Previous surgery (especially prosthetic joints)*
- ○ *Intravenous drug abuse.*

2. ETIOLOGY AND PATHOPHYSIOLOGY
- ○ **Organisms may invade the joint by:**
  - ▪ Direct inoculation,
  - ▪ Contiguous spread from infected periarticular tissue,

264 Currie WJ. The gout patient in general practice. Rheumatol Rehabil. 1978 Nov. 17(4):205-17.

265 Schmitt SK. Reactive Arthritis. Infect Dis Clin North Am. 2017 Mar 11.

- Via the bloodstream (Haematogenous is the most common route).
  o Septic arthritis is caused by invasion of bacteria, viruses or fungi into the synovial membrane of a joint:
    - **Staphylococcus aureus:** is the most common cause in adults. Has specific affinity of synovial structures.
    - **Streptococci:** the second most cause
    - **Haemophilus influenza**: was the most common in children but is now uncommon in areas where Hib vaccination is practiced.
    - **Neisseria gonorrhoea:** in young adults, multiples macules or vesicles seen over the trunk are pathognomonic features.
    - **Escherichia coli:** in elderly, IV Drug users and seriously ill.
    - **M. tuberculosis:** occurs most commonly by direct inoculation, penetrating wound, or direct extension. The most common mechanism of infection is via haematogenous.

3. CLINICAL FEATURES OF SEPTIC ARTHRITIS

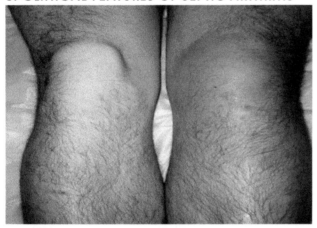

  o A painful, hot, swollen, red joint is the classic presentation. Usually only one joint is affected.
  o Only very limited movement of the joint is possible and it is usually held slightly flexed.
  o The patient may be systemically unwell with fever and rigors. The use of analgesics, steroids, or antibiotics may obscure some of the clinical features. The commonest joint affected is the **knee (50%),** followed by the **hip (20%), shoulder (8%), ankle (7%),** and **wrist (7%).**
  o Detection of septic arthritis in the hip can be very difficult owing to the lack of obvious external findings due to its deep location.
  o *Patients who are intravenous drug-users may have involvement of atypical joints, e.g. vertebral, sacroiliac, or sternoclavicular joints.*

4. INVESTIGATIONS FOR SEPTIC ARTHRITIS
  o **Joint aspiration** and **synovial fluid analysis:** (most important diagnostic test): Fluid should be sent **for gram stain**, **cultures**, **crystal examination**, and **cell count**.
  o **FBC, ESR, and CRP: negative results** do not rule the disease out.
  o **Blood cultures**: useful in identifying the organism but do not help confirm or exclude the diagnosis in the ED.
  o **X-ray**: used as useful baseline, can be initially normal.
  o **Lateral X-rays** may show bone destruction.

5. ED MANAGEMENT OF SEPTIC ARTHRITIS
  o IV Antibiotics: **Flucloxacillin and benzylpenicillin.**
  o **Analgesia**: consider splintage in addition to pharmacological treatment.
  o **Urgent orthopaedic referral**: for joint irrigation/drainage.

IV. GONOCOCCAL ARTHRITIS

- Bacterial septic arthritis is commonly described as either gonococcal or nongonococcal[266]. Neisseria gonorrhoeae remains the most common pathogen (75% of cases) among younger sexually active individuals.
- *Staphylococcus aureus* infection is the cause of the vast majority of cases of acute bacterial arthritis in adults and in children older than 2 years. The increased incidence of this pathogen parallels the increase in presence of prosthetic joints and in the use of immunosuppressive agents. This pathogen is the cause in 80% of infected joints affected by rheumatoid arthritis.
- *Gonococcus* may cause two types of arthritis:
  o *A localized septic arthritis affecting one joint.*
  o *An arthritis-dermatitis syndrome (classic triad is dermatitis, tenosynovitis, and migratory polyarthritis).*

MANAGEMENT OF GONOCOCCAL ARTHRITIS
- It should be managed as any other septic arthritis, with joint irrigation and antibiotics. *Investigations are the same as above but should also include **swabs of the urethra, cervix, throat, and rectum** to help identify the causative agent.*
- Treatment is with broad-spectrum antibiotics until the causative agent is identified. **Cephalosporins** are appropriate once gonococcus is confirmed.
- Open drainage of affected joints is rarely required. Patients should be advised that they and **their partner(s) require** a full sexual health screen.

---

266 *Del Pozo JL, Patel R. Clinical practice. Infection associated with prosthetic joints. N Engl J Med. 2009 Aug 20. 361(8):787-94.*

V. BURSITIS

OVERVIEW

- Bursitis is an inflammation or irritation of the bursae.
- Bursitis can be rapid in onset (acute) or build up slowly over time (chronic).
  - Acute bursitis is often the result of an injury, infection, or inflammatory condition.
  - Chronic bursitis often follows a long period of repetitive use, motion, or compression.
- The olecranon and prepatellar bursae are the most common sites of septic bursitis
- Ultrasound may be helpful but is not diagnostic
- Bursal aspiration is within the scope of practice of emergency physicians and is the most helpful diagnostic tool
- Bursal steroid injection is contraindicated in septic bursitis.

BURSITIS CAUSES

- Injury, such as from a fall or hit; this usually causes bleeding into a bursa. People who take anticoagulant medications (blood thinners) to prevent or treat blood clots are at higher risk for this condition.
- Infection resulting from bacteria entering the body through a cut or scrape in the skin.
- Gout or other crystal diseases.
- Certain types of arthritis, like rheumatoid arthritis or psoriatic arthritis.
- Prolonged pressure, which can result from kneeling, sitting, or leaning on a particular joint for a long period.
- Strain or overuse from repeating the same motion many times
- Joint stress from an abnormal gait; for example, walking unevenly because one leg is shorter than the other

BURSITIS SYMPTOMS

- Pain and/or swelling at the affected site.
- Swelling is less commonly a feature of bursitis that affects deep structures, such as the bursae of the shoulders, hips, and inner knees.
- In acute bursitis, there are often features of inflammation at the bursa. Acute bursitis of a superficial bursa is often accompanied by redness, warmth, and swelling.
- Septic Bursitis:
  - Bursitis caused by an infection is called **"septic bursitis."**
  - Symptoms may include pain, swelling, warmth, and redness around the affected joint. Fever may also be present. This is a potentially serious condition since infection can spread to nearby joints, bone, or the blood.

- Bursitis caused by gout is not infection-related but can mimic septic bursitis in the intensity of inflammation

BURSITIS DIAGNOSIS

- Diagnosing bursitis involves a physical examination, a review of your symptoms, and sometimes tests.
- The diagnostic gold standard for septic bursitis is bursal fluid culture. Negative bursal fluid culture does not exclude the diagnosis of septic bursitis, especially if due to a fastidious organism or when antibiotics precede culture
- A number of other signs are associated with septic bursitis and can be used to support the diagnostic.
- Bursal fluid aspiration should be performed prior to antibiotic use
- X-ray, MRI, or ultrasound are not usually needed to diagnose bursitis. However, it can help in some situations, such as when other problems need to be ruled out (for example, a tear in the cartilage or ligament).

TYPES OF BURSITIS

1. SUBACROMIAL BURSITIS

- Shoulder bursitis causes pain in the shoulder and often extends to the upper arm.
- Pain is often present at rest but increases with movement of the arm, especially with lifting the arms above the head; it also often interrupts sleep. It can be difficult to differentiate shoulder bursitis from other issues such as a rotator cuff tendinitis, rotator cuff tear, shoulder arthritis, or labral tear.

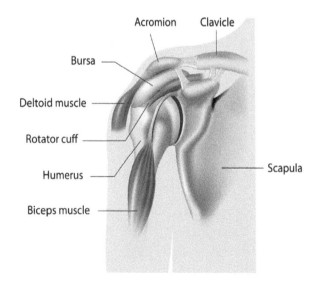

2. SCAPULOTHORACIC BURSITIS

- Upper back bursitis affects the space between the scapula and ribs and can cause pain or a popping sensation. Reaching the arms overhead or doing pushups can make pain worse.

3. OLECRANON BURSITIS

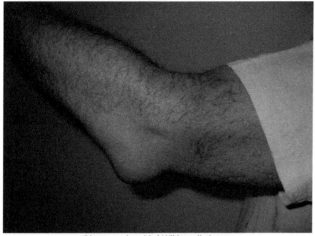

Olecranon bursitis | Wikipaedia image

- The *olecranon* bursa, which is located over the olecranon process of the elbow, is prone to bursitis, or "student's elbow," from trauma, infection, and inflammatory processes[267].
- Athletes, plumbers, carpenters, mechanics, miners, soldiers, and those with chronic disease states such as COPD (leaning on elbows to catch their breath) or requiring hemodialysis are predisposed to olecranon bursitis. Untreated olecranon bursitis can progress to osteomyelitis.
- The superficial location of the olecranon bursa allows for visualization with ultrasound. In a normal bursa this is represented by a thin, hypoechoic layer, with potential septations in the subcutaneous tissues that may be difficult to see in the absence of pathology.
- This is best visualized with the elbow in 90° of flexion with a thick layer of gel and minimal pressure. Imaging may reveal complex fluid, synovial hypertrophy, hyperemia on color Doppler flow, and possibly gas; however, none of these are diagnostic [9]. These findings, particularly gas, should trigger the strong consideration for alternative diagnoses including necrotizing fasciitis

4. GREATER TROCHANTERIC PAIN SYNDROME

- The greater trochanteric bursa is located in the upper outer part of the femur.
- Bursitis in this area is usually associated with inflammation of nearby tendons and can cause pain while lying or sleeping on the affected side of the body.
- Because the primary problem may be more an irritation of the tendons in the area, the term "greater trochanteric pain syndrome" has replaced the former term of "trochanteric bursitis."

- Patient with greater trochanteric pain syndrome also tend to have pain when extending the leg to walk, but not while standing still. Symptoms can be aggravated by an abnormal gait, due to uneven stress on the hips.
- There are many contributing factors, including chronic back pain, contralateral knee pain (knee pain on the opposite side of the body from the bursitis), different leg lengths, and being overweight.

5. ILIOPSOAS BURSITIS

- The iliopsoas bursa abuts the psoas muscle deep in the front of the hip. This type of bursitis causes pain in the groin area, particularly when the hip is flexed against resistance or when climbing stairs.
- It can result from arthritis in the area, overuse (for example, excessive running), or injury.

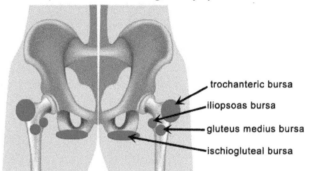

- Because symptoms are similar to those of other hip problems, imaging tests are often required to confirm the diagnosis.
- Psoas abscess can have similar symptoms, although these are usually more severe.

6. KNEE BURSITIS

- **The prepatellar bursa** is located between the patella and the superficial tissues. When inflamed, it is referred to as "housemaid's" or "carpet-layer's" knee.
- This is the most common bursa in the knee to become infected. On ultrasound, it is visualized as a fluid collection directly superficial to the patella[268].
- **The suprapatellar bursa** is located between the femur and the quadriceps tendon and communicates with the knee joint. It is often referred to as the *suprapatellar* recess. This is best visualized in the sagittal plane with the knee flexed to 30°.
- **The infrapatellar bursa** is actually two bursae located at the distal portion of the patellar tendon, near the tibial tuberosity. These are described as superficial and deep, denoting their relative location about the patellar tendon.

267 Zimmermann B 3rd, Mikolich DK, Ho G Jr. Septic bursitis. Semin Arthritis Rheum. 1995; 24:391-410.

268 Ruangchaijatuporn T, Gaetke-Udager K, Jacobson JA, Yablon CM, Morag Y. Ultrasound evaluation of bursae: anatomy and pathological appearances. Skeletal Radiol. 2017;46(4):445-462

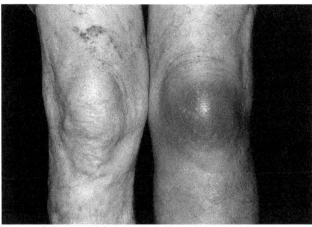

Left Knee Bursitis | science Photo library image

- Inflammation of this bursa is called "clergyman's knee." Ultrasound over the tibial tuberosity will show a focal fluid collection. These views are best obtained with minimal pressure and generous ultrasound gel[268].
- Aspiration of the patellar bursae should be performed with a 2.5-cm, 20-gauge needle and 10-mL syringe held parallel to the extremity and introduced using aseptic technique. Milking the affected bursa during aspiration may help to facilitate removal of fluid in what is often a multi-loculated space. Again, ultrasound may help to guide the needle and evaluate for adequacy of drainage[269].

BURSITIS TREATMENT

- **Pain-relief medication** : NSAIDs can help relieve pain and inflammation.
- **Steroid injections**
- **Protecting the joints** – It is important to protect the affected joints in order to rest the affected area and help the bursae to heal. Bursal protection can also prevent the bursitis from getting worse or recurring. Examples of joint protection include:
  - Avoiding or modifying activities that cause pain
  - The use of pads or cushions for people who have to kneel or sit frequently
  - Modifying footwear to reduce pressure on the back of the heel (eg, cutting a "V"-shaped groove into the back of a shoe; using a pad inside the shoe to lift the heel)
  - Custom-fitted devices worn over the elbows to protect them and prevent fluid from building up again
- **Other measures**
  - Ice , Heat (eg, a heating pad)...
  - Physical therapy

TREATING INFECTION

- All patients suspected of having septic bursitis should be treated with appropriate antibiotic therapy, whether diagnosed clinically or by laboratory findings.
- Therapy should empirically cover *S. aureus* and *Streptococcus* as these are the most common species.
- In reliable, otherwise healthy patients without concern for septic arthritis, immunocompromise, or clinical instability, a trial of outpatient oral antibiotic therapy (up to 14 days) is reasonable for uncomplicated septic bursitis.
- Repeat needle aspiration may improve both symptoms and clinical outcome.
- Follow-up is recommended to assess for improvement.
- In persistent septic bursitis that fails conservative management, surgical intervention with incision and drainage or bursectomy may be required

---

[269] *Gupta N. Treatment of bursitis, tendinitis, and trigger points. In: Roberts JR, Custalow CB, Thomsen TW, eds. Roberts and Hedges' Clinical Procedures in Emergency Medicine and Acute Care. 7th Philadelphia, PA: Elsevier; 2019.*

24. Limb Pain & Swelling
I. DEEP VEIN THROMBOSIS

INTRODUCTION

- Unilateral leg swelling with suspicion of deep venous thrombosis (DVT) is a common emergency department (ED) presentation.
- Proximal DVT (thrombus in the popliteal or femoral veins) can usually be diagnosed and treated at the initial ED encounter.
- Venous thrombosis of the deep venous system, primarily in lower versus upper extremities[270].

PATHOPHYSIOLOGY

- Clot formation in the deep veins due to fibrin production and deposition.
- Inciting mechanisms include venous stasis, venous injury, and hypercoagulability (Virchow's Triad).

ANATOMY

- Lower extremity contains superficial veins (greater and short saphenous veins) and deep veins (common femoral, deep femoral, superficial femoral, popliteal, peroneal, anterior/posterior tibial).
- Proximal DVT forms in the popliteal vein or higher.
- Distal DVT forms in the calf veins (anterior/posterior tibial and peroneal veins).
- DVTs are more common in the left versus right leg due to the left iliac artery crossing over the left iliac vein (compression).
- Upper extremity DVTs are less common but consist of thrombus in the axillary vein.

HISTORY AND EXAM

- Patients often present with nonspecific findings early including calf fullness or cramping[270].
- Symptoms later can include unilateral leg swelling (> 3 cm more than other side), edema, redness, pain for lower DVT. Upper extremity DVTs may present with arm and finger swelling.
- Exam may demonstrate unilateral leg swelling, erythema, warmth, tenderness to palpation, superficial vein dilation.
- **Homan's sign** (painful dorsiflexion of the foot) is not sensitive or specific and should not be relied upon (sensitivity 60-96%, specificity 20-72%).

DIFFERENTIAL: DIAGNOSIS

- Cellulitis,
- Vascular disease,
- Trauma, Compartment syndrome, Fracture,
- Baker's cyst, Gout,
- Necrotizing fasciitis,
- Phlegmasia cerulean dolens,
- Phlegmasia alba dolens,
- Venous gangrene.

DIAGNOSTICS
WELLS SCORE FOR DVT

- Begin with forming pretest probability[271].

CLINICAL FEATURES	POINTS
Active cancer (treatment ongoing, within 6 months, or palliative)	1
Bedridden recently >3 days or major surgery within 12 weeks	1
Calf swelling >3 cm compared to the other leg, Measured 10 cm below tibial tuberosity	1
Collateral (nonvaricose) superficial veins present	1
Entire leg swollen	1
Localized tenderness along the deep venous system	1
Pitting oedema confined to the symptomatic leg	1
Paralysis, paresis, or recent plaster immobilization of the lower extremity	1
Previously documented DVT	1
An alternative diagnosis is at least as likely as DVT	−2
Clinical probability simplified score	
DVT likely	2 points or more
DVT unlikely	1 point or less

- Wells = 0: DVT unlikely (< 5%). Can perform D dimer testing. If negative, ruled out DVT.
- Wells = 1-2: DVT moderate risk; perform D dimer or US. If either negative, ruled out DVT.
- Wells > 3: DVT high risk; perform D dimer and US. If positive D dimer but negative US, require repeat US.

---

[270] BRIT LONG, Deep vein thrombosis [emDocs Online]

[271] MdCalc, Wells' Criteria for DVT [Online]

LABORATORY TESTING

- Obtain FBC and renal function (assists with choosing anticoagulation therapy if DVT is diagnosed)[270].
- **D dimer:** Elevation suggests clot presence. However, many conditions elevate D dimer (malignancy, infection, age, surgery, inflammation, immobilization, MI, new catheter, stroke).
  - If high sensitivity D dimer is negative, can be used to rule out DVT in low to medium risk patients.
  - High risk patients require further testing if the test is negative.

VENOUS DUPLEX ULTRASOUND

- Test of choice, noninvasive, performed rapidly.
- Can use 3-point test (common and superficial femoral veins, popliteal veins) or whole leg.
- Graded compression along path of vein.
  - **Full venous compression with pressure** = no DVT present. Sensitivity and specificity approach 95%.
  - **Low pretest probability**: Negative 3-point or whole leg US rules out DVT.
  - **Moderate to High probability:** Negative whole leg US can rule out DVT. However, negative 3-point US cannot rule out DVT if negative. May add D dimer to 3-point US. If both negative, DVT is ruled out[270].

CT VENOGRAM

- Can be used in conjunction with CT pulmonary angiography for PE. However, this should not be routinely added to CT PE, as interobserver agreement is poor.

MRI

- Limited due to availability, cost, and lack of data.
- May assist in evaluation of vena cava and pelvic veins.

Isolated Distal DVT:

- Unknown significance.
- Most US examinations do not evaluate the distal system; however, the concern is that a distal DVT will extend and become a proximal DVT.
- Risk factors[270] for extension include positive D dimer, > 5 cm in length, multiple veins, close to proximal veins, no reversible provoking factor for DVT, history of DVT/PE, hospital admission, active cancer.

MANAGEMENT

- **Proximal DVT, no history of cancer or active cancer:**
  - Oral anticoagulant (NOAC – Novel oral anticoagulant) preferred over vitamin K antagonist (VKA) (Grade 2B).
  - VKA is preferred over LMWH (Grade 2C).
  - Duration of therapy is 3 months for 1st clot (Grade 1B).

- **Proximal DVT with cancer:**
  - LMWH preferred over NOAC or VKA (Grade 2C).
  - Duration 3 months for 1st clot (Grade 1B).

- **Distal, isolated DVT:**
  - Proximal propagation may occur in up to 25% of distal clots.

- **If no risk factors** for extension and absence of severe symptoms, then serial imaging over 2 weeks is preferred (Grade 2C).
  - No clear role for antiplatelet therapy, but this is reasonable.

- **Presence of risk factors** for extension or severe symptoms:
  - Anticoagulation is preferred over serial imaging (Grade 2C).
  - Same anticoagulation recommendations as for proximal DVT (Grade 1B).

- **Superficial thrombophlebitis:**
  - Clots in the saphenous vein can spread to the deep venous system[270].
  - Treat initially with NSAIDs, warm compresses, compression stockings. Repeat US in 3-5 days.
  - If clot extends or is within 5 cm of the saphenous-femoral junction, may consider anticoagulation.

- **Catheter-directed thrombolysis:**
  - Does not demonstrated benefits in most patients with proximal DVT, increased risk of bleeding. However, patients with iliofemoral DVT may benfit with decreased risk of post-thrombotic syndrome.

- **For phegmasia cerulean dolen:**
  - Consider thrombolytics/thrombectomy with vascular surgery consultation.
  - Anticoagulation with heparin/VKA is needed.

- **Recurrent DVT on anticoagulation:**
  - Consider admission for vascular surgery and hematology consultation, IVC filter, heparin for anticoagulation[270].

- **Rivaroxaban:**
  - This is one of the newer oral anticoagulants.
  - It is a direct inhibitor of factor Xa; it has the advantage over warfarin in not requiring regular monitoring of the INR and not requiring a period of bridging therapy.

- **Thrombolysis:** Thrombolysis of venous clot is an option rarely used in the UK.

- **Aspirin:** Aspirin is not recommended for treatment of DVT.

Mechanical treatments:
- Compression stockings
- Vena caval filters

Other treatment issues:
- **Early ambulation** poses no risk for clot propagation and is encouraged; it may even reduce the risk of post-thrombotic complications.
- Most patients are suitable for outpatient treatment.

COMPLICATIONS
- Pulmonary embolism: (Biggest risk) Of patients with PE, close to 40% will have concomitant DVT.
- Phlegmasia cerulean dolens, Phlegmasia alba dolens,
- Venous gangrene.
- Venous insufficiency may occur due to damage to venous valves. This ranges from varicose veins to postphlebetic syndrome (pain, swelling, ulcerations, increased infection risk).

DISPOSITION
- Most patients with DVT may be discharged home with DOAC or LMWH bridge to warfarin.
- Patients should be ambulatory, hemodynamically stable, low risk of bleeding, have no renal failure, and be able to follow up within several days.
- Consider admission for extensive clot (phlegmasia), ileofemoral DVT, high bleeding risk, significant comorbidities, unable to obtain follow up, renal disease (GFR < 30).
- Patients with negative US who are high risk require repeat US in 3-5 days.

UPPER LIMB DVT
- Upper-extremity deep vein thrombosis (UEDVT) accounts for ≈10% of cases of deep vein thrombosis. The prevalence appears to be increasing, particularly because of an increased use of indwelling central venous catheters[272].
- In the upper extremity the deep veins include the paired radial veins, paired ulnar veins, paired brachial veins, axillary vein, and subclavian vein[273].
- The most common site of UEDVT involves the axillary and subclavian veins; however, the more distal brachial vein may also be involved.

- Primary UEDVT is less common than secondary UEDVT and most typically is effort-induced, known as Paget-Schroetter syndrome (PSS)[274].
- Secondary UEDVT occurs due to thrombosis as a result of indwelling devices such as a central venous catheters (CVC), pacemaker or defibrillator leads, and tunneled central access lines.

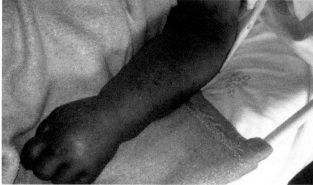

Porto Biomed J. 2016;1:124–5

Upper Limb DVT- Courtesy Elsevier

- The severity of symptoms in UEDVT parallels the degree of venous obstruction.
- Common symptoms include unilateral upper extremity pain, swelling, and arm fatigue.
- If the more proximal superior vena cava (SVC) is involved, facial plethora and chest wall edema may be noted.
- Prominent superficial collateral veins may appear on the shoulder and anterior chest wall, known as Urschel's sign. With increasing venous outflow obstruction, arterial compromise can occur leading to limb threatening phlegmasia cerulea dolens.
- The diagnosis of UEDVT is made by correlating individual history and typical clinical findings with appropriate radiographic imaging. The most commonly use imaging modality in the diagnosis of UEDVT is venous duplex ultrasonography.
- The management of UEDVT depends largely on the etiology; however, in the absence of a contraindication, the cornerstone of treatment is anticoagulation. Treatment should be aimed at obtaining early venous recanalization and attempts to restore vein patency. In primary UEDVT, prompt anticoagulation should be initiated with consideration for more advanced therapeutics including catheter directed thrombolytics (CDT).

[272] Joffe HV, Kucher N, Tapson VF, Goldhaber SZ. Upper-extremity deep vein thrombosis: a prospective registry of 592 patients. *Circulation.* 2004; 110: 1605– 1611.

[273] Ari Mintz ; Michael Shawn Levy, Upper Extremity Deep Vein Thrombosis [American College of Cardiology]

[274] Engelberger RP, Kucher N. Management of deep vein thrombosis of the upper extremity. Circulation 2012;126:768-73.

II. SUPERFICIAL VENOUS THROMBOPHLEBITIS

PREDISPOSING FACTORS[275]

- **Damage to the venous intima** (superficial trauma, drug infusion, intravenous use of illicit drugs),
- **Decreased venous flow** (varices, chronic venous insufficiency, pregnancy, prolonged immobilization),
- **Increased thrombotic tendency** (malignancy, coagulation disorder, hormonal therapy) or a combination of these.
- The condition may also appear without any clear predisposing factor. May be associated with:
  - **Vasculitis**
  - **Polyarteritis nodosa**
  - **Buerger's disease** (i.e. thromboangiitis obliterans), usually affects the small and medium-sized arteries in smokers. Approximately one third of these patients also have superficial venous thrombi. Recurring superficial venous thrombi in a young person who smokes much suggest Buerger's disease.
  - **Behcet's disease**
- Migrating superficial thrombophlebitis (short venous cord, blocked and then cured but recurs in another part) may be a sign of an underlying malignancy, particularly of pancreatic cancer.

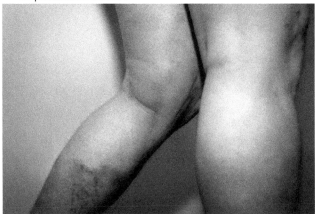

CLINICAL PICTURE

- The affected venous area is painful, reddish and swollen.
- The vein is hard and tender on palpation.
- An extensive phlebitis often is associated with fever and a mild increase of CRP concentration. A superficial venous thrombosis may spread to the deep veins.
- Deep vein thrombosis is the more likely the closer the superficial thrombophlebitis is either to the saphenofemoral junction in the groin or to the perforant veins in the popliteal area.

---

275 EBM Guidelines, Superficial venous thrombophlebitis [Online]

- The clinical picture is often benign and self-limiting.
- The inflammation and the symptoms take usually 3-4 weeks to resolve, but sometimes the condition may become prolonged.
- The thrombosed vein may be felt for months.
- Superficial venous thrombosis may recur, particularly if it was associated with varices.

DIAGNOSIS

- The diagnosis is based on clinical examination.
- The determination of the D dimer concentration is not helpful in the differentiation between superficial and deep venous thrombosis.
- **Ultrasonography** is recommended to confirm the diagnosis and to exclude deep venous thrombosis.

TREATMENT EVD

- The aim of treatment is to alleviate local symptoms as well as to prevent thrombosis from spreading into the deep veins and embolization to lungs.
- Symptoms may be alleviated with **compressive stockings,** cold compresses and by keeping the leg elevated.
- The recommended treatment for a superficial thrombophlebitis of ≥ 5 cm in length is either a mid-treatment dose of **LMWH (e.g. enoxaparin 60 mg once daily)** or with a **prophylactic dose of fondaparinux (2.5 mg once daily) for 6 weeks**.
- Similar treatment is indicated, if the thrombus is located (irrespective of its length) at a distance of less than 3 cm from the saphenofemoral junction located in the groin.
  - Some experts recommend that patients with superficial thrombophlebitis that is located close to the saphenofemoral junction should be given similar anticoagulant treatment as in deep vein thrombosis.
- **Topically applied anticoagulant cream** may alleviate the symptoms of a local venous thrombosis.
- Antimicrobial therapy is not needed and it should only be commenced if the patient clearly has another concomitant infection.
- Superficial thrombophlebitis associated with an intravenous cannula is usually not treated with systemic anticoagulants. First-line treatment consists of removal of the cannula and topical treatment and/or a NSAID if needed.
- The patient is recommended to start **moving around**
- A patient with an extensive or recurring superficial thrombophlebitis should be referred to specialist care.

III. ACUTE LIMB ISCHAEMIA

INTRODUCTION

- Acute limb ischemia (ALI) is an emergent medical condition that is characterized by a precipitous decrease in limb perfusion that threatens the viability of the affected limb, and symptoms that have been present for 14 days or less[276].
- Symptoms suggestive of this condition classically include pain in the effected limb at rest, loss of sensation, impaired motor function, and cyanosis/pallor.
- Irreparable damage can occur in as quickly as 4 to 6 hours with complete arterial occlusion.
- A majority of ALI is caused by thrombosis, with the remainder of cases caused by embolism, 85% and 15% respectively[277]. Immediate initiation of anticoagulation therapy and vascular surgery consultation are mainstays of ED management.

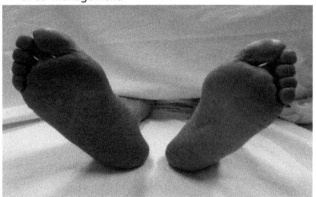

ETIOLOGY

- As stated previously, ALI is a result of either thrombotic or embolic phenomena that either partially or completely occludes a vessel such that adequate perfusion is no longer achieved.
- Consequently, there is a decrease in the metabolism of the tissue supplied in those territories, which can rapidly progress to necrosis. Thrombosis is the most common cause of ALI, accounting for approximately 85%[278].
- Typically, thrombosis presents in the setting of pre-existing peripheral artery disease (PAD).
- As PAD worsens, damage to the arterial endothelium triggers platelet activation, and accumulation in a manner conceptually similar to thrombosis in myocardial infarction.

- Hypercoagulable states increase the risk of thrombi development.
- Symptoms of thrombosis are often more insidious in onset when compared to embolism, and signs/symptoms of prior claudication are almost always present.
- Consequently, there is a greater chance that collateral circulation has developed over time[279].

3. APPROACH TO PATIENT WITH ACUTE LIMB ISCHEMIA

HISTORY

- Obtaining a detailed summary of the events leading to presentation is of critical importance, including **onset, duration, location, intensity of symptoms, any previous history of claudication or associated vascular procedures including vascular repair and arterial bypass**[280].
- Past medical history such as cardiomyopathy, congestive heart failure, renal failure, hypertension, diabetes, malignancy, hypercoagulable states, and/or tobacco use can affect overall morbidity and mortality.
- Suspect embolus when the patient can communicate exact time of onset, has a known embolic source (i.e. atrial fibrillation), no prior history of claudication and/or a normal appearance/examination of the opposite limb.

PHYSICAL EXAMINATION

- Careful examination is necessary to detect signs of ischemia.
- Initial evaluation should include[280]:
  - **External appearance/temperature of the skin**
  - **Peripheral pulses in affected and contralateral limbs**
  - **Neuromotor evaluation for sensation and muscle strength**
- The **6 Ps** (paresthesia, pain, pallor, pulselessness, poikilothermia, paralysis) comprise the classic presentation of acute occlusion in patients without underlying occlusive vascular disease.
- In contrast, signs of chronic insufficiency can be delineated through **examination of hair, skin changes, atrophy of skin and subcutaneous tissues, and muscle**.

276 Braun R, Lin M. Acute limb ischemia: a case report and literature review. J Emerg Med. 2015;49(6):1011-1017. doi:10.1016/j.jemermed.2015.03.008.

277 Acar RD, Sahin M, Kirma C. One of the most urgent vascular circumstances: acute limb ischemia. SAGE Open Med. 2013;1:2050312113516110.

278 Callum K, Bradbury A. ABC of arterial and venous disease: acute limb ischaemia. BMJ. 2000;320(7237):764-767.

279 Blaisdell FW, Steele M, Allen RE. Management of acute lower extremity arterial ischemia due to embolism and thrombosis. Surgery. 1978;84(6):822-834.

280 Daniel Purcell, Matthew Salzberg, and Vincent Kan, Acute Limb Ischemia: Pearls and Pitfalls [Online]

- Physical exam findings of ALI may include **loss of pulses, cool and pale or mottled skin, evidence of ischemic ulcers, and/or gangrene**[280].
- Deoxygenation of stagnated blood and surrounding pallor secondary to vasoconstriction may also be demonstrated by mottling/marbling.

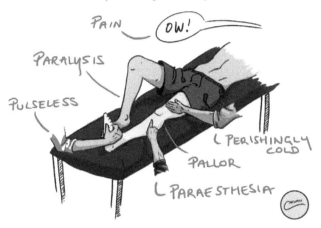

Image source Teachmesurgery

- Vascular evaluation should include palpation/auscultation of Doppler pulses, which allows for determination of perfusion pressure via the ankle-brachial index (ABI) ratio.
- Adequate perfusion pressure is maintained when the ratio exceeds 0.9.

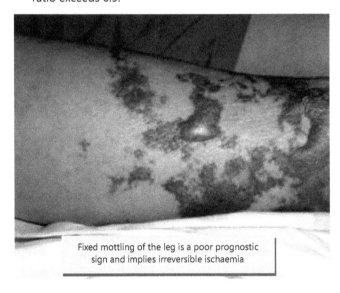

Fixed mottling of the leg is a poor prognostic sign and implies irreversible ischaemia

6. DIFFERENTIAL DIAGNOSIS
- Compartment Syndrome
- Cerebrovascular accident (CVA)
- Deep vein thrombosis (DVT)
- Hypovolaemic Shock
- Acute compressive neuropathyDirect arterial trauma
- Vasospasm

- Blue toe syndrome
- Vasculitis (i.e. Buerger's disease, Takayasu's disease)
- Non-arterial etiology: musculoskeletal trauma, radiculopathy (spinal stenosis, acute disc herniation), spontaneous hemorrhage (hemarthrosis)
- Chronic limb ischemia

7. INVESTIGATION STRATEGIES
- Full blood count, Urea and Electrolytes,
- Glucose,
- Creatinine Kinase
- Clotting,
- Group and Save
- Coagulation studies, and Type and Screen.
- Arterial Blood Gas analysis.
- Obtain an ECG and Chest X-ray and any other potential pre-operative information, and optimize any pre-existing medical conditions for surgical intervention, if necessary. This might diagnose AFib or other cardiac arrhythmias which may be a source of emboli.
- **Imaging:** *The choice of imaging is likely to depend on the local resources available.*

8. ED MANAGEMENT OF ALI
- **Initial management in the Emergency Department**
  - **Analgesia:** *IV morphine.*
  - **Oxygen:** supplemental oxygen to all patients.
  - **HEPARIN:** immediate administration of weight-based IV Heparin bolus (5000units or 80 units/kg) and associated continuous IV infusion (18 units/kg/hr) barring any contraindications intravenous heparin to prevent propagation of thrombosis.
  - **IV FLUIDS:** Careful IV hydration is recommended, as often patients with acute ischemia can be relatively volume depleted. Acute renal failure related to myoglobinuria after revascularization and/or IV contrast from potential radiologic studies may also be reduced by adequate hydration.
  - ***Administration of potassium should be avoided.***
  - The extremity should be placed in a dependent position to maximize perfusion and have any constricting clothing/bandages removed while maintaining the limb at a warm temperature
  - **REFER:** Vascular surgery should be consulted immediately. Any delay may endanger the affected limb, especially in sensorimotor impairment.

IV. SOFT TISSUE INFECTIONS

1. IMPETIGO

DESCRIPTION

o   Impetigo is a superficial bacterial infection of the skin
o   Primary infection: Infection of previously normal skin by direct bacterial invasion[281].
o   Secondary infection: Infection at site of minor skin trauma or previously existing skin lesions
o   Most prevalent in children aged 2-5 yr
o   More common in summer months and warm and humid climates
o   Easily spread among individuals in close contact

PREDISPOSING FACTORS

o   Minor trauma, especially around nose area
o   Burns
o   Insect bites
o   HIV infection
o   Diabetes mellitus
o   Existing skin disease
o   Varicella infection

COMPLICATIONS

o   Acute poststreptococcal glomerulonephritis: 1-5% in patients with nonbullous impetigo
o   Sepsis
o   Cellulitis
o   Endocarditis
o   Toxic shock syndrome
o   Staphylococcal-scalded skin syndrome (SSSS)

ETIOLOGY

o   **Classic (nonbullous) impetigo:**
    ▪   The result of bacteria entering through traumatic skin portal from scratch, abrasion, or insect bite
    ▪   Most common form
    ▪   Caused by *Staphylococcus aureus*, group A β-hemolytic streptococci, or both
    ▪   Often associated with poor hygiene
    ▪   Treatment of both streptococci and *S. aureus*

o   **Bullous impetigo:**
    ▪   Caused by *S. aureus*, phage group II
    ▪   Epidermal cleavage is caused by staphylococcal exfoliative toxins A, B, and D, which are serine proteases that bind and cleave desmoglein 1, an intercellular adhesion molecule in desmosome

CLINICAL FORMS OF IMPETIGO

1. NON-BULLOUS IMPETIGO

•   It is the usual form.
•   Red macules form initially, then golden crusts.
•   It is itchy but not painful.
•   Regional lymphadenopathy is common

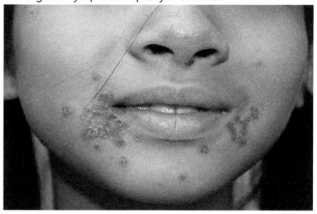

2. BULLOUS IMPETIGO

•   Here there is sloughing of the epidermis due to toxin production.
•   Vesicles/bullae may be on face, buttocks, nappy area or trunk.

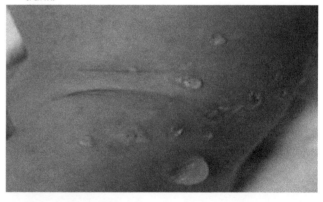

3. FOLLICULITIS

•   It is infection of the hair follicles due to **Staphylococcus aureus.**

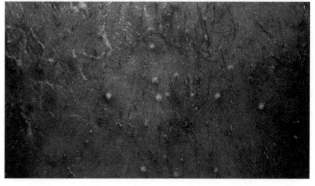

---

[281] *5-Minute Emergency Consult, Impetigo [online]*

4. ECTHYMA
- It is deeper, ulcerating & associated with lymphadenitis.

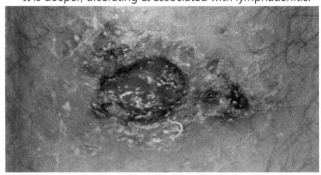

5. IMPETIGINOUS DERMATITIS
- Secondary infection of pre-existing skin disease or traumatized skin

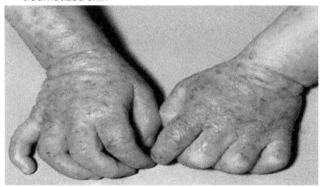

INVESTIGATION
- Impetigo is usually diagnosed on the basis of the clinical appearance
- Poorly responsive or recurrent cases of impetigo should be swabbed for **C&S** to identify possible methicillin-resistant Staphylococcus aureus (MRSA)
- Swabs are best taken from a moist lesion, or, in cases of bullous impetigo from a de-roofed blister

ED MANAGEMENT OF IMPETIGO
General measures
- Provide a patient information leaflet on impetigo
- Cover affected areas where possible
- Wash hands regularly
- Use separate towels and flannels
- Avoid school until the lesions are healed or crusted over, or 48 hours after antibiotics are started

Mild / Local Infections
- Consider hydrogen peroxide 1% cream for people with localised non-bullous impetigo who are not systemically unwell or at high risk of complications
- **Other treatments:**
  o Topical fusidic acid for 7-10 days
  o In cases of fusidic acid resistance use topical mupirocin

More Widespread Infection
- Use a systemic antibiotic for 7 days, either flucloxacillin or erythromycin / clarithromycin if penicillin allergy, or if there are concerns with regards to compliance with flucloxacillin given its unpleasant taste and QDS dosing regime[282].

MRSA infection
- Refer to local guidelines

Persistent or recurrent impetigo
- The nose is one of the most common sites of carriage for Staphylococcus aureus, so treatment of recurrent cases should include the application of **nasal mupirocin up both nostrils BD for 5 days**
- Wash the whole body daily with antibacterial emollient, eg the Dermol range, or anti-septic, eg chlorhexidine
- Consider a prolonged course of oral antibiotics for up to six weeks
- Identify and treat other carriers and possible sources of re-infection - it may be useful to take nasal swabs from other household contacts even if they do not have any cutaneous symptoms

2. CELLULITIS AND ERYSIPELAS
- Cellulitis is an inflammatory skin condition caused by acute infection of the dermal and subcutaneous layers of the skin; it is characterised by a superficial, diffuse, spreading skin infection without underlying collection of pus[283].

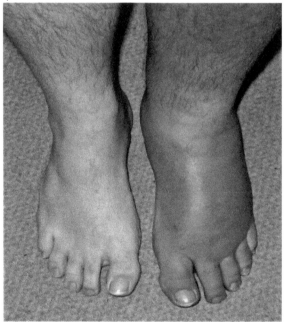

Cellulitis-Image from Health Jade

---

[282] Tim Cunliffe, The Primary Care Dermatology Society.Impetigo [online]

[283] Leanne Atkin. Cellulitis of the lower limbs: incidence, diagnosis and management [pdf document]

RISK FACTORS

- Older age,
- Obesity,
- Venous insufficiency,
- Saphenous venectomy (vein harvest for bypass surgery),
- Trauma,
- Eczema,
- Dermatitis,
- Athletes foot and oedema (Hirschmann and Raugi, 2012a).
- Patients with lymphoedema are especially at risk of developing cellulitis, due to the disturbances in lymph drainage and associated localised impaired host response to infection (Soo et al, 2008)

CLINICAL DIAGNOSIS OF CELLULITIS

- According to the Clinical Resource Efficiency Support Team (CREST) guidelines on the management of cellulitis in adults[284], Cellulitis presents as the acute and progressive onset of a red, painful, hot, swollen and tender area of skin.
- The edge of the erythema may be well demarcated or more diffuse and typically spreads rapidly.
- Constitutional upset with fever and malaise occurs in most cases, and may be present before the localising signs. Blistering/bullae, superficial haemorrhage into blisters, dermal necrosis, lymphangitis and lymphadenopathy may occur.
- The leg is the commonest site and there may be an identifiable portal of entry, for example, a wound, an ulcer or signs of tinea infection.
- Bilateral leg cellulitis is extremely rare.
- The use of simple clinical diagnostic criteria should be encouraged and should avoid over diagnosis and inappropriate investigations and antibiotics .
- The absence of typical clinical features should make one think of the main differential diagnoses, especially:
  - Varicose eczema which is often bilateral with crusting, scaling and itch or other lower leg eczema.
  - DVT with pain and swelling without significant erythema.
  - Acute liposclerosis which may have pain, redness and swelling in the absence of significant systemic upset
- Other differential diagnosis include lower leg oedema with secondary blistering, erythema nodosum, other panniculities or vasculitis and pyoderma gangrenosum. Complications include fasciitis, myositis, subcutaneous abscesses, septicaemia, post streptococcal nephritis and death.

CLINICAL CLASS OF CELLULITIS

- The Eron classification adapted from the CREST guidelines (2005) [285]

Class	Description	Management
I	Patients have no signs of systemic toxicity, have no uncontrolled co-morbidities and can usually be managed with oral antimicrobials on an outpatient basis.	• Oral antibiotic therapy • Identification and management of underlying risk factors
II	Patients are either systemically ill or systemically well but with a co-morbidity such as peripheral vascular disease, chronic venous insufficiency or morbid obesity which may complicate or delay resolution of their infection.	• Requires IV antibiotics. • Admission may not be necessary if there are suitable facilities and expertise in community
III	Patients may have a significant systemic upset such as acute confusion, tachycardia, tachypnoea, hypotension or may have unstable co-morbidities that may interfere with a response to therapy or have a limb threatening infection due to vascular compromise.	• Admit to hospital for IV antibiotics and careful monitoring
IV	Patients have sepsis syndrome or severe life threatening infection such as necrotizing fasciitis.	• Admit to hospital for IV antibiotics and treatment of sepsis.

DIFFERENTIAL DIAGNOSIS OF CELLULITIS

- Post-phlebitic limb
- Panniculitis
- Leg eczema
- Venous insufficiency
- Thrombophlebitis
- Deep Vein Thrombosis

INVESTIGATIONS

Class II-IV	Selected patients
• FBC • U&E • ESR/CRP • Swab any broken skin. • Culture blister fluid.	• Blood cultures only Class III or Class IV infections • Streptococcal serology only in refractory cases where diagnosis is in doubt • Skin biopsy where differential diagnosis includes other non-infectious inflammatory lesions

---

[284] *Clinical Resource Efficiency Support Team (CREST) guidelines on the management of cellulitis in adults [pdf document]*

[285] *Leanne Atkin. Cellulitis of the lower limbs: incidence, diagnosis and management [pdf document]*

ED MANAGEMENT OF CELLULITIS

CREST guidelines on the management of cellulitis in adults

Class	First line	Second line
I	Flucloxacillin 500mg qds po	**Penicillin allergy:** Clarithromycin 500mg bd po
II	Flucloxacillin 2g qds IV Or * Ceftriaxone 1g od IV (OPAT only)	**Penicillin allergy:** Clarithromycin 500mg bd IV or Clindamycin 600mg tds IV
III	Flucloxacillin 2g qds IV	**Penicillin allergy:** Clarithromycin 500mg bd IV or Clindamycin 900mg tds IV
IV	Benzylpenicillin 2.4g 2-4 hourly IV + Ciprofloxacin 400mg bd IV + Clindamycin 900mg tds IV (If allergic to penicillin use Ciprofloxacin and Clindamycin only) NB Discuss with local Medical Microbiology Service	

* Must not be used in penicillin anaphylaxis

Suitable Drug Therapy for Atypical Cellulitis

Class	First line	Penicillin allergy
Human bite	Co-amoxiclav 625mg tds po	Clarithromycin 500mg bd po or Doxycycline 100mg bd po and Metronidazole 400mg tds po
Cat/Dog bite	Co-amoxiclav 625mg tds po	Doxycycline 100mg bd po and Metronidazole 400mg tds po
Exposure to fresh water at site of skin break	Ciprofloxacin 750mg bd po And Flucloxacillin 500mg qds po	Ciprofloxacin 750mg bd po And Clarithromycin 500mg bd po

LOCAL MANAGEMENT OF CELLULITIS

- Management of the locally affected area should include the following:
  - o Adequate analgesia to ensure pain relief
  - o Monitoring and management of any pyrexia
  - o Consider hydration – intravenous/oral
  - o Recording of the site and/or limb affected
  - o Mark off the extent of erythema present on admission
- **If applicable:**
  - o Measurement of the limb
  - o Elevation of the limb
  - o Use of a bed cradle

3. NECROTISING FASCIITIS

- Necrotising fasciitis is a blanket term that is used to describe skin and soft tissue infections caused by one or a number of bacterial species (Schwartz and Kapila, 2004).
- In many cases, the disease progresses rapidly, causing large areas of soft tissue damage, extreme pain for the patient, and systemic sepsis if left untreated.
- Early diagnosis and prompt treatment are essential to halt the progress of the disease[286].

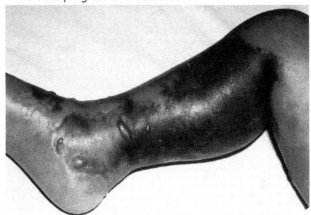

- It is a potentially lifethreatening disorder, in which bacterial toxins invade and destroy large areas of host tissue. The infection has been attributed to a variety of organisms. The most well known of these is the Group A haemolytic streptococcus commonly referred to as Streptococcus pyogenes. It is, however, important to recognise that this bacterium is often not the only one responsible for necrotising soft tissue infection.
- Despite many infections being identified as monomicrobial, some studies have highlighted a number of polymicrobial infections. In such cases, a number of organisms work synergistically to destroy tissue by similar means to a monomicrobial streptococcal infection.

PRESENTATION AND CLINICAL FEATURES

- **Clinical features** as being linked with necrotising infection:
  - o Rapid progression
  - o Poor therapeutic response
  - o Blistering necrosis
  - o Cyanosis
  - o Extreme localised tenderness
  - o Pyrexia
  - o Tachycardia
  - o Hypotension
  - o Altered level of consciousness.

286 *John Timmons, Recognising necrotising fasciitis [pdf document]*

Presentation

- Pain (usually greater than site implies)
- Erythema
- Pyrexia
- Bullae
- Apparent bruising
- Extensive necrosis
- Swelling
- Signs of organ failure (late diagnosis)
- Sweating
- Tachycardia
- Toxic delirium

RISK FACTORS

- Age (greater than fifty)
- Atherosclerosis
- Presence of chronic wound
- Cancer or immunocompromised
- Alcoholic liver disease
- Corticosteroid use
- Diabetes mellitus
- Hypoalbuminaemia
- Intravenous drug abuse
- Renal failure
- Trauma
- Obesity
- Malnutrition
- Occult diverticulitis
- Post-operative infection
- Peripheral vascular disease
- Strangulated femoral hernia
- Use of non-steroidal medication (inconclusive)

DIAGNOSIS

Laboratory screening investigations[287]

- These usually show:
  - WBC count > 15.4 x 109/L
  - Serum sodium < 135 mmoL
  - Raised CRP (> 16 mg/dL)
  - Raised CK level (> 600 U/L)
  - Urea > 18 mg/dL.
- Blood culture, deep tissue biopsy and Gram stain help in identifying the culprit organism(s) and guide the choice of antibiotic.
- If Staphylococcus aureus is detected, MRSA sensitivity test should be done.
- Blood cultures are usually negative for clostridial species.
- Fungal culture should be performed in immunocompromised and trauma patients.

Imaging

- X-ray,
- CT and MRI identify areas of fluid collection, inflammation and gas within the soft tissues.

Laboratory Risk Indicator for Necrotising Fasciitis

- The Laboratory Risk Indicator for Necrotising Fasciitis (LRINEC) is a tool that aids in distinguishing necrotising fasciitis from other tissue infections based on six parameters.
- A score of ≥ 6 favours necrotising fasciitis.
- This test is not appropriate for all cases and is not completely reliable.

LRINEC parameters

- **CRP (mg/L) ≥150:**
  - 4 points
- **WBC count ($\times 10^3$/mm^3):**
  - <15: 0 points
  - 15-25: 1 point
  - >25: 2 points
- **Hemoglobin (g/dL):**
  - >13.5: 0 points
  - 11-13.5: 1 point
  - <11: 2 points
- **Sodium (mmol/L) <135:**
  - 2 points
- **Creatinine (umol/L) >141:**
  - 2 points
- **Glucose (mmol/L) >10:**
  - 1 point

EMERGENCY DEPARTMENT MANAGEMENT

- Obtain intravenous access in the unaffected extremity and
- Begin fluid resuscitation with Crystalloid solution.
- In patients who do not improve with crystalloid resuscitation, norepinephrine is recommended.
- Administer adequate intravenous broad-spectrum antibiotics, as the etiology can be polymicrobial.
- Consider supplemental oxygen and intubation in patients with hypoxia or altered mental status.
- Appropriate analgesic administration is recommended, as patients may have significant analgesic requirements.
- Electrolyte replacement is indicated as needed.
- Immediate surgical consultation is indicated when NSTI is suspected.
- A surgeon should be promptly consulted for definitive management.
- Tetanus status should be assessed and updated, if indicated

---

[287] Vanessa Ngan, Necrotising fasciitis [*Dermanetnz Online*]

V. NON-TRAUMATIC NECK PAIN

INTRODUCTION

- Although most cases of neck pain are related to musculoskeletal trauma, there are some infrequent but potentially serious atraumatic causes for which the ED physician should consider in the differential diagnosis.

RED FLAGS IN SPONTANEOUS NECK PAIN:

- New symptoms below age 20 or above age 55 years
- Trauma,
- Preceding neck surgery,
- Osteoporosis risk,
- Myelopathy,
- History of cancer,
- Unexplained weight loss,
- Constant, progressive, non-mechanical pain
- Fever,
- History of infections (e.g. TB, HIV),
- History of inflammatory arthritis
- Signs of spinal cord compression

CLINICAL ASSESSMENT

History

Points to cover in history and examination:

- Time of onset of pain (spontaneous onset at night or night pain)
- Any associated trauma
- Any relieving or exacerbating factors
- Pain in the occipital condyle (seen in posterior fossa tumours)
- Score the pain on available pain charts
- Duration of pain, whether continuous or intermittent
- Interference with daily activity
- Any history of drugs especially those causing extrapyramidal side effects
- Problems with vision
- Other associated symptoms like headaches, vertigo, vomiting. Unusual neck posturing, that is, hyperflexed position, child trying to splint the neck with their hands.
- These should raise the suspicion of posterior fossa tumours, discitis and spinal cord tumours
- Any gait abnormalities (base of skull tumour and spinal cord tumours) and repeated attendances at the hospital with persistence of symptoms
- This should include timing of the onset of symptoms. Non-traumatic neck pain is always of concern, and the covert causes must be considered, including meningitis, spinal infection and metastatic deposits within the spine.

Examination

- Neck pain in adults is often a manifestation of degenerative disease of the spine whereas in children the commonest causes are trauma and infections.
- A complete physical examination should include examination of the neurological system, spine, and eyes especially eye movements and the cover-uncover test.[288]
- The basis of a proper clinical diagnosis remains the patient's history and physical examination.
- Unusual presentation with neck pain, abnormal neck posturing, gait abnormalities and its persistence should ring a warning bell for other potentially less common but more sinister diagnoses.
- The examiner's index of suspicion is crucial to the completeness of work up of patients with neck pain with/without torticollis.
- With easy access to imaging modalities, conditions like intracranial tumours of the base of skull, intraspinal tumours, congenital abnormalities, and spinal infections can be easily diagnosed and early treatment instituted.

CAUSES OF NON-TRAUMATIC NECK PAIN

- **The more common causes of neck pain include:**
  - Infections[289] (meningitis, pneumonia, otitis media, tonsillitis, cervical adenitis, retropharyngeal abscess, mumps, and cerebral abscess)
  - Ophthalmological conditionssuch as squint.
  - Acute wry neck / torticollis
  - Spondylosis
  - Disc impingement
  - Spinal stenosis

- **The less common causes include:**
  - Metastases
  - juvenile chronic arthritis
  - Infective discitis
  - Myositis ossificans progressiva.
  - Pharyngitis
  - Spinal osteomyelitis
  - Arnold-Chiari malformations

---

[288] Rosenberg NM, Kost S, Dowd MD, et al. The passive and aggressive evaluation of the cervical area. Pediatr Emerg Care1998;14:305–9.

[289] Wang LF, Kuo WR, Tsai SM, et al. Characterizations of life threatening deep cervical space infections: a review of one hundred ninety-six cases. Am J Otolaryngol2003;24:111–17.

1. ACUTE WRY NECK / TORTICOLLIS

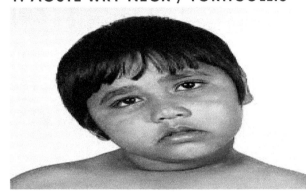

- Torticollis (Latin word meaning "twisted neck") is tilting and rotation of the head to one side with restricted rotation towards the other side. It is a symptom of cervical spine abnormality[290]. This commonly affects adolescents and young adults. The patient presents with the neck held at an angle, in constant pain.
- The pain experienced tends to be localized to the mid cervical region and is unilateral away from the direction of the deformity. The patient often describes a history of a sudden unguarded movement of the neck which causes sudden pain and restricted neck movement.
- There is normally no history of trauma. Treatment is expectant, and NSAID together with heat help to ease it.

2. CERVICAL SPONDYLOSIS

- The aetiology of cervical spondylosis is underlying spontaneous joint degeneration. It is related to age and to wear and tear[291]. However, concordant twin studies note a significant genetic predisposition to development of cervical degeneration, in addition to occupational and activity-related factors.
- Similarly, there appears to be a significant genetic or inherited predisposition to development of cervical spondylotic myelopathy[292].
- Once the degeneration begins (typically in the second or third decade), cervical joint degeneration slowly worsens over the lifetime. The relative roles of daily wear and tear, trauma, and genetics on the rate of degeneration remain unclear, although radiographic spondylosis is generally age related and no known treatments can reverse the process.
- There is no simple, accepted aetiological classification, but symptoms cluster into clinical syndromes.

- Many patients with radiographic cervical spondylosis show no symptoms, so there is commonly dissociation between radiographic studies (i.e., MRI) and presence of symptoms[293].
- In patients with symptomatic cervical spondylosis, there are 3 main clinical syndromes:
  - ○ Axial neck pain
  - ○ Cervical spondylotic radiculopathy (CSR)
  - ○ Cervical spondylotic myelopathy (CSM).
- The last 2 syndromes may overlap and both include degrees of axial neck pain.
- Neck pain may be acute or chronic, is the most common symptom (and most easily treatable), and may occur with or without neurological symptoms due to radiculopathy and/or myelopathy.

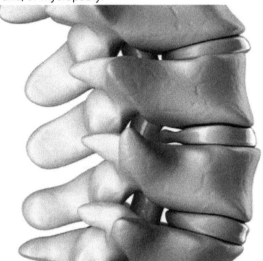

DIAGNOSTIC STUDIES

- **Cervical Xray:** Primarily indicated when trauma suspected or the patient has pain on motion of the neck, and not in the routine, outpatient setting.
- **MRI:** Ordered if neck pain persists for 4 to 6 weeks, radicular pain does not subside with treatments, or more severe deficit suggestive of myelopathy is present. This would normally be the primary study ordered from the clinic setting once these criteria are met.
- **Cervical CT:** An extension to cervical radiographs to obtain more detail about bone structure, such as in trauma setting or instability. Also indicated if an MRI is not possible (e.g., implanted metal).
- **Cervical CT Myelogram:** An extension to cervical radiographs to obtain more detail about bone structure, such as in trauma setting or instability. Also indicated if an MRI is not possible (e.g., implanted metal).

[290] Kuppermann N. Neck stiffness. In: Fleisher GR, Ludwig S, eds. Textbook of Pediatric Emergency Medicine. 4th edn. Philadelphia, PA: WB Sanders, 2000:391–9.

[291] Sherk HH, Watters WC, Zeiger L. Evaluation and treatment of neck pain. Orthop Clin North Am 1982;13:439–52.

[292] Raskas DS, Graziano GP, Herzenberg JE, et al. Osteoid osteoma and osteoblastoma of the spine. J Spinal Disord 1992;5:204–11.

[293] Matsumoto M, Fujimura Y, Suzuki N, et al. MRI of cervical intervertebral discs in asymptomatic subjects. J Bone Joint Surg Br. 1998;80:19-24.

TREATMENT
AXIAL NECK PAIN
- **1st line** – physiotherapy
- **Adjunct** –non-steroidal anti-inflammatory drugs (NSAIDs)
  - Ibuprofen: 300-400 mg orally every 6-8 hours when required, maximum 2400 mg/day **or**
  - Naproxen: 250-500 mg orally twice daily when required, maximum 1250 mg/day **or**
  - Diclofenac potassium: 50 mg orally (immediate-release) twice or three times daily when required **or**
  - Diclofenac sodium: 100 mg orally (extended-release) once daily when required
- **Adjunct** – muscle relaxants
  - Tizanidine: 4 mg orally every 6-8 hours when required initially, increase by 2-4 mg/dose increments according to response, maximum 18 mg/day or
  - Methocarbamol: 1500 mg orally four times daily for 2-3 days initially, then decrease dose according to response, usual dose 4000-4500 mg/day given in 3-6 divided doses or
  - Diazepam: 5-10 mg orally every 8 hours when required
- **Adjunct** – trigger-point and/or facet joint injections
  - Dexamethasone: 4 mg Intra-Articularly/Intrasynovially/Into Tendon Sheath As A Single Dose

CERVICAL SPONDYLOTIC RADICULOPATHY (CSR)
- **1st line** – analgesics
  - Ibuprofen: 400-800 mg orally every 6-8 hours when required, maximum 2400 mg/day or
  - Naproxen: 250-500 mg orally twice daily when required, maximum 1250 mg/day or
  - Diclofenac potassium: 50 mg orally (immediate-release) twice or three times daily when required or
  - Diclofenac sodium: 100 mg orally (extended-release) once daily when required
- **Secondary options**
  - Paracetamol/hydrocodone: 5 mg orally every 4-6 hours when required, maximum 60 mg/day or
  - Oxycodone: 5-10 mg orally (immediate-release) every 4-6 hours when required; 10 mg orally (controlled-release) every 12 hours
- **Adjunct** – Physiotherapy and traction
- **Adjunct** – Oral corticosteroids
  - Prednisolone: 60-80 mg orally once daily for 2-3 days, then taper dose gradually over 10-14 days
- **2nd line** – Epidural anaesthesia or cervical nerve root block

- To be given by a radiologist or pain management anaesthesiologist.
- **3rd line** – surgical nerve decompression
  - If the pain does not resolve and if all symptoms, signs and diagnostic studies indicate pressure on a single nerve root, then surgical nerve decompression may be a helpful treatment in some patients.

CERVICAL SPONDYLOTIC MYELOPATHY (CSM)
- Moderate to severe symptoms: good surgical candidate-**surgical decompression**[294]
- Mild symptoms or poor surgical candidate-**conservative treatment with immobilisation in a hard cervical collar**

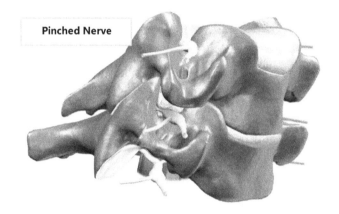

Pinched Nerve

3. DISC HERNIATION
- Cervical disc herniations most commonly occur between C5-C6 and C6-C7 vertebral bodies.
- This, in turn, will cause symptoms at C6 and C7, respectively. History in these patients should include the chief complaint, onset of symptoms, alleviating and aggravating factors, radicular symptoms, and any past treatments. The most common subjective complaints are axial neck pain and ipsilateral arm pain or paresthesias in the associated dermatomal distribution.
- The clinician should assess the patient's range of motion (ROM), as this can indicate the severity of pain and degeneration. A thorough neurological examination is necessary to evaluate sensory disturbances, motor weakness, and deep tendon reflex abnormalities. Careful attention should also focus on any sign of spinal cord dysfunction.

LAB VALUES
- ESR/ CRP
- FBC

[294] Rao RD, Gourab K, David KS. Operative treatment of cervical spondylotic myelopathy. J Bone Surg Am. 2006;88:1619-1640.

IMAGING
- **X-rays:**
  - The first test typically performed
  - Three views (AP, lateral, and oblique)
  - If imaging demonstrates an acute fracture, this requires additional investigation using a computed tomogram (CT) scan or magnetic resonance imaging (MRI).
  - If there is a concern for atlantoaxial instability, the open mouth (odontoid) view may assist in diagnosis.
- **CT Scan:**
  - The most sensitive test to examine the bony structures of the spine.
  - It can also show calcified herniated discs or any insidious process that may result in bony loss or destruction.
  - In patients that are unable to or are otherwise ineligible to undergo an MRI, CT myelography can be used as an alternative to visualize a herniated disc.
- **MRI:**
  - The preferred imaging modality and the most sensitive study to visualize a herniated disc, as it has the most significant ability to demonstrate soft-tissue structures and the nerve as it exits the foramen.

4. SPINAL STENOSIS
- Cervical stenosis is a condition in which the spinal canal is too small for the spinal cord and nerve roots.
- This can cause damage to the spinal cord, a condition called **myelopathy**, or pinch nerves as they exit the spinal canal **(radiculopathy).** Occasionally, damage to the spinal cord and nerve roots may occur, resulting in a condition called **myeloradiculopathy.**

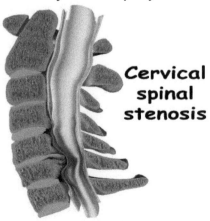

Cervical spinal stenosis

- Men are seen nearly twice as often as women.
- Cervical stenosis is most often caused by a number of factors which combine to cause a critical level of spinal cord compression, at which time symptoms may develop.

- Factors contributing to the development of cervical stenosis include: shorter than average *pedicles* (the bones which form the sides of the spinal canal), degenerative arthritis causing excessive bone growth, increased in size of the *ligamentum flavum* (a ligament which runs down the underside of the roof of the spinal canal), and conditions such rheumatoid arthritis and *ossification* (abnormally turning into bone) of the ligament that forms the floor of the spinal canal.
- Myelopathic findings dominate the physical findings.
- Symptoms of cervical stenosis are related to abnormal compression of the spinal cord and nerve roots. Neck pain, pain in one or both arms, and an electrical sensation that shoots down the back when the head moves are common painful sensations in patients with spinal stenosis. Numbness of the arms can occur, in addition to a feeling that the arms or hands are asleep.
- As the condition progresses, weakness of the arms and hands can occur with loss of coordination. Also, in advanced stages of cervical stenosis, problems with bowel and bladder function can result, in addition to weakness and numbness in the legs and feet, which can cause difficulty walking. Abnormal reflexes such as Babinski and Hoffman are also often present.

5. PHARYNGITIS

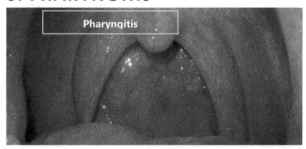
Pharyngitis

- Pharyngitis is defined as an infection or irritation of the pharynx or tonsils. The etiology is usually infectious, with most cases being of viral origin and most bacterial cases attributable to group A streptococci (GAS).
- Other causes include allergy, trauma, toxins, and neoplasia.

SIGNS AND SYMPTOMS
- It is difficult to distinguish viral and bacterial causes of pharyngitis on the basis of history and physical examination alone. Nevertheless, the following factors may help rule out or diagnose GAS pharyngitis:
  - GAS infection is most common in children aged 4-7 years
  - Sudden onset is consistent with GAS pharyngitis; pharyngitis after several days of coughing or rhinorrhea is more consistent with a viral etiology

o   Contact with others who have GAS or rheumatic fever with symptoms consistent with GAS raises the likelihood of GAS pharyngitis

o   Headache is consistent with GAS infection

o   Cough is not usually associated with GAS infection

o   Vomiting is associated with GAS infection

o   Recent orogenital contact suggests possible gonococcal pharyngitis

o   A history of rheumatic fever is important

- **Physical examination includes the following:**
  o   Assessment of airway patency
  o   Temperature, Hydration status
  o   Head, ears, eyes, nose, and throat – Conjunctivitis, scleral icterus, rhinorrhea, tonsillopharyngeal/palatal petechiae, tonsillopharyngeal exudate, oropharyngeal vesicular lesions
  o   Lymphadenopathy (cervical or generalized)
  o   Cardiovascular evaluation
  o   Pulmonary assessment
  o   Abdominal examination
  o   Skin examination

DIAGNOSIS

- Laboratory studies that may be helpful include the following:
  o   Group A beta-hemolytic streptococcal rapid antigen detection test (preferred diagnostic method in ED)
  o   Throat culture (criterion standard for diagnosis of GAS infection [90-99% sensitive])
  o   Mono spot (up to 95% sensitive in children; less than 60% sensitive in infants)
  o   Peripheral smear
  o   Gonococcal culture if indicated by the history
  o   Imaging studies generally are not indicated for uncomplicated viral or streptococcal pharyngitis. However, the following may be considered:
  o   Lateral neck film in patients with suspected epiglottitis or airway compromise
  o   Soft-tissue neck CT if concern for abscess or deep-space infection exists
  o   A throat swab may also be done.

MANAGEMENT

- Emergency measures may include the following:
  o   Assess and secure the airway, if necessary
  o   Assess the patient for signs of toxicity, epiglottitis, or oropharyngeal abscess
  o   Evaluate hydration status, and rehydrate as necessary
  o   Assess for GAS infection if clinically suspected
- First line treatment; **Metronidazole and clindamycin** are effective in combination

6. PERITONSILLAR ABSCESSES

- Peritonsillar abscesses (PTAs) are common infections of the head and neck region, accounting for approximately 30% of soft tissue head and neck abscesses.
- It is a potent cause of neck pain, but is usually associated with ipsilateral ear pain, and obvious swallowing difficulty.
- It usually progresses from tonsillitis to cellulitis and ultimately to abscess formation.
- No definitive studies are required to diagnose PTA.
- The following laboratory tests may be considered:
  - Basic studies, such as Full Blood Count, electrolytes, and C-reactive protein (if the patient has significant comorbidities)
  - Monospot test/heterophile antibody test (to rule out infectious mononucleosis if the etiology is unclear)
  - Culture of fluid from needle aspiration (to guide antibiotic selection or changes)
  - Blood cultures (if the clinical presentation is severe)

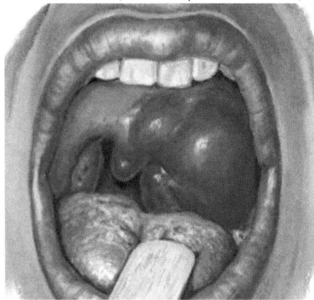

Peritonsillar Abscess|Image Source Quora

MANAGEMENT

- Transport with supplemental oxygen.
- Attention to the ABCs (airway, breathing, and circulation)
- If the patient's airway is compromised, immediate endotracheal intubation or, if this cannot be accomplished, cricothyroidotomy or tracheostomy; alternatively, awake fiberoptic bronchoscopy
- Fluid resuscitation as necessary
- Antipyretics for elevated temperature
- Adequate analgesia for pain
- Empiric antibiotics
- Adjunctive steroids
- ENT referral

7. LUDWIG'S ANGINA

- In Ludwig's angina, the submandibular space is the primary site of infection. This space is subdivided by the mylohyoid muscle into the sublingual space superiorly and the submaxillary space inferiorly.
- The majority of cases of Ludwig's angina are odontogenic in etiology, primarily resulting from infections of the second and third molars.
- The cause is usually a bacterial infection, most often Streptococcal, although other bacteria can also cause this.
- The roots of these teeth penetrate the mylohyoid ridge such that any abscess, or dental infection, has direct access to the submaxillary space.

8. INFECTIVE DISCITIS & SPINAL OSTEOMYELITIS

- Discitis is an inflammation of the vertebral disk space often related to infection. Infection of the disk space must be considered with vertebral osteomyelitis; these conditions are almost always present together, and they share much of the same pathophysiology, symptoms, and treatment.
- Although discitis and associated vertebral osteomyelitis are uncommon conditions, they are often the causes of debilitating neurologic injury.
- Unfortunately, morbidity can be exacerbated by a delay in diagnosis and treatment of this condition.
- The lumbar region is most commonly affected, followed by the cervical spine and, lastly, the thoracic spine[295].
- The most common cause of vertebral osteomyelitis is **Staphylococcus aureus**, accounting for more than 50% of cases in most series from developed countries.
- The relative importance of methicillin-resistant *S. aureus* as a cause of vertebral osteomyelitis has increased as the community and hospital proportion of *S. aureus* strains that are methicillin resistant have increased.
- Other causes of vertebral osteomyelitis include[296]:
  - o Enteric gram-negative bacilli, particularly following urinary tract instrumentation
  - o Nonpyogenic streptococci, including viridans group, milleri group, Streptococcus bovis, and enterococci
  - o Pyogenic streptococci, including groups B and C/G, especially in patients with diabetes mellitus
  - o Pseudomonas aeruginosa, coagulase-negative staphylococci, and Candida spp, especially in association with intravascular access, sepsis, or injection drug use
  - o Tuberculous infection
  - o Brucellosis, especially Brucella melitensis

RISK FACTORS

- Risk factors for vertebral osteomyelitis include:
  - o Injection drug use,
  - o Infective endocarditis,
  - o Advanced age
  - o Degenerative spine disease,
  - o Prior spinal surgery,
  - o Cancer
  - o Organ transplantation
  - o Congenital immunodepression
  - o Diabetes mellitus,
  - o Malnutrition
  - o Corticosteroid therapy, or other immunocompromised state.

CLINICAL PRESENTATION

- The major clinical manifestation of vertebral osteomyelitis is pain; pain is typically localized to the infected disc space area and is exacerbated by physical activity or percussion to the affected area.
- Pain may radiate to the abdomen, leg, scrotum, groin, or perineum.
- The pain is often worse at night; initially, it may be relieved by bed rest. Pain may be absent in patients with paraplegia. Fever is an inconsistent finding.
- Patients whose infections extend posteriorly into the epidural space may present with clinical features of an epidural abscess; this often consists of focal and severe back pain, followed by radiculopathy, then motor weakness and sensory changes (including loss of bowel and bladder control and loss of perineal sensation), and eventual paralysis.
- The risk of severe neurologic deficit is increased in the presence of epidural abscess, especially with thoracic or cervical spinal involvement.

INVESTIGATIONS

- The leukocyte count may be elevated or normal.
- Elevations in the ESR and CRP: > 80%of patients.
- The diagnosis of vertebral osteomyelitis or discitis is established based on positive culture obtained from **CT-guided biopsy** of the involved vertebra(e) and/or disc space.

295 Walters R, Rahmat R, Fraser R, Moore R. Preventing and treating discitis: cephazolin penetration in ovine lumbar intervertebral disc. Eur Spine J. 2006 Sep. 15 (9):1397-403.

296 Lew DP, Waldvogel FA. Osteomyelitis. Lancet 2004; 364:369.

8. CERVICAL SPINE METASTASIS

- Pain is the most common presentation of primary and metastatic lesions of the cervical spine. Axial pain is mechanical in nature; it can be relieved by lying down and worsens with ambulation and axial load.
- Localized pain is attributed to stretching of the vertebral body periosteum and is not responsive to changes in position. Localized pain is the common night time pain seen in cancer patients[297].

DIAGNOSTICS

- **Plain radiograph**
  - First step in imaging the cervical spine and are helpful in identifying tumor-related deformity.
  - Odontoid and swimmer's views should be obtained, depending on the levels involved.

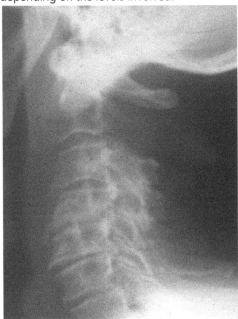

- **MRI** with and without contrast is the gold standard for the imaging evaluation of cervical spine tumors.
- **CT** can be used for surgical planning and to assess the extent of bony destruction. If the primary cause is unknown, or for a presumed primary malignant lesion, then CT of the chest and abdomen can be performed for staging.
- **CT-guided biopsy** is the modality most commonly used for diagnosis. Biopsy is especially critical in patients with a new lesion and no metastases elsewhere
- **Myelography:** useful in finding the cause of pain not found by an MRI or CT.

[297] Mesfin, Addisu MD; Buchowski, Jacob M. MD, MS; Gokaslan, Ziya L. MD; Bird, Justin E. MD Management of Metastatic Cervical Spine Tumors, Journal of the American Academy of Orthopaedic Surgeons: January 2015 - Volume 23 - Issue 1 - p 38-46 doi: 10.5435/JAAOS-23-01-38

- **Total body scans** (eg, positron-emission tomography, bone scan) can be used to study the presence of metastases. Positron-emission tomography can be used to evaluate response to chemotherapy.

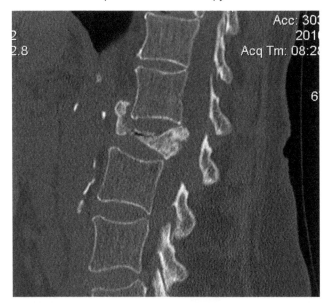

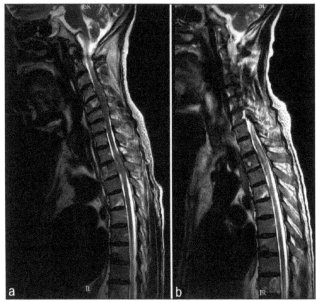

MANAGEMENT

- Analgesia: adequate pain relief
- Management is decided based on the histology of the lesion and the clinical presentation.
- A multidisciplinary team involving the medical oncologist, radiation oncologist, and spine surgeon, along with the patient and family, is necessary.
- Consideration of referral to a spine tumor specialty center may be indicated for appropriate cases, such as patients with neurologic changes resulting from metastatic epidural spinal cord compression..
- **Physiotherapy**

25. Major Incident Management

I. EMERGENCY DEPARTMENT APPROACH

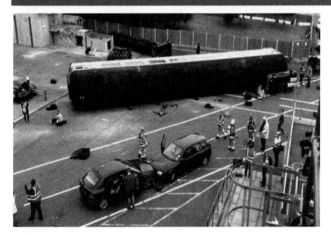

DEFINITION

- A major incident is an incident where the location, number, severity or type of live casualties requires extraordinary resources.
- Incidents can also become major incidents for other agencies – police and fire services, local authorities and public health services among others; a major incident for one agency might not be a major incident for another however.

CLASSIFICATION OF MAJOR INCIDENT

- **Major incidents can be classified as**[298]**:**
  o **Natural or man-made**: e.g. Floods and earthquakes.
  o **Simple**: where the infrastructure is intact
  o **Compound**: where the infrastructure is damaged
  o **Compensated**: load is less than capacity
  o **Uncompensated**

FACTORS INFLUENCING MAJOR INCIDENT

There are lots of factors that might turn an incident into a major incident:

- Location
- Time of the day
- Type of casualties

CATEGORIES OF MAJOR INCIDENT

For hospitals, major incidents can be placed into the following three categories:

- **Category 1: a major external incident** that will involve large numbers of casualties arriving at the hospital. Normal hospital services may have to be stopped or restricted during the incident.
- **Category 2: an external incident** that does not involve large numbers of casualties arriving at the hospital, but does have a significant impact on the normal activities and functions of the hospital.
- **Category 3: an internal incident** (or incidents) that has a significant impact on the normal functions and activities of the hospital. This incident may involve hospital inpatients.

ED APPROACH TO MAJOR INCIDENT

The ambulance service or the police normally warn the relevant services of a possible or definite major incident.

One format for communication of information by relevant personnel is as follows ('**METHANE**')[299]:

- **M**ajor incident standby or declared
- **E**xact location
- **T**ype of incident
- **H**azards
- **A**ccess
- **N**umber of casualties
- **E**mergency services

Once an incident has been identified, the following terms are used to notify hospital staff and all other parties involved:

- **Incident standby:** a potential incident has been identified and the hospital will be required to alert key staff to prepare for an incident.

---

[298] Jamie Sillett, East Midlands Emergency Medicine Educational Media, Major Incident Management [Online]

[299] NHS, Clinical guidelines for use in a trauma major incident or mass casualty event [pdf Online]

- **Incident declared:** a major incident response is implemented. It is declared by an external agency, normally the ambulance service.

- **Incident cancelled:** a standby has been initiated but an incident did not occur.

- **Incident stand down:** a command given to state that the incident is over or that special arrangements can ease.

After a **'declared' status,** a stand down can only be given by the agency calling the alert, and will be communicated to hospital staff by the major incident control centre.

A potential major external incident is alerted to the hospital switchboard, which will proceed according to the appropriate action card.

- The ambulance service uses the phrase **'Major incident – standby'**.
- When the major incident is confirmed, the notification is **'Major incident declared – activate plan'**.
- If a standby was initiated but an incident did not occur, the notification is **'Major incident – cancelled'**.
- Once the last casualty has left the incident site, the ambulance service will use the phrase **'Casualty evacuation complete'**.

- The **ED consultant** on duty needs to be informed immediately to enable participation in the decision to start the major incident procedure.

- **Senior medical, nursing and administrative staff** will set up the hospital's control centre and initiate the full hospital response.

- **All staff in the ED** need to be informed that a major incident has been declared so that the department is cleared of any patients who are not seriously ill or injured and is prepared to receive patients from the major incident. Staff are given action cards as per the major incident plan.

- **All relevant staff** are given labels or tabards for ease of identification of roles. Staff are allocated to small teams, with clear instructions regarding their roles, according to the team leader carrying the tabard and action card.
- The ambulance entrance point could be set up as the triage point.
- The ED can be divided into various areas in terms of the types of patient treated in each area – for example a resuscitation area for the most seriously injured, followed by 'majors' and 'minors' areas.

- Depending on the resources available, clinical decision units or observation wards may be cleared to receive suitable patients.
- Otherwise, a ward needs to be cleared to receive patients from the emergency department.
- Theatres need to be ready to receive patients who need operations.
- This needs to be coordinated by relevant staff as per the major incident action cards.

- **All patients need to be labelled** with a unique major incident number, and this is used on all notes, forms, blood samples and property bags.

TRIAGE IN MASS CASUALTY SITUATIONS

In an external major incident involving a large number of casualties attending the emergency department, a system of triage is used to grade the treatment and environmental needs of each patient:

- ***Priority one casualties (P1)*** *require immediate resuscitation and stabilisation and placement in a critical care area and/or theatre without delay.*
- ***Priority two casualties (P2)*** *have serious injuries that do not pose an immediate threat to life but do require urgent interventions.*
- ***Priority three casualties (P3)*** *have moderate to minor injuries requiring simple measures to treat injuries that can be reviewed later.*
- ***Expectant category (P4):*** *Expectant patients are those whose injuries are so severe that attempting to save them would divert precious resources from other casualties with a greater chance of survival, with no significant chance of a successful outcome. The decision to invoke the expectant category must be taken at silver level and preferably only after discussion with gold command.*

TRIAGE CATEGORIES

	Description	Label colour
1	Immediate	Red
2	Urgent	Yellow
3	Delayed	Green
4	Expectant	Blue
Dead	Dead	White or black

TRIAGE SORT[300]

TRIAGE SORT		
Step 1: Calculate GCS		
A: EYE OPENING	**B: VERBAL RESPONSE**	**C: MOTOR RESPONSE**
Spontaneous 4	Orientated 5	Obeys commands 6
To voice 3	Confused 4	Localises pain 5
To pain 2	Inappropriate 3	Pain withdraws 4
None 1	Incomprehensible 2	Pain flexes 3
	No response 1	Pain extends 2
		No response 1
GCS= A+B+C		
Step 2: Calculate the Triage Sort Score		
X: GCS	**Y: Respiratory Rate**	**Z: Systolic BP**
13-14 ----------- 4	10-29 ----------- 4	≥90----------------- 4
9-12---------------3	**≥30----------------3**	**76-89----------------3**
6-8 ------------- 2	**6-9 ------------- 2**	**50-75 ------------ 2**
4-5 ---------------1	1-5 ---------------1	1-49 ----------------1
3-------------------0	0-------------------0	0 -------------------0
Triage score= X+Y+Z		
Step 3: Assign triage priotity		

12= Priority 3 (P3)
11= Priority 2 (P2)
10= Priority 1 (P1)

STEP 4: Upgrade priority at discretion of senior clinician, dependent on the anatomical injury/ working diagnosis

The key to successful management of an incident is early command and control that is maintained throughout the incident. Hospitals usually use a three-tier command and control system: **strategic, tactical and operational** areas and personnel.

This relates to **Gold, Silver and Bronze Commands:**

- **Gold Command (strategic) – major incident control centre:** This is the focal command point for the management of the incident. All communication issues are handled by the team, consisting of senior management, nursing and medical staff. It is the hospital equivalent of Ambulance Gold Control.
- **Silver Command (tactical) – senior support:** This is provided by a senior manager and a senior nurse, who are able to troubleshoot any immediate problems. This is the hospital equivalent of Ambulance Silver Control.
- **Operational – operational team:** operational teams have specific roles or functions within a defined area or department that is usually familiar to them.

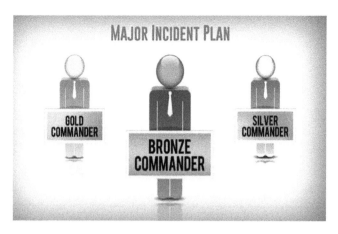

SECURITY DURING A MAJOR INCIDENT

The hospital premises can be vulnerable during a major incident owing to the large volumes of people, patients and staff. Also, other people, such as media personnel, may want to access the hospital, especially if the incident is related to a terrorist or criminal event.

Basic principles need to be applied:

- All hospital entrances will be locked during the incident, except for the emergency department ambulance entrance.
- Identity cards will be worn at all times.
- A police liaison point is situated in the security office.
- Press statements and media interviews are authorized by members of the communications office.
- A special centre for relatives is set up as per the hospital major incident plan.

Police are in overall command at the incident site.

If there is a fire or chemical risk then the fire service take control of the immediate area.

The ambulance service is in control of the medical command.

A medical incident officer (MIO) may be sent from a supporting hospital to the incident site.

The MIO is in charge of all medical and nursing staff at the incident site and ensures supervision of the team, including arrangement of equipment and supplies and breaks.

INCIDENT DEBRIEF

- The review of events and debriefing of all staff involved is an important part of any major incident.
- It is the responsibility of the hospital executive team and senior managers involved in the incident to perform the review and arrange debriefing.
- The debriefing enables staff to discuss what happened and express their feelings.
- Counselling may be required.

---

300 *Wayne Smith, Triage in mass casualty situations [pdf online]*

II. CBRN CHALLENGE

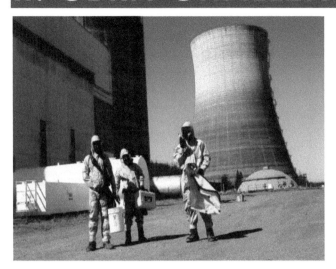

ABSTRACT

- CBRN threats encompass a wide scope of events, including naturally occurring disasters, accidental incidents at hazardous installations or during the transport of dangerous materials, as well as deliberate incidents, among which terrorist acts and state-sponsored uses.
- In this context, considering challenges pertaining to CBRN preparedness and response, the 2009 Commission's Communication presenting the EU CBRN Action Plan advocated starting from an all-hazards approach[301].
- When a **Chemical, Biological, Radiological,** or **Nuclear (CBRN)** event occurs, life or death often is determined within the first few minutes of its onset.
- **An accidental CBRN incident** is an event caused by human error or natural or technological reasons, such as spills, accidental releases or leakages. These accidental incidents are usually referred to as DG or HAZMAT accidents. Outbreaks of infectious diseases, such as SARS, or pandemic influenza are examples of naturally occurring biological incidents.

An intentional CBRN incident includes:
- Criminal acts such as the deliberate dumping or release of hazardous materials to avoid regulatory requirements
- The malicious, but non-politically motivated poisoning of one or more individuals
- Terrorist acts that involve serious violence to persons or property

RESPONDING TO A CHEMICAL, BIOLOGICAL, RADIOLOGICAL, OR NUCLEAR EVENT
- After a CBRN event, hospitals and emergency departments may have only enough resources available for patients who present relatively early after an event. Resource-allocation decisions will need to be made until additional resources become available.
- This means that some patients will receive treatment and others will not. The only option is to make hard resource-allocation decisions with appropriate field triage[302].

SCENE MANAGEMENT
The scene should be **isolated** to mitigate consequences. Effective scene management is required to control access to and from the incident scene, control movement of contaminated victims, provide safe working methods for responders, and contain the release of any substances.
Once first responders approach and arrive at the scene, the following actions will need to be initiated:
a. *Approach scene with caution and upwind;*
b. *Carry out scene assessment;*
c. *Establish incident command (each responding agency);*
d. *Recognize signs and indicators of CBRN incidents;*
e. *Determine whether CBRN or hazardous material incident;*
f. *Estimate the number of casualties/victims;*
g. *Estimate resource requirements;*
h. *Carry out primary triage, decontamination, secondary triage, medical care, and transport; and*
i. *Consider specialist advice/resource requirements*

CBRN CASUALTY MANAGEMENT ZONES
- A CBRN incident site will have three areas. Especially when responding to a chemical accident, one of the first things responders should do is to **establish a clean treatment area**, at least 300 yards upwind of the contaminated area.
- The clean treatment area is referred to as the ***cold zone***, while the contaminated area is called the ***hot zone***.
- Separating the hot and cold zones is the ***warm zone*** where decontamination occurs.

The warm zone should be **several hundred yards upwind** from the contamination and **at least 50 yards from the cold zone.**

---

[301] *European parliament, EU preparedness against CBRN weapons [pdf online]*

[302] *Iserson KV, Sanders AB, Mathieu D. Ethics in Emergency Medicine. 2nd ed. Tucson, AZ: Galen Press, Ltd; 1995.*

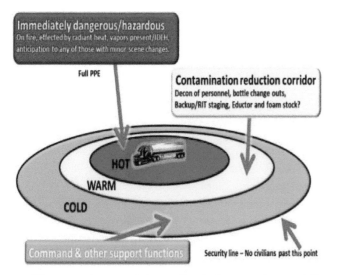

- All responders must leave the hot zone via specially designated pathways into the warm zone where they will be decontaminated[303].

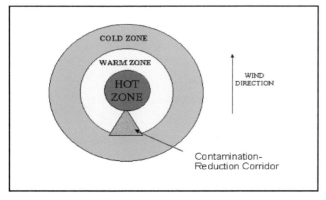

- **The hot line** separating the hot zone from the cold zone is an arbitrarily established line that demarcates the area of liquid-agent contamination from an area that is liquid-agent free. Once established, it should be clearly marked using engineer tape or another marker to ensure that liquid contamination or a person with potential liquid contamination does not cross into the clean area. This might necessitate the use of **concertina wire or armed guards**.
- **The only entrance to the clean treatment area is through the decontamination stations.**
- When the medical facility is set up in a clean area (no liquid contamination), the ground behind the hot line is clean except the holding area for contaminated casualties waiting to be evacuated and the routes traversed by the contaminated evacuation vehicles; these should be far to the side of the contaminated triage and treatment areas.

- In other circumstances, **the clean treatment area will be an oasis surrounded by the hot line.**
- No medical care is provided during this time or during the time spent waiting to begin the decontamination process. Therefore, before leaving the emergency care area, the patient must be stabilized to an extent that his condition will not deteriorate during this time.
- In a contaminated environment, emergency care is given by personnel in the highest level of mission-oriented protective posture, whose capabilities are limited by their protective gear.
- After receiving emergency care, a casualty must go through the decontamination station before receiving more definitive care in a clean environment.
- **Decontamination takes 10–20 minutes.**

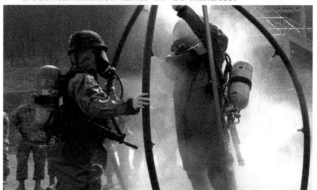

PERSONAL PROTECTIVE EQUIPMENT

All responders must take appropriate measures to protect themselves before entering the contaminated area.

Use of PPE[304] to protect airway, skin, and eyes is an indispensable component of emergency response.

Limitations to the use of PPE are **restriction of physical activity, dehydration, heat-related illness, and psychological effect**. To avoid this, emergency personnel should be trained to use PPE appropriately.

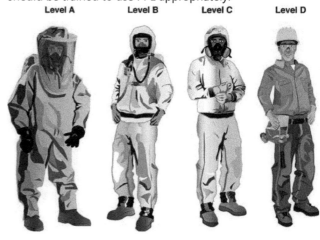

Level A   Level B   Level C   Level D

---

[303] Briggs Susan M, Cronin Michael. *The ABCs of Disaster Medical Response Manual for Providers* 2nd ed. International Trauma and Disaster Institute.

[304] Varela J. *Hazardous Materials Handbook for Emergency Responders.* New York: Van Nostrand Reinhold; 1996.

Level A PPE

- Denotes fully encapsulated suit, with over-gloves and overboots integrated into the suit. Respiratory protection is a self-contained breathing apparatus.
- Level A protection is required for **entry into an unknown hazardous environment**.

Level B PPE

- Denotes a hooded suit, double gloves, overboots, and a self-contained breathing apparatus, and may be used for decontamination procedures for an **unknown substance and for entry into hot zones where the agent is not caustic**.

Level C PPE

- It is similar to Level B, but uses an air-purifying respirator instead of a self-contained breathing apparatus.
- Level C PPE can be used **only after the hazardous substance has been identified**, and **upon verification of adequate oxygen in the environment**.

Level D PPE

- Level D protection consists of: 1. Coveralls 2. Gloves 3. Steel toe and shank boots (chemical-resistant) 4. Boot covers (disposable) 5. Safety glasses 6. Escape mask (optional) 7. Hard hat (optional) 8. Face shield (optional)
- It is used for "nuisance" level contaminants and offers minimal protection to the employer.

CBRN CASUALTIES TRIAGE

- The casualties can be initially triaged into **ambulatory** and **nonambulatory groups**. Ambulatory Casualties most often are classified as **minor** or **delayed.** However, even these casualties triaged as minor or delayed must be observed for worsening signs and symptoms.
- Victims may be classified as **expectant** when they have serious signs and symptoms after initial therapy or are **unresponsive** to antidotes.

TRIAGE ZONES

- In CBRN mass casualty incident, the site should be divided into zones/sectors and, in addition to the appointment of an overall triage officer, triage officers should be appointed for each of the identified zone.
- Field medical triage must be conducted at three levels:
  1. *On-site triage (Level 1)*
  2. *Medical triage (Level 2)*
  3. *Evacuation triage (Level 3)*

1. ON-SITE TRIAGE HOT ZONE (LEVEL 1)

- This is a rapid categorization of victims with potentially severe injuries needing immediate medical care "where they are lying" or at a triage site.

- Personnel are typically first responders from the local population or local emergency medical personnel. Patients are characterized as **"acute" or "non-acute"**. Simplified color coding may be done if resources permit: Acute = **Red**; Non-Acute = **Green**.
- During the initial response phase, first responders can use the **START Protocol** for the Primary Triage. "START" stands for Simple Triage and Rapid Treatment.
- The START protocol is intended to provide a simple technique to be used in conducting *Primary Triage* by the first rescuers arriving on scene. This will assist in quickly identifying those patients in need of *immediate treatment and transportation*.
- **Triage takes priority over emergency treatment.**
- All victims will need to be tagged. Emergency care administered by START teams is restricted to opening airways, controlling severe hemorrhage, and elevating patient's feet.
- Casualties will be tagged according to the seriousness of their conditions and placed into one of the following categories[305]:
  a. **Immediate (critical) = red tag =** Ventilations present after positioning the airway or ventilations are over 30 per minute or capillary refill greater than 2 seconds or no radial pulse or cannot follow simple command.
  b. **Delayed (urgent) = yellow tag =** Any patient not in the immediate or minor categories. These patients are generally non-ambulatory.
  c. **Minor (ambulatory) = green tag =** Any patient requiring medical attention who is not immediate or delayed and who is able to walk.
  d. **Deceased (expired) = black tag =** No ventilations present after the airway is opened.

2. MEDICAL TRIAGE COLD ZONE (LEVEL 2)

- Rapid categorization of victims at a casualty site by the most experienced medical personnel available to identify the level of medical care is needed.
- Personnel assigned to the treatment areas will perform a secondary exam and complete any required information on the triage tag. Emergency personnel are not required to follow the START protocol during secondary and subsequent triage. "The greatest good for the greatest number of people" has to be kept in mind.
- Knowledge of the medical consequences of various injuries (e.g., burn, blast, or crush injuries or exposure to chemical, biological, or nuclear weapons) is critical.

---

[305] *EMS Response for a Mass Casualty. Kootenai County M.C.I.Plan Protocol #108. 2006 Mar 31;*

- **Color coding may be used:**
  - o Casualties who require immediate life-saving interventions (airway, breathing, circulation): **Urgent.**
  - o Casualties who do not require immediate life-saving interventions and for whom treatment can be delayed: Delayed.
  - o Individuals who require minimal or no medical care: **Minor**[306].
  - o Casualties who are not expected to survive due to the severity of injuries complicated by the conditions and lack of resources: **Expectant/Deceased.**

I. RADIOLOGICAL ATTACK CONCERNS

Effects of a radiological dispersion device (RDD), also known as a "**dirty bomb,**" would produce injuries from heat, force of the explosion, debris, and radiological dust. A dirty bomb consists of radioactive material attached to a conventional bomb. Upon confirming the initial fatalities after an explosion, the future radiation can be determined.

This will be dependent upon the grade of radioactive material and the amount that has been released[307].

The health risks of exposure to radioactive material are dependent upon several factors: the amount of radiation received, known as the dose, and the length of time over which the dose is received. Radiation generally penetrates the body when exposed to beta particles and gamma rays.

- **Beta particles** can be a hazard to both bare skin and eyes by causing **burns.** If ingested or inhaled, **damage to internal organs** will occur in its victims.
- **Gamma radiation** travels hundreds of meters in open air and penetrates most objects. Gamma rays penetrate tissue farther than do beta or alpha particles. Gamma rays **can cause death**.
- **Alpha particles** do not damage living tissue when outside the body; however, when alpha emitting atoms are inhaled or swallowed, they especially are damaging because they transfer relatively large amounts of ionizing energy to living cells. **Damage to internal organs** will occur in these victims.

2. BIOLOGICAL ATTACK CONCERNS

- Biological weapons are weapons that achieve their intended effects by infecting people with disease-causing microorganisms and other replicative entities, including viruses, infectious nucleic acids and prions.
- The chief characteristic of biological agents is their ability to multiply in a host over time.

- The disease they may cause is the result of the interaction between the biological agent, the host (including the host's genetic constitution, nutritional status and the immunological status of the host's population) and the environment (e.g., sanitation, temperature, water quality, population density). Biological agents are commonly classified according to their taxonomy (e.g., fungi, bacteria, viruses).
- **The infectivity of an agent** is its capability to enter, survive and multiply in a host, and may be expressed as the proportion of persons exposed to a given dose who become infected.
- **Virulence** is the relative severity of the disease caused by a microorganism (i.e., the ratio of clinical cases to the number of infected hosts). Different strains of the same microorganism may cause diseases of different severity.
- **Lethality** is the ability of an agent to cause death in an infected population.
- **Pathogenicity** is the capacity of a microorganism to cause disease, and is measured by the ratio of the number of clinical cases to the number of exposed persons.
- The incubation period is the time between exposure to an infective agent and the first appearance of the signs and symptoms of disease. The incubation period can be affected by many variables, such as the initial dose, virulence, route of entry, rate of replication, and the immunological status of the host.
- For those infections that are contagious, a measure of their contagiousness is the number of secondary cases following exposure to a primary case in relation to the total number of exposed susceptible secondary contacts.
- The mechanisms of transmission involved may be direct (i.e., direct contact between an infected and an uninfected person) or indirect. (i.e., through inanimate material that has become contaminated with the agent, such as soil, blood, bedding, clothes, surgical instruments, water, food or milk).
- Infections may also be through airborne droplets (i.e., through coughing or sneezing) or through vectors, such as biting insects. The distinction between types of transmission is important in selecting control measures.
- For example, direct transmission can be interrupted by appropriate handling of infected persons, while interrupting indirect transmission requires other approaches, such as adequate ventilation, chlorination of water, or vector control.
- **Stability** is the ability of the agent to survive the influence of environmental factors such as air pollution, sunlight and extreme temperatures or humidity.

---

[306] Ryan JM Eur J Trauma Emerg Surg. 2008 Oct; 34(5):427.

[307] Hrdina CM, Coleman CN, Bogucki S, Bader JL, Hayhurst RE, Forsha JD, Marcozzi D, Yeskey K, Knebel AR Prehosp Disaster Med. 2009 May-Jun; 24(3):167-78.

3. CHEMICAL ATTACK CONCERNS

- Chemical weapons are those that are effective because of their toxicity: that is, their chemical action can cause death, permanent harm or temporary incapacity.
- Delaying medical care for casualties who are categorized into "delayed" group may not change or affect adversely the outcome of progress.
- Therefore, taking basic life support measures for this triage category and then providing the discharge to treatment centers can be beneficial for other chemical casualties with severe injuries in immediate category to improve the survival rate[308]. Weapons that use chemicals as propellants, explosives, incendiaries or obscurants are not chemical weapons, even though the chemicals in them may also have toxic effects. Only weapons whose main goal is to have toxic effects are considered chemical weapons.
- Some toxic chemicals, such as **phosgene, hydrogen cyanide and tear gas,** may be used for both civil and peaceful, and hostile purposes. When they are used for hostile purposes, they are considered chemical weapons.
- A common way to classify chemical agents is according to the degree of effect (e.g., harassing, incapacitating or lethal).
- **A harassing agent** disables exposed people for as long as they remain exposed. They are acutely aware of discomfort, but usually able to remove themselves from exposure to it unless they are otherwise constrained. They usually recover fully a short time after exposure ends, and do not require medical treatment.
- **An incapacitating agent** also disables, but people exposed to it may not be aware of their predicament (e.g., certain psychotropic agents), or may be unable to function or move away from the exposed environment. The effect may be prolonged, but recovery may not require specialized medical aid.
- **A lethal agent causes** death for those exposed. This approach to classifying chemical agents is not particularly precise because the effects of chemical agents will depend on the dose received, and on the health and other factors that affect how susceptible people are to the agent. For example, tear gas is usually a harassing agent, but it can be lethal if a person is exposed to a large quantity in a small closed space.
- On the other hand, **nerve agents** are usually lethal, but may only incapacitate people who are exposed to a low concentration for a short time. If it is not possible to totally protect people from the chemical weapons, protective measures should try to reduce their effect. For example, the use of pre-treatment and antidotes in a nerve gas victim is unlikely to provide a complete "cure", but may reduce what would have been a lethal effect to an incapacitating one.

- Another form of classifying chemical agents is based on their effects on the body:
  o **Nerve agents** gain access to the body usually through the skin or lungs, and cause systemic effects.
  o **Respiratory agents** are inhaled and either cause damage to the lungs, or are absorbed there and cause systemic effects.
  o **Blister agents** are absorbed through the skin, either damaging it (e.g., mustard gas) or gaining access to the body to cause systemic effects (e.g. nerve agents), or both.
- A further classification is based on the duration of the hazard:
  o **Persistent agents** remain in the area where they are applied for long periods (sometimes up to a few weeks). They are generally substances of low volatility that contaminate surfaces and have the potential to damage the skin if they come into contact with it. A secondary danger is inhalation of any vapours that may be released. **Mustard gas and VX** are persistent agents.
  o **Non-persistent agents** are volatile substances that evaporate or disperse quickly, and may be used to cause casualties in an area that the group using the weapons wants to occupy soon after. Surfaces are generally not contaminated. The primary danger is from inhalation, secondary from skin exposure. Respirators are the main form of protection required. Protective clothing may not be necessary if concentrations are below skin toxicity levels. Hydrogen cyanide and phosgene are typical non-persistent agents.
- Chemical agents are often grouped according to their effect on the body, based on the primary organ system affected by exposure. Typical classes include:
  o Nerve agents or "gases" (e.g., SARIN, VX, VR)
  o Blood gases or systemic agents (e.g., hydrogen cyanide)
  o Vesicants or skin blistering agents (e.g., mustard gas, lewisite)
  o Lung irritants, asphyxiants or choking agents (e.g., chlorine, phosgene)

3. EVACUATION TRIAGE-LOADING ZONE (LEVEL 3)
There are several indications for evacuation in a disaster:
a. To decompress the disaster area;
b. To improve care for most critical casualties by removal to off-site medical facilities; and
c. To provide specialized care for specific casualties, such as those with burns and crush injuries

There are also several reasons to delay or defer evacuation of some casualties. These include:
a. Contaminated casualties;
b. Casualties with transmissible diseases; and
c. Unstable casualties

---

308 Briggs Susan M, Cronin Michael. *The ABCs of Disaster Medical Response Manual for Providers* 2nd ed. International Trauma and Disaster Institute. [Cited in 2010]. Available from: http://www.hospitalesseguros.crid or cr/pdf/abc_2nd_edition.pdf .

26. Observational Medicine

OVERVIEW

- Observation ward is a short stay ward
- Integral part of the emergency department
- Staffed by the emergency department
- Has defined admission and discharge criteria
- Admission of specific diagnostic related groups
- Has a focused multidisciplinary approach

PRINCIPLES OF OBSERVATION MEDICINE

- The defining characteristic of emergency medicine is "time," or the acuity of disease presentation.
- Observation, like resuscitation, involves the management of time-sensitive conditions.
- In the ED there is a continuum of time-sensitive conditions. This continuum extends from resuscitation on one end to observation on the other.
- When performed well, observation services have been shown to improve diagnostic accuracy, improve treatment outcomes, decrease costs, and improve patient satisfaction.
- For the subset of ED patients who would have been inappropriately discharged or unnecessarily admitted, the observation unit (OU) has become a safety net of the ED itself. Like EDs, OUs have progressed from being poorly managed areas of the hospital to the cutting edge of acute health care.
- The principles developed through past experience and research provide a framework for future developments in emergency medicine.
- Observation medicine encompasses the management of selected patients for a timeframe of 6 to 24 hours to assess their need for inpatient admission. This service is best provided in a dedicated observation unit, ideally in the Emergency Department. Relative to traditional admission, studies have shown this alternative to have several beneficial health care outcomes:
  - *Improved patient satisfaction*
  - *Lower health care costs*
  - *Shorter length of stays*
  - *Improved use of hospital resources*
  - *Less diagnostic uncertainty*
- Across the country, hospital emergency departments are being stretched beyond capacity. Increased emergency room admissions lead to bottlenecking, overcrowding, longer wait times, and inefficient use of resources.

- Observation medicine involves the assessment and care of patients who do not meet criteria for inpatient status, but need further evaluation and treatment with anticipated stays of up to 24 hours.
- Ideally, observation medicine is offered in a dedicated unit under the direction of the emergency department.

DIAGNOSES APPROPRIATE FOR OBS WARD

Specific diagnosis related groups (DRGs) examples

- Minor head injury
- Drug overdose
- Intoxication
- Renal colic
- Mild-moderate pyelonephritis
- Musculoskeletal low back pain
- Elderly patients not suitable for discharge at night, but no other barriers to discharge

ADVANTAGES FOR THE HOSPITAL

- Shorter admission time: On average, the admission rates from ED to inpatient services are 13.3%.[309]
- Thus, cost savings and decreased average length of stay
- Acts as a safety net
- Decreased incorrect discharge and thus decreased litigation

ADVANTAGES FOR THE ED

- Streamed lined treatment pathway
- Decompression of ED
- Assessment for intoxicated patients

ADVANTAGES FOR THE PATIENT

- Access to experts in DSH and Psychiatry
- Crisis intervention
- Prevents inappropriate discharge for example elderly late at night

DISADVANTAGES

- Fragmentation of care of patients who will require admission
- Inappropriate admission
- Problematic discharge, d/c with inadequate assessment and community social support
- Resources for ED diverted

---

[309] *Centers for Disease Control and Prevention. Fast stats. Centers for Disease Control and Prevention. [Online]*

27. Oncology Emergencies
I. MULTIPLE MYELOMA

DEFINITION

- Multiple myeloma (MM) is a debilitating malignancy that is part of a spectrum of diseases ranging from monoclonal gammopathy of unknown significance (MGUS) to plasma cell leukemia.
- Multiple myeloma is the most common primary bone tumor in people over 40 years old, and peak incidence occurs in the seventh decade of life. It represents 10-15% of hematologic neoplasms and 1% of all cancer deaths[310].
- MM is characterized by a proliferation of malignant plasma cells and a subsequent overabundance of monoclonal paraprotein (M protein).
- Bone marrow aspirate demonstrating plasma cells of multiple myeloma. Note the blue cytoplasm, eccentric nucleus, and perinuclear pale zone (or halo).

SIGNS AND SYMPTOMS

- Bone pain, Pathologic fractures
- Spinal cord compression (from pathologic fracture)
- Weakness, malaise
- Bleeding, anemia, Infection (often pneumococcal)
- Hypercalcemia, Renal failure, Neuropathies

DIAGNOSIS

- **HEENT examination:** Exudative macular detachment, retinal hemorrhage, or cotton-wool spots
- **Dermatologic evaluation:** Pallor from anemia, ecchymoses or purpura from thrombocytopenia; extramedullary plasmacytomas (most commonly in aerodigestive tract but also orbital, ear canal, cutaneous, gastric, rectal, prostatic, retroperitoneal areas)
- **Musculoskeletal examination:** Bony tenderness or pain without tenderness
- **Neurologic assessment:** Sensory level change (ie, loss of sensation below a dermatome corresponding to a spinal cord compression), neuropathy, myopathy, positive Tinel sign, or positive Phalen sign
- **Abdominal examination:** Hepatosplenomegaly
- **Cardiovascular evaluation:** Cardiomegaly

Diagnostic criteria

In 2003, the International Myeloma Working Group agreed on diagnostic criteria for symptomatic myeloma, asymptomatic myeloma and MGUS, which was subsequently updated in 2009:

- Symptomatic myeloma (all three criteria must be met):
  1. Clonal plasma cells >10% on bone marrow biopsy or (in any quantity) in a biopsy from other tissues (plasmacytoma)
  2. A monoclonal protein (Myeloma protein) in either serum or urine (except in cases of true non-secretory myeloma)
  3. Evidence of end-organ damage felt related to the plasma cell disorder (related organ or tissue impairment, commonly referred to by the acronym "CRAB"):
     - Hyper**C**alcemia (corrected calcium >2.75 mmol/l, >11 mg/dl)
     - **R**enal insufficiency attributable to myeloma
     - **A**nemia (hemoglobin <10 g/dl)
     - **B**one lesions (lytic lesions or osteoporosis with compression fractures)

- ❖ Emergency physicians should suspect multiple myeloma based on pathologic fractures, back or bone pain at rest, normocytic anemia, and renal failure in an older patient. On exam, signs of amyloid deposition such as macroglossia, retinal hemorrhage, cotton wool spots, macular detachment, carpal tunnel compression, and cardiomegaly suggest the diagnosis, however these are usually late findings[311].

In patients with MM and amyloidosis, the characteristic examination findings include the following:

- Shoulder pad sign
- Macroglossia
- Typical skin lesions
- Post-proctoscopic peripalpebral purpura (eyelid purpura may also follow coughing, vomiting, the Valsalva maneuver, or forced expiration during spirometric testing)
- Carpal tunnel syndrome
- Subcutaneous nodules

---

[310] Hillman RS, Ault KA. Hematology in clinical practice. 5th ed. New York: McGraw-Hill Medical; 2011.

[311] Moses MDS. Multiple Myeloma. Family Practice Notebook. [Online]

Testing

- Serum and urine assessment for monoclonal protein (densitometer tracing and nephelometric quantitation; immunofixation for confirmation)
- Serum free light chain assay (in all patients with newly diagnosed plasma cell dyscrasias)
- Bone marrow aspiration and/or biopsy
- Serum beta2-microglobulin, albumin, and lactate dehydrogenase measurement
- Standard metaphase cytogenetics
- Fluorescence in situ hybridization
- Skeletal survey
- MRI

Routine laboratory tests include the following:

- Full blood count and differential
- Erythrocyte sedimentation rate
- Comprehensive metabolic panel (eg, levels of total protein, albumin and globulin, BUN, creatinine, uric acid)
- 24-hour urine collection for quantification of the **Bence Jones protein** (ie, lambda light chains), protein, and creatinine clearance; proteinuria greater than 1 g/24 hr is a major criterion
- C-reactive protein
- Serum viscosity in patients with CNS symptoms, nosebleeds, or very high M protein levels

Imaging studies

- **Simple radiography** for the evaluation of skeleton lesions; skeletal survey, including the skull, long bones, and spine

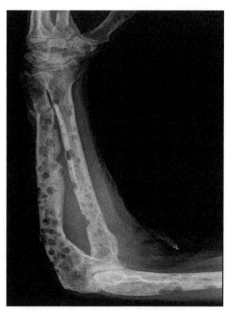

X-ray of the forearm, with lytic lesions.

- **MRI** for detecting thoracic and lumbar spine lesions, paraspinal involvement, and early cord compression.

- **PET scanning** in conjunction with MRI potentially useful

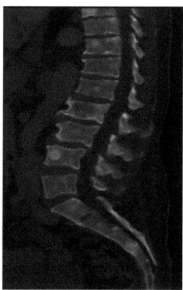

CT scan of the lower vertebral column in a man with multiple myeloma, showing multiple osteoblastic lesions.
These are more radiodense (brighter in this image) than the surrounding cancellous bone, in contrast to osteolytic lesions which are less radiodense.

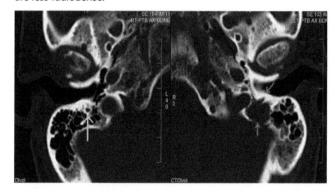

A CT of the brain revealed a lytic lesion in the left temporal bone(right side of image), and petroustemporal bones involving the mastoid segment of the facial nerve canal. Red arrows: lesion; green arrow: normal contralateral facial nerve canal. The lesions are consistent with a myeloma deposit.

- These lytic lesions and compressions fractures are often the cause of back pain in multiple myeloma patients. Cord compression can present without any significant neurologic deficit, and the progression to irreversible paraplegia can be abrupt. Emergency physicians must maintain a low threshold for obtaining a spinal MRI and emergent surgical consultation in the multiple myeloma patient with suspected epidural involvement.
- **Initial management** of cord compression includes initiation of steroids (dexamethasone 16 mg IV or PO daily) and emergent neurosurgical consultation for laminectomy or decompression

II. METASTATIC SPINAL CORD COMPRESSION

INTRODUCTION

- Metastatic spinal cord compression (MSCC) is one of the ominous causes of back pain where there is a compression of the thecal sac and its components by tumour mass. This is a true spinal emergency, and if the pressure on the spinal cord is not relieved quickly, it may result in irreversible loss of neurologic function.
- The most important prognostic factor for functional outcome is neurologic function before treatment[312]. Hence, any delay could result in poorer functional outcome and decreased quality of life, with increased dependence on healthcare resources. There is a need for improving awareness among all clinicians so as to make prompt diagnosis and referral of MSCC a reality[313].

CLINICAL PRESENTATION

- The most common presenting feature for spinal metastases is increasing **back pain**.
- The pain may be localised or generalised and is due to compression, pathological fractures, or axial pain from mechanical instability. It often increases in recumbent position or with activities such as sneezing or coughing secondary to distension of the epidural venous plexus.
- **Radicular pain** may develop due to nerve root compression by the tumour or secondary to vertebral collapse. It is important however to bear in mind that patients might present with backache totally unrelated to MSCC and some patients with MSCC experience no backache

When to think of metastatic spinal cord compression:

Low index of suspicion	High index of suspicion
• Persistent back pain localised to an area • No neurological signs • No cancer diagnosis • No bowel or bladder symptoms	• Known cancer diagnosis with bone metastases • Night-time pain during movements • Band-like bilateral nerve root pain/radiculopathy • Unsteadiness of gait • Progressive weakness of limbs • Bowel and bladder symptoms

- Usually the progression to sensori-motor deficits and

bladder and bowel dysfunction occurs slowly. Heaviness or clumsiness of limbs may be an early sign of motor deficits. Sensory deficits include anaesthesia, hyperaesthesia, or paraesthesia in the involved dermatomes. Autonomic dysfunction with bowel and bladder problems is associated with a poorer prognosis and irreversibility of functional recovery.

- In patients with undiagnosed cancers, using detailed history taking and physical examination coupled with awareness of red flags would increase chances of detection of suspected cases of MSCC. One needs to explore other cancer symptoms such as anorexia, weight loss, lymphadenopathy, cough, and bowel and bladder symptoms.
- **Physical examination** findings may vary from isolated spinal tenderness with no definite neurology to hard neurological signs with deficits.

INVESTIGATIONS

Laboratory tests:
- Urinalysis
- FBC, U&Es, LFT, ESR,

Imaging studies:
- Plain radiography
- MRI is the imaging modality of choice.

Plain films of the spine frequently demonstrate associated vertebral blastic or lytic lesions. However, gadolinium-enhanced MRI provides the best definition of spinal lesions. Magnetic resonance imaging not only shows cord compression caused by extra dural masses but also shows paravertebral masses, intramedullary disease, and bone metastasis. Magnetic resonance imaging of the entire spine should be ordered, because approximately 10% to 30% of patients with clinical symptoms of SCC have multiple lesions. **Lumbar puncture** is contraindicated because removal of cerebrospinal fluid may worsen the MSCC.

TREATMENT

Treatment is palliative in most cases, but goals are relief of pain and maintenance or restoration of neurologic function. Other goals include spinal column stabilization and local tumor control.

Dexamethasone is started to reduce the edema and cord compression caused by the tumor mass and to thereby relieve the pain.

Refer to medical oncologist:
- Radiation Therapy
- Chemotherapy

---

312 Bach F, Larsen BH, Rohde K, et al. (1990) Metastatic spinal cord compression. Occurrence, symptoms, clinical presentations and prognosis in 398 patients with spinal cord compression. Acta Neurochir **107**(1–2):37–43.

313 Husband DJ (1998) Malignant spinal cord compression: prospective study of delays in referral and treatment. BMJ **317**(7150):18–21.

III. SPINAL METASTASIS

INTRODUCTION

- Spinal metastasis is common in patients with cancer[314]. The spine is the third most common site for cancer cells to metastasize, following the lung and the liver.
- This amounts to 70% of all osseous metastases.
- Approximately 5-30% of patients with systemic cancer will have spinal metastasis; some studies have estimated that 30-70% of patients with a primary tumor have spinal metastatic disease at autopsy. Spinal metastases are slightly more common in men than in women and in adults aged 40-65 years than in others.
- Fortunately, only 10% of these patients are symptomatic, and approximately 94-98% of those patients present with epidural and/or vertebral involvement.
- Intradural extramedullary and intramedullary seeding of systemic cancer is unusual; they account for 5-6% and 0.5-1% of spinal metastases, respectively.

HISTORY

- **Bone pain at night** in a patient with systemic cancer is always an ominous symptom. In fact, it is the most ominous symptom in patients with metastatic disease to the spine. Not all spinal metastasis result in neurological deficit, only 50% of these patients have sensory and motor dysfunction, and 50% have bowel and bladder dysfunction.
- A small group of (5-10%) of patients with cancer present with cord compression as their initial symptom. Among those who present with cord compression, 50% are nonambulatory at diagnosis, and 15% are paraplegic. Cord compression is commonly seen as a preterminal event in cancer patients.

IMAGING STUDIES

- In patients with rapidly progressing symptoms, chest radiography and physical examination is all that is warranted.
- Plain radiography and, whenever possible, a CT of the entire spine should then be performed, followed by MRI with and without contrast enhancement.
- **Plain radiography** is used to show erosion of the pedicles or the vertebral body. Owl-eye erosion of the pedicles in the anteroposterior (AP) view of lumbar spine is characteristic of metastatic disease and is observed in 90% of symptomatic patients.

- However, radiologic findings become apparent only when bone destruction reaches 30-50%.
- Osteoblastic or osteosclerotic changes are common in prostate cancer and Hodgkin disease; they are occasionally seen in breast cancer and lymphoma.
- **CT scanning** is useful in determining the integrity of the vertebral column, especially when surgery is anticipated.
- **CT myelography** is used if MRI is not available. CT also allows for an examination of paraspinal soft tissues and paraspinal lymph nodes.
- **Emergency myelography** is still used in situations where an MRI is not available.
- The advantage of an MRI is its noninvasive nature, whereas myelography allows for cerebrospinal fluid (CSF) sampling. CSF sampling should be deferred if evidence of near-complete or complete spinal block is noted. The risk of neurologic deterioration after myelography is about 14% but is less likely with C1-2 puncture. With MRI, the sagittal scout image is used for rapid screening of the entire spinal axis and its surrounding soft tissues.
- **MRI** is the imaging modality of choice. Contrast-enhanced fat-suppressed images help to differentiate metastasis from degenerative bone marrow. Diffusion-weighted images distinguish metastasis from osteoporotic bone. Osteoporotic fractures are hypointense, and metastases are hyperintense. See the image below.
- **Bone scanning:** Bone scans are positive in 60% of patients but they are not specific. Lesions that activate bone metabolism increase technetium-99m uptake.
- **Nuclear studies** are useful to determine cancer burden and are effective in scanning the entire axial and appendicular skeleton.
- The use of single photon emission CT (SPECT) and positron emission tomography (PET)-CT allow for rapid screening and staging of systemic disease.
- In many ways, this PET-CT is a standard modality to stage systemic disease and tumor burden, and it is extremely useful in guiding the aggressiveness of surgical management of metastatic disease to the spine.

ED MANAGEMENT

- **Spinal cord compression** is an oncological emergency and treatment should be started within 24 hours.
- Most patients will be given **steroids** and will need **radiotherapy or surgery**.
- Patients with a risk of spinal instability should be nursed flat in neutral alignment.

---

[314] Abeloff MD, Armitage JO, Niederhuber JE, Kastan MB, McKenna WG. Abeloff's *Clinical Oncology. 4th edition. Philadelphia, Pa, USA: Churchill Livngstone Elsevier; 2008.*

IV. SVC COMPRESSION SYNDROME

A 48-year-old woman presents with a 2-week history of progressive dyspnea on exertion, neck swelling, decreased appetite, and fatigue. There is no history of syncope or dysphagia. She smokes 20 cigarettes a day for 22 years.

The physical examination reveals a heart rate of 105 beats per minute, a respiratory rate of 20 breaths per minute, and superficial vascular distention over the neck, chest, and upper abdomen. Stridor is not present.

How should his case be evaluated and managed?

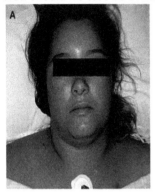 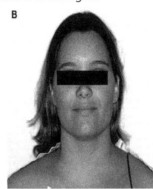

The Superior Vena Cava Syndrome.

ANATOMY AND PHYSIOLOGY

- The SVC transports blood from the head and neck, upper extremities, and parts of the chest toward the heart.
- It carries approximately one third of the total venous return to the heart. SVC compression can be caused by tumor masses in the middle or anterior mediastinum, usually to the right of the midline.
- Cardiac output may be transiently diminished due to acute SVC obstruction, but within a few hours usually an increased venous pressure and collaterals achieve a novel steady state of blood return. Hemodynamic compromise is usually a result of mass effect on the heart rather than the SVC compression[315].
- Because of its relatively thin wall, compared to the aorta or trachea, and the low venous pressure, the SVC is among the first of the mediastinal structures to be obstructed. If the SVC becomes obstructed, blood flows through multiple smaller collaterals to the azygos vein or the inferior vena cava.
- These venous collaterals usually become dilated over several weeks, so that the upper body venous pressure is markedly elevated initially, but decreases over time[316].

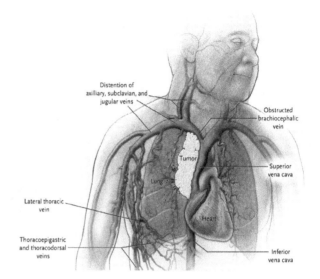

ETIOLOGIC FACTORS

- Mainly due to infectious disease (syphilis and tuberculosis) for several centuries, the primary cause of SVCS changed to malignancies some 25 years ago, and malignancies now account for up to 90% of all SVCS[317].
- In recent years thrombotic complications have increasingly occurred, reflecting the increased use of intravascular devices such as catheters, port-a-caths, pacemakers, and implantable defibrillators[318].
- Malignant Causes of the Superior Vena Cava Syndrome:

Tumor type	%	Suggestive clinical features
Non small-cell lung cancer	50	Hx of smoking, Often age >50yr
Small-cell lung cancer	22	Hx of smoking, Often age >50yr
Lymphoma	12	Adenopathy outside the chest, often age < 65yr
Metastatic cancer	9	Hx of malignant condition (usually breast Ca)
Germ-cell cancer	3	Usually, male sex Age < 40yr; elevated levels of β HCG or α-fetoprotein
Thymoma	2	Characteristic radiographic appearance on the basis of the location of the thymus; frequently associated with the parathymic syndromes
Mesothelioma	1	Hx of asbestos exposure

[315] Wilson LD, Detterbeck FC, Yahalom J. Clinical practice. Superior vena cava syndrome with malignant causes. N Engl J Med 2007;**356**(18):1862–1869.

[316] Trigaux JP, Van BB. Thoracic collateral venous channels: normal and pathologic CT findings. J Comput Assist Tomogr 1990;**14**(5):769–773.

[317] Chen JC, Bongard F, Klein SR. A contemporary perspective on superior vena cava syndrome. Am J Surg 1990;**160**(2):207–211.

[318] Rice TW, Rodriguez RM, Light RW. The superior vena cava syndrome: clinical characteristics and evolving etiology. Medicine (Baltimore) 2006;**85**(1):37–42.

CLINICAL EVALUATION

Symptoms and Signs Associated with the **Superior Vena Cava Syndrome:**

- *Facial edema*
- *Arm edema*
- *Distended neck veins*
- *Distended chest veins*
- *Facial plethora*
- *Visual symptoms*
- *Dyspnoea, Cough*
- *Hoarseness, Stridor*
- *Headaches, Dizziness, Syncope*
- *Confusion, Obtundation*

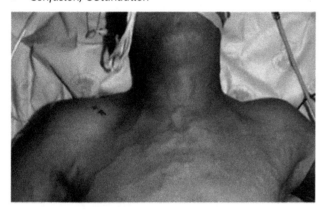

- Clinical diagnosis of obstruction of the superior vena cava is made on the basis of signs and symptoms above.
- The history taking should attend to the duration of symptoms, previous diagnoses of malignant conditions, or previous intravascular procedures.
- In most cases, symptoms are progressive over several weeks, and in some cases, they may improve as collateral circulation develops. The severity of the symptoms is important in determining the urgency of intervention.

IMAGING

Patients presenting with overt superior vena cava syndrome (SVCS) may be diagnosed by means of physical examination alone. However, subtle presentations necessitate diagnostic imaging.

Chest radiography:

- CXR may reveal a widened mediastinum or a mass in the right side of the chest.

Computed tomography (CT)

- CT has the advantage of providing more accurate information on the location of the obstruction and may guide attempts at biopsy by mediastinoscopy, bronchoscopy, or percutaneous fine-needle aspiration. It also provides information on other critical structures, such as the bronchi and the vocal cords.
- **A CT scan of the chest** is the initial test of choice to determine whether an obstruction is due to external compression or due to thrombosis.

- The additional information is necessary because the involvement of these structures requires prompt action for relief of pressure.

Gallium Single-Proton Emission CT (SPECT)

- SPECT may be of value in select cases.

Magnetic Resonance Imaging (MRI)

- MRI has not yet been sufficiently investigated in this setting, but it appears promising.
- It has several potential advantages over CT, in that it provides images in several planes of view, allows direct visualization of blood flow, and does not require iodinated contrast material (an especially important characteristic when stenting is anticipated).
- MRI is an acceptable alternative for patients with renal failure or those with contrast allergies.

Venography

- Invasive contrast venography is the most conclusive diagnostic tool (see the image below).
- It precisely defines the etiology of obstruction.
- It is especially important if surgical management is being considered for the obstructed vena cava.

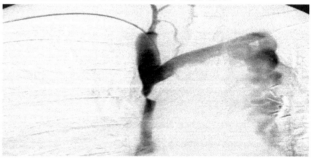

Radionuclide Technetium-99m Venography

- It is an alternative minimally invasive method of imaging the venous system.

MANAGEMENT

- In the management of superior vena cava syndrome (SVCS), the goals are to relieve symptoms and to attempt cure of the primary malignant process.
- Only a small percentage of patients with rapid-onset obstruction of the superior vena cava (SVC) are at risk for life-threatening complications.
- Patients with clinical SVCS often gain significant symptomatic improvement from conservative treatment measures, including **elevation of the head of the bed and supplemental oxygen**.
- **Corticosteroids and diuretics** are often used to relieve laryngeal or cerebral edema, although documentation of their efficacy is questionable.
- **Radiotherapy** has been advocated as a standard treatment for most patients with SVCS. **Chemotherapy** may be preferable to radiation for patients with chemosensitive tumors.

V. RAISED ICP IN CANCER

INTRODUCTION

- Increased intracranial pressure due to metastatic brain disease is one of the oncological emergencies.
- It may cause herniation or insufficient brain blood flow; thus, it is a life-threatening condition.
- In patients with cancer, a frequent neurologic emergency is the development of elevated intracranial pressure (ICP).
- When it is not appropriately managed, elevated ICP rapidly results in irreversible neurologic deficits and death. Cerebral perfusion pressure is equal to the difference between the mean arterial pressure and intracranial pressure; hence, elevated ICP if left untreated results in cerebral ischemia[319].
- A rise in ICP also places patients at risk for herniation since it leads to the development of a pressure gradient, which the brain attempts to normalize by shifting the contents of one compartment into the adjacent, lower pressure, compartment[320].
- Nevertheless, with ICP over 200-250 mm any further volume increase is followed by disproportionate rise of pressure.
- The consequence may be impaired **cerebral perfusion pressure** (CPP = mean blood pressure – ICP), described as plateau waves when lasting over 5 minutes. Unless they last longer than 30-40 minutes the prognosis is not getting worse.
- With ICP over 40-50 mm Hg cerebral blood flow becomes insufficient leading to permanent brain damage.
- The immediate reason for herniation is the gradient in the intracranial compartmental pressure. It causes parenchymal tissue shifts with impairment of different structures depending on location.
- Ischemia or infarction from vascular compression may cause oedema and further deterioration in compliance.

  o Normal ICP: 10-20mmHg
  o CPP is closely linked to ICP
  o CPP=MAP-ICP
  o Normal CPP=70 to 100
  o A CPP of less than 50 results in permanent brain damage

[319] Stocchetti N, Maas AI, Chieregato A, van der Plas AA. Hyperventilation in head injury: a review. Chest. 2005;127:1812–1827.

[320] Gower DJ, Baker AL, Bell WO, Ball MR. Contraindications to lumbar puncture as defined by computed cranial tomography. J Neurol Neurosurg Psychiatry. 1987;50:1071–1074.

ETIOLOGY

Five primary tumours account for 80% of brain metastases:
1. Lung cancer
2. Renal cell carcinoma
3. Breast cancer
4. Melanoma
5. Colorectal carcinoma
6. Thyroid

Primary factors that influence elevated ICP include:
- Blood pressure
- Heart function
- Intra-abdominal/Intrathoracic
- Temperature
- Pain
- Carbon Dioxide/Acidosis
- Hypoxia

SYMPTOMS

- **Patient Presentation:**
  o Decreased LOC (subtle)
  o Decreased Motor function
  o Increased Restlessness
  o Nausea & vomiting
  o Sensory deficits
  o Headache
  o Visual changes
  o Seizures
  o Pupil changes

- **Vital Signs:**
  o Elevated BP with no obvious cause
  o Rising systolic pressure
  o Widening pulse pressure
  o Bradycardia

Cushing's Triad:
o Hypertension
o Bradycardia
o Irregular respirations

HEADACHE AND RAISED ICP

- Features of headache that suggest raised intracranial pressure are: **headache which is worse on bending down or lying down, so tends to be worse on waking.**
- Valsalva manoevres, exertion, coughing, vomiting and straining may all exacerbate the headache.
- Associated symptoms that suggest raised intracranial pressure are: lethargy, nausea, fluctuating level of consciousness (GCS), visual obscurations, diplopia and pulsatile tinnitus.

- Visual obscurations (photopsias) are brief (seconds) episodes of loss of vision associated with manoevres that increased ICP, such as bending over. They are thought to be due to critical ischaemia of the optic nerve head.
- Any symptoms suggestive of a brain tumour would also support a diagnosis of raised intracranial pressure (either from a primary tumour or from metastases). This would include symptoms of personality change, abnormal behaviour, seizure or neurological deficit. Systemic symptoms of malignancy, such as weight loss, bone pain and night sweats should also be elicited, as should any previous history of malignancy or HIV infection.

DIAGNOSIS

- The most important diagnostic tools are the history and clinical examination. With the initial presumption and the patient stabilised neuroimaging should be obtained.
- **Cranial computed tomography (CT)** is preferred over Magnetic Resonance Imaging (MRI) due to availability and speed of imaging. CT Scan is often the first line of imaging, contrast enhanced CT was previously thought to be equivalent to MRI for the detection of metastases. However, current MRI technology has been shown to be more sensitive than CT and is the preferred imaging of choice.
- Raised intracranial pressure is suggested by the following CT features:
  - Signs of mass effect, including effacement of the anterior horns of the lateral ventricles and effacement of the sulci. (These signs all indicate loss of CSF -containing spaces, ie a "tight" brain. At the level of the brainstem, reduction in the size of the basilar cisterns may also be seen).
  - In addition there is some loss of grey-white differentiation. This reflects global brain ischaemia due to reduced cerebral perfusion pressure secondary to raised ICP.

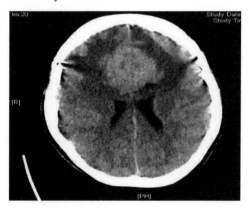

- **MRI and MR venography** can accurately diagnose cerebral sinus thrombosis in cancer patients.
- **Lumbar puncture** allows CSF pressure measurement.

Intracranial hypertension is defined as a sustained (>5 min) elevation of the ICP of >20 mmHg. However, there are no indications for ICP monitoring in cancer patients.

- Lumbar puncture is a necessity in certain clinical situations like making an **accurate diagnosis of cryptococcal meningitis**
- Contraindication for lumbar puncture is **compartmentalisation,** revealed by CT scan.
- Compartmentalisation is a result of obstructive hydrocephalus or obliteration of basal cisterns due to herniation. Thus, CT inevitably precedes while there is a serious risk of initiating or exacerbating the herniation.
- **Transcranial Doppler ultrasonography** is helpful in monitoring cerebral perfusion in patients with increased ICP. Management While increased intracranial pressure occurs as a heterogenous group of conditions, treatment of acute hypertension requires a thorough understanding of its pathophysiology.

ED MANAGEMENT

Symptomatic treatment

- Start with assessment for adequate **A**irway, **B**reathing, **C**irculation and **D**isability
- Patient's **head should be elevated to 30 degrees** in order to facilitate cerebral venous drainage.
- **Hyperthermia** is treated with antipyretics.
- Correct hyponatraemia
- Control Blood pressure: **labetalol, esmolol and nicardipine** are recommended, whereas phenylephrine, norepinephrine and dopamine can be used to raise BP.
- **Corticosteroid therapy** is initiated for vasogenic oedema resulting from brain tumours, abscesses or non-infectious neuroinflammatory conditions with a starting dose of **4–8 mg/day of dexamethasone**. If patients exhibit severe symptoms higher doses such as 16 mg/day or more are considered.
- **Monitoring of serum osmolality** is required with a target level of **300 to 320 mOsm per litre** with adjustment to the clinical circumstances. Only after the ICP drops the osmolality can be normalised, in order to prevent the rebound effect ensuing reverse of water gradient. If HTS with a concentration of more than 3% is chosen a central venous catheter should be inserted.
- **20% mannitol solution** at initial doses of 0.25 g/ kg to 1 g/kg body weight. It can be followed by lower doses every 3-6 hours.
- Arterial hypotension (systolic blood pressure < 90 mm Hg) should be avoided.
- The levels of serum sodium or serum osmolarity, blood urea nitrogen and serum creatinine should be measured regularly.
- Refer to **neurosurgery/ Oncology**

VI. NORMAL PRESSURE HYDROCEPHALUS

DEFINITION

- Normal pressure hydrocephalus (NPH) is an abnormal buildup of cerebrospinal fluid (CSF) in the brain's ventricles, or cavities[321].
- It occurs if the normal flow of CSF throughout the brain and spinal cord is blocked in some way. This causes the ventricles to enlarge, putting pressure on the brain.

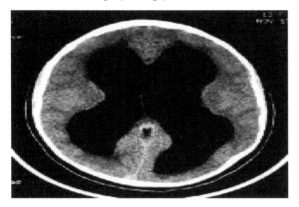

PREDISPOSING FACTORS

- Normal pressure hydrocephalus can occur in people of any age, but it is most common in the elderly.
- It may result from:
  - Meningitis
  - Intraventricular Hemorrhage (sah)
  - Meningomyelocele (Spina bifida)
  - Head trauma,
  - Tumor,
  - Complications of surgery.
- However, many people develop NPH even when none of these factors are present. In these cases the cause of the disorder is unknown

SYMPTOMS OF NPH

- Include progressive mental impairment and dementia, problems with walking, and impaired bladder control.
- The person also may have a general slowing of movements or may complain that his or her feet feel "stuck." Because these symptoms are similar to those of other disorders such as Alzheimer's disease, Parkinson's disease, and Creutzfeldt-Jakob disease, the disorder is often misdiagnosed.

- **Symptoms**
  - Headache
  - Vomiting
  - Limb weakness
  - Incoordination

- **Signs**
  - Classic Triad of Normal Pressure Hydrocephalus
    - Dementia of subcortical type
    - Gait disturbance
    - Incontinence
  - Abulia
  - Papilledema
  - Eyes displaced downward

CAUSES OF NPH

- Nonobstructive (ex vacuo)
  - Alzheimer's Disease
  - Pick's Disease
  - Multiple Cerebral Infarctions
  - Huntington's Disease
- Obstructive (Incomplete except in Acute Hydrocephalus)
  - Adult: Communicating (Extraventricular Blockage)
    - Post-Subarachnoid Hemorrhage
    - Post-Meningitis
    - Idiopathic Normal Pressure Hydrocephalus

IMAGING

- Cranial Ultrasound (Infants)
- CT Head
- MRI Head (preferred)

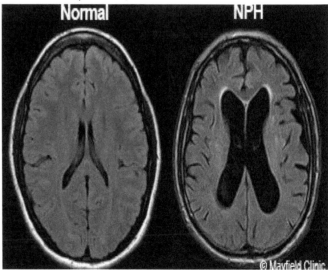

MANAGEMENT

- Surgical: Ventriculoperitoneal Shunt
- Non-Surgical: Indicated when surgery not possible
  - **Acetazolamide (Diamox)**: Decreases CSF production
    - Child: 10-25 mg/kg/day PO divided tid
    - Adult: 250 mg PO tid
  - Serial Lumbar Puncture (Temporize until surgery)

---

321 *NINDS, Normal Pressure Hydrocephalus [Online]*

VII. NEUTROPENIC SEPSIS

OVERVIEW

Definition

- Diagnose neutropenic sepsis in patients having anticancer treatment whose neutrophil count is 0.5×10^9 per litre or lower and who have either[322]:
  - A temperature higher than 38°C **or**
  - Other signs or symptoms consistent with clinically significant sepsis.
- Neutropenic patients with sepsis or severe sepsis may not have a fever (e.g. elderly, patients on corticosteroids)

Key points

- Rapid empirical initiation of broad-spectrum IV antibiotics and source control is essential
- The optimal antibiotic regime remains controversial
- Non-infectious causes of fever are common in patients with haematological malignancy but often difficult to distinguish from infective causes acutely

INFECTIVE ORGANISMS

Organisms of primary concern include:

- Gram negative bacilli
- Coagulase-negative Staphylococci
- Staphylococcus aureus (MSSA)
- Streptococcus viridans

Others:

- Resistant organisms in some patient groups / institutions (e.g. MRSA, VRE, ESBL, Pseudomonas, Stenotrophomonas, Acinetobacter)
- Fungal infection

Note that gram-positive cocci (GPC) (Staphylococcus, Streptococcus, Enterococcus) now predominate due to the ubiquity of long-term vascular access devices and use of fluoroquinolone prophylaxis in patients with neutropaenia.

RISK FACTORS

Risk factors for febrile neutropaenia include:

- Post-chemotherapy
- Post-transplantation
- Chronic granulomatous disease
- Clozapine-induced agranulocytosis

ASSESSMENT

History and examination

- Suspect neutropaenia in any haematology/ oncology patient that has received chemotherapy (oral or intravenous) within the last 14 days or has a history of recurrent neutropenia.
- **Assess:**
  - Upper respiratory tract for otitis media and sinusitis
  - Oropharynx for dental abscess and mucositis
  - Lower respiratory tract for signs of pneumonia, including Pneumocystis *pneumonia* (cough, tachypnoea, hypoxia, interstitial infiltrate on CXR)
  - Abdomen for signs of *Clostridium difficile* colitis (generalised abdominal tenderness) or typhlitis (tenderness over caecum)
  - Skin for cellulitis or vesicular lesions
  - Perineum and perianal area for anal fissure, cellulitis or abscess
  - CVAD for signs of tunnel/exit site infection
  - Signs of anaemia and/or thrombocytopenia
- Do not perform a rectal examination

INVESTIGATIONS

- Take blood cultures from a peripheral site in addition to each lumen of all pre-existing intravascular devices before administering antibiotics
- FBC, U&E and LFTs (including albumin), CRP and lactate
- If clinically indicated:
  - **CXR** (there may be no changes while neutropenic)
  - **Nasal swab** (throat swab if thrombocytopenic), for respiratory virus PCR
  - **Sputum MCS**
  - **Stool culture and viral studies** (diarrhoea); C. difficile *toxin assay if recent treatment with antibiotics*
  - **Bacterial swab** of skin, vascular access site or mouth lesions
  - **Viral swab** of vesicular lesions and mouth ulcers for HSV and VZV PCR
  - **CTB and lumbar puncture** (neurological symptoms)
  - **CT "pan scan"** (suspected occult infection source)
  - **Echocardiography** (endocarditis)

MASCC score

- ❖ The Multinational Association for Supportive Care in Cancer risk index is a validated tool for measuring the risk for neutropenic fever-related medical complications. The MASCC risk index may be used as an alternative to the clinical risk assessments described above.

---

[322] *Nice clinical guideline, Neutropenic sepsis: prevention and management in people with cancer, 19 September 2012 [NICE CG151]*

MANAGEMENT
Nice CG151[323]

- Offer beta lactam monotherapy with piperacillin with tazobactam as initial empiric antibiotic therapy to patients with suspected neutropenic sepsis who need intravenous treatment unless there are patient-specific or local microbiological contraindications.
- Do not offer an aminoglycoside, either as monotherapy or in dual therapy, for the initial empiric treatment of suspected neutropenic sepsis unless there are patient-specific or local microbiological indications.

Emergency treatment and assessment
- Treat suspected neutropenic sepsis as an acute medical emergency and offer empiric antibiotic therapy immediately.
- Include in the initial clinical assessment of patients with suspected neutropenic sepsis:
  o History and examination
  o Full blood count, kidney and liver function tests (including albumin), C-reactive protein, lactate and blood culture.

Further assessment
- After completing the initial clinical assessment (see above) try to identify the underlying cause of the sepsis by carrying out:
  o additional peripheral blood culture in patients with a central venous access device if clinically feasible
  o urinalysis in all children aged under 5 years.
- Do not perform a chest X-ray unless clinically indicated.

Immediate care
- Resuscitation
  o Address life threats such as septic shock
  o E.g. IV fluid resuscitation, vasopressor support and invasive haemodynamic monitoring
- Early IV antibiotics (within 30 minutes if sepsis/ unwell, always within 1 hour)
  o See antibiotic choice above
  o Seek expert advice regarding duration, influenced by:
    ▪ Patient's response
    ▪ Isolation of a causative organism
    ▪ Rate of neutrophil recovery
- Early source identification and control
  o Discuss with hematology before removing any intravascular devices, required if:
    ▪ CLABSI due to *S. aureus, P. aeruginosa*, fungi, or mycobacteria

323 Nice clinical guideline, Neutropenic sepsis: prevention and management in people with cancer, 19 September 2012 [NICE CG151]

- ▪ Port pocket site infection
- ▪ Endocarditis
- ▪ Septic thrombosis
- ▪ Septic shock
- ▪ Tunnel infection
- ▪ Persistence of bloodstream infection even after 72h of appropriate antibiotic treatment

ENVIRONMENTAL PRECAUTIONS
- Protective isolation
- Hand hygiene
- Full barrier precautions (e.g. Mask, gown, gloves, overshoes)

G-CSF
- Increases neutrophil count
- Reduces rate of serious infections
- Decreased mortality in bmt or dose-intensive chemotherapy
- Don't use in acute leukaemia (may stimulate leukaemic clone)
- Cease once neutrophils > 1.0×10^9/L
- Adverse effects: rash, injection site pain, bone pain, influenza-like symptoms and splenic rupture (rare)

SUPPORTIVE CARE AND MONITORING
Disposition
- Early consultation with hematology (refer after administering first dose of antibiotics)
- A subgroup of low-risk neutropenic patients may be able to be managed (at home) with oral therapy

PROGNOSIS
General
- prognosis proportional to the number of organ failures involved as opposed to underlying malignancy
- outcomes following ICU admission not as dismal as traditionally thought

Factors improving ICU survival:
- Better patient selection
- Early admission before the onset of multi-organ failure
- Overall improved prognosis in haematological and solid malignancy
- Use of non-invasive ventilation (NIV)
- Use of diagnostic bronchoscopy
- Improved survival rates in septic shock

High risk patients are those with comorbidities and prolonged (>7 days) and profound neutropaenia.

28. Pain Management-Adult

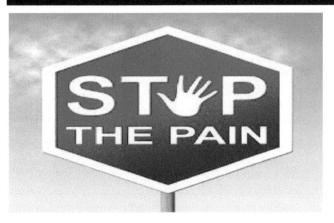

PAIN ASSESSMENT

- Pain is commonly under-treated and treatment may be delayed. Recognition and alleviation of pain should be a priority when the treating ill and injured.
- This process should start at the triage, be monitored during their time in the ED and finish with ensuring adequate analgesia at, and if appropriate, beyond discharge. The pain ladder contains objective and subjective descriptions with a numerical scale.
- The experience of the member of staff triaging will help in estimating the severity of the pain.

ASSESSMENT OF ACUTE PAIN IN THE ED [324]

Pain score	No pain 0	Mild Pain 1-3	Moderate Pain 4-6	Severe Pain 7-10
Suggested route & Type of Analgesia	No Action	Oral analgesia	Oral analgesia	IV Opiates or PR NSAID
Initial assessment	Within 20 min of arrival	Within 20 min of arrival	Within 20 min of arrival	Within 20 min of arrival
Re-evaluation	Within 60 min of initial assessment	Within 60 min of analgesia	Within 60 min of analgesia	Within 30 min of analgesia

- Using this method of pain scoring it should be possible to adequately assess into one of four categories and treat pain appropriately. Once the category has been established, appropriate analgesia may be prescribed according to the flow chart. In all cases it is important to think of using other non-pharmacological techniques to achieve analgesia, which may include measures such as **applying a dressing or immobilising a limb** etc.

324 RCEM, Management of Pain in Adults, December 2014 [pdf online]

- Following reassessment if analgesia is still found to be inadequate, stronger / increased dose of analgesics should be used along with the use of nonpharmacological measures.
- It is important to re-assess the pain control within **30-60 minutes** in severe and moderate pain.

HOW TO MANAGE PAIN IN THE ED

- Patients in severe pain should be transferred to an area where they can receive appropriate intravenous or rectal analgesia within 20 minutes of arrival at the Emergency Department.
- Patients in severe pain should have the effectiveness of analgesia re-evaluated within 30 minutes of receiving the first dose of analgesia.
- Patients in moderate pain should be offered oral analgesia at triage / assessment.
- Patients with moderate pain should have the effectiveness of analgesia re-evaluated within 60 minutes of the first dose of analgesia.
- Documentation of the above on the ED card is essential.
- **Patients in severe pain**
  o Should be transferred to an area where they can receive appropriate **intravenous or rectal analgesia within 20 minutes of arrival.**
  o Should have the effectiveness of analgesia re-evaluated **within 30 minutes of receiving the first dose of analgesia**.
- **Patients in moderate pain**
  o Should be offered **oral analgesia at triage / assessment**.
  o Should have the effectiveness of analgesia re-evaluated **within 60 minutes of the first dose of analgesia.**
- When patients first present to the ED the diagnosis may be unclear and it is important that the lack of diagnosis does not delay administration of appropriate analgesia.
- Emergency physicians are sometimes placed in the very difficult position of having to decide whether a patient's pain is genuine or not (i.e. is the patient displaying 'drug seeking' behaviour?). Careful decision making is required to balance the embarrassment of 'being tricked' by a drug seeker as opposed to denying a patient with genuine pain appropriate and adequate analgesia.
- Being **'wise after the event'** and instituting appropriate measures is likely to be preferable.

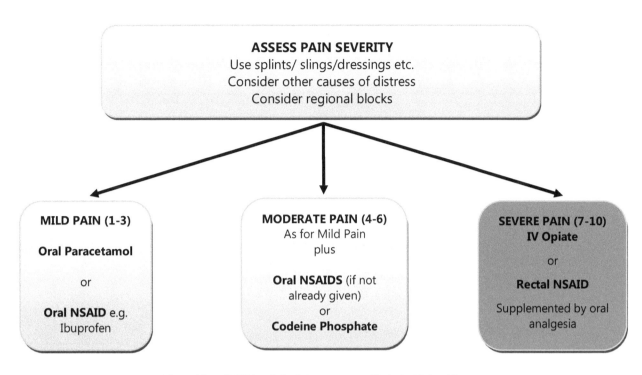

ASSESS PAIN SEVERITY
Use splints/ slings/dressings etc.
Consider other causes of distress
Consider regional blocks

MILD PAIN (1-3)

Oral Paracetamol

or

Oral NSAID e.g.
Ibuprofen

MODERATE PAIN (4-6)
As for Mild Pain
plus

Oral NSAIDS (if not
already given)
or
Codeine Phosphate

SEVERE PAIN (7-10)
IV Opiate

or

Rectal NSAID

Supplemented by oral
analgesia

Adapted fromRCEM website ([Management of Pain in Adult pdf](#))

- **WHEN PRESCRIBING FOR THE ELDERLY**[325]
  - It is worth remembering that **Paracetamol** *(including intravenous) is a safe first line treatment with a good safety profile.*
  - **NSAIDS** should be used with caution and at the lowest possible dose in older adults in view of gastrointestinal, renal and cardiovascular side effects as well as drug-drug interactions and the effects on other co-morbidities.
  - **Opiate medication** in the elderly, an appropriate dose reduction should be used as well as anticipating any other drug interactions; particularly those acting on the central nervous system which may increase the likelihood of respiratory depression.

- **WHEN PRESCRIBING IN PREGNANCY**
  - The general rule is try to avoid any medication; however, this is not always practical.
  - **Paracetamol** is considered safe in all three trimesters,
  - **Ibuprofen** is best avoided and can only be used **during the second trimester** (if essential).
  - **Morphine and codeine** can be used in all three trimesters if necessary but should be avoided during delivery.

1. PARACETAMOL
- Available as oral, rectal and intravenous preparations.
- **The standard oral** and IV dose for adults is **1gram qds** however when administering the IV preparation the dose must be adjusted for those patients weighing less than 50Kg (adults 40-49kg 750mg qds, 35-39kg 500mg qds).
- **The IV route** is particularly useful when patients need to be kept nil by mouth and rapid mild-moderate analgesia is required.
- **The rectal preparation** is probably best avoided due to variable and slow absorption in adults.
- Before prescribing paracetamol, inquiry must be made regarding previous paracetamol use (including preparations such as co-codamol and OTC preparations e.g. cold relief powders as well as paramedic use prior to arrival in the ED).

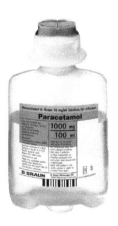

---

325 RCEM, Management of Pain in Adults, December 2014 [pdf online]

2. NON-STEROIDAL ANTI-INFLAMMATORY DRUGS (NSAIDS) [326]

o Available as oral, rectal, intravenous and intra-muscular preparations (although it should be noted **IM Diclofena**c has been associated with sterile abscesses following IM use).

o **Ibuprofen 400mg PO tds**; fewer side effects than other NSAIDs, good analgesic but relatively weak anti-inflammatory properties.

o **Naproxen 500mg PO initially then 250mg every 6-8hrs** in acute musculoskeletal disorders; stronger anti-inflammatory properties than ibuprofen but with relatively fewer side-effects compared to other NSAIDs.

o **Diclofenac 50mg PO tds, 100mg PR**; particularly useful for the treatment of renal colic pain via the rectal route however in recent years' concern has been raised regarding increased risk of thrombotic events (incl. MI) and Clostridium difficile and it is **contra-indicated in IHD, PVD, CVD and heart failure.**

o Avoid NSAIDS in **asthmatics** who are known to get worsening bronchospasm with NSAIDS, also avoid in patients with previous or **known peptic ulcer disease**.

o NSAIDs should be **used with caution in the elderly** (risk of peptic ulcer disease) and **women who are experiencing fertility issues**.

o It should also be **avoided in pregnancy**, particularly during the third trimester.

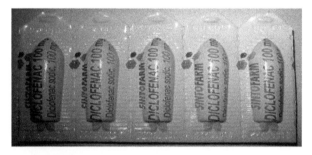

3. OPIATES

o **Codeine Phosphate** is available as oral and IM preparations, **30-60mg qds** are typical adult doses however consider lower doses in the elderly.

o Codeine prescribed in combination with paracetamol is significantly more effective than codeine when prescribed alone.

o **Morphine** is available as oral, intravenous and intra-muscular preparations (due to its relatively slow onset of action the oral preparation is not recommended for acute pain control in the ED, unless the patient is already taking the drug in which case this might be a reasonable alternative).

o **Morphine 0.1-0.2mg/kg IV** is a typical adult dose, however a titrated dose to provide the desired response is recommended; consider lower doses in the elderly.

o Use with caution if **risk of depression of airway, breathing or circulation.**

o The routine **prescription of an anti-emetic with an opiate is not recommended**, and only required if patient is already experiencing nausea / vomiting. It should be noted that the use of opioids in abdominal pain does not hinder the diagnostic process.

4. ENTONOX

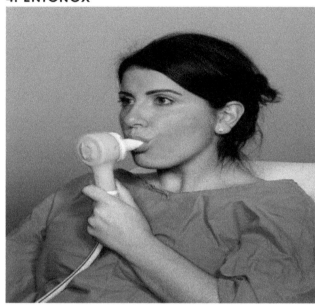

Image source hey.nhs.uk

o **Entonox, a 50% mixture of nitrous oxide and oxygen**, is very useful for short term relief of severe pain and for performing short lasting uncomfortable procedures.

o It should not be viewed as a definitive analgesic and EDs need mechanisms in place to ensure rapid assessment and institution of appropriate analgesia when paramedics bring patients to the ED who are using Entonox as their sole source of analgesia.

o **Entonox should be avoided in patients with:**
  - *Head injuries,*
  - *Chest injuries,*
  - *Suspected bowel obstruction,*
  - *Middle Ear disease,*
  - *Early pregnancy and*
  - *B12 or folate deficiency*

---

326 RCEM, Management of Pain in Adults, December 2014 [pdf online]

29. Palpitations
I. TACHYCARDIA

ADULT TACHYCARDIA (WITH PULSE) ALGORITHM

Adapted from Resuscitation Council Uk (G2015 Tachycardia in Adults pdf) [327]

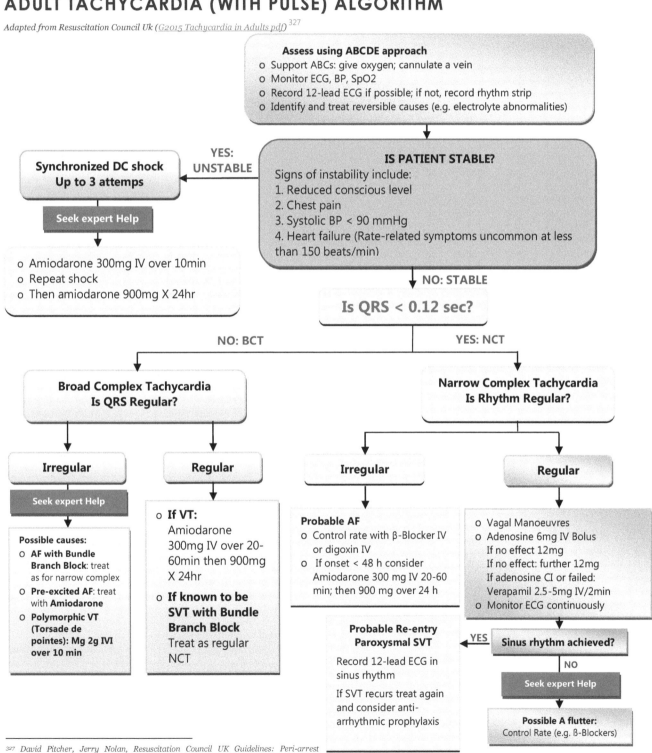

[327] David Pitcher, Jerry Nolan, Resuscitation Council UK Guidelines: Peri-arrest arrhythmias 2015 [pdf Online]

1. BROAD COMPLEX TACHYCARDIA

1.1. IRREGULAR BCT

- This is most likely to be atrial fibrillation (AF) with bundle branch block, but careful examination of a 12-lead ECG (if necessary by an expert) may enable confident identification of the rhythm. [328]
- Other possible causes are AF with ventricular pre-excitation (in patients with Wolff-Parkinson-White [WPW] syndrome), or polymorphic VT (e.g. torsade de pointes), but sustained polymorphic VT is unlikely to be present without adverse features.
- Seek expert help with the assessment and treatment of irregular broad-complex tachyarrhythmia.

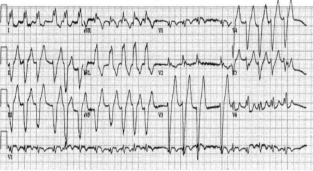

Irregular Broad Complex tachycardia

A. ATRIAL FIBRILLATION

- The atrial fibrillation gives rise to an irregular rhythm and the variable conduction down the accessory pathway gives rise to QRS complexes which do change in morphology due to the presence or absence of **Delta waves** giving a similar appearance to Torsade's de pointes.
- **Treatment of AF:**
  - o Once atrial fibrillation is identified as the underlying arrhythmia, it should be treated as such the treatment of atrial fibrillation is discussed in detail in the relevant module.

B. POLYMORPHIC VENTRICULAR TACHYCARDIA

- **Polymorphic ventricular tachycardia (PVT)** is a form of ventricular tachycardia in which there are multiple ventricular foci with the resultant QRS complexes varying in amplitude, axis and duration.
- The commonest cause of PVT is myocardial ischaemia.
- **Torsades de pointes (TdP)** is a specific form of polymorphic ventricular tachycardia occurring in the context of QT prolongation; it has a characteristic morphology in which the QRS complexes "twist" around the isoelectric line.

- For TdP to be diagnosed, the patient has to have evidence of both PVT *and* QT prolongation.
- Bidirectional VT is another type of polymorphic VT, most commonly associated with digoxin toxicity.

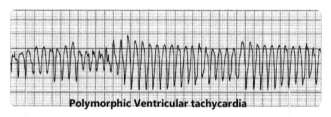

Polymorphic Ventricular tachycardia

- **TREATMENT OF POLYMORPHIC VT:**
  - o Treat torsade de pointes VT immediately by stopping all drugs known to prolong the QT interval.
  - o Do not give amiodarone for definite torsade de pointes. Correct electrolyte abnormalities, especially hypokalaemia. Give magnesium sulfate 2 g IV over 10 min (= 8 mmol, 4 mL of 50% magnesium sulfate).
  - o Obtain expert help, as other treatment (e.g. overdrive pacing) may be indicated to prevent relapse once the arrhythmia has been corrected.
  - o If adverse features are present, which is common, arrange immediate synchronised cardioversion. If the patient becomes pulseless, attempt defibrillation immediately (ALS algorithm)

1.2. REGULAR BCT

A. VENTRICULAR TACHYCARDIA

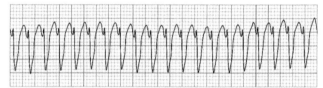

Ventricular tachycardia

- A regular broad-complex tachycardia is likely to be ventricular tachycardia (VT) or a regular supraventricular rhythm with bundle branch block[329].
- In a stable patient, if the broad-complex tachycardia is thought to be VT, treat with amiodarone 300 mg IV over 20–60 min, followed by an infusion of 900 mg over 24 h.
- If a regular broad-complex tachycardia is known to be a supraventricular arrhythmia with bundle branch block (usually after expert assessment of previous episodes of identical rhythm) and the patient is stable use the strategy indicated for regular, narrow-complex tachycardia (below).
- Where there is uncertainty, seek urgent expert help whenever possible.

---

[328] David Pitcher, Jerry Nolan, Resuscitation Council UK Guidelines: Peri-arrest arrhythmias 2015 [pdf Online]

[329] David Pitcher, Jerry Nolan, Resuscitation Council UK Guidelines: Peri-arrest arrhythmias 2015 [pdf Online]

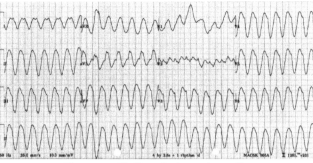
Monomorphic Ventricular tachycardia

- **TREATMENT OF MONOMORPHIC VT**
  o **If compromised:** DC cardioversion.
    - Synchronised DC cardioversion at **200 joules** (monophasic) or **100 joules (biphasic)**.
    - If unsuccessful repeat the cardioversion up to a **maximum of 3 attempts** before giving **amiodarone**.
    - Changing the paddle position may be helpful in resistant cases.
  o **If stable**:
    - **IV Amiodarone** (in a dose of 5mgs/kg up to a maximum of 300mgs) administered over 20-60 minutes is the treatment of choice. If unsuccessful, **DC cardioversion** should be considered. However, **amiodarone** is poorly effective in the treatment of acute VT.
    - **Sotalol** appears more effective in the treatment of stable VT (compared with lignocaine, which was the ALS recommendation at that time).
    - **Procainamide** has class IIa evidence supporting its usage in this situation but is slow to work.
  o **DC cardioversion** is reasonable as first-line treatment of stable VT.
  o **Correction of any underlying abnormalities** that might be precipitating the arrhythmia (e.g. hypo/hyperkalaemia and hypomagnesaemia) is also required.

B. SUPRAVENTRICULAR TACHYCARDIA WITH BBB
DIFFERENCE BETWEEN VT & SVT WITH BBB
1. If the patient is **>50** and/or has a **history of structural or ischaemic heart disease**, assume the rhythm is VT. If there is any doubt whatsoever, treat a regular broad complex tachycardia as VT.

2. a. The following are suggestive of VT:
  o *Dissociated P waves*
  o *Fusion/Capture beats*
  o *A bizarre axis*
  o *QRS >140 msec*
  o *Concordance of the QRS complexes in the chest leads.*

2. b. Features suggestive of BCT of supraventricular origin[330]:
  o *Young patient (age < 35)*
  o *Rate =150 beats/min*
  o *Rate >200 beats/minute and patient asymptomatic*
  o *QRS Duration < 140 msec*
  o *Axis normal*
  o *Absence of independent atrial activity or concordance*

3. Brugada Criteria
- *The following should be noted:*
1. *Is there an absence of RS complexes in all the chest leads?*
2. *Is the R-S interval (interval between the tip of the R wave and the lowest part of the S wave) > 100mS in any V lead?*
3. *Are there capture beats, fusion beats, or evidence of AV dissociation?*
4. *Does the morphology of the QRS complex in leads V1/ V6 suggest VT?*

MORPHOLOGIC CRITERIA SUGGESTIVE OF VT
1. LBBB morphology

RS wave
- **V1:**
  o R wave > 30 msec wide
  o RS wave > 60 msec wide
- **V6**:
  o QR wave
  o QS wave

2. RBBB morphology

RS interval
- **V1:**
  o Monophasic R wave
  o QR wave
  o RS wave
- **V6:**
  o Monophasic R wave
  o QR wave
  o R wave smaller than the S wave

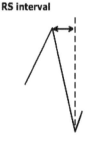

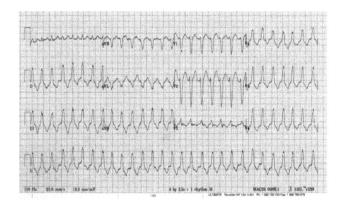

[330] Elizabeth Docherty, Francis P Morris , RCEM Learnig, Broad Complex Tachycardias [RCEMLearning Online]

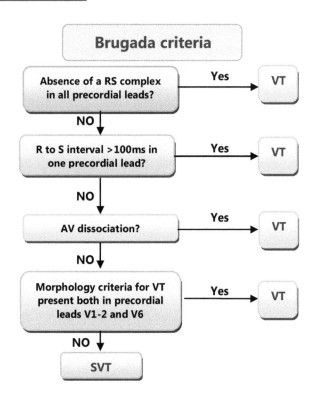

- If the answer to **any** of these questions is **YES**, then the diagnosis is VT.
- If the answer to **all** of these questions is **NO**, then the diagnosis is SVT with a bundle branch block.

TREATMENT:

o **Vagal manoeuvres and Adenosine** (a short acting purine) may be used diagnostically (to help identify BCT which is supraventricular in origin) and therapeutically (to terminate the arrhythmia).

o Detailed management of supraventricular tachycardia is discussed in a separate module.

2. NARROW COMPLEX TACHYCARDIA
2.1. IRREGULAR NCT

- An irregular narrow-complex tachycardia is most likely to be **AF** with an uncontrolled ventricular response or, less commonly, **atrial flutter with variable AV block.**
- The three main causes are:
  o *Atrial Fibrillation*
  o *Atrial flutter with variable block*
  o *Multifocal Atrial Tachycardia*

Synchronised cardioversion[331]

- If the patient is conscious, carry out cardioversion under sedation or general anaesthesia.
- Ensure that the defibrillator is set to synchronised mode.

o For a broad-complex tachycardia or atrial fibrillation, start with 120-150 J and increase in increments if this fails.
o Atrial flutter and regular narrow-complex tachycardia will often be terminated by lower energies: start with 70-120 J.

- **Atrial fibrillation:** there is no evidence of any organised atrial activity. Beware labelling coarse AF as flutter – the clue is the 'flutter' rate not being sufficiently fast. True flutter is demonstrated by atrial activity every 200 msec (i.e. every large square).
- **Atrial flutter with variable block:** Look hard for regular flutter waves. Note flutter with variable block is much rarer than AF (and not necessarily treated differently)
- **Multifocal atrial tachycardia:** Look for varying and irregular atrial activity – P waves of 3 different morphologies are needed to make the diagnosis. It is typically seen in **patients with decompensated lung disease.** The treatment is geared towards resolving the respiratory embarrassment rather than the tachycardia itself. Once atrial fibrillation is identified as the underlying arrhythmia, it should be treated as such the treatment of atrial fibrillation is discussed in detail in the relevant module.

2.2. REGULAR NCT

- **Narrow complex tachycardias**[332] are always supraventricular, as a normal QRS width indicates that conduction is down the Bundle of His in the normal antegrade manner.
- Examine the ECG to determine if the rhythm is regular or irregular.
- Regular narrow-complex tachycardias include:
  o sinus tachycardia
  o AV nodal re-entry tachycardia (AVNRT) – the commonest type of regular narrow-complex tachyarrhythmia
  o AV re-entry tachycardia (AVRT) – due to WPW syndrome
  o atrial flutter with regular AV conduction (usually 2:1).

A. SINUS TACHYCARDIA

- Sinus tachycardia is not an arrhythmia. This is a common physiological response to stimuli such as exercise or anxiety. In a sick patient, it may occur in response to many conditions including pain, infection, anaemia, blood loss, and heart failure.

---

[331] *David Pitcher, Jerry Nolan, Resuscitation Council UK Guidelines: Peri-arrest arrhythmias 2015 [pdf Online]*

[332] *David Pitcher, Jerry Nolan, Resuscitation Council UK Guidelines: Peri-arrest arrhythmias 2015 [pdf Online]*

- Treatment is directed at the underlying cause.
- Trying to slow sinus tachycardia that has occurred in response to most of these conditions will usually make the situation worse.
- *Do not attempt to treat sinus tachycardia with cardioversion or anti-arrhythmic drugs.*

B. SUPRAVENTRICULAR TACHYCARDIA

- AV nodal re-entry tachycardia is the commonest type of paroxysmal supraventricular tachycardia (SVT), often seen in people without any other form of heart disease.
- It is rare in the peri-arrest setting. It causes a regular, narrow-complex tachycardia, often with no clearly visible atrial activity on the ECG.
- The heart rate is commonly well above the typical range of sinus rhythm at rest (60-100/min).
- It is usually benign (unless there is additional, co-incidental, structural heart disease or coronary disease) but it may cause symptoms that the patient finds frightening.
- AV re-entry tachycardia occurs in patients with the WPW syndrome, and is also usually benign, unless there is additional structural heart disease.
- The common type of AVRT is a regular narrow-complex tachycardia, usually having no visible atrial activity on the ECG.

C. ATRIAL FLUTTER WITH REGULAR AV CONDUCTION (OFTEN 2:1)

- This produces a regular narrow-complex tachycardia. It may be difficult to see atrial activity and identify flutter waves in the ECG with confidence, so the rhythm may be indistinguishable, at least initially, from AVNRT or AVRT. Typical atrial flutter has an atrial rate of about 300/min, so atrial flutter with 2:1 conduction produces a tachycardia of about 150 /min. Much faster rates (>160/min) are unlikely to be caused by atrial flutter with 2:1 conduction. Regular tachycardia with slower rates (e.g. 125-150/min) may be due to atrial flutter with 2:1 conduction, usually when the rate of the atrial flutter has been slowed by drug therapy.

TREATMENT OF REGULAR NCT

- If the patient is **unstable (compromised)**: **Synchronised DC cardioversion**.
- It is reasonable to apply **vagal manoeuvres** and/or give **adenosine** to an unstable patient with a regular narrow-complex tachycardia while preparations are being made urgently for synchronised cardioversion.

- Do not delay electrical cardioversion if adenosine fails to restore sinus rhythm.
- **In the absence of adverse features (Not compromised):**
  - Start with **vagal manoeuvres**.
  - If the arrhythmia persists and is not atrial flutter, give **Adenosine 6 mg as a rapid IV bolus.**
  - If there is no response (i.e. no transient slowing or termination of the tachyarrhythmia) to adenosine 6 mg IV, **give a 12 mg IV bolus**.
  - If there is no response give one further **12 mg IV bolus**.
  - If adenosine is contra-indicated, or fails to terminate a regular narrow-complex tachycardia without demonstrating that it is atrial flutter, consider giving **Verapamil 2.5–5 mg IV over 2 min.**

- ❖ Vagal manoeuvres or adenosine will terminate almost all AVNRT or AVRT within seconds.
- ❖ Failure to terminate a regular narrow-complex tachycardia with adenosine suggests an atrial tachycardia such as **atrial flutter** (unless the adenosine has been injected too slowly or into a small peripheral vein).

OTHER DRUGS IN SVT:

- Amiodarone
- Beta blockers
- Sotalol
- Flecainide
- Digoxin - not in uni or multifocal atrial tachycardia or AV dependent arrhythmias
- Verapamil - **not in AV node re-entry tachycardia.**

ADENOSINE CONTRAINDICATIONS:

- Hypersensitivity
- 2nd or 3rd degree AV block (except those on pacemakers),
- Sick Sinus Syndrome,
- Atrial Fibrillation,
- V-Tach
- Bronchoconstrictive or Bronchospastic Lung Disease (e.g., asthma)

II. BRADYCARDIA

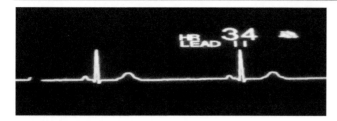

1. INTRODUCTION

- Bradycardia is defined as a heart rate of less than **60 beats per minute**[333].
- Causes include:
  - o Physiological (e.g. During sleep, in athletes)
  - o Cardiac causes (e.g. Atrioventricular block or sinus node disease)
  - o Non-cardiac causes (e.g. Vasovagal, hypothermia, hypothyroidism, hyperkalaemia)
  - o Drugs (e.g. Beta-blockade, diltiazem, digoxin, amiodarone) in therapeutic use or overdose.

TYPES OF BRADYCARDIA[334]

- **Narrow complex bradydysrhythmias**
  - o **Regular**
    - Sinus bradycardia
    - Junctional bradycardia
    - Complete AV block (junctional escape)
    - Atrial flutter with high degree block
  - o **Irregular**
    - Sinus arrhythmia, pause or arrest
    - Sinoatrial exit block (second degree)
    - Atrial fibrillation with slow ventricular response
    - Atrial flutter with variable block
    - Second degree AV block, type I
    - Second degree AV block, type II
- **Wide complex bradydysrhythmias**
  - o **Regular**
    - Idioventricular rhythm
    - Complete AV block (ventricular escape)
    - Sinoventricular rhythm
    - Regular bradycardias with aberrancy or bundle branch block
  - o **Irregular**
    - Second degree AV block, type I
    - Second degree AV block, type II
    - Sinoatrial exit block (second degree) with bundle branch block
    - Irregular bradycardias with bundle branch block

1. ATRIOVENTRICULAR BLOCK

- AV blocks are conduction delays or a complete block of impulses from the atria into the ventricles.
- AV block may be due to increased vagal tone that may be elicited during sleep, athletic training, pain, or stimulation of the carotid sinus[335].
- Damage of the conduction system secondary to hereditary fibrosis or sclerosis of the cardiac skeleton are known as idiopathic progressive cardiac conduction disease. Ischemic heart disease causes 40% of AV blocks.
- AV blocks are also seen in cardiomyopathies, myocarditis, congenital heart diseases, and familial diseases. A plasma potassium concentration above 6.3 mEq/L may also cause AV block.
- They may be iatrogenic, from medications such as Verapamil, Diltiazem, Amiodarone, and Adenosine, or from cardiac surgeries and catheter ablations for arrhythmias. AV blocks are further classified according to the degree of blockage and include first degree AV block, second degree AV block, and third-degree AV block.

1. FIRST DEGREE AV BLOCK

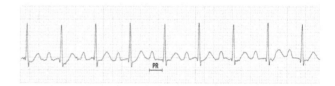

First degree AV Block

- Prolongation of the PR interval of more than 200 milliseconds is considered to be a first-degree AV block.
- These can be due to structural abnormalities within the AV node, an increase in vagal tone, and drugs that slow conduction such as digoxin, beta-blockers and calcium channel inhibitors. It is important to note that in first degree AV block, no actual block occurs.

2. SECOND DEGREE AV BLOCK

- The QRS remains narrow but atrial impulses fail to conduct normally to the ventricles in one of the following ways:

A. MOBITZ TYPE I (WENCKEBACH)
- o Mobitz type I (Wenckebach) occurs when there is a progressive lengthening of PR interval with eventual dropped ventricular conduction.

---

333 David Pitcher, Jerry Nolan, Resuscitation Council UK Guidelines: Peri-arrest arrhythmias 2015 [pdf Online]

334 Chris Nickson, Life in the fast lane, Bradycardia [Online]

335 Carrus Health, ACLS Carer cert, Atrioventricular Blocks [Online]

o This causes an absent impulse into the ventricles, reflected by the disappearance of the QRS complex in the ECG.

o Mobitz type I is a benign condition that rarely causes hemodynamic instability; asymptomatic patients need no further treatment. Symptomatic patients will require a pacemaker.

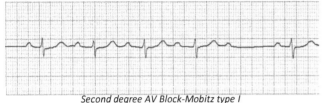

Second degree AV Block-Mobitz type I

B. MOBITZ TYPE II

o The Mobitz type II AV block occurs when there is a constant PR interval but some P waves fail to conduct to the ventricles

o The Mobitz type II AV block is secondary to a disease involving the His-Purkinje system, in which there is a failure to conduct impulses from the atria into the ventricles. A block occurs after the AV node within the bundle of His, or within both bundle branches. The His-Purkinje system is an all-or-none conduction system; therefore, in Mobitz type II, there are no changes in the PR interval, even after the non-conducted P wave[336].

o Because of this, Mobitz type II has a higher risk of complete heart block compared to Mobitz type I.

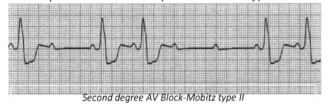

Second degree AV Block-Mobitz type II

3. THIRD DEGREE AV BLOCK (COMPLETE HEART BLOCK)

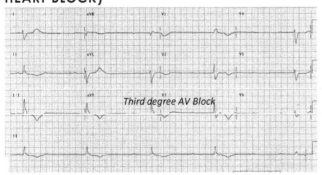

Third degree AV Block

• A complete failure of the AV node to conduct any impulses from the atria to the ventricles is the main feature of third-degree AV block.

• There is AV dissociation and escape rhythms that may be junctional or ventricular, which represent perfusing rhythms.

• This is due to AV nodal disease or a disease involving the His-Purkinje system caused by coronary artery disease, enhanced vagal tone, a congenital disorder, underlying structural heart disease such as myocardial infarction, hypertrophy, inflammation or infiltration, Lyme disease, post-cardiac surgery, cardiomyopathies, rheumatologic diseases, autoimmune diseases, amyloidosis, sarcoidosis, or muscular dystrophy. At any time, the patient may suffer ventricular standstill that may result in sudden cardiac death. Pacemaker insertion is necessary to provide needed perfusion[337].

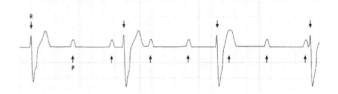

4. BIFASCICULAR BLOCK

• Bifascicular block is the combination of **RBBB with either LAFB or LPFB.**

• Conduction to the ventricles is via the single remaining fascicle.

• The ECG will show typical features of RBBB plus either left or right axis deviation.

• **RBBB + LAFB** is the most common of the two patterns.

• Bifascicular block is a sign of extensive conducting system disease, although the risk of progressing to complete heart block is thought to be relatively low (1% per year in one cohort study of 554 patients).

⤸ *NB. Some authors also consider LBBB to be a 'bifascicular block', because both fascicles of the left bundle branch are blocked (see image below).*

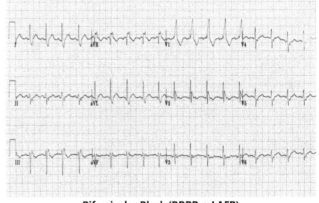

Bifascicular Block (RBBB + LAFB)

[336] *Carrus Health, ACLS Carer cert, Atrioventricular Blocks [Online]*

[337] *Carrus Health, ACLS Carer cert, Atrioventricular Blocks [Online]*

Main Causes of Bifascicular Block:

- Ischaemic heart disease (40-60% cases)
- Hypertension (20-25%)
- Aortic stenosis
- Anterior MI (occurs in 5-7% of acute AMI)
- Primary degenerative disease of the conducting system (Lenegre's / Lev's disease)
- Congenital heart disease
- Hyperkalaemia (resolves with treatment)

5. TRIFASCICULAR BLOCK[338]

Trifascicular block (TFB) refers to the presence of conducting disease in all three fascicles:

- **Right bundle branch (RBB)**
- **Left anterior fascicle (LAF)**
- **Left posterior fascicle (LPF)**

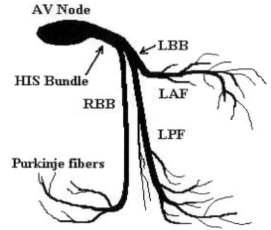

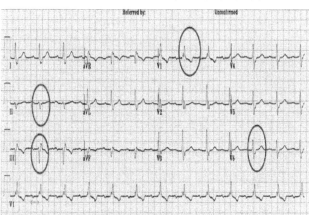

*This ECG record of a **trifascicular block** contains the combination of LAFB (red), RBBB (blue) and the **first-degree AV block** (indicated by the **green arrow** in lead V1).*

INCOMPLETE VS COMPLETE TFB

Trifascicular block can be *incomplete* or *complete*, depending on whether all three fascicles have completely failed or not.

A. INCOMPLETE TRIFASCICULAR BLOCK

- Incomplete ("*impending*") trifascicular block can be inferred from one of two electrocardiographic patterns:
  - Fixed block of two fascicles (i.e. bifascicular block) with delayed conduction in the remaining fascicle (i.e. 1st or 2nd degree AV block).
  - Fixed block of one fascicle (i.e. RBBB) with intermittent failure of the other two fascicles (i.e. alternating LAFB / LPFB).

Example 1

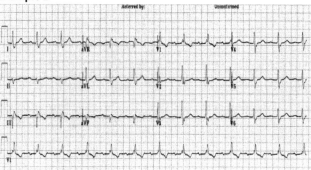

Incomplete Trifascicular Block :

- *Right bundle branch block*
- *Left axis deviation (= left anterior fascicular block)*
- *First degree AV block*

Example 2

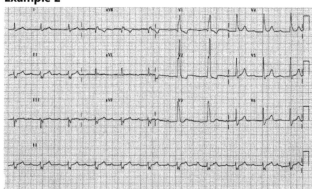

Incomplete Trifascicular Block :

- Right bundle branch block
- Left axis deviation (= left anterior fascicular block)
- First degree AV block

B. COMPLETE TRIFASCICULAR BLOCK

- Complete trifascicular block produces 3rd degree AV block with features of bifascicular block.
- This is because the escape rhythm usually arises from the region of either the left anterior or left posterior fascicle (distal to the site of block), producing QRS complexes with the appearance of RBBB plus either LPFB or LAFB respectively.

- *The most common pattern referred to as "trifascicular block" is the **combination of bifascicular block with 1st degree AV block**.*

---

338 *Ed Burns, Life in the fast lane, Trifascicular Block [Online]*

Example 3

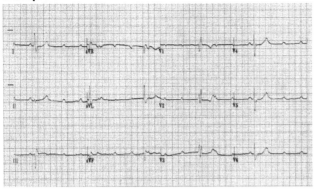

Complete Trifascicular Block :

- *Right bundle branch block*
- *Left axis deviation (Left anterior fascicular block)*
- *Third degree heart block*

Incomplete trifascicular block

- Bifascicular block + 1st degree AV block (most common)
- Bifascicular block + 2nd degree AV block
- RBBB + alternating LAFB / LPFB

Complete trifascicular block

- Bifascicular block + 3rd degree AV block

⚓ *NB. For patients with the combination of bifascicular block plus 1st or 2nd degree AV block it is usually impossible to tell from the surface ECG whether the AV block is at the level of the remaining fascicle (a "true" trifascicular block) or at the level of the AV node (i.e. not technically a trifasicular block).*

CLINICAL IMPLICATIONS

- Incomplete trifascicular block may progress to complete heart block, although the overall risk is low.
- Patients who present with syncope and have an ECG showing incomplete trifascicular block usually need to be admitted for a cardiology work-up as it is possible that they are having episodes of complete heart block. Some of these patients will require insertion of a permanent pacemaker (class II indication).
- *Asymptomatic* bifascicular block with first degree AV block is not an indication for pacing (class III).

MAIN CAUSES

- Ischaemic heart disease
- Hypertension
- Aortic stenosis
- Anterior MI
- Primary degenerative disease of the conducting system (Lenegre's / Lev's disease)
- Congenital heart disease
- Hyperkalaemia (resolves with treatment)
- Digoxin toxicity

PACEMAKER RHYTHMS

Red Arrows are referring to Pacing Spikes

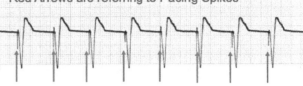

There are multiple types of pacemaker rhythms:

- Normal Single Chamber Pacemaker
- Normal Dual Chamber Pacemaker
- Failure to Capture
- Failure to Pace
- Failure to Sense
- Pacemaker Rhythm Sample Tracing

Categories of Pacemaker Rhythms

1. Normal Single Chamber Pacemaker

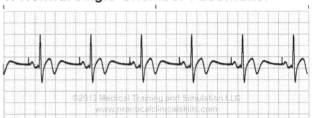

2. Failure to Capture

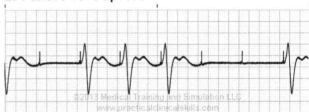

Failure to capture means that the ventricles fail to response to the pacemaker impulse. On an ECG tracing, the pacemaker spike will appear but it will not be followed by a QRS complex.

3. Failure to Pace

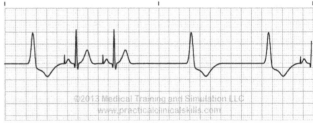

Failure to pace occurs when the pacemaker does not generate an electrical impulse. On an ECG tracing, pacemaker spikes will be missing.

4. Failure to Sense

- Failure to sense occurs when the pacemaker does not detect the patient's myocardial depolarization. This can often be seen on an ECG tracing as a spike following a QRS complex too early.

ADULT BRADYCARDIA ALGORITHM

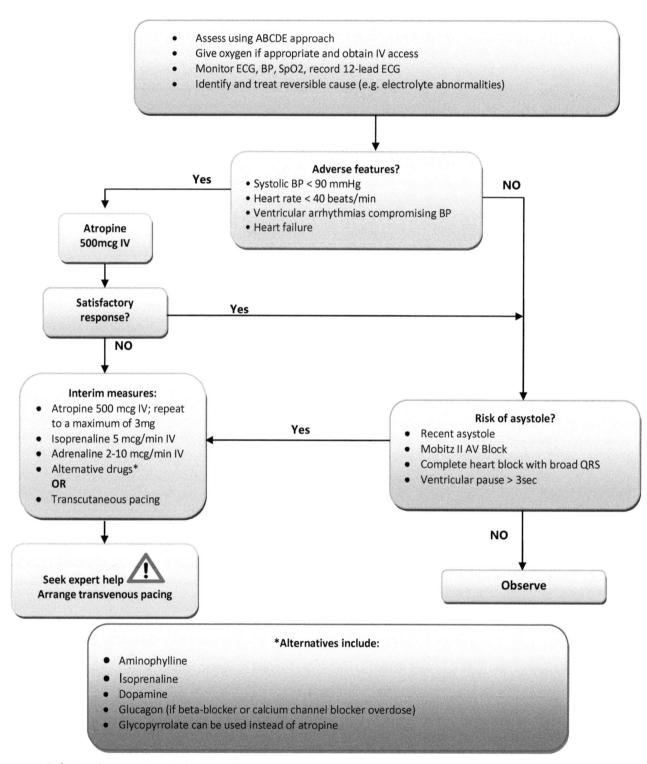

- Assess using ABCDE approach
- Give oxygen if appropriate and obtain IV access
- Monitor ECG, BP, SpO2, record 12-lead ECG
- Identify and treat reversible cause (e.g. electrolyte abnormalities)

Adverse features?
- Systolic BP < 90 mmHg
- Heart rate < 40 beats/min
- Ventricular arrhythmias compromising BP
- Heart failure

Yes

Atropine 500mcg IV

Satisfactory response?

Yes

NO

NO

Interim measures:
- Atropine 500 mcg IV; repeat to a maximum of 3mg
- Isoprenaline 5 mcg/min IV
- Adrenaline 2-10 mcg/min IV
- Alternative drugs*
  OR
- Transcutaneous pacing

Yes

Risk of asystole?
- Recent asystole
- Mobitz II AV Block
- Complete heart block with broad QRS
- Ventricular pause > 3sec

NO

Seek expert help
Arrange transvenous pacing

Observe

*Alternatives include:
- Aminophylline
- Isoprenaline
- Dopamine
- Glucagon (if beta-blocker or calcium channel blocker overdose)
- Glycopyrrolate can be used instead of atropine

Reference Source: Resuscitation Council UK

III. INTRAVENTRICULAR BLOCKS

A. RIGHT BUNDLE BRANCH BLOCK

1. "COMPLETE" RBBB
- **Diagnostic Criteria**
  - Broad QRS > 120 ms
  - RSR' pattern in V1-3 ('M-shaped' QRS complex)
  - Wide, slurred S wave in the lateral leads (I, aVL, V5-6)
- **Associated Features**
  - ST depression and T wave inversion in the right precordial leads (V1-3)
- **Variations**
  - Sometimes rather than an RSR' pattern in V1, there may be a broad monophasic R wave or a qR complex.

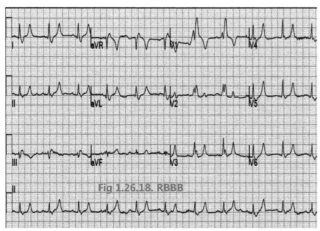

Fig 1.26.18. RBBB

Lead 1	Lead aVF	Quadrant	Axis
POSITIVE	POSITIVE		**Normal Axis** (0 to +90°)
POSITIVE	NEGATIVE		****Possible LAD** (0 to -90°)
NEGATIVE	POSITIVE		**RAD** (+90° to 180°)
NEGATIVE	NEGATIVE		**Extreme Axis** (-90° to 180°)

- The frontal plane QRS axis in RBBB should be in the normal range (i.e., -30 to +90 degrees).
  - If left axis deviation is present, think about **left anterior fascicular block**
  - If right axis deviation is present, think about **left posterior fascicular block** in addition to the RBBB.

2. "INCOMPLETE" RBBB
- QRS duration of **0.10 - 0.12s** with the same terminal QRS features.
- This is often a normal variant.
- The "normal" ST-T waves in RBBB should be oriented opposite to the direction of the terminal QRS forces; i.e., in leads with terminal R or R' forces the ST-T should be negative or downwards; in leads with terminal S forces the ST-T should be positive or upwards.
- If the ST-T waves are in the *same direction* as the terminal QRS forces, they should be labelled **primary *ST-T wave abnormalities***

ECG DIAGNOSIS OF BUNDLE BRANCH BLOCK

- ***QRS > 0.12 sec***
- ***Look at V1:***
  - ***Terminal R*** *= RBBB as excitation spreading from left to right*
  - ***Terminal S*** *= LBBB as excitation spreading away from right*
- ***Confirm I: (& aVL V5 & 6)***
  - ***Terminal S*** *= RBBB as excitation going away from left side*
  - ***Terminal R*** *= LBBB as excitation heading towards left*
  - *The above equates to pattern recognition of **MaRrow/ WiLliam** in V1-6.*
  - *With LBBB associated ST/T opposite to QRS, poor R progression in V1-6, RS in V5, 6 left axis deviation.*

B. LEFT BUNDLE BRANCH BLOCK

1. "COMPLETE" LBBB"
- **Diagnostic Criteria**
  - QRS duration of > 120 ms
  - Dominant S wave in V1
  - Broad monophasic R wave in lateral leads (I, aVL, V5-V6)
  - Absence of Q waves in lateral leads (I, V5-V6; small Q waves are still allowed in aVL)
  - Prolonged R wave peak time > 60ms in left precordial leads (V5-6)

- **Associated Features**
  - Appropriate discordance: the ST segments and T waves always go in the opposite direction to the main vector of the QRS complex
  - Poor R wave progression in the chest leads
  - Left axis deviation

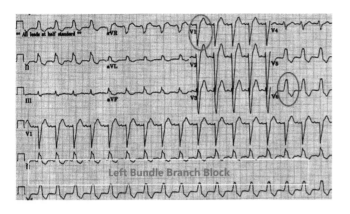

Left Bundle Branch Block

2. "INCOMPLETE" LBBB:

o Looks like LBBB but QRS duration = **0.10 to 0.12s**, with less ST-T change.
o This is often a progression of LVH.
o Increased QRS voltage in the limb leads

- **Diagnosing AMI in LBBB**
  o The Sgarbossa criteria only apply in LBBB (see rules below)
  o In true LBBB, there must not be any Q wave in the lateral leads

SGARBOSSA CRITERIA

- **Of acute MI with LBBB (any of following)**
  o *ST elevation ≥ 1mm concordant with QRS*
  o *ST depression ≥ 1mm in V1-3*
  o *ST elevation ≥ 5mm discordant with QRS*

C. WOLFF-PARKINSON-WHITE

o QRS complex represents a **fusion** between two ventricular activation fronts:
  - Early ventricular activation in region of the accessory AV pathway **(Bundle of Kent)**
  - Ventricular activation through the normal AV junction, bundle branch system.

o **ECG criteria include all of the following:**
  - Short PR interval (< 0.12s)
  - Initial slurring of QRS complex **(delta wave)** representing early ventricular activation through normal ventricular muscle in region of the accessory pathway
  - Prolonged QRS duration (usually > 0.10s)
  - Secondary ST-T changes due to the altered ventricular activation sequence.

o QRS morphology, including polarity of delta wave depends on the particular location of the accessory pathway as well as on the relative proportion of the QRS complex that is due to early ventricular activation (i.e., degree of fusion).

o **Delta waves,** if negative in polarity, may mimic infarct Q waves and result in false positive diagnosis of myocardial infarction.

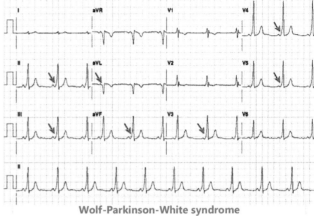

Wolf-Parkinson-White syndrome

D. ATRIAL FIBRILLATION & ATRIAL FLUTTER IN WPW

- Atrial fibrillation can occur in up to 20% of patients with WPW.
- Atrial flutter can occur in up to 7% of patients with WPW.
- The accessory pathway allows for rapid conduction directly to the ventricles bypassing the AV node.
- Rapid ventricular rates may result in degeneration to **VT** or **VF**.

- **ECG features of Atrial Fibrillation in WPW are:**
  o Rate > 200 bpm
  o Irregular rhythm
  o Wide QRS complexes due to abnormal ventricular depolarisation via accessory pathway
  o QRS Complexes change in shape and morphology
  o Axis remains stable unlike **Polymorphic VT**

- *Atrial Flutter results in the same features as AF in WPW except the rhythm is regular and may be mistaken for **VT**.*

- **TREATMENT OF AF WITH WPW**
  o **In a haemodynamically unstable** patient urgent synchronised DC cardioversion is required.
  o Medical treatment options in a **stable patient** include **Procainamide or Ibutilide,** although DC cardioversion may be preferred.
  o Treatment with AV nodal blocking drugs e.g. **adenosine, calcium-channel blockers, beta-blockers may increase conduction via the accessory pathway** with a resultant increase in ventricular rate and possible degeneration into **VT** or **VF**.

IV. ATRIAL FIBRILLATION

1. DEFINITION

o Atrial fibrillation (AF) is the **most common atrial arrhythmia worldwide** and the overall incidence is expected to rise in the future. AF is also the **most frequently diagnosed arrhythmia in emergency departments** (ED) [339].

o In the normal heart, impulses originate from the sinus node, followed by regular atrial and ventricular activation and contraction. In AF, the impulses are not regular and it is these irregular beats that cause **ineffective atrial contraction, which can lead to clot formation in the left atrial appendage, causing potential for stroke**. The irregular beats can also **occasionally lead to dangerous tachycardias.**

o AF can be divided into five main categories based on its presentation and duration. This includes **first diagnosis, paroxysmal, persistent, long-standing persistent, and permanent AF**.

o Paroxysmal AF usually terminates on its own within 48 hours but may continue up to seven days, while persistent AF is present for longer than 7 days and typically requires treatment.

o Long standing AF is defined as lasting longer than one year and permanent AF is defined as the presence of continuous AF that is accepted by both the patient and his or her physician.

2. CLINICAL ASSESSMENT

• Patients with AF usually present to the ED because of symptoms as a result of an irregular, rapid heart rate.

• These symptoms will vary, and some patients may even be asymptomatic. Typically, symptoms of AF include **palpitations, chest pain, shortness of breath, lightheadedness, or syncope**. Some may be considered hemodynamically unstable, showing signs of shock, pulmonary edema, angina or myocardial infarction. However, most patients who present to the ED with AF or AFL will be alert with a normal, perfusing blood pressure. Careful evaluation of both stable and unstable AF/AFL patients is critical, as treatment and disposition will depend on each patient's diagnosis and hemodynamic stability[339]

• Some patients present with what has often been called **"Fast AF."** This is a misnomer since all patients in AF have chaotic atrial electrical activity with no discernible pattern, so the description "fast" which implies a contradistinction to "slow" is incorrect.

• The correct description is **AF with a fast /slow / controlled ventricular response.**

3. CAUSES OF ATRIAL FIBRILLATION

CARDIAC PRECIPITANTS	NON-CARDIAC PRECIPITANTS
o Ischaemic heart disease	o Hyperthyroidism
o Heart failure	o Pulmonary embolus
o Hypertension	o Sepsis
o Valvular heart disease (commonly mitral)	o Alcohol excess or withdrawal
o Sick sinus syndrome	o Hypokalaemia
o Pericarditis	o Hypothermia
o Cardiomyopathy	o Drug use (cocaine)

4. NICE GUIDANCE ON STROKE RISK STRATIFICATION CHA2DS2 VASC SCORE[340]

THROMBOEMBOLIC/STROKE RISK		
	Condition	Point
C	Congestive heart failure (or Left ventricular systolic dysfunction)	1
H	Hypertension: blood pressure consistently above 140/90 mmHg (or treated hypertension on medication)	1
A_2	Age ≥75 years	2
D	Diabetes Mellitus	1
S_2	Prior Stroke or TIA or thromboembolism	2
V	Vascular disease (e.g. peripheral artery disease, myocardial infarction, aortic plaque)	1
A	Age 65-74 years	1
Sc	Sex category (i.e. female sex)	1

❖ **A score of 0 in men or 1 in female:** low risk and no anticoagulation is required.

❖ **A score of 1 in men only**: moderate risk, anticoagulant should be considered.

❖ **If the score is 2 or greater (male and female):** the patient is high risk, and the patient should be anticoagulated if there are no contraindications.

❖ Anticoagulation may be with **Apixaban, Dabigatran Etexilate, Rivaroxaban** or **Warfarin**

❖ **Do not offer Aspirin** monotherapy solely for stroke prevention to people with atrial fibrillation.

---

[339] *Jennifer Robertson, More Atrial Fibrillation Management Pearls in the ED, [emDocs]*

[340] *Clinical guideline [CG180], Atrial fibrillation: management [Online]*

HAS BLED SCORE

RISK OF BLEEDING

	Condition	Points
H	**Hypertension:** (uncontrolled, >160 mmHg systolic)	1
A	**Abnormal renal function:** Dialysis, transplant, Cr >2.26 mg/dL or >200 µmol/L	1
	Abnormal liver function: Cirrhosis or Bilirubin >2x Normal or AST/ALT/AP >3x Normal	1
S	**Stroke**: Prior history of stroke	1
B	**Bleeding:** Prior Major Bleeding or Predisposition to Bleeding	1
L	**Labile INR:** (Unstable/high INRs), Time in Therapeutic Range <60%	1
E	**Elderly:** Age > 65 years	1
D	Prior Alcohol or **Drug Usage History** (≥ 8 drinks/week)	1
	Medication Usage Predisposing to Bleeding: (Antiplatelet agents, NSAIDs)	1

❖ **A score of 3 or more:** indicates an increased risk of bleeding when anticoagulated that warrants caution or more regular review of the patient.

INVESTIGATION

o Full blood count, coagulation, U&E, LFT, TFT, Inflammatory markers
o Chest X ray, ECG
o ECHO to document LA diameter, LV systolic function, any evidence of valvular abnormality, or cardiac pathology

NICE CG180 A.FIB RECOMMENDATIONS[341]

- For a patient with AF, it is desirable to restore sinus rhythm within the 48-hour time period (from onset). In this instance, **no further anticoagulation or further in-hospital intervention is required.**
- However, where the AF has continued for longer than 48-hours, restoration of sinus rhythm **risks dislodging thrombi from the left atrial appendage.** In this instance, treatment is limited to **determining stroke risks and controlling the ventricular rate.**

RATE AND RHYTHM CONTROL

o Sign of life-threatening haemodynamic instability: DC Cardioversion stat
o No sign of life-threatening haemodynamic instability:
  ▪ Less than 48hrs: offer rate or rhythm control
  ▪ More than 48 hours or is uncertain: start rate control

WHEN TO OFFER RATE OR RHYTHM CONTROL[342]

- OffeOffer rate control as the first-line strategy to people with atrial fibrillation, except in people:
  o Whose atrial fibrillation has a reversible cause
  o Who have heart failure thought to be primarily caused by atrial fibrillation
  o With new-onset atrial fibrillation
  o With atrial flutter whose condition is considered suitable for an ablation strategy to restore sinus rhythm
  o For whom a rhythm control strategy would be more suitable based on clinical judgement. **[new 2014]**

RATE CONTROL

- Offer either a standard **beta-blocker** (that is, a beta-blocker other than sotalol) or a rate-limiting **calcium-channel blocker** as initial monotherapy to people with atrial fibrillation who need drug treatment as part of a rate control strategy. Base the choice of drug on the person's symptoms, heart rate, comorbidities and preferences when considering drug treatment.
- Consider **digoxin monotherapy** for people with non-paroxysmal atrial fibrillation **only if they are sedentary** (do no or very little physical exercise).
- If monotherapy does not control symptoms, and if continuing symptoms are thought to be due to poor ventricular rate control, consider combination therapy with any 2 of the following: **A beta-blocker, Diltiazem and Digoxin.**
- **Do not offer amiodarone** for long-term rate control.

IV Route		PO Route	
Metoprolol	2.5-5mg IVI	Bisoprolol	2.5-10mg PO,
		Atenolol	25-100mg PO
Verapamil	5mg IVI	Diltiazem	60-360mg PO tds
Digoxin	0.5-1mg IVI	Digoxin	0.125-0.5mg PO

RHYTHM CONTROL

- Consider **pharmacological and/or electrical rhythm control** for people with atrial fibrillation whose symptoms continue after heart rate has been controlled or for whom a rate-control strategy has not been successful.
- If pharmacological cardioversion has been agreed on clinical and resource grounds for new-onset atrial fibrillation, offer:
  o **Flecainide or Amiodarone** to patient with no evidence of structural or ischaemic heart disease
  o **Amiodarone** if evidence of structural heart disease

---

341 *Clinical guideline [CG180], Atrial fibrillation: management* [Online]

342 *Clinical guideline [CG180], Atrial fibrillation: management* [Online]

WHEN TO OFFER EMERGENCY CARDIOVERSION?

- Carry out emergency electrical cardioversion, without delaying to achieve anticoagulation, in people with **life-threatening haemodynamic instability caused by new-onset atrial fibrillation.**

CARDIOVERSION

- For people having cardioversion for atrial fibrillation that has persisted for longer than 48 hours:
  - o Offer electrical (rather than pharmacological) cardioversion.
  - o Consider **amiodarone therapy starting 4 weeks before** and continuing for **up to 12 months** after electrical cardioversion to maintain sinus rhythm, and discuss the benefits and risks of amiodarone with the person.

- For people with atrial fibrillation of greater than 48 hours' duration, in whom elective cardioversion is indicated:
  - o Both **transoesophageal echocardiography-guided cardioversion and conventional cardioversion** should be considered equally effective
  - o A transoesophageal echocardiography-guided cardioversion strategy should be considered:
    - Where experienced staff and appropriate facilities are available and
    - Where a minimal period of precardioversion anticoagulation is indicated due to the person's choice or bleeding risks.

ANTICOAGULATION

- **Do not offer aspirin monotherapy** solely for stroke prevention to people with atrial fibrillation.
  - o In people with **new-onset atrial fibrillation** who are receiving no, or subtherapeutic, anticoagulation therapy:
    - In the absence of contraindications, **offer heparin at initial presentation**
    - Continue heparin until a full assessment has been made and appropriate antithrombotic therapy has been started, based on risk stratification.

  - o In people with a **confirmed diagnosis of atrial fibrillation of recent onset** (less than 48 hours since onset), offer oral anticoagulation if:
    - Stable sinus rhythm is not successfully restored within the same 48-hour period following onset of atrial fibrillation or
    - There are factors indicating a high risk of atrial fibrillation recurrence

  - o In people with new-onset atrial fibrillation where there is uncertainty over the precise time since onset, **offer oral anticoagulation as for persistent atrial fibrillation.**

- ❖ **Consider amiodarone for people with left ventricular impairment or heart failure**
- ❖ Do not offer class 1c antiarrhythmic drugs such as **flecainide or propafenone** to people with known ischaemic or structural heart disease.
- ❖ The combination of **WPW and atrial fibrillation** can potentially be fatal, especially if AV blocking agents are given (remember **"ABCD"** for **A**denosine or **A**miodarone, **B**eta-blockers, **C**alcium channel blockers and **D**igoxin)

V. TORSADES DE POINTES

1. BACKGROUND

o Torsade de pointes (TdP) is a form of polymorphic ventricular pro-arrhythmia.

o Associated with QT interval prolongation and prominent U waves on resting ECG

o ECG = prolonged re-polarisation and so, early after depolarisation (EAD)

o Can be congenital

o Usually acquired due to **potassium channel dysfunction**.

o It may degenerate to ventricular fibrillation.

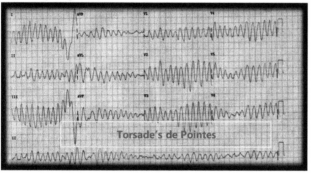

2. PHYSIOLOGY

o Ventricular re-polarisation is initiated by exodus of intracellular K+.

o Drugs can block this K+ channel - delaying repolarisation (prolonging Q-T interval).

o Other factors are
  ▪ Female
  ▪ ↑ Age
  ▪ Electrolyte disturbance
  ▪ CCF, Bradycardia, Ischaemia Congenital
  ▪ Main drug culprits

3. DRUG CAUSES

o Antiarrhythmics especially Class Ia and III.

o Phenothiazines and butyrophenones.

o Tricyclic antidepressants.

o Non-sedative antihistamines.

o Some antibiotics especially macrolides and antifungals.

o Organophosphates.

o Cocaine

o Electrolyte abnormalities (hypokalaemia, hypomagnesaemia)

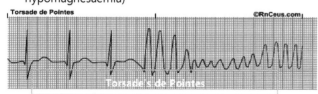

4. TREATMENT

o To treat haemodynamic compromise immediately.

o To alter the after-depolarisation effect.

o To shorten the QT interval.

o **Haemodynamic compromise: immediate DC cardioversion:** 150-200J

o **Magnesium**, at a dose of **2g magnesium sulphate IV over 1-2min**, is used to suppress EAD`s in the emergency situation. The serum magnesium level need not be known prior to treatment.

o **Correction of hypokalaemia** to a serum K+ concentration of > 4.5 mmol/l also helps suppress EAD`s.

o **Lignocaine** has been used. However, its effect is inconsistent with a reported success rate of only 50%.

o **Cardiac pacing at 100-140/min is the treatment of choice**. The basic heart rate should be accelerated, as there is an inverse relationship between rate and the re-polarisation duration.

o **Isoprenaline** should only be a temporising measure as in can promote EADs. Involve a cardiologist early.

5. TdP SECONDARY TO HYPOKALAEMIA

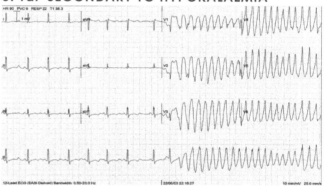

*Sinus rhythm with **inverted T waves**, **prominent U waves** and a **long Q-U interval** due to severe hypokalaemia (K+ 1.7). A premature atrial complex (beat #9 of the rhythm strip) lands on the end of the T wave, causing 'R on T' phenomenon and initiating a paroxysm of polymorphic VT. Because of the preceding long QU interval, this can be diagnosed as TdP.*

❖ **Polymorphic ventricular tachycardia (PVT)** is a form of ventricular tachycardia in which there are multiple ventricular foci with the resultant QRS complexes varying in amplitude, axis and duration. The commonest cause of PVT is **Myocardial Ischaemia.**

❖ **Torsade's de pointes (TdP)** are a specific form of polymorphic ventricular tachycardia occurring in the context of QT prolongation; it has a characteristic morphology in which the QRS complexes "twist" around the isoelectric line. For TdP to be diagnosed, the patient has to have **evidence of both PVT and QT prolongation.**

❖ **Bidirectional VT** is another type of polymorphic VT, most commonly associated with digoxin toxicity.

VI. WELLENS' SYNDROME

- Wellens' syndrome is a **preinfarction stage of coronary artery disease and heralds an impending extensive myocardial infarction of the anterior wall**.
- It is typified by **anginal chest pain**, **characteristic ECG changes** that usually occur after chest pain has resolved, and **negative cardiac biomarkers**.
- Wellens' syndrome presents as one of two characteristic T-wave abnormalities **seen in leads V2 and V3** on ECG:

TYPE A WELLENS' SYNDROME

Type A (approximately 25% of cases) shows **biphasic T-waves**, with an initial positive deflection, and terminal negative deflection.

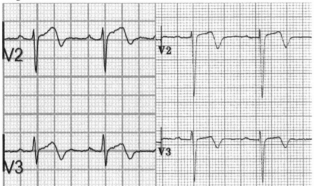

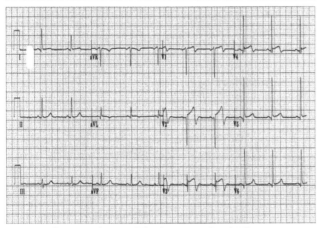

Type A wellen's syndrome: Biphasic T-waves in V2-V3

TYPE B WELLENS' SYNDROME

Type B (approximately 75% of cases) shows **deeply inverted and symmetric T-waves**.

- The ST segment is seldom involved, but when it is, consists of ST elevation of less than 1 mm.
- These changes are always **seen in leads V2 and V3**, but can be seen commonly in V4, less often in V1, and only occasionally seen in leads V5 and V6.

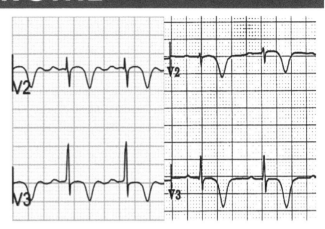

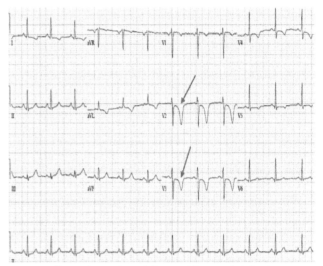

Type B well's syndrome: Deeply inverted T waves in V2-V3

- Patients presenting with Wellens' syndrome will generally have signs and symptoms of typical anginal chest pain and **usually respond well to drug therapy** (nitrates and morphine).
- *What is unusual is that the **ECG changes that are typical of Wellens' syndrome typically appear after chest pain has resolved**.*
- ***In fact, during an acute attack of chest pain, the T-wave abnormalities will normalize or become ST-segment elevation.***
- Left untreated, the patient presenting with Wellens' syndrome has a significant risk of **severe myocardial infarction and death**.
- In de Zwaan et al's initial study, of the patient's presenting with this ECG pattern who had myocardial infarction, the infarction occurred within 1 to 23 days (mean of 8.5 days) of admission.

VII. BRUGADA SYNDROME

- **Brugada Syndrome** is an abnormal ECG (**Right Bundle Branch Block Pattern with coved ST elevation over the right precordial leads**), which leads to ventricular fibrillation (VF) and sudden cardiac death (SCD) in patients with structurally normal hearts.
- It has been recognized as a clinical entity since 1992.
- Why should all ED physicians know about this entity? Although a rare syndrome, it is often mistaken as a STEMI and more importantly the clinical spectrum can be asymptomatic to SCD.

- **WHO GETS BRUGADA SYNDROME?**
  o Males > Females in a 8 – 10: 1 ratio
  o Ages 20 – 40 years (There are case reports of age 2 days all the way up to 84 years)
  o Asian > US populations
  o Typically occurs at night, when there is a predominance of vagal activity.

- **HOW COMMON IS BRUGADA SYNDROME?**
  o Worldwide 4 – 12% of all sudden deaths
  o Type 1 Brugada occurs in 12/10,000 people
  o Type 2 and 3 Brugada occurs in 58/10,000 people
  o Prevalence of Brugada Pattern ECG: Asia (0.36%), Europe (0.25%), and in the USA (0.03%)
  o ECG pattern can wax and wane, making the true incidence underestimated
- **Sodium channel defect** that leads to impaired fast upstroke of phase 0 of the action potential.

AETIOLOGY

- ECG changes can be transient with Brugada syndrome and can also be unmasked or augmented by multiple factors:
  o Fever/ Ischaemia/ Hypokalaemia/ Hypothermia
  o Post DC cardioversion
  o Multiple Drugs
    - Sodium channel blockers e.g.: Flecainide, Propafenone
    - Calcium channel blockers
    - Alpha agonists/ Beta Blockers/ Nitrates
    - Cholinergic stimulation/ Cocaine/ Alcohol
- **ECG**
  o ECG changes may be intermittent and transient
  o Unusual or saddle-shaped ST elevation (>2mm) in leads V1 - V3
  o Partial or complete RBBB (+ T inversion)
  o J point elevation

DIAGNOSTIC CRITERIA

- Coved ST segment elevation >2mm in >1 of V1-V3 followed by a negative T wave is the only ECG abnormality that is ***potentially*** diagnostic.
- ***This has been referred to as Brugada sign.***

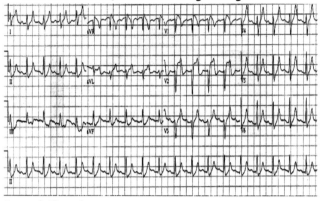

Brugada Type 1

- **WHERE IS THE MOST LIKELY ARRHYTHMOGENIC SUBSTRATE OF BRUGADA SYNDROME?**
  o Right Ventricular Outflow Tract (RVOT)
  o Only cardiac structure lying underneath 2nd and 3rd intercostal spaces
  o Brugada pattern may be absent in typical 4th intercostal space of leads V1 – V3.

RISK STRATIFY PATIENTS WITH BRUGADA SYNDROME

o Symptomatic patients with recurrent syncope, agonal respirations at night during sleep, or unknown seizures are at the highest risk of dying.
o Asymptomatic patients have an annual cardiac event rate of 0.25%, therefore there is little value in a risk stratification strategy to identify high risk patients.

TREATMENT OPTIONS FOR BRUGADA SYNDROME

o **Quinidine** is the only medication that has shown benefit in prevention of VF and reduction of AICD shocks (Only 67% of patients can tolerate drug due to side effects)
o **Implantable Cardiac Defibrillator (ICD):** Class 1 Indication in symptomatic patients (past history of VT/VF or syncope)
o Defibrillator Versus ß-Blocker in Unexplained Death in Thailand (DEBUT) Trial: Showed 0% death rate after ICD versus 18% in Beta Blocker group.
o **Leadless ICDs:** 98% termination rate of VF/VT, but less pocket infection and lead revisions.
o **Catheter Ablation:** Performed in 14 patients with no recurrent VF/VT with a median 32 months follow up.

VIII. LONG QT SYNDROME (LQTS)

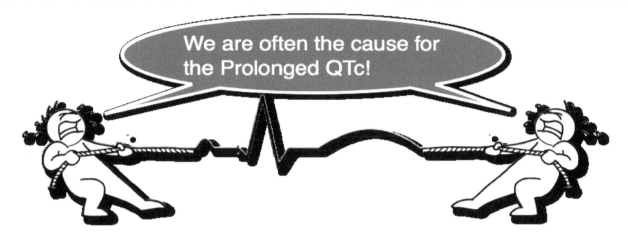

- Prolonged ventricular re-polarisation = prolongation of the QT interval
- Risk of Torsade de pointes and sudden death

CAUSES OF A PROLONGED QTC (>440MS):
- **4H Must Raise Cardiac Pressure with Drugs**
  - o **H**ypokalaemia
  - o **H**ypomagnesaemia
  - o **H**ypocalcaemia
  - o **H**ypothermia
  - o **M**yocardial ischemia
  - o **Raised** intracranial pressure
  - o **C**ongenital long QT syndrome
  - o **P**ost-cardiac arrest
- **DRUGS: Triple AAA Tears First Endothelium**
  - o **A**ntihistaminics
  - o **A**nticholinergics
  - o **A**ntiarrythmics (specially Quinidine and Sotalol)
  - o **T**CAS
  - o **F**luoroquinolones
  - o **E**rythromycin
- **Other drugs are**: Chloroquine, Mefloquine, Haloperidol, Risperidone, Methadone, and HIV protease Inhibitors.

- **Congenital**
  - o Romano-Ward syndrome - autosomal dominant.
  - o Lange-Nielsen syndrome - autosomal recessive (assoc congenital deafness.)
  - o F > M, usually childhood or adolescence.
- Once identified, first degree relatives should be screened.

- **CLINICAL PRESENTATION**
  - o Palpitations, syncope or near syncope, seizures, or cardiac arrest.

- o These patients are susceptible to lethal ventricular tachyarrhythmias, increasing their risk for sudden cardiac death.
- **ECG FINDINGS**
  - o **QTc** = QT/R-R^{-2}. **>0.45 sec abnormal**
  - o Abnormal T-wave (notched or biphasic)
  - o T-wave alternans

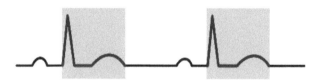

Normal QT interval

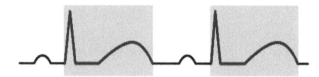

Prolonged or abnormal QT interval

- **TREATMENT**
  - o "Lifestyle modifications," (avoidance competitive sports and of all drugs known to prolong QT interval) (See above list).
  - o Treat with **ß-blockers** (shorten the QT interval, reduce risk of Torsade and sudden death).
  - o High risk patients - **Implantable Cardioverter-Defibrillators (ICDs).**
  - o Left cervicothoracic sympathectomy (Block sympathetic to heart so reduce event rate).

30. Poisoning

I. GENERAL ED MANAGEMENT

INTRODUCTION

Acute poisoning accounts for >100 000 hospital admissions per year in the UK with in excess of 4000 deaths reported in England and Wales per annum. Although the majority of poison-related deaths occur in the community, reduction of in-hospital morbidity and mortality remains an important challenge. A recent report indicated that 85% of poisonings occur in the home. Drugs accounted for the majority, but industrial chemicals and household products were involved in a significant number. Only one-third of cases were deliberate. The medications most commonly taken were Paracetamol, NSAIDs, and antidepressants.

Poisoning should be considered in any patient exhibiting bizarre behaviour, a reduced conscious level, or unexplained metabolic, cardiovascular, or respiratory instability.

All cases are managed as acute medical emergencies using an ABC approach regardless of the agent used.

Rare exceptions include patients poisoned with organophosphates, where health-care workers first need to protect themselves from the agent, and cyanide poisoning, where the antidote for cyanide is immediately required.

All cases require: A focused and detailed poisoning history and examination are required to identify specific physical signs of poisoning followed by the selective use of antidotes and laboratory tests (Table 1).

Most poisoned patients require supportive treatment only.

- *Resuscitation;*
- *Risk assessment;*
- *Substance identification;*
- *Specific treatment (if available);*
- *A period of observation.*

A risk assessment should be performed by obtaining specific information from ambulance personnel or witnesses regarding the nature, timing, and amount of drug or poison. One-third of cases involve more than one toxin and alcohol is a common contributing factor. The patient's clothing should be checked for notes or blister packets, which may give a clue to quantity and type of drug ingested.

In cases of deliberate self-harm, there may be previous hospital admissions to aid diagnosis. The patient's general practitioner should be contacted for previous history as family or witness sources are often unreliable.

SPECIFIC SIGNS IN POISONING & OVERDOSE

Toxidrome	Drug	Common Findings	Potential Treatments
Anticholinergic	Scopolamine, Atropine	Altered mental status, Dilated pupils, Urinary retention, Hyperthermia, Dry mucous membranes	**Physostigmine** Sedation with Benzodiazepines Cooling, Supportive management
Cholinergic	Organophosphates Carbamates	Salivation, Lacrimation, Sweating, Nausea, Vomiting, Urination, Defaecation, Muscle weakness, Bronchorrhoea	Airway protection & IPPV **Atropine,** **Pralidoxime**
Opioid	Heroin, Morphine	CNS and respiratory depression, Small pupils	Airway protection, IPPV **Naloxone**
Salicylates	Aspirin	Altered mental status, Respiratory alkalosis, Metabolic acidosis, Tinnitus, Hyperpnoea, Tachycardia, Sweating	**Multi-dose AC,** Alkalinization of urine, K^+ repletion, **Haemodialysis** Hydration
Serotonin Syndrome	Meperidine; MAOI, SSRI, TCA	Altered mental status, Increased muscle tone, Hyperreflexia, Hyperthermia	Cooling, Benzodiazepines
Sympathomimetic	Cocaine; Amphetamine	Agitation, Dilated pupils, Excessive sweating, Tachycardia, Hypertension, Hyperthermia	Cooling, Sedation with benzodiazepines Hydration

SUPPORTIVE CARE AND MONITORING

Patients suspected of being exposed to a poison or drug should be monitored in an appropriate clinical environment. Where coma is inevitable, patients should be intubated pre-emptively or at the first sign of deterioration in level of consciousness.

Tracheal intubation will protect the airway and allow early administration of activated charcoal (AC) via a nasogastric tube if required.

Patients who are at risk of cardiac instability and acidosis should have continuous ECG and invasive arterial pressure monitoring with regular blood gas analysis.

Body temperature and serum glucose should be checked and I.V. dextrose administered if required.

INVESTIGATIONS

- **Paracetamol levels** are considered mandatory in all cases of adult overdose and should be taken 4 h post-exposure.
- **Salicylate levels** are not recommended in the asymptomatic patient. Screening for substances of abuse can be achieved quickly with readily available commercial urine kits.
- Other laboratory tests include: FBC, U&Es, Lactate, LFT and coagulation studies.
- Where poisoning is caused by specific agents, for example, **Methanol or carbamazepine plasma levels** are taken 4 hourly to allow refinement of risk assessment and to gauge the response to enhanced elimination techniques.
- **A chest radiograph** may indicate pulmonary oedema, which is suggestive of poisoning with narcotics or salicylates.
- **Abdominal radiographs** can identify packets of drugs smuggled in **'body packers'**.
- Radiological investigations are otherwise rarely required in the setting of acute poisoning.

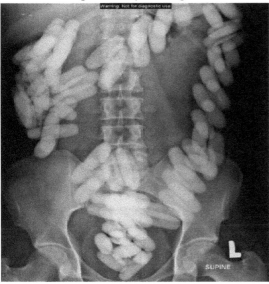

GASTRIC DECONTAMINATION

There is much debate regarding the use of the so-called **'decontamination triangle'** of forced emesis, gastric lavage, and single-dose AC.

Decontamination strategies are not without side-effects and the risk: benefit ratio should be considered before administration.

1. INDUCED EMESIS

- **Ipecac** induces vomiting by both direct gastrointestinal effects and central nervous system actions.
- It is administered at a dose of **30 ml in adults followed by water 240 ml.** Emesis typically occurs within 20 min and persists for 30-120 min.
- Several studies have compared ipecac with single-dose AC. Ipecac conveys no benefit, whether given alone or combined with AC.
- **Side-effects include** prolonged time in the ED and increased incidence of aspiration pneumonitis.
- **Its use is no longer recommended.**

2. GASTRIC LAVAGE

- Gastric lavage is performed by placing a large-bore orogastric tube (30-40 F), instilling and re-aspirating several litres of water to wash out the stomach contents.
- This is continued until no more pill fragments are identified in gastric contents.
- Patients **must be able to protect their own airway**.
- Drug absorption is not reduced if lavage is commenced 1 h or more after drug ingestion.
- Paradoxically, one study suggested that gastric lavage promotes post-pyloric transfer of poison into the small intestine where it is more rapidly absorbed.
- There are no data demonstrating improved clinical outcome with gastric lavage and its use is associated with significant morbidity and mortality.
- **Complications** include **GIT perforation** and **aspiration**.

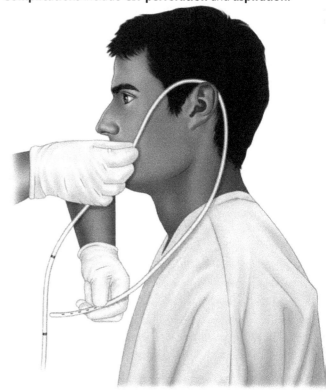

CONTRAINDICATIONS
- Vomiting
- Unintubated patients with potential to lose airway protective reflexes
- Ingestion of a xenobiotic with aspiration potential (e.g., hydrocarbon) without intubation
- Ingestion of caustic substances (alkali or acidic)
- Ingestion of sharp metals
- Ingestion of a foreign body (e.g., drug packet)
- Risk for hemorrhagic gastrointestinal perforation
- Ingestion of xenobiotic in a form known to be too large to fit into the lumen of the orogastric tube
- Nontoxic ingestions

COMPLICATIONS
- Vomiting
- Esophageal tears or perforation after orogastric tube insertion
- Inadvertent tracheal intubation and/or airway trauma
- Aspiration pneumonitis

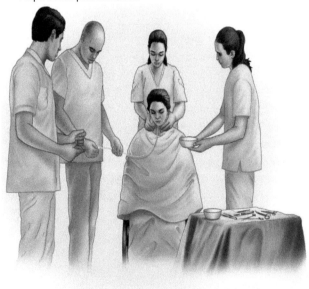

3. ACTIVATED CHARCOAL (AC)
- Most drugs and chemicals are absorbed by AC.
- It creates weak van der Waals forces that bind with the substance in the gastrointestinal tract.
- The numerous charcoal particles provide a large enough surface area to prevent further absorption.
- AC should be administered orally or nasogastrically via a 16 F tube in the intubated patient.
- The charcoal to toxin ratio is 10:1 with a usual dose of **25–50 g or 1 g/kg in a child**.
- This dose should be given within 1 h of poison ingestion.
- Its efficacy is time-dependent, with nearly 90% reduction in absorption 30 min after drug ingestion decreasing to 30% at 1 h.

- It has been shown to reduce Paracetamol absorption up to 2 h after ingestion.
- AC is unpalatable and can cause vomiting, thus in children it can be mixed with ice cream. Patients should also be warned that it will make their stools black.
- Multiple doses interrupt the enterohepatic circulation of the drug, reducing the plasma levels, and there are data that this reduces the duration of toxicity.
- A major but rare adverse effect from repeat doses is acute bowel obstruction from charcoal concretions, which is particularly likely in the presence of an anticholinergic ileus.

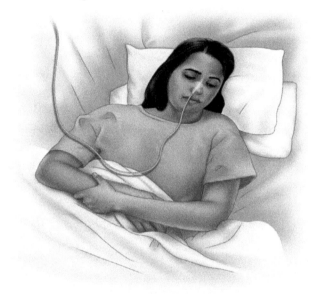

DIALYSABLE TOXINS
STUMBLED
- **S**alicylates
- **T**heophylline
- **U**remia
- **M**etformin/methanol
- **B**arbiturates
- **L**ithium
- **E**thylene glycol
- **D**epakote (valproic acid—in massive overdose)

Multiple-Dose Activated Charcoal Therapy (MDAC)
- Repeated doses of **25 g per 4–6 hourly** can be of benefit for poisoning with slow release formulations, for example: **CDD-PQ-ST**
  - Carbamazepine
  - Digoxin
  - Dapsone
  - Phenobarbital
  - Quinine
  - Salicylate (Controversial)
  - Theophylline

- **It does not work for poisonings by:**
  - Cyanide
  - Iron
  - Lithium
  - Corrosive agents,
  - Organophosphates
  - Inorganic salts (K^+)
  - Alcohols,
  - Glycoles (ethylene glycol)
  - Metals (Mercury, Arsenic)
  - Fluoride

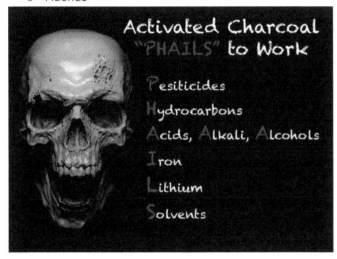

CONTRAINDICATIONS

- **Absolute**
  - Gastric perforation
  - Gastrointestinal ileus, obstruction, or diminished peristalsis
  - Nonintubated patients with the potential of losing protective airway reflexes
  - Intestinal obstruction
  - Ingestion of:
    - Corrosives
    - Petroleum distillates

- **Relative**
  - Altered or decreased level of consciousness unless intubated.
  - Vomiting.
  - Xenobiotic has limited toxicity at almost any dose.
  - Dose ingested is less than the dose expected to produce significant illness.
  - Presentation many hours after ingestion.
  - Minimal signs or symptoms of poisoning.
  - Ingested xenobiotic has a highly efficient antidote.
  - Administration of charcoal may increase the risk of aspiration (i.e., hydrocarbons).

COMPLICATIONS

- Aspiration pneumonitis
- Transient constipation
- Intestinal bezoars
- Bowel obstruction
- Diarrhea, dehydration, hypermagnesemia, and hypernatremia with coadministered cathartics or MDAC
- Vomiting
- Corneal abrasion if spilled in the eyes
- Mother may adversely affect the fetus.

4. WHOLE BOWEL IRRIGATION

- Whole bowel irrigation (WBI) aims to reduce the time for ingested substances to be absorbed.
- It requires the administration of **Polyethylene Glycol (PEG)** 1.5-2 litres solution per hour and is best administered through a 12 F feeding tube.

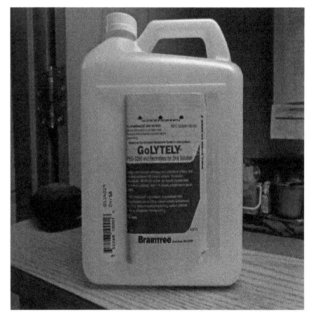

- The head of the bed should be elevated to 45° to prevent aspiration. If emesis occurs, then the infusion should be discontinued for 30 min and restarted at half the normal rate. **Metoclopramide** can be helpful as an antiemetic due to its prokinetic effects.
- Current recommendations are that the PEG is administered until the effluent is clear. The technique is not used routinely but may be considered where poisoning includes sustained release or enteric coated tablets.
- It may also be used for drugs for which charcoal is known to be ineffective, for example, **alcohols, boric acid, cyanide, iron, lithium, hydrocarbons, acids, and alkalis.**
- It has been used with some success in the treatment of **body packers, heavy metal, and battery ingestion**.

CONTRAINDICATIONS

- **Absolute**
  - Bowel obstruction
  - Bowel perforation
  - Ileus
  - Hemodynamic instability
  - Compromised or unprotected airway
  - Intractable vomiting

- **Relative**
  - Concurrent or recent administration of activated charcoal (may decrease the effectiveness of activated charcoal)

COMPLICATIONS

- Nausea, vomiting, and bloating
- Misplacement of the NG tube
- Esophageal perforation owing to NG tube placement
- Aspiration pneumonitis in the unprotected airway

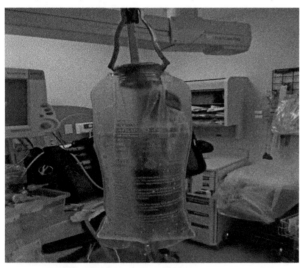

5. INCREASED ELIMINATION

- **Alkaline diuresis** enhances the elimination of weak acids such as salicylates and some herbicides.
- **Sodium bicarbonate** is administered and the pH of the urine measured to keep the urinary pH 7.5-8.5.
- Weak acids become charged in alkaline urine resulting in a concentration gradient drawing more toxin into the renal tubular system. **Hypokalaemia** can result from this technique and should be corrected aggressively.
- Alkaline diuresis should be used with caution in patients with **renal impairment or cardiac disease.**

6. HAEMODIALYSIS

- Haemodialysis is helpful in **ethylene glycol, methanol, lithium, theophylline, and salicylate poisoning**.
- The usefulness of this technique depends on the pharmacological properties of the ingested drug.
- The drug or poison should have a low volume of distribution (<1 litre/kg), a low molecular weight (<500 Da), low protein binding, and low water solubility.

COMMON ANTIDOTES

Poison	Antidote
Benzodiazepines	Flumazenil
Ethylene glycol, Methanol	Fomepizole Ethanol (10% for I.V. use)
Digoxin	Digibind
Methaemoglobinaemia	Methylene blue
Opiate	Naloxone
Paracetamol	N-Acetylcysteine or Mucomyst/ Methionine
Warfarin	Prothrombin Complex Concentrate (PCC) or Vit K
Beta-Blockers	Glucagon
Calcium Channel Blockers	Calcium; Anticholinergics
Dabigatran (Pradaxa)	Idarucizumab, Dialysis
Cyanide	Hydroxycobalamin, Na^+/Amyl Nitrite Dicobalt Edetate, Na^+ Thiosulfate
Iron	Deferoxamine
Heparin	Protamine Sulfate
Organophosphates	Atropine, Pralidoxime
Potassium	Insulin + Glucose, Kayexalate
Sodium channel blockers (TCAs), Salicylates	Sodium Bicarbonate
Local anesthetics	Intralipid Fat emulsion
Carbone Monoxide	Oxygen Hyperbaric Oxygen
Heavy metals	Dimercaprol, Penicillamine, Na^+ channel edetate
Paraquat	Charcoal, Fuller's earth
Antidepressants	Diazepam for convulsion, Bicarbonate for arrhythmia
Aspirin	Hemodialysis
Lithium	Gut decontamination, Hydration, Dialysis

INDICATIONS, CONTRAINDICATIONS, & COMPLICATIONS OF GASTROINTESTINAL DECONTAMINATION PROCEDURES

GASTRIC LAVAGE	
Indications	• Rarely indicated • Consider for recent (<1 hour) ingestion of life-threatening amount of a toxin for which there is no effective treatment once absorbed
Contraindications	• Corrosive/hydrocarbon ingestion • Supportive care/antidote likely to lead to recovery • Unprotected airway • Unstable, requiring further resuscitation (hypotension, seizures)
Complications	• Aspiration pneumonia/hypoxia • Water intoxication • Hypothermia • Laryngospasm • Mechanical injury to GIT • Time consuming, resulting in delay instituting other definitive care

Activated Charcoal	Adults 50 grams orally, Children 1 g/kg orally
Indications	• Ingestion within the previous hour of a toxic substance known to be adsorbed by activated charcoal, where the benefits of administration are judged to outweigh the risks
Contraindications	• Nontoxic ingestion • Toxin not adsorbed by AC • Recovery will occur without administration of activate charcoal • Unprotected airway • Corrosive ingestion • Possibility of upper gastrointestinal perforation
Complications	• Vomiting • Aspiration of the activated charcoal • Impaired absorption of orally administered antidotes

Whole-Bowel Irrigation	Polyethylene glycol 2 L/h in adults, Children 25 mL/kg per hour (maximum 2 L/h)
Indications	• (potential) Iron ingestion >60 milligrams/kg with opacities on abdominal radiograph • Life-threatening ingestion of diltiazem or verapamil • Body packers or stuffers • Slow-release potassium ingestion • Lead ingestion (including paint flakes containing lead) • Symptomatic arsenic trioxide ingestion

	• Life-threatening ingestions of lithium
Contraindications	• Unprotected airway • Gastrointestinal perforation, obstruction or ileus, hemorrhage • Intractable vomiting • Cardiovascular instability
Complications	• Nausea, vomiting • Pulmonary aspiration • Time consuming; possible delay instituting other definitive care

INDICATIONS, CONTRAINDICATIONS, & COMPLICATIONS OF ENHANCED ELIMINATION PROCEDURES

Multidose Activated Charcoal	Initial dose: 50 grams (1 gram/kg children), Repeat dose 25 grams (0.5 g/kg children) every 2 hours
Indications	• Carbamazepine coma (reduces duration of coma) • Phenobarbital coma (reduces duration of coma) • Dapsone toxicity with significant methemoglobinemia • Quinine overdose • Theophylline overdose if hemodialysis/hemoperfusion unavailable
Contraindications	• Unprotected airway • Bowel obstruction • Caution in ingestions resulting in reduced gastrointestinal motility
Complications	• Vomiting • Pulmonary aspiration • Constipation • Charcoal bezoar, • Bowel obstruction/perforation

URINARY ALKALINIZATION	
Indications	• Moderate to severe salicylate toxicity not meeting criteria for hemodialysis • Phenobarbital (multidose activated charcoal superior) • Chlorophenoxy herbicides (2-4-dichlorophenoxyacetic acid and mecoprop): requires high urine flow rate 600 mL/h to be effective • Chlorpropamide: supportive care/IV dextrose normally sufficient
Contraindications	• Preexisting fluid overload • Renal impairment • Uncorrected hypokalemia
Complications	• Hypokalemia • Volume overload • Alkalemia • Hypocalcemia (usually mild)

II. TREATMENT FOR SPECIFIC POISONS

1. PARACETAMOL

OVERVIEW

- Paracetamol is responsible for 30,000 UK hospital admissions a year and results in 345 deaths per annum.
- Paracetamol is the most common drug to be taken in overdose (48% of poisoning related admissions).
- Can be fatal if not treated appropriately (between 100-200 deaths per year).
- Assessment for risk factors for hepatotoxicity is no longer required.
- Paracetamol induced hepatic injury is most likely to occur after ingestions of >10g or >200mg/kg.
- Ingestion of ≥**75mg/kg** is considered a significant ingestion and needs further investigation.

SIGNS AND SYMPTOMS

- Initially asymptomatic
- End-organ toxicity often does not manifest until 24-48 hours after an acute ingestion.

3. MANAGEMENT OF PARACETAMOL OD IN THE ED

- The earliest and most sensitive indicator of liver damage is a **prolonged INR**, which starts to rise at around **24 hours after overdose**.
- **LFTs** are usually normal **until around 16 hours after overdose**.
- **AST and ALT levels** then sharply rise and can reach > 10,000 units/L by **72-96 hours** after overdose.
- **Bilirubin** levels rise more slowly and reach their maximum at around **5 days**.
- Do bloods immediately unless ingestion <4 hours ago then **delay bloods until 4 hours post-ingestion**[343].

- **Start NAC immediately, if:**
  - Single ingestion >15 hours ago
  - Staggered ingestion
  - Timing of overdose uncertain
  - Ingestion >4 hours ago and bloods results will not be known within 8 hours of ingestion

- **Give activated charcoal, if:**
  - Ingestion <1 hour ago AND dose >150mg/kg

- **Wait for blood results before prescribing NAC, if:**
  - Ingestion >4 hours ago and blood results will be known with 8 hours of ingestion

1. MANAGEMENT OF ADULT PATIENTS WHO PRESENT WITHIN 1-4 HOUR OF INGESTION[344].

- Consider **charcoal** if more than 150 mg/kg body weight taken, presentation within 1 hour of ingestion and able to control the airway.
- **Take blood for plasma paracetamol concentration at 4 hours post ingestion**.
- Assess whether at high risk of severe liver damage (see above).
- Confirm timings of ingestion.

2. MANAGEMENT OF ADULT PATIENTS WHO PRESENT WITHIN 4-8 HOURS OF INGESTION

- **Do not** start NAC immediately.
- Wait until 4 hours post ingestion and take Paracetamol/salicylates levels.
- Start NAC if level taken at 4 hours is in the appropriate treatment range.
- If the paracetamol concentration result is not available within 8 hours of ingestion (> 150 mg/kg or > 12 g in total) **start NAC immediately.**
- It can be stopped later if subsequent level well below treatment line.

3. MANAGEMENT OF ALL PATIENTS WHO PRESENT 8-15 HOURS AFTER INGESTION.

- Urgent action is required (antidote efficacy drops sharply).
- **Give NAC immediately** without waiting for the result of the plasma paracetamol concentration measurement if it is thought that more than 150 mg/kg body weight or a total of 12 g or more has been ingested.
- Take Paracetamol/Salicylates levels, INR, Creatinine and ALT.
- If the paracetamol concentration result is not available within 8 hours of ingestion (> 150 mg/kg or > 12 g in total) **start NAC immediately.**
- In patients already receiving NAC, only discontinue NAC if the plasma paracetamol concentration is below the treatment line on the graph and there is no abnormality of the INR, plasma creatinine or ALT and the patient is asymptomatic.
- Continue the infusion if there is any doubt as to the timing of the overdose.
- At the end of NAC infusion **check INR and plasma creatinine concentration**.

---

343 *RCEM Guidance, paracetamol overdose [RCEM Online]*

344 *Dr Neil Long,Paracetamol toxicity [Life in the fast lane]*

o Patients who are symptomatic or in whom the INR and/or plasma creatinine are abnormal require further monitoring.
o **Vitamin K** should be given if the INR is increased.
o **FFP / clotting factors** are only indicated **for active bleeding.**

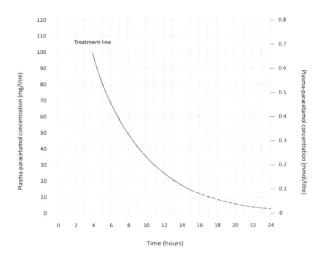

4. MANAGEMENT OF PATIENTS WHO PRESENT 15-24 HOURS AFTER INGESTION:

o **Start NAC immediately.**
o Measure the plasma paracetamol concentration on admission.
o The infusion may be stopped and the patient discharged from medical care if each of the following criteria is met:
  ▪ The patient is asymptomatic.
  ▪ The INR and plasma creatinine are normal.
  ▪ The plasma paracetamol concentration is **less than 10 mg/L** (0.07 mmol/L) 24 hours after ingestion.
o Patients in whom the INR and/or plasma creatinine are abnormal or whose plasma paracetamol concentrations exceed 10 mg/L at 24 hours after ingestion require further monitoring and contact with a hepatologist.

5. MANAGEMENT OF PATIENTS WHO PRESENT LONGER THAN 24 HOURS AFTER INGESTION:

o All should have their **INR, Plasma Creatinine concentration, ALT and Venous pH** (or hydrogen ion / bicarb concentration) determined.
o We recommend that they **all** be discussed with a poison's information centre or a specialist liver or poisons unit.

6. SPECIALIST ADVICE ON THOSE WITH LIVER DISEASE

• Liver transplantation is occasionally needed for liver failure secondary to paracetamol overdose for patients who presented or were treated late.

KING'S COLLEGE CRITERIA FOR ACETAMINOPHEN/PARACETAMOL TOXICITY

The presence of one of the following should prompt a referral/transfer to a liver transplantation center[345]:

• Acidosis (admission arterial pH < 7.30) OR
• Hepatic encephalopathy (grade III or IV), AND coagulopathy (PT > 100 s), AND acute kidney injury (creatinine > 3.4 mg/dL), OR
• Hyperlactatemia (4-hour lactate > 3.5 mmol/L, or 12-hour lactate > 3.0 mmol/L), OR
• Hyperphosphatemia (48-96 hour phosphate > 3.7 mg/dL) in patients with acetaminophen-induced fulminant hepatic failure.

1. N- ACETYLCYSTEINE (NAC)[346]

• Acetylcysteine should be administered by intravenous infusion preferably using **Glucose 5%** as the infusion fluid.
• **Sodium Chloride 0.9% solution** may be used if Glucose 5% is not suitable.
• The full course of treatment with acetylcysteine comprises of 3 consecutive intravenous infusions.
• Doses should be administered sequentially with no break between the infusions.
• The patient should receive a total dose of **300 mg/kg body weight over a 21-hour period**.

ADULTS & CHILDREN >40Kg

• Weigh the patient to determine the correct weight band.
• If the patient weighs less than 40kg use the paediatric dosage table.
• Ampoule volume has been rounded up to the nearest whole number.
• **First infusion**
  o 150mg/kg NAC in 200 mL of DW 5% over 1 hour.
• **Second infusion**
  o 50mg/kg NAC in 500 mL of DW 5% over 4 hours.
• **Third infusion**
  o 100mg/kg NAC in 1000 mL of DW 5% over 16 hours.

CHILDREN

• Children are treated with the same doses and regimen as adults. However, the quantity of intravenous fluid used has been modified to take into account age and weight, as fluid overload is a potential danger.
• Doses should be administered sequentially using an appropriate infusion pump.

---

[345] King's College Criteria for Acetaminophen Toxicity [MdCalc Online]
[346] RCEM Guidance, paracetamol overdose [RCEM Online]

- Preparation and administration of paediatric infusions
- Weigh the child to determine the correct weight band.
- Read off the table the total infusion volume required for each dose according to the weight of the child and make up the solutions according to the directions below.

First Infusion

- Prepare a **50 mg/mL** solution by diluting each 10 mL NAC (200 mg/mL) with **30 mL** glucose 5% or sodium chloride 0.9% to give a total volume of **40 mL** over 1 hr.

Second Infusion

- Prepare a **6.25 mg/mL solution** by diluting each 10 mL NAC (200 mg/mL) with **310 mL** glucose 5% or sodium chloride 0.9% to give a total volume of **320 mL** over 4 hours.

Third Infusion

- Prepare a **6.25 mg/mL** solution by diluting each 10 mL NAC (200 mg/mL) with **310 mL** glucose 5% or sodium chloride 0.9% to give a total volume of **320 mL** over 16 hours.

For example, for a child weighing 12 kg, the first infusion would be 38 mL infused at 38 mL/h over 1 hour, the second infusion would be 100 mL infused at 25 mL/h over 4 hours and the third infusion is 208 mL infused at 13 mL/h over 16 hours.

2. ANAPHYLACTOID REACTION

- N-Acetylcysteine can cause **anaphylactoid reactions** with vomiting, flushing, urticaria, angioedema, bronchospasm and rarely shock.
- Very rarely it can also cause respiratory depression, acute kidney injury and DIC.
- Reactions occur in around **20% of patients** and are more likely in **women, brittle asthmatics** and those **with low paracetamol levels**.
- Reactions can usually be controlled by **simply stopping the infusion.**
- If the reaction persists **10 mg IV chlorphenamine can be given and salbutamol nebulisers** added if bronchospasm is present.
- Previous reactions are no longer considered a contraindication to the use of acetylcysteine.

2. SALICYLATES

OVERVIEW

- Salicylate poisoning is a relatively common cause of poisoning and effective early treatment can prevent organ damage and death.
- Poisoning can be classified as mild, moderate or severe depending upon the plasma salicylate level:
  - *Mild poisoning* = < 450 mg/L
  - *Moderate poisoning* = 450-700 mg/L
  - *Severe poisoning* = > 700 mg/L

CLINICAL FEATURES INCLUDE:

- Nausea and Vomiting
- Tinnitus and Deafness
- Sweating and Dehydration
- Hyperventilation
- Cutaneous flushing
- Hyperpyrexia (particularly children)
- Hypoglycaemia (particularly children)
- Severe poisoning can cause convulsions, cerebral oedema, coma, renal failure, non-cardiogenic pulmonary oedema and cardiovascular instability.

INVESTIGATIONS SHOULD INCLUDE:

- Plasma salicylate level
- Arterial blood gas: **Primary respiratory alkalosis** may occur, followed by concomitant **primary metabolic acidosis (RALMAC)**
- Blood glucose level
- Urea and electrolytes
- Clotting profile
- ECG

ECG ABNORMALITIES IN SALICYLATE OD:

- Widening of the QRS complex
- AV Block
- Ventricular Arrhythmias

TREATMENT

- Initial Management[347]
  - Basics: ABC's, IV, O2 (if hypoxic), cardiac monitor
  - GI decontamination: activated charcoal if patient awake and alert to tolerate
  - Alkalinization with Sodium Bicarbonate
    - Goal in treatment is to increase pH of both serum and urine to shift towards charged state to prevent neurotoxicity and enhance elimination through the urine. (Goldfrank 2015)

---

[347] *Anand Swaminathan, Salicylate Toxicity [RebelEM]*

- Start with 1-2 mEq/kg bolus followed by a drip ("1 amp" of bicarbonate is equal to 50mL of 8.4% sodium bicarbonate 1mEq/mL, or 50mEq of NaHCO3⁻)
  - Bicarb drip can be made with 3 ampules of NaHCO3⁻ (150 mEq) in one liter of D5W
  - Do not make bicarb drip with normal saline because this will be hypertonic solution due to sodium in sodium bicarbonate
  - Run bicarb drip at 1.5-2X maintenance fluid rate. These patients are fluid down and need to replace losses
  - Goal serum pH around 7.55, urine pH 8.0
  - No benefit of forced diuresis
- Treat hypo or normoglycemia to prevent neuroglycopenia (Thurston 1970, Kuzak 2007)
  - No human studies showing a "goal" serum glucose concentration
  - If patient is altered, consider glucose supplementation regardless of serum glucose concentration
- Treat hypokalemia to goal K of 5.5 mEq
  - If hypokalemia, renal tubules will reabsorb potassium ions in exchange for hydrogen ions
  - This prevents alkalinization of the urine

- **Airway and Respiratory Management (Mosier 2015)**
  - Tachypnea alone is not an indication for intubation
    - Tachypnea and hyperpernea leads to respiratory alkalosis (This is necessary compensation for the metabolic acidosis)
  - Avoid intubation if possible
    - Hypoventilation during the apneic period causes respiratory acidosis
    - Associated with peri-intubation period morbidity and possible cardiac arrest (Stolbach 2008)
  - Indications for airway management include hypoxia, pulmonary edema, hypoventilation/tiring out, worsening acidosis despite appropriate therapy
  - Give bicarb 1-2 mEq/kg bolus peri-intubation
  - Consider awake intubation or ketamine facilitated intubation to minimize or eliminate apneic time
  - Ventilator settings very important post-intubation
    - Need to match minute ventilation of patient pre-intubation to prevent respiratory acidosis
    - High tidal volumes and high rate needed
  - Frequent blood gas monitoring post-intubation, as well as need for frequent BMP, salicylate concentrations. Consider A-line placement
  - If unable to appropriately alkalinize and eliminate salicylate with bicarbonate, Hemodialysis may be indicated

3. BENZODIAZEPINES

Deaths associated with benzodiazepine overdose are due to mixed overdoses, especially alcohol and other drugs. Clinical manifestations are associated with drowsiness, respiratory depression, dysarthria, and ataxia. Coma is not common but is most often seen in the elderly or patients who have ingested alcohol or other drugs.
Treatment is supportive.

FLUMAZENIL
The use of **flumazenil** is controversial as it has many side-effects and is rarely indicated. Adverse effects include ventricular tachycardia, raising intracranial pressure, withdrawal in chronic abusers, and seizures if used in the presence of tricyclic antidepressants. It can be used to reverse benzodiazepine coma so as to avoid intubation, but this should be limited to situations of benzodiazepine overdose where no other drugs have been taken.

4. OPIATES

Increasing doses of opioids progressively produce euphoria, pinpoint pupils, sedation, respiratory depression, and apnoea. Complications include hypotension, convulsions, non-cardiogenic pulmonary oedema, and compartment syndrome from prolonged immobility.
Where this is suspected, **serum CK and urinary myoglobin** should be measured to look for evidence of rhabdomyolysis.

NALOXONE
Naloxone should be given in **100 µg boluses I.V.** to a maximum of **2 mg** with the aim of reversing the opiate effect and reversing respiratory depression.
This antidote can precipitate an acute agitated withdrawal state and when giving it staff should be mindful of their own safety. Naloxone can be administered I.V., I.M., S.C., or via the tracheal route. It has a short half-life (20 min if given i.v.) and therefore may be needed as an infusion since respiratory depression may reoccur.
It can rarely cause ventricular dysrhythmias and hypertension and drowsiness at very high doses.
Continuous IV infusion (Off-label)
- For use in patients exposed to long acting opioids (eg, methadone), sustained release products
- Calculate dose/hr based on effective intermittent dose used and duration of adequate response seen.
- Alternatively, **use two-thirds of initial effective naloxone bolus** on an hourly basis (0.25-6.25 mg/hr); administer one-half of initial bolus dose 15 min after initiating continuous IV infusion to prevent drop in naloxone levels

5. TRICYCLIC ANTIDEPRESSANTS

- Any overdose of amitriptyline > **10 mg/kg** is potentially life-threatening.
- An overdose > **30 mg/kg** will result in severe toxicity, cardiotoxicity and coma.
- The toxic effects of TCAs are mediated by several pharmacological effects:
  - *Anticholinergic effects*
  - *Direct alpha-adrenergic blockade*
  - *Blockade of noradrenaline reuptake at the preganglionic synapse*
  - *Blockade of sodium channels*
  - *Blockade of potassium channels*

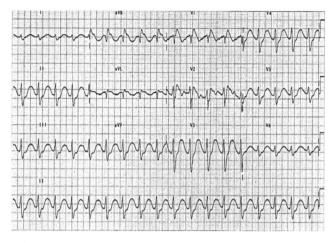

CLINICAL EFFECTS

Anticholinergic	• Dry mouth, • Dry Skin • Constipation, • Urinary retention • Mydriasis • Blurred vision • Aggravation narrow angle glaucoma
Anti-alpha adrenergic	• Orthostatic hypotension
Antihistaminic	• Sedation
Cardiac	• Tachycardia, • Hypotension • Palpitation, • Chest pain.
CNS	• Decrease mental status, • Respiratory depression, • Drowsiness, Confusion, • Convulsion, Coma.

- The cardiotoxic effects of TCAs are mediated by the blockade of **Na+ channels,** which causes QRS broadening, and blockade of **K+ channels**, which causes QT interval prolongation.
- The degree of QRS broadening correlates with adverse events:
  - *QRS > 100 ms is predictive of **seizures***
  - *QRS > 160 ms is predictive of **ventricular arrhythmias***
- **The ECG changes seen in TCA overdose include:**
  - *Sinus tachycardia (very common)*
  - *Prolongation of the PR interval & Broadening of QRS complex*
  - *Prolongation of the QT interval & Ventricular arrhythmias (severe toxicity)*

ED MANAGEMENT OF TCAs POISONING[348]

- **Airway protection**
  - Patients with GCS ≤8 should undergo rapid sequence induction at the earliest opportunity (Grade C).
  - Some patients with GCS >8 may also need intubation, particularly in the presence of airway compromise, hypoventilation or refractory seizures (Grade C).
  - Benzodiazepines may be considered to control agitation following TCA overdose (Grade E).
- **Gastric decontamination**
  - Activated charcoal may be considered for use within 1 hour of TCA ingestion but only in patients with an intact or secured airway.
  - The potential risk of aspiration should be strongly considered before use (Grade D).
  - Multiple dose activated charcoal should not be considered (Grade D).
  - Gastric lavage may be considered for potentially life-threatening TCA overdoses only when it can be delivered within 1 hour of ingestion and the airway is protected (Grade D).
- **Initial assessment**
  - An ECG should be recorded at presentation to the ED following TCA overdose (Grade B).
  - The ECG should be used to risk stratify patients with TCA overdose and to guide subsequent therapy (Grade B).
  - Serial ECG recordings should be examined for the presence of QRS prolongation (>100ms), QTc prolongation (>430ms) and R/S ratio >0.7 in lead aVR.
  - These changes identify patients at high risk of developing complications following TCA overdose (Grade B).

---

[348] *Guideline for the Management of Tricyclic Antidepressant Overdose by RCEM [RCEM website]*

- **Blood pH for risk stratification**
  - Blood gas analysis is an important part of the initial assessment and monitoring of patients who have taken a TCA overdose (Grade E).
  - Venous sampling for blood gas analysis is an acceptable alternative to arterial sampling unless hypoxia or hypoventilation are suspected (Grade D).
- **Treatment of haemodynamic instability**[349]
  - A bolus of intravenous fluids should be considered as a first-line therapy to treat hypotension induced by TCA overdose (Grade D).
  - Sodium bicarbonate is indicated for the treatment of dysrhythmias or hypotension associated with TCA overdose. (Grade C).
  - Sodium bicarbonate may be considered for the treatment of QRS prolongation (>100ms) associated with TCA overdose (Grade E).
  - The treatment of dysrhythmias or hypotension should include alkalinisation to a serum pH of 7.45 to 7.55. (Grade E).
  - Vasopressors should be used for hypotension following TCA overdose that has not responded to initial treatment (including sodium bicarbonate and intravenous fluids). (Grade D).
  - Epinephrine may be superior to norepinephrine for treating refractory hypotension and preventing arrhythmias. (Grade D).
  - It is not unreasonable to administer 10mg intravenous glucagon to treat life-threatening hypotension or arrhythmias refractory to other measures (Grade D).
  - Magnesium sulphate may be considered for the treatment of TCA-induced dysrhythmias when other treatments have been unsuccessful. (Grade D).
- **Management of seizures**[350]
  - Phenytoin should be avoided in patients with TCA overdose (Grade D).
  - Benzodiazepines should be used to control seizures following TCA overdose (Grade E).
- **Observation of asymptomatic patients**
  - Following TCA overdose asymptomatic, stable patients with no significant ECG abnromalities six hours after ingestion may be safely discharged (Grade B).

---

[349] *Guideline for the Management of Tricyclic Antidepressant Overdose by RCEM [RCEM website]*

[350] *Guideline for the Management of Tricyclic Antidepressant Overdose by RCEM [RCEM website]*

6. METHANOL & ETHYLENE GLYCOL

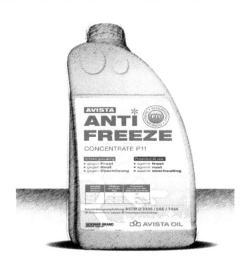

- The toxic alcohols are rapidly absorbed following ingestion, and then slowly metabolized by **alcohol dehydrogenase** to either **glycolaldehyde** (in the case of ethylene glycol) or **formaldehyde** (in the case of methanol). The aldehydes are then rapidly metabolized further by **aldehyde dehydrogenase** and other enzymes – the secondary metabolites are predominantly acids and are responsible for the toxic effects.
- Both of the antidotes **(ethanol and fomepizole)** act on the initial rate-limiting step as competitive inhibitors of alcohol dehydrogenase to prevent the development of the toxic metabolites. Since ethylene glycol requires metabolism before the toxic effects develop, the clinical presentation can vary with time from ingestion:
  - **Early (<12 hours):** inebriation, mild depression in consciousness, nausea and vomiting, focal fits, ataxia, nystagmus, and decreased tone and reflexes
  - **Middle (12–24 hours):** tachycardia, tachypnoea, hypertension and cardiac failure
  - **Late (>24 hours):** renal failure and hyperkalaemia, abdominal pain, tetany, convulsions, coma, hypocalcaemia, arrhythmias, and hypomagnesaemia

CLINICAL ASSESSMENT
This should follow the standard ABCDE approach:
- Ensure a patent airway (provide adjuncts as necessary).
- Provide supplemental oxygen as per BTS guidelines.
- Assess breathing, including respiration rate and auscultation for equal air entry and added sounds. Attach pulse oximetry.
- Take the pulse, measure the blood pressure and look for signs of shock. Apply cardiac monitoring and request a 12-lead ECG.
- Obtain intravenous access.
- Obtain a blood glucose.

- Assess the formal GCS.
- Expose the patient but maintain a comfortable environment. Check for any signs of obvious injury, especially to the head. Look for any alert badges and signs of chronic disease (e.g. liver disease, intravenous drug use and sites of insulin injection).
- Perform a brief neurological examination, including pupils, eye movements, reflexes and plantars.

INVESTIGATIONS

- FBC, U&E, LFT, calcium, magnesium and albumin. Consider paracetamol levels.
- Perform **ABG:** Patients presenting late with ethylene glycol poisoning have a **raised-anion-gap metabolic acidosis** that is due to the metabolism of the parent alcohol to a number of organic acids.
- Calculate the **osmolal gap OG** as the difference between the measured and calculated serum osmolalities, i.e.

  OG = measured osmolality – calculated osmolarity
  (all in mosmol/kg), where the calculated osmolality is given by:

  Calculated osmolarity = 2 Na + Glucose + Urea

  with Na+, glucose and urea in mmol/L.
  An OG > 10 mosmo/kg is a strong indicator for toxic alcohol ingestion.

- Measurement of ethylene glycol in the serum is rarely performed in practice.
- The presence of **calcium oxalate crystals** in the urine is diagnostic for ethylene glycol poisoning.
- Ethylene glycol has no specific cardiac effects and the ECG will likely show a sinus tachycardia.
- Request a **chest X-ray** to look for signs of aspiration.

Causes of raised-anion-gap metabolic acidosis: 'MUDPILES'
- **M**ethanol
- **U**raemia
- **D**iabetic ketoacidosis
- **P**araldehyde
- **I**soniazid, iron
- **L**actic acidosis
- **E**thanol, ethylene glycol
- **S**alicylate, starvation, solvents

Causes of raised osmolal gap: 'ME DIE O'
- **M**ethanol
- **E**thylene glycol
- **D**iuretics (mannitol)
- **I**sopropanol
- **E**thanol
- **O**ther (ketoacidosis, multiple organ failure)

ED MANAGEMENT

- The management of ethylene glycol poisoning should follow the standard pattern for any toxicological emergency.
- **Gut decontamination**
  - Gastric lavage may be considered if ingestion may have been within the last hour.
  - Activated charcoal is of no benefit, because it does not adsorb alcohols.
- **Symptomatic and supportive**
  - This is along the ABCDE lines as detailed above.
  - Control seizures with intravenous lorazepam.
  - Rehydrate with intravenous fluids.
  - Consider bicarbonate to correct the metabolic acidosis. High doses may be required, and U&E and ABG need to be regularly monitored.
- **Enhanced elimination techniques**
  - Haemodialysis may be used in severe toxic alcohol poisoning (including ethanol).
- **Antidotes**
  - The specific antidote for use in ethylene glycol poisoning is **ethanol.**
  - This should be given where there is a strong suspicion of ethylene glycol poisoning and at least two objective indicators:
    - pH < 7.3
    - Serum bicarbonate < 20 mmol/L
    - Osmolal gap > 10 mosmol/kg
    - Urinary oxalate crystals
    - Severe symptoms
    - Ethylene glycol levels > 200 mg/L
- Ethanol may be given orally or intravenously and is commenced as a loading dose equivalent to **800 mg/kg of 100% ethanol** followed by maintenance therapy based on the clinical situation.
- **Serum ethanol levels** need to be taken at least every 2 hours; the aim of therapy is to achieve a level of 1-1.5 g/L (100-150 mg/dL).
- **Fomepizole** is given intravenously. Although it is more expensive than ethanol, it does not require regular biochemical monitoring. It must be obtained from the NPIS, who will also advise on the dosing regime.
- **Fomepizole** blocks the metabolism of methanol and ethanol and can be injected 12 hourly. It is expensive and not widely available. Folate deficiency in primates is predictive of poor outcome in methanol toxicity and it is suggested that **folate be given in a dose of 1 mg/Kg/day for 48 h.**

7. DIGOXIN TOXICITY

OVERVIEW

o Digoxin is a cardiac glycoside that primarily works by inhibiting the **Na+/K+ ATPase** in the myocardium.

o This results in **a slowing of the ventricular response** and **a positively inotropic effect**.

o Digoxin has a long half-life and maintenance doses need to be given only once daily. It should be monitored to ensure that the correct dosage is being given and to ensure that factors that can provoke toxicity (e.g. **renal dysfunction and hypokalaemia**) are not developing.

o Regular monitoring of plasma digoxin concentrations during maintenance treatment is not necessary once steady state has been achieved unless problems are suspected. In atrial fibrillation, the best monitor of response to treatment is the ventricular rate.

o A target range of **1.0-1.5 nmol/L** should be aimed for but concentrations of **2 nmol/L** may be required.

o The plasma concentration alone cannot indicate toxicity reliably, but the likelihood of toxicity rises dramatically at levels above 2 nmol/L.

o **Hypokalaemia** predisposes to digoxin toxicity and can be managed by co-administration of a **potassium-sparing diuretic or potassium supplementation**.

THE CLINICAL FEATURES

o **General:** Weakness, Fatigue, General Malaise

o **Cardiac:** almost any arrhythmia or heart block

o **Neurological:** Headache, Facial Pain, Dizziness, Confusion, Delirium, Psychoses and Hallucinations

o **Gastrointestinal**: Anorexia, Nausea, Vomiting and Abdominal Pain.

o **Visual:** Blurred Vision, Xanthopsia (**yellow vision**)

Digoxin Effect on ECG

- Digoxin effect on ECG is not a marker of digoxin toxicity
- It merely indicates that the patient is taking digoxin
- The QRS-ST morphology is described as:
"slurred" , "sagging" , "scooped" , "reverse tick" , "hockey stick" or "Salvador Dali's moustache"

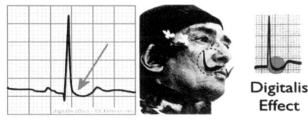

Digitalis Effect

ECG FEATURES OF DIGOXIN TOXICITY:

o **PR** interval Prolonged

o **QRS** Prolonged

o **QT** Shortened

o **ST** depression (**reverse tick/check sign**)

o **T** wave inversion

o Bradycardia

o AV Block or dissociation

o Ventricular ectopics

ED MANAGEMENT OF DIGOXIN TOXICITY

o Stop the digoxin

o Involve the cardiology team and/or the Poisons Information Service

o Monitor pulse, blood pressure and cardiac rhythm

o Check urea and electrolytes, magnesium, and digoxin levels

o Correct serum potassium

o Correct serum magnesium

o Monitor ECG and treat arrhythmias as appropriate

DIGIBIND

o Digoxin-specific antibody Fab is the antidote used for digoxin poisoning.

o The digoxin-specific antibody fragments have a higher affinity for digoxin than the receptor in the body.

o It is expensive and rarely needed and its use should be reserved for cases of severe poisoning only.

8. LITHIUM OVERDOSE

- Lithium is commonly used as a maintenance treatment for bipolar affective disorder. Lithium poisoning occurs relatively frequently as it is used in a population that is at high-risk for overdose. Poisoning can also occur accidentally due to therapeutic overdosage due to its relatively **narrow therapeutic index.**

- The usual therapeutic range for lithium is **0.4-0.8 mmol/l** (but the range may vary between laboratories).

- Toxic effects are often seen at **levels > 1.5 mmol/l.**

- **There are three main categories of lithium poisoning:**
  o **Acute poisoning:**
    ▪ Occurs in patients recently started on lithium.
    ▪ The main symptoms are **GIT upset** (nausea, vomiting, abdominal pain and diarrhoea).
    ▪ More severe cases progress to **tremor, ataxia and confusion**.
    ▪ In severe cases there can be **convulsions, coma and renal failure**.
  o **Acute-on-chronic poisoning**:
    ▪ Occurs in patients taking lithium regularly that increased their dose or taken too much.
    ▪ Symptoms are similar to acute poisoning but serum levels can be difficult to interpret.
  o **Chronic poisoning:**
    ▪ Occurs in patients on long-term lithium patients and is usually precipitated by the introduction of a new medication that has impaired renal function.

- Symptoms are primarily neurological.
- Mental status is often altered and can progress to coma and seizures if the diagnosis is unrecognized.
- These patients are very difficult to treat.

INVESTIGATIONS
○ U&E
○ Lithium level

> ✦ *Patients with lithium overdose should have their **urea and electrolyte levels** measured due to the risk of renal impairment and **a lithium level checked** (which is sent in a plain tube, not a lithium heparin tube).*

MANAGEMENT
○ Admit all with symptoms of toxicity or levels **> 2mmol/l**
○ Observe All patients tor at least 24 hours.
○ **Gastric lavage** if presents within 1 hour of overdose
○ **WBI** for an overdose of slow-release tablets.
○ **Haemodialysis**: treatment of choice for severe poisoning.
○ **Activated charcoal**: does not absorb lithium.

9. IRON POISONING
BACKGROUND
In iron poisoning, the important consideration is the amount of elemental iron ingested, not the amount of iron salt.

ASSESSMENT
Patients Requiring Assessment
- Ingestion **of > 40mg/kg elemental iron**.
- Ingestion of an unknown quantity.
- Any symptomatic children.

History and Examination
Classic stages and time course of iron toxicity:
- **0-6 hours:** vomiting, diarrhoea, haemetemesis, melena, abdominal pain. Significant fluid losses may lead to hypovolemic shock
- **6-12 hours:** gastrointestinal symptoms wane and the patient appears to be getting better. During this time iron shifts intracellularly from the circulation
- **12-48 hours:** Cellular toxicity becomes manifest as vasodilative shock and third-spacing, high anion gap metabolic acidosis (HAGMA) and hepatorenal failure
- **2-5 days:** acute hepatic failure, although rare mortality is high
- **2-6 weeks:** chronic sequelae occur in survivors, cirrhosis and gastrointestinal scarring and strictures

INVESTIGATIONS
Asymptomatic Children:
- If tablet ingestion
  ○ Abdominal X-ray (AXR) (if negative, no further investigation or observation are required)
- If unknown amount or >40 mg/kg ingested
  ○ Measure **serum iron concentrations 4 hourly until falling.**

All symptomatic patients should have the following investigations:
- AXR (if tablet ingestion)
  ○ AXR may also be helpful in evaluating gastrointestinal decontamination after whole bowel irrigation (WBI)
- Blood gas (acidosis)
- Glucose (hyperglycaemia)
- FBC (leukocytosis)
- U&E, LFTs
- Clotting (reversible early coagulopathy and late coagulopathy secondary to hepatic injury)
- Blood group and cross-match
- Serum iron concentration
  ○ Should be performed immediately and repeated 4-6 hours after ingestion since concentration usually peaks at 4-6 hours after ingestion.
  ○ Concentrations taken after 4-6 hours may underestimate toxicity because the iron may have either been distributed into tissues or be bound to ferritin.
  ○ In the case of slow release or enteric coated tablets, concentrations should be repeated at 6-8 hours as absorption may be erratic and delayed.
  ○ Once **desferrioxamine** is commenced, iron concentrations are not accurate at most labs using automated methods (including RCH)

ACUTE MANAGEMENT
Resuscitation
- Supportive treatment to maintain adequate blood pressure and electrolyte balance is essential.
- I.V. fluid resuscitation 20 mL/kg for hypovolaemia or hypotension
- Potassium and glucose administration as necessary.

DECONTAMINATION
- Activated charcoal does not bind to iron and is not indicated.
- Decontamination of choice is **whole bowel irrigation (WBI)**
  ○ WBI is indicated if the AXR reveals tablets or capsules ingested and more than 60mg/kg ingested

- o Discuss with a toxicologist for advice before performing WBI
- o Usual protocol is nasogastric colonic lavage solution 30mL/kg/hr until rectal effluent clear. This is an extremely resource-intensive processing requiring 1-1 nursing.
- o WBI is contraindicated if there are signs of bowel obstruction or haemorrhage

ONGOING CARE AND MONITORING
ANTIDOTE - DESFERRIOXAMINE
- Consider desferrioxamine if:
  - o Serum iron concentrations **> 90 micromol/L**.
  - o Concentration **60 - 90 micromol/L** and tablets visible on AXR or symptomatic (nausea, vomiting, diarrhoea, abdominal pain, haematemesis, fever).
  - o The patient has significant symptoms of altered conscious state, hypotension, tachycardia, tachypnoea, or worsening symptoms irrespective of ingested dose or serum iron concentration.
  - o **Do not wait for iron concentration** if altered conscious state, shock, severe acidosis (pH <7.1), or worsening symptoms. If serum iron concentration is not readily available, a fall in serum bicarbonate concentration is a reasonable surrogate marker of systemic iron poisoning. Commence desferrioxamine without delay, in consultation with a toxicologist.
- **Desferrioxamine dose**
  - o **15mg/kg/hr intravenous**
  - o The rate is reduced after 4-6 hours so that the total intravenous dose does not exceed 80mg/kg/24 hours.
- **Duration**
  - o Significant poisoning usually requires administration for 12 -16 hours, however it is recommended to continue desferrioxamine until:
    - The patient is asymptomatic
    - Decontamination complete
    - Anion-gap acidosis resolved
    - Serum iron concentration <60 micromol/L
- Desferrioxamine has been associated with pulmonary toxicity and should be used with caution if indications persist >24 hours
- Desferrioxamine-iron complex is renally excreted. If oliguria or anuria develop, **peritoneal dialysis or haemodialysis** may become necessary to remove ferrioxamine.

When to admit:
- Ingestions of **>40mg/kg or unknown quantities**.
- Admission should be considered for all children and young people with an intentional overdose

- Consult ICU being considered for desferrioxamine or with worsening symptoms.

When to consider transfer to a tertiary centre:
- Desferrioxamine and/or whole bowel irrigation is required
- Significantly decreased conscious stage or conscious state not improving as expected.
- Need for respiratory support

DISCHARGE CRITERIA
- If <40mg/kg ingestion and negative AXR (if tablet ingestion) can discharge if asymptomatic 6 hours post ingestion.
- If ingestion of >40mg/kg, discharge only if remains asymptomatic and serum iron concentration falling and <60micromol/L on two measurements 4 hours apart

- *Remember in severe iron poisoning, there is often **6-24-hour latent period** when initial symptoms resolve, before overt systemic toxicity declares.*
- *Thus, improvement over this time may be a result of actual improvement or be proceeding deterioration.*

10. CARBON MONOXIDE POISONING
OVERVIEW
- Carbon monoxide (CO) is a colourless, odourless gas produced by incomplete combustion of carbonaceous material. CO poisoning may be acute or chronic.
- Exposure is most commonly from suicide attempts using car exhaust, and accidental exposures from incomplete combustion in charcoal burners, faulty heaters, fires, and industrial accidents.
- Chronic CO poisoning may have an insidious presentation (e.g. intermittent headaches), and a high index of suspicion is required in at-risk groups (e.g. fires inside the home)

TOXICODYNAMICS
- Carbon monoxide has **~210 times** the affinity for haemoglobin than oxygen.
- Binding therefore renders haemoglobin oxygen carrying capacity and delivery to the tissues. This can result in tissue **hypoxia and ischaemic injury**.
- CO also binds to intracellular cytochromes, impairing aerobic metabolism.
- **Typical clinical symptoms and signs relative to COHb (Normal = 0.5%):**
  - o **<10%**: Nil, commonly found in smokers.
  - o **10 – 20%**: Nil or vague nondescript symptoms.
  - o **30 – 40%**: Headache, tachycardia, confusion, weakness, nausea, vomiting, collapse.

- o **50 – 60%**: Coma, convulsions, Cheyne-Stokes breathing, arrhythmias, ECG changes.
- o **70 – 80%**: Circulatory and ventilatory failure, cardiac arrest, Death.

CLINICAL FEATURES

- **Acute poisoning**
  - o The **cherry red skin** colour produced when carboxyhaemoglobin (COHb) concentrations exceed about 20% is rarely seen in life.
  - o **CNS:** Headache, Nausea, Dizziness, Confusion, Mini Mental Status Examination Errors, Incoordination, Ataxia, Seizures and finally Coma.
  - o **CVS:** Dysrhythmias, Ischaemia, hyper or hypotension (exacerbated in patients with anaemia or underlying cardiovascular disease)
  - o **GI:** Abdominal Pain, N+V, Diarrhoea
  - o **RESP:** Dyspnoea, Tachypnoea, Chest Pain, Palpitation
  - o **Other:**
    - Non-cardiogenic pulmonary oedema
    - Lactic acidosis, Rhabdomyolysis
    - Hyperglycaemia, DIC
    - Bullae, Alopecia
    - Sweat gland necrosis

- **Chronic exposures**
  - o May have similar effects to acute poisoning, but often with a gradual, insidious onset, and symptoms may fluctuate with varying levels of exposure to CO over time.
  - o Compared with acute exposures, they typically involve a lower dose of carbon monoxide for a long period, which increases the risk of developing neurological complications.
  - o Symptoms are usually non-specific but can include Headache, Personality changes, Poor Concentration, Dementia, Psychosis, Parkinsonism, Ataxia, Peripheral Neuropathy and Hearing loss.

INVESTIGATIONS

- **Bedside**
  - o **ABG**
    - HbCO: Elevated levels are significant, but low levels do not rule out exposure.
    - Lactate (Tissue Hypoxia)
    - PaO2 should be normal, SpO2 only accurate if measured (not calculated from PaO2)
    - MetHb (exclude)
  - o **ECG:** Sinus Tachycardia, Ischaemia
  - o **Urinalysis**: Positive for albumin and glucose in chronic intoxification; **β-HCG** for pregnancy.

- **Laboratory**
  - o **FBC** (Mild Leukocytosis)
  - o **BSL** (Hyperglycaemia)
  - o **U&E** (Hypokalaemia, Acute renal failure from myoglobinuria)
  - o **CK** (Rhabdomyolysis)
  - o **LFT** derangement (ischaemia)
  - o **Ethanol level** (Polypharmacy OD)
  - o **Cyanide level** (Industrial fire, Cyanide exposure)

- **Imaging**
  - o **CT/MRI brain:** may demonstrate cerebral oedema, cerebral atrophy, basal ganglia injury or cortical demyelination
  - o **CXR**: pulmonary symptoms

ED MANAGEMENT OF CO POISONING

- **Resuscitation**
  - o FiO2 1.0 (continue until patient asymptomatic or CO level < 10%)
  - o Cardiac monitoring
  - o Intubate the comatose patient

- **Specific Treatment**
  - o **High flow O2 via non-rebreather mask** until asymptomatic
    - Or for 24 hours while foetal wellbeing is assessed if pregnant
  - o **Hyperbaric oxygen (HBO)**
    - Role is uncertain
    - 3 atmospheres will decrease the half-life of carboxyHb **from 6 hours to ~ 24 minutes**

    - **INDICATIONS OF HBO:**
      - *All pregnant patients*
      - *Significant LOC*
      - *Signs of ischaemia*
      - *Significant neurological deficit*
      - *Metabolic acidosis*

    - **CONTRA-INDICATIONS OF HBO**
      - *Chest trauma*
      - *Serious drug overdose,*
      - *Severe burns*
      - *Uncooperative patient*

    - **COMPLICATIONS OF HBO**
      - *Decompression sickness*
      - *Rupture of tympanic membranes*
      - *Damaged sinuses*
      - *Oxygen toxicity*
      - *Problems due to lack of monitoring*

  - o Supportive care and monitoring

- o Seek and treat cause and complications
  - Address suicidality if present
  - Treat coexistent cyanide toxicity if suspected (e.g. House fire)
  - Seek and treat ischaemic complications and neurological sequelae.

6. DISPOSITION
- o Depending on severity:
  - *Home,*
  - *Ward environment,*
  - *ICU and/or*
  - *Hyperbaric chamber*
- o Consider transfer to hyperbaric facility if severe intoxication or persistent symptoms after 4h
- o Suicidality requires a psychiatric referral/ admission
- o Work or home environment assessment
- o Check if other household members are affected
- o **FOLLOW UP**
  - Anyone with a neurological deficit will require **neuropsychiatric testing in 1-2 months**
  - Complications are present in 30% of survivors at 1 month and 6-10% at 12 months

7. PREGNANCY
- Significant CO poisoning in the mother often results in foetal death or neurological damage
- The foetus is thought to be especially susceptible to CO poisoning due to:
  - o Low oxygen pressures
  - o High affinity of foetal haemoglobin for CO.
  - o Much longer half-life of CO in the foetal circulation.

- **There may be an added benefit from HBO in this setting**
  - o HBO shortens the half-life of CO
  - o Allows delivery of oxygen to the tissues independent of haemoglobin
  - o HBO appears to be safe in pregnancy

11. CYANIDE POISONING
OVERVIEW
- Cyanide is a potentially lethal toxic agent that can be found in liquid and gaseous form.
- Average lethal dose of prussic acid (hydrogen cyanide, HCN) taken by mouth between 60 and 90 mg (adult), this corresponds to about 1 teaspoonful of a 2% solution of hydrocyanic acid and to about 200 mg of potassium cyanide

SOURCES
Include:
- **Smoke inhalation** (fires burning plastics, wools, silk and other natural and synthetic polymers)
- **Cyanogenic glycosides** such as amygdalin (e.g. almonds, apricot kernels and other *Prunus* species such as peach, apple, cherry and plum)
- **Sodium nitroprusside**
- **Industrial exposure** (e.g. cyanide salts used in metal extraction and refining, electroplating, photography and fumigation)
- **Acetonitrile** (industrial solvent used as cosmetic remover and in laboratories)
- **Chemical warfare and acts of terrorism** (e.g. deliberate contamination of medications and food)
- **Poison for feral animal control** (e.g. rodenticide)
- **Alternative medicines** (e.g. derived from apricot kernels)
- **Fumigant** in airplanes, buildings, ships

TOXICODYNAMICS
Mechanisms of toxicity include:
- Binds the ferric (Fe^{3+}) ion of cytochrome oxidase causing **'histotoxic hypoxia' and lactic acidosis.**
- Stimulates biogenic amine release causing pulmonary and coronary vasoconstriction, which results in pulmonary edema and heart failure
- Stimulates neurotransmitter release, such as N-methyl-D-aspartate (NMDA), causing neurotoxicity and seizures

TOXICOKINETICS
- **Absorption**
  - o Cyanide is rapidly absorbed and taken up into cells
- **Metabolism**
  - o Cyanide is metabolised via the liver enzyme rhodanese (named before international enzyme nomenclature was standardised, hence -ese not -ase!)
  - o Rhodanese catalyses the reaction of CN + thiosulfate to form thiocyanate and sulphite.
  - o Thiocyanate is non-toxic (unless it accumulates with high levels) and is excreted in the urine.
  - o The body's supply of thiosulfate is limited so it is the rate limiting step in cyanide metabolism
- **Elimination**
  - o The elimination half-life of cyanide is 2-3 hours

CLINICAL FEATURES
Acute inhalation or ingestion
- Rapid loss of consciousness and seizures with inhalation
- Onset of symptoms over ~30 minutes with ingestion

Milder exposures result in non-specific features including:

- Nausea, vomiting, headache, dyspnoea, increased respiratory rate, hypertension, tachycardia, altered level of consciousness and seizures

Severe exposures:
- Progressive features will result from end-organ damage secondary to anaerobic respiration and histotoxic hypoxia
- Hypotension, bradycardia, reduced GCS and respiratory depression, cardiovascular collapse
- Hyperlactaemia
- May appear **'pink'** due to high SvO2 following oxygen administration
- Smell of **bitter almonds** may be present (not everyone can detect or recognise this smell!)

↓ *Consider cyanide toxicity as the diagnosis in patients who collapse with a raised lactate level*

INVESTIGATIONS
- **Blood gas**
  - Lactate >10 mmol/L
    - In patients without severe burns, this corresponds to a cyanide level of > 40 micromol/L
    - Sensitivity of 87% and a specificity of 94% (positive likelihood ratio of 14.5 and a negative likelihood ratio of 0.14)
  - High SvO2 with oxygen administration (poor oxygen extraction)
  - COHb (suspect coexistent carbon monoxide poisoning if smoke inhalation)
- **Cyanide levels**
  - Help confirm the diagnosis in retrospect (take blood in a heparinsed tube), turn around times mean they are not useful in the acute setting
  - Cyanide is concentrated 10-fold by RBCs, therefore whole blood levels give the best information on the potential for a toxic level.
  - Levels correlate with clinical severity
    - **>20 microM** – symptomatic
    - **>40 microM** – potentially toxic
    - **>100 microM** – lethal

MANAGEMENT
- **Removal from the source**
- **Personal protection**
  - Cyanide is a potential danger to healthcare workers through the dermal route and through inhalation
  - Patient vomitus can liberate hydrogen cyanide gas
  - Avoid mouth-to-mouth/nose ventilation
- **Resuscitation**
  - Attend to ABCs and administer high flow oxygen
  - Provide haemodynamic support
    - Inotropes/ vasopressors

- Consider extracorporeal support
  - Give antidote if suspected toxicity
    - Hydroxocobalamin then sodium thiosulfate is generally preferred if available (see below)
- **Supportive care and monitoring**
  - Cases that survive to hospital will typically recover with supportive care, even in the absence of antidotal therapy
- **Seek and treat underlying causes and complications**
  - Address suicidality if appropriate
  - Address burns and injuries if due to smoke inhalation
- **Decontamination**
  - Remove any contaminated clothing and bag these
  - Wash contaminated skin with soap and water
  - Avoid activated charcoal unless intubated
- **Enhance elimination**
  - Nil
- **Antidotes**
  - Hydroxocobalamin
  - Na Thiosulfate
  - Dicobalt edetate
  - Amyl nitrite (inhaled), Sodium nitrite (IV) and Dimethyl Aminophenol (IV/IM)
- **Disposition**
  - Asymptomatic patients with normal blood gases can be discharged at 6 hours
  - Critically ill patients will require ICU admission
  - Consult a clinical toxicologist early

ANTIDOTE DOSAGE
- Administer 5g hydroxocobalamin diluted in 200 mL of 5% dextrose IV over 30 minutes (binds 100mg cyanide – use a larger inital dose if necessary)
- Dicobalt edetate is administered 300 mg IV (7.5 mg/kg in children) over 1 minute followed by 50 mL of 50% glucose.
- This is repeated up to 3 times if an immediate clinical response is not seen.

Further reading:
1. Toxbase: https://www.toxbase.org/
2. Life In The Fast lane:
   a. https://litfl.com/approach-to-acute-poisoning/
   b. https://litfl.com/paracetamol-toxicity/
3. RCEM Guidance webpage
4. Rebel EM: https://rebelem.com/salicylate-toxicity/
5. Uptodate: https://www.uptodate.com/contents/cyanide-poisoning

III. TOXIDROMES (DRUG INDUCED HYPERTHERMIA)

1. INTRODUCTION

- Drug poisoning, either accidental or intentional, accounts for one of the most common causes of admission to the emergency department and intensive care unit (ICU).
- The most common causes of poisoning reportedby In France, 19 of 20 most common medications involved in the reported exposures by the Poison Control Centre of Paris are psychotropics[351].

2. LABORATORY INVESTIGATIONS TO BE CONSIDERED INCLUDE:

- FBC (leucocytosis is common in NMS), U&E, Lactate
- CK (elevated in NMS and for detection of rhabdomyolysis as a complication)
- Clotting, Toxicology screen
- CT head and lumbar puncture to be considered if central nervous system aetiologies are suspected

3. GENERAL MANAGEMENT OF DRUG-INDUCED HYPERTHERMIA IN THE ED

- **Discontinue** causative agent.
- Ensure **adequate ABC**: Airway protection, Breathing and Circulation
- Consider administration of **activated charcoal if within 1 hour** of ingestion and patient able to protect own airway.
- **Control hyperthermia** by reducing excessive muscle activity from agitation, seizures or shivering with the use of **benzodiazepines for sedation.**
- In severe cases (temperature **>41.1^{0}C**) the patient is likely to **require intubation and paralysis.**
- **External cooling measures** e.g. cooling blankets, ice packs, ice water submersion, cool water mist and fans.
- **Volume replacement** as indicated.
- Patients with moderate to severe symptoms will require treatment in a **HDU or intensive care setting.**
- Treat complications: Respiratory dysfunction, seizures, vomiting and diarrhoea, rhabdomyolysis, acute kidney injury, hepatic injury, DIC, multi-organ failure and death

[351] Villa A, Cochet A, Guyodo G. Poison episodes reported to French poison control centers in 2006. Rev Prat 2008;58:825-31. (In French)

1. MALIGNANT HYPERTHERMIA

- It is a life-threatening complication of anaesthesia.

PATHOPHYSIOLOGY

- Following exposure to a trigger, excessive jaw rigidity, excessive carbon dioxide production, hyperthermia and tachycardia develop.
- As ATP is used up, lactate production increases with a resulting **metabolic acidosis.**
- Muscle breakdown leads to potentially fatal **Hyperkalemia.**
- Triggering agents include **inhalational anaesthesia (Halothane, Enflurane, Desflurane, Sevoflurane, Isoflurane)** and the **depolarising agent suxamethonium**. Previous exposure to known triggering agents does not rule out the disease.
- Excessive exercise in warm conditions can also trigger a reaction in those who are susceptible.
- During a reaction, there are significant increases in noradrenaline and increased survival has been demonstrated with alpha-blockade in animal models.
- Elevated levels of serotonin appear during malignant hyperthermia and serotonergic drug have exaggerated responses in susceptible swine but serotonin antagonists have not been shown to be effective.

TREATMENT OF MALIGNANT HYPERTHERMIA

- **General management:** as above
- **Specific management:**
  - **Dantrolene 1mg/kg IV every 5 minutes to a maximum dose of 10mg/kg.**
  - **Treatment of hyperkalaemia** accordingly.
- Patient who have thought to have had an episode of malignant hyperthermia need to be referred to a malignant hyperthermia centre for investigation and genetic counselling.

2. NEUROLEPTIC MALIGNANT SYNDROME

- NMS is a rare idiosyncratic reaction occurring in patients that are taking neuroleptic drugs or after sudden withdrawal of dopamine agonists.

PATHOPHYSIOLOGY

- Neuroleptic syndrome can occur at any time; even after years of therapy but is more likely to develop **within 10 days.** Drug levels are often found to be therapeutic in neuroleptic malignant syndrome.

o Butyrophenones and phenothiazines are most commonly implicated though at least 25 agents have been identified as triggers.
o Some patients will develop neuroleptic malignant syndrome with any dopamine agonist, some will develop neuroleptic malignant syndrome with specific dopamine agonists whilst others can be treated with the same drug without any ill effect.

CLINICAL FEATURES

o Hyperthermia, Altered mental status, Skeletal muscle rigidity, Autonomic dysfunction. A temperature of 38^{0}C or above is a key diagnostic feature.
o Autonomic dysfunction manifests as tachycardia, hypotension or hypertension and diaphoresis.
o Mental status changes often precede muscle rigidity.
o It is often difficult to differentiate between neuroleptic malignant syndrome and serotonin syndrome in patients presenting with muscular rigidity, hyperthermia and autonomic instability.

o Patients with serotonin syndrome present **within 24 hours of starting the medication**, whilst those with neuroleptic malignant syndrome present at any time with peak symptoms not occurring for days.

DRUGS CAUSING NMS

Atypical Antipsychotics	Typical Antipsychotics	Antiemetics
Chlorpromazine	Clozapine	Domperidone
Fluphenazine	Olanzapine	Metoclopramide
Haloperidol	Quetiapine	Prochlorperazine
Perphenazine	Risperidone	Promethazine
Thioridazine	Paliperidone	Triperidol
Thiothixene	Aripiprazole	

ED MANAGEMENT OF NMS

o **General management:** as above
o **Specific management:**
  - **Bromocriptine** (a dopamine agonist) **2.5-10 mg 6 hourly**
  - **Amantadine 100 mg orally** has been used as an alternative to bromocriptine
  - Coagulopathy should be treated with **FFP and platelets**
  - **Dantrolene 1-2.5 mg/kg up to a maximum of 10 mg/kg/day.**
  - This is the treatment for malignant hyperthermia but its use has been described in NMS.

3. SEROTONIN SYNDROME

- Serotonin syndrome is a predictable consequence of excess serotonergic agonism of central nervous system receptors and peripheral serotonergic receptors.
- It is not an idiopathic drug reaction. Most cases occur with a therapeutic concentration, not overdoses.
- The commonest drugs that precipitate serotonin syndrome are **Venlafaxine, Fluoxetine, Citalopram, Pethidine and Tramadol.**
- **Ondansetron** blocks serotonin post synaptic receptors and cannot induce this syndrome.
- **Clinical features:** The clinical picture includes[352]:
  o **Neurological disorders** including agitation, confusion, hallucinations, myoclonus, tremor, pyramidal syndrome, seizure, coma;
  o **Autonomic disorders** such as mydriasis, sweating, tachycardia, tachypnea, hyperthermia, chills, hypotension, diarrhea or even respiratory arrest;
  o **Biological abnormalities** such as hyperglycemia, leukocytosis, hypokalemia, hypocalcemia, disseminated intravascular coagulation, lactic acidosis and rhabdomyolysis.
  o In moderate intoxication, a core temperature of 40^{0}C is not uncommon.
  o Physical examination includes mydriasis, hyperactive bowel sounds, diaphoresis with normal skin colour.
  o Clonus (inducible, spontaneous and ocular) is the most important finding in establishing the diagnosis.
  o Hyperthermia and hypertonicity occur in life threatening cases.

ED MANAGEMENT OF SS

o **General management:** as above
o **Specific management:**
  - **Antidote: Cyproheptadine 12 mg orally or via NG tube**
  - Patients with serotonin syndrome with severe hypertension and tachycardia should be treated with short acting cardiovascular agents such as **Esmolol or Nitroprusside.**
  - Longer acting agents such as propranolol should be avoided due to the autonomic instability in this group of patients.
  - Other agents such as olanzapine, chlorpromazine, bromocriptine or dantrolene are not recommended for use in the treatment of serotonin syndrome.

---

[352] Boyer EW, Shannon M. The serotonin syndrome. N Engl J Med 2005;352:1112-20.

4. ANTICHOLINERGIC SYNDROME

- The combination of increased muscle activity causing increased heat production and the impaired ability to sweat leads to hyperthermia.
- Anticholinergic agents are associated with hyperthermia at both therapeutic and toxic doses.
- Symptoms arise as result of the blockade of both the central and peripheral muscarinic acetylcholine receptors.

- **Symptoms resulting from central muscarinic receptor blockade:**
  - o Altered mental status, confusion, restlessness, seizures, coma
  - o Coma is usually not profound without focal signs and is associated with pyramidal signs and restlessness. A deep coma with quick progression (< 6h) is suggestive of poor prognosis [353].

- **Symptoms resulting from peripheral muscarinic receptor blockade:**
  - o Impaired sweat gland function, Dry mouth, Dry axillae, Mydriasis, Tachycardia
  - o Flushing, Urinary retention
- The onset of anticholinergic symptoms depends upon the drug but usually occurs **within a couple of hours of ingestion**.
- **Agents:** Antipsychotics, TCAs, Atropine, Antihistamines and Amphetamines

ED MANAGEMENT OF ANTICHOLINERGIC SYNDROME

- o **Physostigmine 0.5-2 mg over 5 minutes** with continuous cardiac monitoring.
- o Most patients with anticholinergic syndrome improve with **supportive care alone.**
- o Supportive and general measures as previously described including **benzodiazepines** for the management of agitation and seizures.
- o **Phenothiazines** and **butyrophenones** are themselves anticholinergic so their use should be avoided in anticholinergic toxicity.
- o **Sodium bicarbonate** should be used in the case of arrhythmias or prolonged QRS intervals related to the anticholinergic poisoning.

5. CHOLINERGIC SYNDROME

- It is mainly related to poisoning with anticholinesterase pesticides including organophosphates or carbamates [354].
- **NMJ:** weakness, Flaccid paralysis
- **Parasympathetic: DUMBELS: D**iarrhoea, **U**rination, **M**iosis, **B**ronchospasm, **E**mesis, **L**acrimation, **S**alivation
- **Sympathetic:** Mydriasis, sweating, increased HR and BP
- **CNS:** agitation, confusion, Fits
- **Agents:** Organophosphates, Donepezil, Nerve agents, Neostigmine and Physostigmine
- **Treatment:**
  - o Personal Protective Equipment
  - o Supportive: Secretion Management
  - o **Atropine 2-5mg IV every 5 min till sign of atropinisation appear**
  - o **Pralidoxime 1-2g IV infusion over 15-20min**

6. SYMPATHOMIMETIC SYNDROME

- Sympathomimetic agents can cause life-threatening hyperthermia although the exact mechanism is unknown.
- Sympathomimetics cause a central increase in the concentrations of norepinephrine, dopamine and serotonin whilst peripherally causing a vasoconstriction, increased muscle activity and impaired behavioural responses. The degree of hyperthermia is not directly related to drug, mode of administration or duration.
- The agents which are most commonly associated with hyperthermia are **Amphetamine, Methamphetamine, MDMA and Cocaine.** Symptoms of sympathomimetic syndrome include agitation, altered mental status, hallucinations, coma, and seizures.
- Hyperthermia caused by sympathomimetics can also exacerbate these symptoms.

MANAGEMENT IN THE ED

- o General measures and supportive treatment as described previously. There **is no specific antidote** to treat the hyperthermia in sympathomimetic poisoning.
- o Treatment should aim for control of hyperthermia by reducing excessive muscle activity and supportive care to normalise vital signs.
- o Treatment might also be required for associated features such as hyponatraemia, hypertension and myocardial ischaemia. Sympathomimetics such as cocaine and MDMA might also cause serotonin toxicity.
- o If there are features of serotonin toxicity as suggested by the Hunter diagnostic criteria, then consider treatment with **cyproheptadine** alongside supportive measures.

[353] Hulten BA, Adams R, Askenasi R, Dallos V, Dawling S, Volans G, et al. Predicting severity of tricyclic antidepressant overdose. J Toxicol Clin Toxicol 1992;30:161-70.

[354] Eddleston M, Buckley NA, Eyer P, Dawson AH. Management of acute organophosphorus pesticide poisoning. Lancet 2008;371:597-607.

31. Pre-Hospital Care in UK

INTRODUCTION

- Emergency medical services (EMS) is defined as the system that organizes all aspects of care provided to patients in the pre-hospital or out-of-hospital environment[355].
- Hence, EMS is a critical component of the health systems and is necessary to improve outcomes of injuries and other time-sensitive illnesses.
- Still there exists a substantial need for evidence to improve our understanding of the capacity of such systems as well as their strengths, weaknesses, and priority areas for improvement in low-resource environments.
- Throughout the United Kingdom, doctors and other healthcare professionals respond to requests for assistance from the ambulance service on a voluntary basis. These practitioners respond to a wide variety of incidents both medical and traumatic.
- West Midlands Ambulance Service's (WMAS) catchment area covers approximately 5.3 million people: from April 2009 to April 2010, doctors tasked by WMAS responded to 953 incidents[356].
- The role of such practitioners in the prehospital environment has yet to be fully defined: no formal skill set is established, with practitioners coming from a wide range of medical and nursing backgrounds.
- This variation in base clinical competencies can lead to disparities in the standard of care delivered, as well as leading to practitioners working outside of their established clinical skill set

1. PRE-HOSPITAL CARE TODAY

- Pre-hospital care today is an emerging multidisciplinary field.
- While pre-hospital medical care used to be solely the responsibility of the ambulance service, prehospital care today encompasses any specialised medical care delivered outside of the hospital.
- This care may be provided by first aiders, police officers, fire and rescue services, first responders and physicians, each of whom are trained to varying levels.
- It is no longer the case that the first medical aid to reach a patient will come from ambulance personnel.

CHALLENGES TO DELIVERY

- Many obstacles exist to the introduction of structured and standardised prehospital care in the UK.
- With no nationally agreed standards for provider competencies, training and revalidation, it is impossible to provide standardised patient care or indeed monitor the delivery of this care. Providers work in a wide range of environments, over a widespread geographical area, often working in isolation, these limitations make a thorough governance system difficult to deliver.
- The lack of a central governing body means that there is difficulty reporting and acting on equipment failures, hazards or other risk-management issues.
- The majority of prehospital care providers in the UK are volunteers; they provide their time for free on an ad hoc basis, providing medical cover for their local community.
- This arrangement means minimum standards (which take both time and money) are difficult to establish or indeed implement.

CHANGES IN THE AMBULANCE SERVICE

- Many ambulance services across the UK have now introduced tiered levels of expertise. These will range from volunteer first responder basic aid to advanced paramedics such as the HEMS and critical care-trained paramedics.
- Advanced/critical care paramedics are trained beyond Joint Royal Colleges Ambulance Liaison Committee (JRCALC) guidelines and are the main providers of enhanced care in the pre-hospital setting.
- The formation of the physician–paramedic partnership has produced the highest level of enhanced care that the pre-hospital environment can provide.

2. PRE-HOSPITAL TRANSPORT

- EMS is defined as the system that organizes all aspects of medical care provided to patients in the pre-hospital or out-of-hospital environment[357].
- Unique to the field of pre-hospital care is the need for practitioners to consider how best to get to the incident and how best to get the patient to definitive care.
- With the range of transport modes at the potential disposal of the pre-hospital care team, it is essential to have a basic understanding of the limitations of each.

355 Mehmood, A., Rowther, A.A., Kobusingye, O. et al. Assessment of pre-hospital emergency medical services in low-income settings using a health systems approach. Int J Emerg Med 11, 53 (2018). https://doi.org/10.1186/s12245-018-0207-6

356 Tim Nutbeam, Clinical governance and prehospital care in the UK [Researchgate]

357 Mistovich JJ, Hafen BQ, Karren KJ. Prehospital emergency care. USA: 8th ed: Brady Prentice Hall Health; 2007.

- The decision-making process about the mode of transport is as crucial as the clinical interventions provided to the patient on-scene. Both are integral to the delivery of gold-standard care in the pre-hospital setting.
- The effects of the mode of transport on the patient, the medical equipment and in limiting possible medical interventions, must all be considered.

1. LAND AMBULANCE

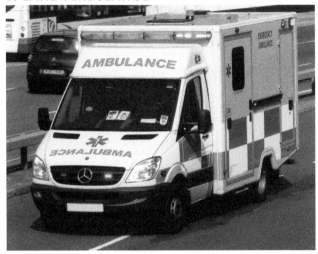

Land ambulances are responsible for the delivery to hospital of the majority of patients in the pre-hospital care setting.

1. **Advantages:**
   i. Generally, readily available;
   ii. Larger area to work in compared with air transport;
   iii. Easy to pull over if patient deteriorates.

2. **Disadvantages:**
   i. Potentially slower than air transport;
   ii. In spinal injury cases, uneven roads and routes may have a detrimental effect.

2. HELICOPTERS

- Several different types of helicopter are used in UK pre-hospital practice by air ambulance services.
- The differences between the types of helicopter used are beyond the scope of this text. However, the same principles apply irrespective of which model of helicopter is used.

1. **Advantages:**
   i. Short transport times;
   ii. Ability to land in remote environments.

2. **Disadvantages:**
   i. Landing sites can be restricted at night-time (only some units in the UK are able to fly at night);
   ii. Difficulty in assessing patients in-flight (noise makes auscultation of chest impossible, for example);
   iii. Unable to fly in adverse weather conditions;

iv. Unsuitable for transport of certain patient groups, e.g. psychiatrically unstable;
v. Potentially unsafe for unstable patients as able to perform very few interventions in-flight;
vi. Require regular servicing;
vii. Some patients have fear of flying;
viii. Monitoring equipment, e.g. ECG and pulse oximetry affected by heavy vibrations in-flight;
ix. May not be possible to land close to the patient – a road vehicle may have better access.

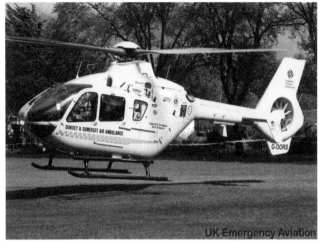

LANDING SITES

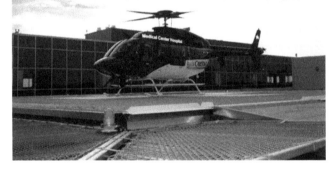

The pilot(s) has the ultimate decision regarding the selection of landing site. Some criteria for the identification of suitable landing sites are listed below:
- A landing site should be twice the diameter of the rotating blades
- The ground must be firm and flat
- The site must be away from power or telephone lines and free of debris
- The site should be clear of people (this may necessitate making several low passes over the landing site with flashing lights in order to encourage people to move away)

3. FIXED WING AIRCRAFT

- Fixed wing aeromedical retrieval is uncommon in UK pre-hospital care practice.
- **The main advantage** of a fixed wing aircraft over a helicopter is the distance it is able to travel.
- With the UK being geographically much smaller than countries such as Australia or the USA, **the disadvantage** of fixed wing aircraft – that they require an airfield to land – significantly outweighs the benefit.
- Around the world, however, fixed wing aircraft are being used regularly for retrieval.

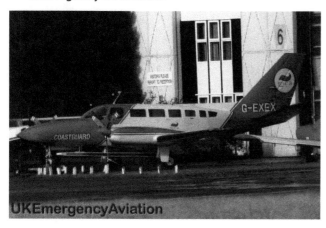

3. SCENE SAFETY

IMPORTANCE OF SCENE SAFETY

- The mantra at the forefront of the mind of any pre-hospital care practitioner has always been: is it safe to approach? Although scene control is primarily the responsibility of the fire and police crews, it is no help to the casualty or the other rescuers if any harm comes to the medics, and so every practitioner must be personally vigilant for hazards. Always think of your own safety first, then the safety of other rescuers and bystanders, and finally the safety of the patient. This is the 1-2-3 of safety.

INITIAL APPROACH & ARRIVAL AT THE SCENE

- On arriving at the scene, assess it thoroughly for hazards to your team and to other rescuers.
- One should communicate with crew members already on the scene to obtain as much information about current and former dangers. If the scene has not yet been made safe, then this should be left to the fire and police crews.
- It is vital to understand that the scene is a *dynamic* environment. Factors in scene safety may include the following: cutting of vehicles, movement of power cables, leaking fuel and live rail tracks.
- What was once judged to be safe may become decidedly – and sometimes unpredictably – unsafe. Assessment of scene safety is a dynamic process.

PERSONAL PROTECTIVE EQUIPMENT

- Pre-hospital care practitioners have to be able to work in a diverse range of environments, from the roadside, to water, to areas with chemical or nuclear hazards.
- As a result, rescuers are exposed to risks from multiple sources, and so require a full range of PPE and the training to use it effectively:
  1. Helmet
  2. Eye protection
  3. Ear protection
  4. Facemasks Gloves
  5. A high visibility jacket
  6. Robust safety boots

4. PRINCIPLES OF RAPID INITIAL ASSESSMENT

- The primary survey forms the rapid initial assessment of the acutely unwell patient in any context, and in the case of major trauma is directed exclusively at identifying and treating immediately life-threatening injuries.
- The systematic, stepwise approach of **C-ABCDE** ensures that pathology is addressed in the order of speed of fatality; airway compromise will kill more quickly than hypoglycaemia.
- Equally as important is the need to reassess the patient constantly from the beginning each time an intervention is made, as pathology rapidly evolves. Initial assessment is a repeated dynamic process.

IMMEDIATELY LIFE-THREATENING CHEST PATHOLOGY

Condition	Findings (affected side)	Management
Tension pneumothorax	Asymmetrical chest movement Hyper-resonance Absent breath sounds	Needle decompression Thoracostomy
Open chest wound	Bubbling blood from open chest defect	Three-sided occlusive dressing
Massive haemothorax	Asymmetrical chest movement Dullness to percussion Absent breath sounds	Good vascular access, Thoracostomy
Flail chest	Paradoxical chest wall segment movement	Good analgesia Intubation and Ventilation if respiratory compromise

SITES OF MAJOR INTERNAL HAEMORRHAGE

Site	Example injury	Specific management
Chest	Pulmonary artery dissection causing massive haemothorax	Tube thoracostomy Resuscitative thoracostomy with lobar compression
Abdomen	Splenic rupture, liver laceration	REBOA*/urgent transfer for damage control surgery
Pelvis	Open book pelvic fracture	Pelvic binder
Long bones	Femoral shaft fracture	Fracture reduction and traction splint

5. CONTROL OF MAJOR HAEMORRHAGE

THE PROBLEM OF MAJOR HAEMORRHAGE IN TRAUMA

- Uncontrolled haemorrhage has been shown to be the most common cause of preventable deaths in trauma and is responsible for 40% of early in-hospital trauma mortality. Observational studies have shown that 25% of trauma patients also have an established coagulopathy on arrival in the emergency department and that this is associated with a fourfold increase in mortality.
- The so-called **'lethal triad of death'** describes the mutually perpetuating combination of **acute coagulopathy, hypothermia and metabolic acidosis**.
- These are seen in exsanguinating trauma patients.
- Hypoperfusion results in reduced oxygen delivery and the consequent switch to anaerobic metabolism results in lactate production and therefore metabolic acidosis.

DAMAGE CONTROL RESUSCITATION

- While pre-hospital teams are vital in the initial management of major haemorrhage, surgery is the definitive intervention in the context of severe blood loss and scene times must therefore be limited. The concept of 'damage control resuscitation' has emerged in recent years. It involves the following key components:
  - **Haemostatic resuscitation:** this describes the very early use of blood and blood products as primary resuscitation fluids.
  - **Permissive hypotension:** this is a relatively new concept whereby the target blood pressure is set as low as is necessary to ensure adequate organ perfusion, but no higher. Higher blood pressures are associated with haemodilution and clot disruption. Target systolic pressure is **80–100 mmHg** (radial pulse should be palpable).

  - **Damage control surgery:** this is the definitive way of controlling major haemorrhage and is surgery limited to what is needed to control haemorrhage.
- Pre-hospital efforts should be focused on limiting time delays on-scene to allow rapid transport to hospital for definitive surgical intervention once the patient has sufficient physiological reserve.

THE LADDER APPROACH TO PRE-HOSPITAL HAEMORRHAGE CONTROL

- Under normal circumstances, major external haemorrhage may be controlled by the stepwise application of basic techniques – the so-**called haemostatic ladder**[358].

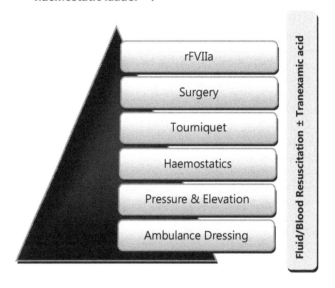

The first step on the ladder is a **basic wound dressing.**

6. CERVICAL SPINE INJURIES

- Patients with C-spine injuries have the highest reported early mortality rate in spinal trauma as, owing to the anatomy, trauma to this section of the spine commonly causes cord damage.
- Prompt spinal immobilisation and detection of these injuries is paramount in avoiding additional spinal cord injury.
- Fractures of the odontoid peg of C2 are also extremely common.
- Four key mechanisms of injury – often in combination – are responsible: **hyperflexion, hyperextension, rotation and compression of the spine**.
- Half of all Cspine injuries follow road traffic accidents, in which these four mechanisms are often involved.

---

[358] *A diagram illustrating the steps to stop bleeding in an injured patient. By Tom Mallinson*

ASSESSING THE CERVICAL SPINE

- **Manual immobilisation** of the C-spine should be commenced immediately in *all* trauma patients while the initial assessment is undertaken.

History

- The mechanism of injury is important in determining whether spinal cord injury is likely to have occurred as well as the nature of the damage.
- Road traffic accidents, falls, and sporting injuries are responsible for most C-spine fractures, and the mechanism can often be deduced from the incident, e.g. hyperextension and then hyperflexion in rapid deceleration collisions.
- The patient may also report midline spinal pain.

Examination

- C-spine tenderness can be elicited by palpating the back of the neck in the midline, while maintaining manual immobilisation.
- A rapid assessment of movement and sensation in all four limbs should also be carried out during the primary survey.

Cervical spine clearance

- Identification and assessment of C-spine injury in the field may be challenging if patients present with a reduced GCS.
- This may be because of concomitant head injury or intoxication (alcohol, sedative or analgesic medication). Furthermore, high levels of circulating catecholamines and endogenous opioids in trauma patients conspire to mask spinal fractures.
- C-spine immobilisation can often make it more difficult to deliver certain interventions (e.g. endotracheal intubation), and in some situations cause direct harm to the patient.
- Clinical decision rules have thus been formulated to guide the practitioner as to when C-spine immobilisation can be safely discontinued.
- **The NEXUS guidelines and Canadian C-Spine Rule** both have a high sensitivity but low specificity.
- This means that they can be used safely to rule out significant C-spine injury and allow appropriate spinal immobilisation.
- Initially used in the emergency department as a means to clear patients with suspected spinal injury without radiological assessment, these guidelines are also used reliably in the pre-hospital environment.
- It is important to remember, however, that spinal immobilisation, and *not* spinal clearance, is the priority in multiple trauma.

Securing the cervical spine

- The principle of minimal movement, maximum safety applies to all spinal injuries. The use of a **scoop stretcher,** the practice of scoop-to-skin immobilisation and 10° tilts all minimise further spinal cord damage. As well as these, there are specific measures to stabilise the C-spine:

1. Manual in-line stabilisation (MILS)

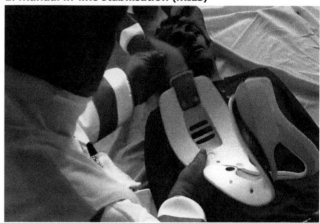

- It is performed on an upright or supine patient.
- The practitioner stands behind or above the patient and holds the patient's head in a neutral position while locking their own elbows or resting them on the ground to stabilise them.
- This should prevent any side-to-side head movement. Two centimetres of padding placed under the head in healthy, supine patients can optimise the neutral position of the head relative to the body. MILS should be initiated immediately on reaching the patient.

- **Rigid cervical collars (RCCs)** reduce C-spine movement by 80–90% but only when used in combination with blocks and tape; MILS should be performed until such **'three-point immobilisation' is applied**.
- C-spine mobility is reduced by 90-95% when three-point immobilisation is used with an extrication device or a spinal board.

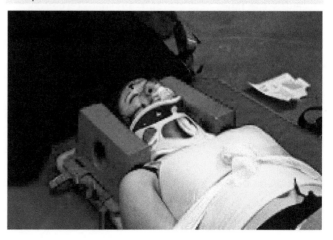

CAVEATS IN IMMOBILISATION

There are some situations in which the risks of MILS and RCC can outweigh the benefits:

1. MILS drastically reduces the quality of the view on laryngoscopy, impeding intubation in difficult airways. A bougie should be used routinely to minimise unnecessary manipulation of the C-spine.

2. RCCs have been shown to increase intracranial pressure by up to 4 mmHg by restricting venous outflow from the head.

3. RCCs may be detrimental in those with spinal deformities and the elderly (both groups have kyphosis, for example). Padding should be used to splint the neck in the position found.

4. Vomiting and aspiration is a serious risk of immobilisation.

5. There is some evidence to suggest that **RCCs may restrict breathing, contribute to dysphagia,** cause skin ulceration and pain, but these events are rare.

7. THE DIFFICULT AIRWAY

ASSESSING THE AIRWAY

The following mnemonic (MOANS) helps to predict those patients in whom BVM ventilation may be difficult.

❖ **M** – Mask seal difficulty, i.e. blood, facial injuries and facial hair

❖ **O** – Obesity and Obstruction: obese and pregnant patients are more difficult to ventilate due to excess tissue/oedema

❖ **A** – Age > 55: elderly patients are more difficult to ventilate due to decreased upper airway compliance

❖ **N** – No teeth

❖ **S** - Stiff lungs or stiff chest wall, snoring

The following mnemonic, LEMON helps to predict those patients/scenarios in whom difficult laryngoscopy and intubation may be expected.

❖ **L** – Look for obesity, receding jaw, short muscular neck, burns, facial trauma or macroglossia

❖ **E** - Evaluate the 3-3-2 rule (Figure 14.2) to estimate the size of the oral cavity

❖ **M** – Mallampati score (Figure 14.3) may not be particularly useful in the prehospital setting as it is assessed in a conscious, seated patient

❖ **O** - Obstruction with blood, vomitus, oedema, a mass or foreign body

❖ **N** – Neck mobility – may be restricted. With appropriate manual C-spine stabilisation, it is acceptable to undo a cervical collar during intubation

❖ **S** - Space (confined or restricted), scene (location and lighting) and skill of the operator

PREHOSPITAL RAPID SEQUENCE INTUBATION

• The decision to place a definitive airway is based on clinical judgment and the understanding that a stable patient may deteriorate rapidly, requiring frequent reassessment of their airway, ventilatory and neurologic status, as well as vital signs.

Common indications for intubation include:

• Decreased level of consciousness (GCS <8)–at risk for increased intracranial pressure and need for hyperventilation

• Patients at risk for aspiration secondary to impaired airway-protective reflexes

• Massive facial fractures/injuries, burn patients with risk or evidence of inhalation injury

• Apnea

• Failure to maintain a patent airway and oxygenation by other means.

A definitive airway is meant to represent an ETT that is placed in the trachea, past the vocal cords. A balloon, located distally, serves to protect against aspiration when inflated. The airway can be placed orally, nasally or surgically in the form of a cricothyroidotomy or tracheostomy.

8. SPINAL INJURIES

• Spinal cord injuries (SCI) can have a devastating impact on long-term mobility and independence. The most commonly affected group are young males between 16 and 30 years old, as they are most likely to be the victims of trauma. Road traffic collisions account for half of all SCI. However, the ageing population means that rising numbers of active elderly people are becoming involved in trauma and are particularly vulnerable to SCI.

• This is because of comorbidities such as osteoporosis, osteoarthritis of the spine and cervical spondylosis. As a result, SCI are a growing problem with an increasingly diverse demographic picture.

PATHOPHYSIOLOGY OF CORD INJURY

• There are four main mechanisms of blunt injury: hyperflexion, hyperextension, rotation and compression.

• These may be seen in high-speed road traffic collisions or sporting incidents. The cord is most likely to be damaged at the points of transition (cervicothoracic, thoracolumbar, lumbosacral junctions), for it is at these points that the prevailing mobility of the spine changes.

PRIMARY SPINAL CORD INJURY

• Primary SCI occurs at the time of impact, and can be due to either blunt or penetrating injury.

• The functional sequelae of primary SCI depends on the vertebral level of the lesion as well as the tracts that are affected.

- In terms of the latter, four key syndromes exist: anterior cord, posterior cord, central cord and Brown-Séquard syndromes.

SECONDARY SPINAL CORD INJURY

- Secondary SCI is caused by further mechanical disruption, hypoxia and hypoperfusion of the cord after the initial injury.
- These three factors can extend the area of primary injury through causing oedema with resultant ischaemia of the cord. SCI management in the pre-hospital phase and beyond is aimed at preventing secondary SCI.

SPINAL SHOCK

- Spinal shock is a transient reflex depression of cord function. Within 24-72 hours of the primary injury, there is loss of anal tone, bladder and bowel function, and sustained priapism.

NEUROGENIC SHOCK

- Neurogenic shock refers to a triad of hypotension, bradycardia and hypothermia. This is due to vasodilation which results from loss of sympathetic outflow and unopposed vagal parasympathetic tone. This occurs in **significant injuries at T6 or above.**

MANAGEMENT OF SPINAL CORD INJURY

- The treatment of SCI should be aimed at minimising secondary SCI. SCI should otherwise be managed using an ABCDE approach:

  1. Airway: ensure airway is patent without unnecessary manipulation of the Cspine. Always use a bougie and be prepared to settle for a view of the arytenoids.

  2. Breathing: spinal cord is neurological tissue and may suffer secondary hypoxic neurological damage in the same way as the brain. Titrate oxygen saturations to 100%. If the patient is complaining of being - or appears - short of breath, look for diaphragmatic breathing, as this may indicate a high cervical lesion (C3-C5).
  Have a low threshold for intubation in these patients, especially if there is concurrent chest trauma.

  3. Circulation: hypotension (<100 mmHg) should be corrected by fluid resuscitation. If SCI is confirmed - and all other causes of hypotension excluded - inotropic support may be initiated.

  4. Disability: check blood glucose and administer dextrose if patient is hypoglycaemic.

  5. Exposure: consider that SCI patients will lose the ability to thermoregulate if autonomic function is impaired, and so should be kept warm. Expose the patient and carry out a full top-to-toe examination, but restrict the duration of full exposure to the minimum required in order to lessen the potential for hypothermia.

9. LIMB INJURIES

- Limb injuries are commonplace and range from minor sprains to traumatic amputations.
- Pre-hospital care practitioners should be prepared to treat the entire range of limb injuries whilst maintaining appropriate overall clinical priority.

PRIMARY SURVEY

- **The ABCDE approach** should always be adopted as initial management.
- The exception to this is massive external haemorrhage where time spent performing assessment of airway and breathing would put the patient at risk of death from exsanguination.
- In this case, **stop the haemorrhage first** by progressing up the haemostatic ladder and then transfer the patient urgently to the nearest trauma centre with an appropriate pre-alert message.

SECONDARY SURVEY

- Having addressed any life-threatening issues in the primary survey, the secondary survey should be carried out.
- Full exposure of the patient is important. This will allow for complete assessment of all four limbs for injury.

WOUND CARE

- Any abrasion or laceration may represent an open (compound) fracture. Any gross contamination should be washed away with normal saline.
- The wound should be dressed with sterile, saline-soaked, dressings.
- Tetanus injections are not given in the pre-hospital environment, and antibiotics may or may not be given depending on local pre-hospital protocols.

• FRACTURES AND DISLOCATIONS

- Limb deformity should be identifiable from rapid assessment, signifying long bone fractures or dislocations.
- Remove all jewellery from the injured limb before swelling occurs. The distal neurovascular status of the affected limb should be determined immediately and documented.
- If compromised, urgent realignment of the limb to the anatomical position ought to be performed after provision of adequate analgesia with or without sedation depending on the presence of enhanced care teams.
- The limb can be manipulated using longitudinal traction and manual correction. Distal neurovascular status must be rechecked after realignment and once again documented.

ANALGESIA

- Before any manipulation of an injured limb, appropriate analgesia must be given. Options for analgesia can include **Entonox, opiates and procedural sedation.**
- Procedural sedation must be delivered by an enhanced care team led by a prehospital care physician.
- Drugs considered for sedation include **ketamine and midazolam**. During the procedure, appropriate monitoring must be attached.

SPLINTAGE AND PACKAGING

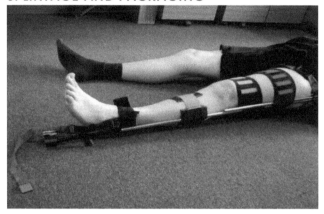

- Bringing deformed limbs back into anatomical alignment prevents further haemorrhage and neural damage from the mobile ends of fractured bones damaging blood vessels and nerves, and also minimises the area into which any torn blood vessels can bleed.
- Immobilisation reduces pain by eliminating unnecessary movement at fracture sites.
- **Splintage** is a means of maintaining fractured limbs in the anatomical arrangement and preventing unstable fractures or dislocations from slipping back into their original positions.

- It also may be necessary in cases where the current position of the displaced limb or joint is impeding patient packaging and transport.
- There is a variety of methods for splinting injured limbs. Upper limb injuries may be splinted most easily by the patient holding their limb in the most comfortable position; a triangular bandage can be used to support the limb.
- In forearm and lower limb fractures, specialised splints exist, each with different indications. The advantages and disadvantages of each are explained opposite.

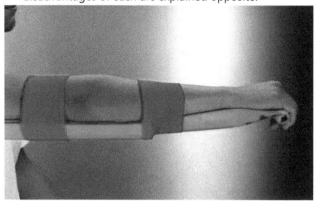

- Finally, the patient should be transferred to the hospital that best serves their clinical needs. For instance, a patient with an open fracture and significant soft tissue injury or an amputation should be treated at a centre with plastic and orthopaedic surgical expertise.

32. Penile Conditions

I. PARAPHIMOSIS

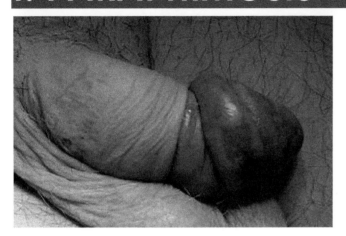

INTRODUCTION

- Paraphimosis is a urologic emergency in which the retracted foreskin of an uncircumcised male cannot be returned to its normal anatomic position.
- It is important for clinicians to recognize this condition promptly, as it can result in gangrene and amputation of the glans penis. Prompt urologic intervention is indicated. Paraphimosis occurs when the foreskin of an **uncircumcised or partially circumcised** male is retracted for an extended period of time. This in turn causes venous occlusion, edema, and eventual arterial occlusion. The foreskin is unable to be reduced easily over the glans owing to this progressive edema.
- The condition represents a urologic emergency, as compromise of the arterial flow to the glans and constriction can cause gangrene and amputation of the glans penis. Paraphimosis differs from **Phimosis,** a nonemergent condition in which the foreskin cannot be retracted behind the glans penis[359].

ETIOLOGY

- **Children** whose foreskins have been forcefully retracted or who forget to reduce their foreskin after voiding or bathing
- **Adolescents or adults** who present with paraphimosis in the setting of vigorous sexual activity.
- **Men** with chronic balanoposthitis
- **Patients** with indwelling catheters in whom caretakers forget to replace the foreskin after catheterization or cleaning

- **More unusual causes of paraphimosis include the following:**
  - Self-infliction, such as piercing with a penile ring into the glans[360]
  - Placement of a preputial bead
  - Erotic dancing
  - Plasmodium falciparum infection[361]
  - Contact dermatitis (eg, from the application of celandine juice to the foreskin)
  - Haemophilus ducreyi infection (chancroid) [362]

CLINICAL PRESENTATION

- Adult patients with symptomatic paraphimosis most often report **penile pain.**
- In the pediatric population, paraphimosis may manifest as **acute urinary tract obstruction** and may be reported as obstructive voiding symptoms.
- On examination, the glans penis is enlarged and congested with a collar of edematous foreskin.
- A constricting band of tissue is noted directly behind the head of the penis. The remainder of the penile shaft is unremarkable. An indwelling urethral catheter is often present. Simply removing the catheter may help treat paraphimosis caused by an indwelling urethral catheter.
- If paraphimosis is left untreated for too long, **necrosis of the glans penis** can occur.
- **Partial amputation of the distal penis** has been reported.

ED MANAGEMENT

- When diagnosed early, paraphimosis can be remedied easily with **simple manual reduction** in combination with other conservative measures.
- Patients with severe paraphimosis that proves refractory to conservative therapy will require a **bedside emergency dorsal slit procedure** to save the penis.
- Formal circumcision can be performed in the operating room at a later date.

359 Bragg BN, Leslie SW. Paraphimosis. 2017 Jun.

360 Jones SA, Flynn RJ. An unusual (and somewhat piercing) cause of paraphimosis. British Journal of Urology. Nov 1996. 78:80-804.

361 Gozal D. Paraphimosis apparently associated with Plasmodium falciparum infection. Transactions of the Royal Society of Tropical Medicine and Hygiene. July-August 1991. 85:443.

362 Harvey K, Bishop L, Silver D, Jones T. A case of chancroid. The Medical Journal of Australia. 1977. 26:956-957.

Pain control

- Paraphimosis is a painful condition and care should be taken to ensure patient comfort by providing **adequate analgesia and local anesthesia** using a dorsal penile nerve block and circumferential penile ring block with lidocaine, bupivicaine, or a combination of the two.
- Epinephrine should never be injected. In additional, topical application of lidocaine or prilocaine creams and direct injection of anesthetic into the foreskin can be used.

Reduction

- Once pain control is adequate, manual reduction by attempting to circumferentially compress the foreskin and holding for 2-10 minutes to "squeeze" the edematous fluid along the penile shaft may be attempted.

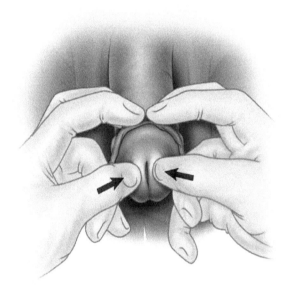

- After this fluid has passed proximally, the foreskin is reduced by placing both thumbs on the glans and using the remaining fingers to pull the foreskin back over the glans into the anatomic location.
- There are many variations of this technique, all using the same principle of traction on the foreskin and countertraction on the glans.
- In addition, reduction can include the use of forceps and clamps to pull the foreskin. Those instruments must be used cautiously, however, as they can crush the skin and cause necrosis of this tissue due to devascularization.
- The use of a 25-gauge needle to make several small stab incisions as an outlet for edema fluid has also been described[363].

Adjuncts to reduction

- Ice, osmotic agents such as sugar, and compression wrapping with Coban® have been used as adjuncts to manual reduction and can be considered.
- Ice and osmotic agents may require 1-2 hours to take effect, however, so they should not be used when arterial compromise is suspected.

Dorsal slit

- After adequate local anesthesia (with or without sedation) or general anesthesia, the plane between the dorsal foreskin and the corona is identified.
- Normally, when performing a dorsal slit, the operator then uses a hemostat to crush the foreskin at the 12 o'clock position, which is also the midline of the dorsal foreskin. This is left in place for 30-60 seconds, to provide hemostasis. The crushed area is then sharply incised with scissors. The edges are often oversewn with an interrupted or running stitch, using a dissolvable suture such as chromic.
- However, when performing a dorsal slit for paraphimosis, one should identify the dorsal midline of the rolled preputial skin. Make a vertical incision at the junction of the rolled foreskin (identified as the point between the mucosal, smooth skin and the preputial thicker, dull skin). This should release the contricting tissue. Mobilize the foreskin so that it can slide over the glans and back and then oversew the cut edges[364].
- Regardless of the method used, urologic evaluation acutely in the emergency department and then following the acute interaction for consideration of circumcision are crucial.

CONTRAINDICATIONS

- Do not consider circumcision in a neonate with hypospadias, a dorsal hood deformity, or a small penis.
- Refer the neonate to a urologist.

---

363 Pohlman GD, Phillips JM, Wilcox DT. Simple method of paraphimosis reduction revisited: Point of technique and review of the literature. Journal of Pediatric Urology. Feb 2013. 9:104-107.

364 Julian Wan. Dorsal Slit. Joseph Smith Jr, Stuart Howards, Glenn Preminger. Hinman's Atlas of Urologic Surgery. Third Edition. Philadephia, PA: Elsevier-Saunders; 2012. 145-146.

II. PRIAPRISM & ASSOCIATED CONDITIONS

DEFINITION

- Prolonged, pathologic erection of the penis for > 4 hours in the absence of sexual desire. It is usually painful and it is unrelated to sexual stimulation and unrelieved by ejaculation. Priapism is frequently idiopathic in etiology but it is a known complication of a number of important medical conditions and pharmacologic agents[365].

ETIOLOGY

- Priapism can be idiopathic or can be secondary to a variety of diseases, conditions, or medications.
- The most common cause of priapism in the pediatric population is **sickle cell disease (SCD),** which is responsible for 65% of cases. Leukemia, trauma, and idiopathic causes are the causes in 10% of patients. Pharmacologically induced priapism is the etiology in 5% of children[366].

SECONDARY CAUSES OF LOW-FLOW PRIAPISM:

- **Thromboembolic/hypercoagulable states:** Sickle cell anemia, Thalassemia, Fabry disease, Dialysis, Vasculitis, Fat embolism
- **Neurologic diseases:** Spinal cord stenosis (ie, trauma to the medulla), Autonomic neuropathy and cauda equina compression
- **Neoplastic disease:** Prostate cancer, Bladder cancer, Hematologic cancer (leukemia), Renal carcinoma, Melanoma
- **Pharmacologic causes:**
  - **Intracavernosal agents** - Papaverine, phentolamine, prostaglandin E1
  - **Intraurethral pellets** (ie, medicated urethral system for erection with intracavernosal prostaglandin E1)
  - **Antihypertensives** - Ganglion-blocking agents (eg, guanethidine), arterial vasodilators (eg, hydralazine), alpha-antagonists (eg, prazosin), calcium channel blockers
  - **Psychotropics** - Phenothiazine, butyrophenones (eg, haloperidol), perphenazine, trazodone, selective serotonin reuptake inhibitors (eg, fluoxetine, sertraline, citalopram)
  - **Anticoagulants** - Heparin, warfarin (during rebound hypercoagulable states)
  - **Recreational drugs** - Cocaine

- **Hormones** - Gonadotropin-releasing hormone (GnRH), tamoxifen, testosterone, androstenedione for athletic performance enhancement
  - **Herbal medicine** -Ginkgo biloba with concurrent use of antipsychotic agents
  - **Miscellaneous agents** - Metoclopramide, omeprazole, penile injection of cocaine, epidural infusion of morphine and bupivacaine[367].
- Only rare case reports have associated phosphodiesterase-5 enzyme inhibitors such as sildenafil with priapism. In fact, several reports suggest sildenafil as a means to treat priapism and as a possible means of preventing full-blown episodes in patients with sickle cell disease.

CAUSES OF HIGH-FLOW PRIAPISM:

- High-flow priapism may result from the following forms of genitourinary trauma:
  - Straddle injury
  - Intracavernous injections resulting in direct cavernosal artery injury

RARE CAUSES OF PRIAPISM INCLUDE THE FOLLOWING:

- Amyloidosis (massive amyloid infiltration)
- Gout (one case report)
- Carbon monoxide poisoning
- Malaria
- Black widow spider bites[368].
- Asplenia
- Fabry disease (rare association, occasionally noted to be priapism of the high-flow type)
- Vigorous sexual activity
- Mycoplasma pneumoniae infection (mechanism is thought to be a hypercoagulable state induced by the infection)

SIGNS AND SYMPTOMS

Low-flow priapism

- This condition is generally painful, although the pain may disappear with prolonged priapism. Characteristics of low-flow priapism include the following:
  - Rigid erection
  - Ischemic corpora: As indicated by dark blood upon corporeal aspiration
  - No evidence of trauma

---

[365] Dubin J, Davis JE. Penile emergencies. Emerg Med Clin North Am. 2011 Aug. 29(3):485-99.

[366] Donaldson JF, Rees RW, Steinbrecher HA. Priapism in children: a comprehensive review and clinical guideline. J Pediatr Urol. 2013 Sep 8. pii: S1477-5131(13):00214-3.

[367] Ruan X, Couch JP, Shah RV, Liu H, Wang F, and Chiravuri S. Priapism - A Rare Complication Following Continuous Epidural Morphine and Bupivacaine Infusion. Pain Physician. Sep 2007. 10(5):707-711.

[368] Quan D, Ruha AM. Priapism associated with Latrodectus mactans envenomation. Am J Emerg Med. 2009 Jul. 27(6):759.e1-2.

High-flow priapism

- This type of priapism is generally not painful and may manifest in an episodic manner. Characteristics of high-flow priapism include the following:
  - Adequate arterial flow
  - Well-oxygenated corpora
  - Evidence of trauma: Blunt or penetrating injury to the penis or perineum (straddle injury is usually the initiating event)

DIFFERENTIAL DIAGNOSIS

- Normal sexual arousal
- Penile trauma
- Urethral foreign bodies
- Spinal cord injury
- Peyronie's disease
- Penile implant

MANAGEMENT

Low-flow priapism

- **Intracavernosal phenylephrine** (Neo-Synephrine) is the drug of choice and first-line treatment for low-flow priapism because it has almost pure alpha-agonist effects and minimal beta activity.
- Following pharmacologic therapy, the next step in the treatment of low-flow priapism is **aspiration of the corpora cavernosa** followed by **saline irrigation** and, if necessary, **injection of an alpha-adrenergic agonist** (eg, phenylephrine). If the aforementioned interventions are unsuccessful, a diluted solution of phenylephrine may be used for irrigation. If medical treatment fails, the condition **warrants surgical intervention.**
- Key steps in the management of low-flow priapism caused by SCD include the following:
  - Oxygenation
  - Analgesics (eg, intravenous morphine)
  - Hydration
  - Alkalization
  - Exchange transfusions
  - Emergent surgical decompression: Advocated by most experts when conservative management fails

High-flow priapism

- Once the causative fistula has been located, it can be obliterated by selective **arterial embolization**, using an autologous blood clot, gelatin sponge, microcoils, or chemicals[369].
- Refer to Urology

CONTRAINDICATIONS

- **To cavernosal aspiration/irrigation**
  - Nonischemic ("high-flow") priapism
  - Overlying cellulitis
  - Uncontrolled bleeding disorder
  - Skin infection at the site of injection
- **To intracavernosal injection of vasoactive agents (α-adrenergic sympathomimetics)**
  - Severe hypertension
  - Dysrhythmias
  - Monoamine oxidase inhibitor use

COMPLICATIONS

- **Of cavernosal aspiration/irrigation**
  - Hematoma (at puncture site)
  - Infection (at insertion site or systemic)
  - Thrombosis
  - Arteriovenous fistula
  - Pseudoaneurysm formation
  - Traumatic puncture of dorsal penile or urethra
- **Of intracavernosal injection of vasoactive agents (α-adrenergic sympathomimetics)**
  - Fibrosis of the corpora, pain, penile necrosis, urinary retention
  - Phenylephrine toxicity
  - Acute hypertension, headache, reflex bradycardia, tachycardia, palpitations, cardiac arrhythmia.

SICKLE CELL DISEASE

- Key steps in the management of sickle cell disease-associated priapism include oxygenation, analgesics (eg, intravenous morphine), hydration, alkalization, and exchange transfusions.
- Although conservative management has commonly been advocated in the literature, several studies have questioned its efficacy, and most experts advocate emergent surgical decompression when conservative management fails.
- Ekong and colleagues reported successful use of automated red cell exchange transfusion (ARCET) in five patients with sickle cell disease who were experiencing severely affected by stuttering priapism.
- Immediately after undergoing ARCET, with a target post-transfusion HbS level below 10%, all five became completely free of stuttering priapism.
- All five experienced recurrences as their HbS percentage increased towards the end of the ARCET cycle, but with subsequent cycles, most of the patients remained essentially free of stuttering priapism[370].

---

[369] Kulmala RV, Lehtonen TA, Tammela TL. Preservation of potency after treatment for priapism. Scand J Urol Nephrol. 1996 Aug. 30(4):313-6.

[370] Ekong A, Berg L, Amos RJ, Tsitsikas DA. Regular automated red cell exchange transfusion in the management of stuttering priapism complicating sickle cell disease. Br J Haematol. 2016 Oct 10.

III. PENILE TRAUMA

1. PENILE FRACTURE

- Penile fracture is the traumatic rupture of the **corpus cavernosum.** Traumatic rupture of the penis is relatively uncommon and is considered a urologic emergency[371].
- Sudden blunt trauma or abrupt lateral bending of the penis in an erect state can break the markedly thinned and stiff tunica albuginea, resulting in a fractured penis.
- One or both corpora may be involved, and concomitant injury to the penile urethra may occur. Urethral trauma is more common when both corpora cavernosa are injured[372].

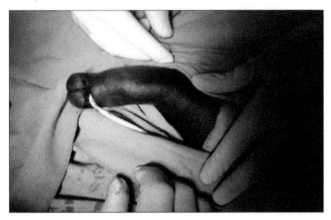

- Penile rupture can usually be diagnosed based solely on history and physical examination findings; however, in equivocal cases, **diagnostic cavernosography or MRI** should be performed.
- Concomitant urethral injury must be considered; therefore, **preoperative retrograde urethrographic studies** should generally be performed.

ETIOLOGY

- Sexual intercourse
- Industrial accidents,
- Masturbation,
- Gunshot wounds, or
- Any other mechanical trauma that causes forcible breaking of an erect penis.
- Additional rare etiologies include:
  - Turning over in bed,
  - A direct blow,
  - Forced bending, or hastily removing or applying clothing when the penis is erect.

PRESENTATION
HISTORY

- Most affected patients report penile injury coincident with sexual intercourse. Patients usually report that the female partner was on top, straddling the penis. During sexual relations, the penis slipped out, hitting the perineum or the pubis of the female partner.
- Patients sometimes report that they were having sexual relations on a desk (with the patient on top) and the penis slipped out, hitting the edge of the desk. Patients describe a **popping, cracking, or snapping sound** with immediate detumescence[373]. They may report minimal to severe sharp pain, depending on the severity of injury.
- Upon physical examination, evidence of penile injury is self-evident. In a typical penile fracture, the normal external penile appearance is completely obliterated because of significant penile deformity, swelling, and **ecchymosis (the so-called "eggplant" deformity).**

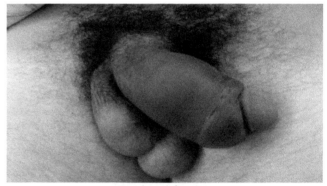

Eggplant deformity.

PHYSICAL EXAMINATION

- Upon inspection, significant soft tissue swelling of the penile skin, penile ecchymosis, and hematoma formation are apparent.
- The penis is abnormally curved, often in an S shape. The penis is often deviated away from the site of the tear secondary to mass effect of the hematoma.
- If the urethra has also been damaged, blood is present at the meatus. If the Buck fascia is intact, penile ecchymosis is confined to the penile shaft.
- If the Buck fascia has been violated, the swelling and ecchymosis are contained within the Colles fascia.
- In this instance, a **"butterfly-pattern" ecchymosis** may be observed over the perineum, scrotum, and lower abdominal wall.
- The fractured penis is often quite tender to the touch.

---

[371] *Mahapatra RS, Kundu AK, Pal DK. Penile Fracture: Our Experience in a Tertiary Care Hospital. World J Mens Health. 2015 Aug. 33 (2):95-102.*

[372] *Bhoil R, Sood D. Signs, symptoms and treatment of penile fracture. Emerg Nurse. 2015 Oct 9. 23 (6):16-7.*

[373] *Kitrey ND (Chair), Djakovic N, Kuehhas FE, et al. European Association of Urology Guidelines on Urological Trauma. uroweb.org.*

- Because of the severity of pain, a comprehensive penile examination may not be possible. However, **a "rolling sign"** may be appreciated when a judicious examination is performed on a cooperative patient.
- **A rolling sign** is the palpation of the localized blood clot over the site of rupture. The clot may be felt as a discreet firm mass over which the penile skin may be rolled.
- **Patients with a rupture of the deep dorsal vein** of the penis can present with findings similar to those of a penile fracture. Associated swelling and ecchymosis of the penis **("eggplant" sign)** is present. Injury commonly occurs during sexual intercourse. However, the patient does not typically hear a crack or popping sound.
- In addition, detumescence does not immediately occur. However, because of similar physical examination findings, a deep dorsal vein rupture should be surgical explored, as it is often difficult to differentiate from penile fracture. Patients with **concomitant urethral trauma** report hematuria upon postinjury voiding.
- Approximately 30% of men with penile fractures demonstrate blood at the meatus. Some patients may also report dysuria or experience acute urinary retention. Retention may be secondary to urethral injury or periurethral hematoma that is causing a bladder outlet obstruction. Urinary extravasation may be a late complication of unrecognized urethral injury. Successful voiding does not exclude urethral injury; therefore, retrograde urethrography is required whenever urethral injury is suspected.

ED MANAGEMENT
1. Conservative management:
- Fluid resuscitation
- Analgesia: Anti-inflammatory medications,
- Antibiotherapy if surgery is delayed
- Cold compresses, Pressure dressings,
- Penile splinting,
- Fibrinolytics,
- Suprapubic urinary diversion with delayed repair of urethral injuries.

Complications of conservative management:
- Missed urethral injury,
- Penile abscess,
- Nodule formation at the site of rupture,
- Permanent penile curvature,
- Painful erection, Erectile dysfunction,
- Painful coitus,
- Corporourethral fistula,
- Arteriovenous fistula, and
- Fibrotic plaque formation.

2. Surgical repair:
Advantages:
- Fewer complications,
- Increased patient satisfaction,
- Shorter hospital stays,
- Better outcomes.

2. PENILE AMPUTATION
- Penile amputation involves the complete or partial severing of the penis. A complete transection comprises severing of both corpora cavernosa and the urethra.
- Amputation of the penis may be accidental but is often self-inflicted, especially during psychotic episodes in individuals who are mentally ill.

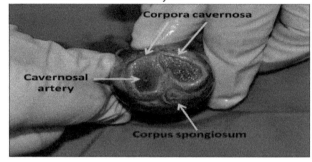

ETIOLOGY
- Mental illness: 87%
- Attempt at gender conversion.
- Assault: enraged wives amputated the penises of their adulterous husbands in Thailand.

PRESENTATION
- Diagnosis of the amputated penis is obvious on physical examination. A thorough history must be taken to determine the **patient's mental state** and if self-mutilation is responsible for the amputation.
- Many patients present to the hospital for evaluation because of the alarming, although seldom life-threatening, volume of blood loss. Determination of the psychiatric state helps with operative planning.
- The literature suggests that, in cases of self-amputation, resolution of the acute psychotic episode and treatment of the underlying mental illness typically results in a desire for penile preservation. The only exception may involve men who have repeatedly attempted amputation. The risks of future self-mutilation must be weighed against the effects of no penile replacement.
- Examination of the penis and remnant (if available) is important to determine the possible reconstructive options. The condition of the graft bed is closely inspected. Destruction of the amputated segment precludes reimplantation, and the patient should be prepared for future phallic reconstruction.

- Patients with adequate penile stumps may avoid reimplantation altogether, although this is typically a less desirable outcome.

MEDICAL THERAPY

- Pretreatment of the patient with an amputated penis has unique requirements.
- In the face of an acute psychotic episode, **psychological stabilization is required,** often with the aid of a psychiatrist. Management of the amputated penile remnant is imperative to a successful reimplantation.
- The severed penis should be **cleaned of debris** and **wrapped in sterile, saline-soaked gauze**. The wrapped penis should be placed into a sealed bag and placed inside a second container filled with an ice-slush mix. This helps to reduce the ischemic injury to the severed penis. **Reimplantation** should be performed as quickly as possible.

SURGICAL MANAGEMENT

- Penile amputation is a surgical emergency. Imaging studies are not necessary.
- The patient should be taken to the operating room for penile replantation or revision of the penile stump, with or without plans for future phallic reconstruction

3. PENETRATING INJURY

- Penetrating injury is the result of ballistic weapons, shrapnel, or stab injuries to the penis.
- Penetrating injuries are most commonly seen in wartime conflicts and are less common in civilian medicine. Penetrating injuries can involve one or both corpora, the urethra, or penile soft tissue alone.

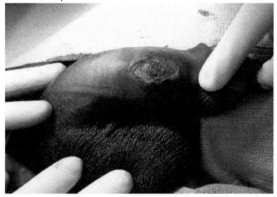

PRESENTATION

- Diagnosis of a penetrating penile injury is obvious based on both history and physical examination findings.
- Care must be paid to the patient's other **associated injuries**, which can be life-threatening and should take precedence over genital injuries.
- Significant associated injuries are present in 50-80% of cases.

- The patient must be medically stabilized prior to surgical repair of the injured penis.
- Blood in the meatus can indicate urethral injury and should be suspected in any penetrating trauma to the penis.
- The authors routinely perform retrograde **urethrography** to evaluate for urethral injury. Penetrating injuries to the corpora cavernosa often have a hematoma that overlies the defect and have a **"rolling sign"** similar to that of penile fracture.

MANAGEMENT

- The signs of penetrating penile injury should be an **indication for surgical exploration**.
- The only contraindication to surgery is medial instability due to other associated injuries.

4. PENILE SOFT TISSUE INJURY

- Penile soft tissue injury can result through multiple mechanisms, including infection, burns, human or animal bites, and degloving injuries that involve machinery.
- The corpora, by definition, are not involved.

PRESENTATION

- Examination of the penis reveals soft tissue loss. Those who have undergone laceration secondary to a human bite usually present in a delayed fashion because of embarrassment of the injury. This places them at increased risk for infection, which may be seen in the form of abscess, cellulitis, or tissue necrosis.

MEDICAL THERAPY

Bite injuries to the penis require extra care, as they have the potential for infection with unique organisms.

Dog bites, the most common animal bite, consist of multiple pathogens such as:

- Staphylococcus and Streptococcusspecies,
- Escherichia coli, and
- Pasteurella multocida.

Antibiotic treatment should generally include oral **dicloxacillin or cephalexin.**

Patients with possible *Pasteurella* resistance can be treated with **penicillin V**. Chloramphenicol has also been shown to have good efficacy. Human bites are considered infected by definition and should not be closed. They can be treated with antibiotics similar to those used in animal bites despite the fact that bacterial cultures may differ.

MANAGEMENT

- Surgical repair of soft tissue loss to the penis should be undertaken quickly. Prolonged exposure of the denuded penis increases the risk of secondary infection.

IV. BALANITIS & POSTHITIS

- **Balanitis** is inflammation of the glans penis, **Posthitis** is inflammation of the prepuce, and **Balanoposthitis** is inflammation of both.
- Balanitis usually leads to Posthitis except in circumcised patients.
- Inflammation of the head of the penis has both infectious and noninfectious causes. Often, no cause can be found.

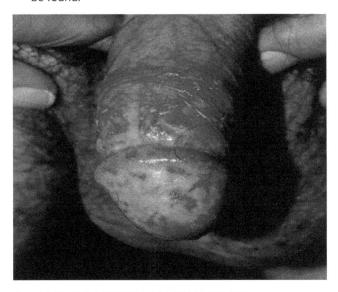

CAUSES OF PENILE INFLAMMATION

CATEGORY

INFECTIOUS	NONINFECTIOUS
• Candidiasis	• Balanitis xerotica obliterans
• Chancroid	
• Chlamydial urethritis	• Contact dermatitis
• Gonococcal urethritis	• Fixed drug eruptions
• Herpes simplex virus infection	• Lichen planus
	• Lichen simplex chronicus
• Molluscum contagiosum	• Psoriasis
• Scabies	• Reactive arthritis
• Syphilis, primary or secondary	• Seborrheic dermatitis
• Trichomoniasis	

RISK FACTORS

- Balanoposthitis is predisposed to by:
  o Diabetes mellitus
  o Phimosis (tight, nonretractable prepuce)
- Phimosis interferes with adequate hygiene.
- Subpreputial secretions may become infected with anaerobic bacteria, resulting in inflammation.

- **Chronic balanoposthitis** increases the risk of:
  o Balanitis xerotica obliterans
  o Phimosis
  o Paraphimosis
  o Cancer

SYMPTOMS AND SIGNS

- Pain, irritation, and a subpreputial discharge often occur 2 or 3 days after sexual intercourse.
- Phimosis, superficial ulcerations, and inguinal adenopathy may follow.

DIAGNOSIS

- Clinical evaluation and selective testing. History should include investigation of latex condom use.
- The skin should be examined for lesions that suggest a dermatosis capable of genital involvement.
- Patients should be tested for both infectious and noninfectious causes, especially **candidiasis**.
- **A swab** may be taken if the diagnosis is uncertain.
- Blood should be tested for **glucose.**

TREATMENT[374]

- **Good hygiene** and gentle cleaning of the area
- Treatment of specific causes (**Clotrimazole** if candidal infection is suspected)
- Sometimes subpreputial irrigation
- Sometimes circumcision

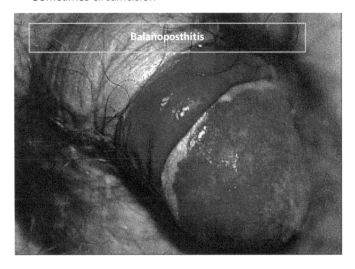

Balanoposthitis

---

374 Patrick J. Shenot, Balanitis, Posthitis, and Balanoposthitis [Msd manuals]

V. ACUTE URINARY RETENTION

INTRODUCTION

- Acute urinary retention (AUR) is the inability to voluntarily pass urine. It is the most common urologic emergency[375].
- In men, AUR is most often secondary to benign prostatic hyperplasia (BPH); AUR is rare in women[376].
- Symptoms and signs of obstruction are often mild, occurring over long periods of time and requiring a high index of suspicion for diagnosis.
- Early recognition and treatment are the keys to preventing renal loss.

SIGNS AND SYMPTOMS

Most acute obstructive uropathies are associated with significant pain or abrupt diminution of urine flow; however, chronic urinary obstruction is insidious and requires a careful history and a high index of suspicion. The following may be noted in urinary obstruction:

- Pain (most common symptom in acute obstruction but typically absent with slowly obstructing conditions)
- Altered patterns of micturition
- Acute and chronic renal failure
- Gross or microscopic hematuria
- Recurrent urinary tract infection (UTI)
- New-onset or poorly controlled hypertension secondary to obstruction and increased renin-angiotensin
- Polycythemia secondary to increased erythropoietin production in the hydronephrotic kidney
- History of recent gynecologic or abdominal surgery

COMMON CAUSES OF ACUTE URINARY RETENTION

- Benign prostatic hypertrophy
- Bladder calculi
- Bladder clots
- Meatal stenosis
- Neoplasm of the bladder
- Neurogenic etiologies
- Paraphimosis and Phimosis
- Penile trauma
- Prostate cancer
- Prostatic trauma/avulsion
- Prostatitis
- Urethral foreign body
- Urethral inflammation
- Urethral strictures

DIAGNOSIS

Physical exam

The physical examination should include the following:

- Evaluation for signs of dehydration and intravascular volume depletion; peripheral edema, hypertension, and signs of congestive heart failure from fluid overload may be observed in obstruction from renal failure
- Palpable kidney or bladder (indicative of a dilated urinary collection system)
- Rectal or pelvic examination to help determine whether enlargement of pelvic organs is a possible source of urinary obstruction.
- Examination of the external urethra for phimosis or meatal stenosis

LAB STUDIES

Laboratory studies that may be helpful include the following:

- **Urinalysis** (Dipstik) and examination of sediment
- **Urinary diagnostic indices** (eg, sodium, creatinine, osmolality)
- **FBC, U&Es, CMP, Uric Acid** and albumin

IMAGING STUDIES

- **CT KUB:** (especially without contrast) rapidly is replacing kidneys-ureters-bladder (KUB) x-rays as the first step in the radiologic evaluation of the urinary system
- **MRI** - Where available, MRI quickly is becoming the imaging study of choice for urinary obstruction
- **IV pyelography (IVP)** - IVP is the procedure of choice for defining the extent and anatomy of obstruction
- **Invasive pyelography** - This modality provides the same information as IVP without depending on renal function and can be used when the risks of IVP are considered too great
- **Ultrasonography** - This is the procedure of choice for determining the presence of hydronephrosis

ED MANAGEMENT

- The overriding therapeutic goal is reestablishment of urinary flow.
- Before specific therapy for obstruction is initiated, the **life-threatening complications of obstructive uropathy** must be investigated and treatment started.
- Once urinary obstruction is under consideration, a **transurethral bladder catheter** should be placed:
- **A urologist** should be consulted when a transurethral catheter cannot provide adequate bladder drainage

---

[375] Marshall JR, Haber J, Josephson EB. An evidence-based approach to emergency department management of acute urinary retention. Emerg Med Pract 2014; 16:1.

[376] Jacobsen SJ, Jacobson DJ, Girman CJ, et al. Natural history of prostatism: risk factors for acute urinary retention. J Urol 1997; 158:481.

INDWELLING URINARY CATHETERS

- Acute urinary retention should be managed by immediate and complete decompression of the bladder through catheterization. Standard transurethral catheters are readily available and can usually be easily inserted.
- If urethral catheterization is unsuccessful or contraindicated, the patient should be referred immediately to a physician trained in advanced catheterization techniques, such as placement of a firm, angulated Coude catheter or a suprapubic catheter[377].
- An indwelling urinary catheter is inserted in the same way as an intermittent catheter, but the catheter is left in place. The catheter is held in the bladder by a water-filled balloon, which prevents it falling out. These types of catheters are often known as **Foley catheters.**

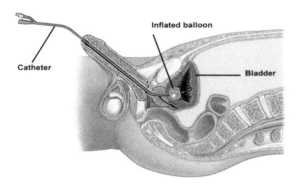

- Urine is drained through a tube connected to a collection bag, which can either be strapped to the inside of your leg or attached to a stand on the floor.
- Indwelling catheters are sometimes fitted with a valve. The valve can be opened to allow urine to be drained into a toilet, and closed to allow the bladder to fill with urine until drainage is convenient.
- Most indwelling catheters need to be changed at least every three months.

INDICATIONS FOR CATHETERISATION
- **Diagnostic indications include the following:**
  o Collection of uncontaminated urine specimen
  o Monitoring of urine output
  o Imaging of the urinary tract

- **Therapeutic indications include the following :**
  o Acute urinary retention (eg, benign prostatic hypertrophy, blood clots)
  o Chronic obstruction that causes hydronephrosis
  o Initiation of continuous bladder irrigation
  o Intermittent decompression for neurogenic bladder
  o Hygienic care of bedridden patients

---

377 Curtis LA, Dolan TS, Cespedes RD. Acute urinary retention and urinary incontinence. Emerg Med Clin North Am. 2001;19(3):591–619.

CONTRAINDICATIONS
- Presence of traumatic injury to the lower urinary tract (eg, urethral tear).
- **Signs that increase suspicion for injury are:**
  o A high-riding or boggy prostate,
  o Perineal hematoma, or blood at the meatus.
- When any of these findings are present in the setting of possible trauma, a **retrograde urethrogram** should be performed to rule out a urethral tear prior to placing a catheter into the bladder.

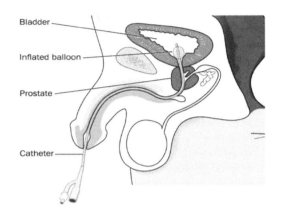

COMPLICATIONS OF INDWELLING CATHETERISATION (IDC)
- **Insertion**
  o Malposition
  o Trauma – false passage, urethral stricture (delayed), haemorrhage, balloon inflation in urethra
  o Pain
  o Failure (e.g. meatal, urethral or prostatic stricture – may require SPC or dilation)
- **When in situ**
  o Infection – 100% colonised at 1 week, 5% risk of septic complication per day, 8% bacteraemia, 1-3% UTI
  o Paraphimosis
  o Bladder irritation and erosion
  o Haemorrhage post-decompression (if >1 litre bladder)
  o Concretion formation
- **Removal**
  o Traumatic removal (e.g. Balloon not deflated, concretions)
  o Unable to remove (e.g. balloon won't deflate, concretions)
- **OTHER INFORMATION**
  o Administer antibiotics prior to IDC insertion if infection suspected
  o Review ongoing need for IDC daily and monitor for infection.

VI. TESTICULAR PAIN & SWELLING

SCROTAL SWELLING: PAINLESS VS PAINFUL

PAINFUL	PAINLESS
• Testicular torsion	• Testicular tumour
• Torsion of Appendix testis	• Hydrocele
• Trauma	• Varicocele
• Inguinal Hernias	• Spermatocele
• Fourniers gangrene	
• Epididymitis	
• Epidydimal cyst	
• Referred pain: Renal colic, AAA	

1. EPIDIDYMITIS

BACKGROUND

- Acute epididymitis is an infection of the epididymis.
- Epididymitis is a significant cause of morbidity and is the fifth most common urologic diagnosis in men aged 18-50 years[378].
- Epididymitis must be differentiated from testicular torsion, which is a true urologic emergency.

CLINICAL

- Pain in the scrotum usually develops quite quickly.
- The patient may notice a rapid swelling of the affected hemiscrotum. Irritative voiding symptoms and fever may also be present.
- On exam, the hemiscrotum is usually visibly enlarged and the overlying skin reddened. The affected epididymis is quite tender. At first the indurated epididymis may be distinguishable from the testicle but as the inflammatory process continues the epididymis and testicle become one inflammatory mass.
- A reactive hydrocele may also develop.
- **Rectal exam** should be done to rule out prostatitis as the source of infection.

INVESTIGATIONS

- The patient may have an elevated **white count and positive urinalysis** but this is not always the case.
- Urine should be routinely sent for **culture and sensitivity.**

ED MANAGEMENT

- The diagnosis is often difficult to make because of the similar presentation of testicular torsion.

- If there is any possibility that torsion exists then a urologist should be consulted. **A Doppler ultrasound** or **Testicular Flow Scan** can sometimes be helpful in distinguishing the two conditions but imaging studies should not be done if they will delay surgical treatment.
- In a young man a **sexual transmitted organism** is the most likely cause.
- If Sexually-Transmitted infection suspected treatment is typically: **PO Doxycycline 100mg BD 10-14days + IM Ceftriaxone 500mg STAT**.
- Refer to a sexual health specialist for follow up and contact tracing, with abstinence until sexual partners have been traced and treated.
- If gonorrhoea is the suspected pathogen seek specialist sexual health advice.
- If infection suspected secondary to enteric organism treatment is typically: **PO Ciprofloxacin 500mg BD 10 days** (be cautious of tendonitis) or PO Co-amoxiclav 625mg TDS for 10days

2. TESTICULAR TORSION

o Testicular torsion refers to the torsion of the spermatic cord structures and subsequent loss of the blood supply to the ipsilateral testicle.

o This is a urological emergency; early diagnosis and treatment are vital to saving the testicle and preserving future fertility[379]. The rate of testicular viability decreases significantly after 6 hours from onset of symptoms[380].

o Testicular torsion is primarily a disease of adolescents and neonates. It is the most common cause of testicular loss in these age groups. However, torsion may occasionally occur in men 40-50 years old[381].

o The patient typically develops acute onset severe unilateral testicular pain.

o The pain may also radiate to the lower abdominal with nausea and vomiting.

Examination reveals that the:

❖ *Scrotal skin oedematous and erythematous*
❖ *Testis too tender to touch*
❖ *Affected testis lies high in scrotum (Deming's sign)*
❖ *Opposite testis lies horizontally (Angel's sign)*

---

[379] Ta A, D'Arcy FT, Hoag N, D'Arcy JP, Lawrentschuk N. Testicular torsion and the acute scrotum: current emergency management. Eur J Emerg Med. 2015 Aug 11. 37-41.

[380] Barbosa JA, Denes FT, Nguyen HT. Testicular Torsion-Can We Improve the Management of Acute Scrotum?. J Urol. 2016 Jun. 195 (6):1650-1.

[381] Acute Scrotum. American Urological Association. Available at https://www.auanet.org/education/acute-scrotum.cfm. July 2016; Accessed: November 22, 2016.

[378] Taylor SN. Epididymitis. Clin Infect Dis. 2015 Dec 15. 61 Suppl 8:S770-3.

❖ *Pain not relieved by elevating testis (**Negative Prehn's sign**)*

❖ *Absence of cremasteric reflex*

o Scrotal elevation relieves pain in epididymo-orchitis but not in torsion (**Prehn's sign**). This sign may be difficult to test reliably in children

- **The cremasteric reflex** has 100% sensitivity and 66% specificity (the cremasteric reflex can be absent in neonates and in people with neurological disorders).

- **The cremasteric reflex (L1/L2 spinal nerves)** - gentle pinching or stroking of the inner thigh while observing the scrotal contents.

- The normal response, owing to shared innervations, is for the cremasteric muscle to contract, resulting in elevation of the ipsilateral testicle.

DIFFERENTIAL DX

- Problems to be considered in the differential diagnosis of testicular torsion include the following:
  o Torsion of testicular or epidydimal appendage
  o Epididymitis, orchitis, epididymo-orchitis
  o Hydrocele
  o Testis tumor
  o Idiopathic scrotal oedema
  o Idiopathic testicular infarction
  o Traumatic rupture
  o Traumatic hematoma

ED MANAGEMENT OF TESTICULAR TORSION

- This requires an **urgent urology consult**.

- If the diagnosis of torsion is suspected **surgical exploration** is necessary.

- The spermatic cord must be untorted **within 6 hours** if the testicle is to be saved.

- Whether or not the testicle has undergone torsion it should be sutured down to the scrotal skin to preclude any subsequent torsion and any uncertainty over the diagnosis should the pain recur.

- Once the testicle has been surgically tacked down it should never twist again.

- The opposite testicle should also be sewn down since the anatomic abnormality that caused torsion on one side may be present bilaterally.

- If, however, the testicle does not appear viable intra operatively **it should be removed.**

- It has been shown that leaving a non-viable testicle in situ **will significantly decrease the patient's future fertility**. This is most likely due to an **autoimmune phenomenon** which occurs as the body is exposed for the first time the its own sperm.

3. TORSION OF TESTICULAR APPENDAGE

- Torsion of testicular appendages can result in the clinical presentation of acute scrotum. Two such appendages are the appendix testis, a remnant of the paramesonephric (müllerian) duct, and the appendix epididymis, a remnant of the mesonephric (wolffian) duct. The most common cause of acute scrotum in prepubertal boys is torsion of the testicular or epididymal appendages[382]. Torsion of testes presents with severe pain, vomiting and an abnormal high riding transverse lie.

- **The appendix testis** is by far the most common of the appendages to twist. It presents as acute onset unilateral scrotal pain in the adolescent.

- Usually a **tender pea-sized nodule** can be palpated at the upper pole of the ipsilateral testis.

- If the appendix testis has infarcted, a **small blue dot** can sometimes be seen through the scrotal skin "**BLUE DOT SIGN**".

- Torsion of the testicular appendix presents with pain that is less severe, usually of a slower onset and can sometimes be visualised and palpated through the

- scrotum. On transillumination the appendix torsion appears as a "blue dot".Torsion of the testicular appendix is a benign condition that resolves within 2-3 days and is treated with simple analgesia. A testicular torsion can result in infarction. If there is any diagnostic doubt an ultrasound or surgical exploration must be performed.

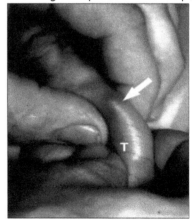

- Torsion of the appenages cause no damage to the testis and can be managed conservatively with NSAIDs, ice and support. Pain typically lasts a week and is self-limiting. It is important to reassure parents. This is clearly a diagnosis of exclusion.

- Surgical exploration is usually required.

382 *Lev M, Ramon J, Mor Y, Jacobson JM, Soudack M. Sonographic appearances of torsion of the appendix testis and appendix epididymis in children. J Clin Ultrasound. 2015 Oct. 43 (8):485-9.*

- If an infarcted appendix is found it should simply be excised. However, in the acute setting, differentiating testicular torsion from torsion of the appendix is often impossible, and **scrotal exploration** should be performed whenever the diagnosis is uncertain.

4. MUMPS ORCHITIS

- Viral orchitis is most often caused by mumps infection but can also be caused by a nonspecific inflammatory process in the testes.
- Approximately 20% of prepubertal patients (younger than 10 years) with mumps develop orchitis. Unilateral testicular atrophy occurs in 60% of patients with orchitis[383].
- Mumps is characterised by fever, malaise, headache and parotid swelling. Symptoms last approximately 7-10days.
- This typically occurs 10-14 days after the parotid gland becomes inflamed. The treatment is supportive therapy.
- Mumps is a notifiable disease in the UK.
- Discussion must take place with Public Health.
- Mumps is usually diagnosed clinically but can be confirmed with saliva or serum samples.
- It is highly contagious and you would be concerned about a possible outbreak in a community e.g. a school in a patient of this age group. A vaccination history should also be sought in this patient to see if they had their MMR immunisation

5. ACUTE PROSTATITIS

- Acute prostatitis is a common disease amongst men over 50 years of age. According to the National Institute of Health (NIH)[384], prostatitis can be grossly subdivided into acute/chronic bacterial and nonbacterial prostatitis.
- The more prevalent type is bacterial prostatitis with E-coli being the most common pathogen.
- Acute prostatitis presents with a wide range of symptoms.
- Systemically, it can present with features of sepsis such as fever or arthralgia. Urinary symptoms include dysuria, penile discharge, frequency or urgency.
- Urinary retention is a characteristic often encountered in prostatitis accompanied by abscess formation.
- Lower abdominal pain is a frequent manifestation (suprapubic region, scrotal and genito-rectal). Common signs include a swollen and tender prostate upon digital rectal examination as well as sigs of bacteraemia such as pyrexia, tachycardia or a decrease in blood pressure.

RISK FACTORS

- Long term catheterisation,
- Compromised immune system (e.g HIV)
- Unprotected intercourse.

ASSESSMENT

- History should include a detailed travel and sexual background.
- Examination comprises the ABC approach with an additional abdominal,scrotal and digital rectal examination.
- Bed side tests include a urinary dipstick and culture, FBC, CRP, U+E and blood cultures.
- Additional blood tests can include an HIV test, STI screen, semen culture, penile swab and PSA.
- Imaging can aid the diagnosis of prostatitis. Abdominal x-ray can help to exclude alternative differentials such as bowel obstruction.
- US of the scrotum and urinary tract can be performed to exclude anomalies.
- CT abdomen/pelvis and trans-rectal US will ultimately show an inflamed prostate. However, the diagnosis of prostatitis will rely on clinical judgement and diagnosed based on imaging.

MANAGEMENT

- Initial steps include rest, analgesia, laxatives, NSAIDS and adequate rehydration.
- If the patient displays signs of sepsis, admit to hospital. Catheterise the patient, however if the they are symptomatic with acute urinary retention, opt for a suprapubic catheterisation to avoid germ spreading.
- Empirical antibiotics should be started and switched to culture sensitive antibiotics once blood culture results have returned.
- The choice of antibiotics should follow local recommendations, however a suitable regime would be;
- Broad spectrum (cephalosporin) plus gentamycin if patient is systemically unwell.
  - If oral antibiotics are appropriate, use
    - Ciprofloxacin 500mg BD for 28 days or
    - Ofloxacin 200mg BD for 28 days
    - If patient is allergic to quinolones, consider trimethoprim (200mg BD for 28days) as an alternative.
    - It is possible to add on an alpha blocker such as tamsulosin which has been proven as an beneficial adjunct for symptom relief.
    - A referral to the Urology Team should be made upon discharge.

[383] Gazibera B, Gojak R, Drnda A, et al. Spermiogram part of population with the manifest orchitis during an ongoing epidemic of mumps. Med Arh. 2012. 66(3 Suppl 1):27-9.

[384] Krieger JN, Nyberg L Jr, Nickel JC. NIH consensus definition and classification of prostatitis. JAMA. 1999. 282:236-7.

33. Pregnancy in the ED
I. PELVIC PAIN

INTRODUCTION

- **Acute pelvic pain** is defined as pelvic pain lasting for less than three months. It is more common in women than men. Most women experience mild pelvic pain at some time during menstrual periods, ovulation or sexual intercourse. It is the most common reason for urgent laparoscopic examination in the UK.
- In a randomized trial of women of reproductive age presenting with nonspecific abdominal pain, a diagnosis during hospitalization was established in only 45 percent of the women randomized to the observation arm compared with 79 percent of the women randomized to the laparoscopy arm[385].
- Multiple organ systems can contribute to pelvic pain: Gastrointestinal, genitourinary, and musculoskeletal systems all must be considered in patients who present with this symptom. It is a common presentation in primary care.

HISTORY

- The medical history should include previous abdominal and gynecologic surgeries. Past gynecologic problems should be elicited; in one study, 53 percent of patients with ovarian torsion had a known history of ovarian cyst or mass[386].
- Evaluate the location, duration (constant or intermittent), onset, radiation, associated symptoms, severity, quality (sharp or dull ache), alleviating and aggravating factors and previous history of similar pain.
- **Relevant organ system symptoms** (urinary, gastrointestinal and musculoskeletal) should also be reviewed as there are many non-gynaecologic causes of pelvic pain.
- **A detailed sexual history** is of paramount importance in the evaluation of acute pelvic pain, as pelvic inflammatory disease and ectopic pregnancy are major considerations.
- In male patients, it is important to ask about testicular pain and urethral discharge.

- **Past medical and surgical histories** are also important. Any history of abdominal surgery increases the risk of bowel obstruction. Adnexal pathology (ovarian or paratubal cyst, hydrosalpinx) is a risk factor for adnexal torsion.
- **Social history** may be important, especially if there is any substance abuse, history of domestic violence or high-risk behaviour.
- **Family history** may be relevant (history of coagulation disorders or sickle cell disease).

SEXUAL HISTORY

- It is often difficult to approach the patient regarding a sexual history. You may wish to introduce the subject in the following way:

'I need ask some questions about your sexual health that, although they may seem very personal, are very important for me know so that I can help you. I ask these questions to all my patients, regardless of age, gender or marital status. All the information that you give will be treated in the strictest of confidence. Do you have any questions?'

Ask about the '6 Ps' of a sexual history[387]:

1. Partners:

- *Are you sexually active?*
- *Do you have sex with men or women?*
- *How many sexual partners have you had in the last 2 months – male and/or female?*
- *How may sexual partners have you have had in the last 12 months – male and/or female?*
- *Were the partners long-term or casual?*
- *Were the partners sex workers?*
- *Did the partners have any risk factors for STD and HIV?*

2. Protection from pregnancy:

- *Are you trying to get pregnant?*
- *Are you concerned about getting pregnant?*
- *What kind of contraception do you normally use?*

3. Protection from STD:

- *How do you protect yourself from STD and HIV?*
- *Do you and your partner use any barrier contraception?*
- *How often do you use protection?*

---

385 Morino M, Pellegrino L, Castagna E, Farinella E, Mao P. Acute nonspecific abdominal pain: A randomized, controlled trial comparing early laparoscopy versus clinical observation. Ann Surg. 2006;244(6):881–888.

386 Houry D, Abbott JT. Ovarian torsion: a fifteen-year review. Ann Emerg Med. 2001;38(2):156–159..

387 CDC, A Guide To Aking A Sexual History [pdf Online]

4. Practices:
- *Have you had vaginal (penis in vagina) intercourse in the last month and did you use any barrier protection?*
- *Have you had anal (penis in rectum or anus) sex in the last month and did you use any barrier protection?*
- *Have you had oral (mouth to penis, vagina or anus) sex in the last month and did you use any barrier protection?*

5. Previous history of STD:
- *Have you or your partner ever had an STD?*
- *When was it diagnosed?*
- *How was it treated?*

6. Predisposition to HIV and hepatitis B &C:
- *Have you or a partner ever injected drugs?*
- *Have you or a partner ever had an HIV test?*
- *Have you or a partner ever had sex with a sex worker?*

⨁ **Complete the sexual history by asking the patient if there is anything else about their sexual health that may be helpful.**

Possible causes

Pregnancy related
- Miscarriage
- Ectopic pregnancy
- Rupture of corpus luteal cyst
- Causes in later pregnancy include premature labour, placental abruption and (rarely) uterine rupture.

Gynaecological
- Ovulation (mid-cycle, may be severe pain)
- Dysmenorrhoea
- Pelvic inflammatory disease
- Rupture or torsion of ovarian cyst
- Degenerative changes in a fibroid
- The possibility of a pelvic tumor or pelvic vein thrombosis should also be considered.

Non-gynaecological
- Diverticulitis
- Appendicitis
- Prostatitis
- Epididymo-orchitis
- Bowel obstruction
- Adhesions
- Strangulated hernia
- Urolithiasis
- Musculoskeletal
- Vascular - pelvic vein thrombosis
- Pelvic (testicular) tumour
- Neurogenic - herpes zoster, impingement by arthritis, tumours, syphilis
- Multiple sclerosis
- Functional somatic syndromes
- Pelvic floor muscle dysfunction

EXAMINATION
- The physical examination should focus on the vital signs, and abdominal and pelvic examination. The pelvic examination is the most important part and is required for any woman with abdominal or pelvic pain. ED Physicians should acknowledge the limitations of a pelvic examination when assessing the adnexa[388].
- In women, pelvic examination should be performed besides abdominal examination. The external genitalia should be visually inspected for lesions first.
- The vagina and cervix should be visualised by speculum examination. The bladder, vaginal walls, and levator muscles should be palpated with 1 or 2 fingers after the speculum examination to assess for tenderness in these regions. In men, examination of genitalia and prostate should be performed. In both sexes, the hernia orifices should be examined along with DRE if history suggests.
- Pelvic floor muscles and thigh muscles should also be examined. Body habitus plays a role in the quality of examination as palpation of pelvic organs may be limited by obesity.

INVESTIGATIONS
- Urine dipsticks/MSU
- Full blood count
- Urine pregnancy test and transvaginal ultrasound (if suspected pelvic mass) in women
- Endometrial pipette sampling or hysteroscopy (suspected endometrial pathology)
- Nucleic acid amplification tests for chlamydia and gonococcus
- In systemically unwell patients, urgent diagnostic laparoscopy

MANAGEMENT
- Management is based on identifying and treating the cause.
- Empirical use of antibiotics and analgesia without a clear diagnosis should be avoided.
- Referral is required if the diagnosis cannot be established or if there is no response to treatment in primary care.

INDICATIONS FOR REFERRAL
Emergency referral
- Suspected ectopic pregnancy or premature labour
- Suspicion of placental abruption or uterine rupture
- Evidence of strangulated inguinal or femoral hernia
- Pain in a haemodynamically unstable patient with signs of sepsis, for example appendicitis, peritonitis

Urgent outpatient referral
- Suspected gynaecological, gastroenterological or urological malignancy.

---
[388] *Padilla LA, Radosevich DM, Milad MP. Accuracy of the pelvic examination in detecting adnexal masses. Obstet Gynecol. 2000;96(4):593–598.*

II. INTIMATE EXAMINATIONS & CHAPERONES

1. INTIMATE EXAMINATIONS[389]

- Intimate examinations can be embarrassing or distressing for patients and whenever you examine a patient you should be sensitive to what they may think of as intimate.
- This is likely to include examinations of **breasts, genitalia and rectum**, but could also include any examination where it is necessary to touch or even be close to the patient.
- In this guidance, we highlight some of the issues involved in carrying out intimate examinations.
- This must not deter you from carrying out intimate examinations when necessary.
- You must follow this guidance and make detailed and accurate records at the time of the examination, or as soon as possible afterwards.

Before conducting an intimate examination, you should:

1. Explain to the patient why an examination is necessary and give the patient an opportunity to ask questions
2. Explain what the examination will involve, in a way the patient can understand, so that the patient has a clear idea of what to expect, including any pain or discomfort
3. Get the patient's permission before the examination and record that the patient has given it
4. Offer the patient a chaperone (see below). If dealing with a child or young person:
   a. You must assess their capacity to consent to the examination
   b. If they lack the capacity to consent, you should seek their parent's consent
5. Give the patient privacy to undress and dress, and keep them covered as much as possible to maintain their dignity; do not help the patient to remove clothing unless they have asked you to, or you have checked with them that they want you to help.

During the examination, you must follow the guidance in *Consent: patients and doctors making decisions together*. In particular you should:

1. Explain what you are going to do before you do it and, if this differs from what you have told the patient before, explain why and seek the patient's permission
2. Stop the examination if the patient asks you to
3. Keep discussion relevant and don't make unnecessary personal comments.

INTIMATE EXAMINATIONS OF ANAESTHETISED PATIENTS

- Before you carry out an intimate examination on an anaesthetised patient, or supervise a student who intends to carry one out, you must make sure that the patient has given consent in advance, usually in writing.

2. CHAPERONES

INTRODUCTION

- The Emergency Department is an environment in which the entire range of physical examinations may be clinically necessary, and so a hospital should recognise the need for a clear chaperone policy tailored to the Emergency Department setting.
- This should involve increased use of chaperones for all examinations of Sensitive Areas to ensure compliance with defence organisations advice and GMC guidelines.
- Any patient undergoing a Sensitive Area examination or procedure in the ED should be offered the opportunity to have a chaperone present, regardless of the patient's age or gender.

CHAPERONES

A chaperone should be a trained and impartial practitioner, health professional or volunteer, who will act to protect the patient from inappropriate conduct by the examining practitioner as well as protecting the examining clinician from allegation of inappropriate behaviour or action. An exemplary chaperone will:

- Be familiar with the examination or procedure being carried out.
- Be respectful to the patient and sensitive to their dignity and confidentiality.
- Be present throughout the entirety of the examination.
- Be positioned so that they have a clear view of what the doctor is doing, as well as being able to hear clearly everything the doctor is saying to the patient.
- Be prepared to raise concerns regarding a doctor's behaviour or actions, remembering that abuse can exist in both auditory and visual forms and it is not necessarily tactile.
- Reassure the patient if necessary.
- Pay attention to whether the examining clinician is spending an excessive amount of time on a particular examination of a sensitive area.

Ideally, the managerial lead should be responsible for making sure that all healthcare professionals, staff or volunteers who might act as chaperones in the ED are appropriately trained to act as chaperones, ensuring that they are capable of fulfilling the above criteria.

---

[389] *General medical Council, Intimate examinations and chaperones [GMC online]*

It is a managerial responsibility to provide resource, and to ensure compliance. Friends or family members of the patient are not regarded as impartial and therefore cannot act as formal chaperones, however efforts should be made to comply with reasonable requests to have these people present also. Chaperones should have a low threshold for, and be empowered to, raising of concerns regarding:

- A less than professional manner.
- Over-exposure of a patient's body.
- Inappropriate comments or gestures.
- Inappropriate facial expressions.

In the scenario that a chaperone identifies a problem with a clinician's conduct, it is essential that a chaperone should inform the most senior member of the team as soon as possible. This should ensure that problems are dealt with efficiently and avoids confusion or muddled facts when attempting to recount the sequence of events subsequently. The ED is a place of urgency and the relentless time pressures leave it vulnerable to practitioners not complying with their responsibility to offer and provide a chaperone to patients. To avoid this frequently encountered problem, the onus is on the hospital to ensure that there are sufficient numbers of trained staff or volunteers readily available at all times. It is appreciated that in some departments, resources could limit full compliance, however if this is the case, this should be identified as a departmental risk, and managerial responsibility clarified.

SENSITIVE AREA EXAMINATIONS

A Sensitive Area examination or procedure should be considered to be any examination or procedure that will occur below the level of the clavicles or above the level of the mid-thigh. This encompasses all of the intimate examinations (of breasts, anus, genitalia) as well as targeting body regions that are in close proximity to intimate areas, such as the axilla or the inner thigh and groin. It should be noted that a patients definition or appreciation of what constitutes a sensitive area examination may differ from this. For vulnerable patients, (e.g. those that are known to have been victims of abuse in the past or those that a clinician perceives to be particularly anxious or sensitive to examination), any examination should be treated as a Sensitive Area examination. Consideration should be given for chaperone presence for all patient interaction in some cases. If no history is available, clinical judgement and common sense must be used to identify these patients by determining a perceived level of patient anxiety as well as considering any views expressed by the patient during the assessment. For all examinations conducted in the presence of a chaperone, the clinician must converse in a language that is comfortably understood by both the patient and chaperone unless language barriers dictate otherwise.

In the U.K. this will almost entirely refer to English, however if the patient cannot easily understand English and the practitioner is able to speak a language more familiar to them, then this acceptable, provided:

- There is no chaperone present that can also understand the preferred language.
- The practitioner diligently relates, exactly what is being communicated between patient and practitioner so that the chaperone can hear and understand.

All Sensitive Area examinations must be performed with the area of the body being examined completely exposed, to ensure that clothing does not obscure the chaperone's view of the practitioner's hand. The presence or absence of a chaperone should be documented clearly in the notes.

DECLINED CHAPERONE

It is the patient's right to decline a chaperone if offered.
If this is the case it must be documented that a chaperone was offered and declined before physical examination.

- A practitioner may feel uncomfortable performing the examination without a chaperone. This might occur because the patient is behaving in a sexualised way, or because the patient is known to file complaints against practitioners. If a doctor feels uncomfortable to proceed without a chaperone the care of the patient should be handed to the most senior member of the team.
- The patient's clinical needs should always take precedence. If delaying the examination or procedure could adversely affect the patient's well-being then the practitioner should continue without a chaperone, taking special care to document that one was offered and declined. This situation is unlikely to occur in the Emergency Department; in the acute setting presence of other staff is often required for the unwell patient.

DOCUMENTATION

- The Emergency Department record could contain a section specific to chaperoning that should be completed alongside the assessment of every patient.
- Such a section could include the following details: presence of chaperone, name, full job title, date and whether any issues or concerns were raised.
- Exemplary documentation would be completed by chaperone and include both the time that the chaperone arrived to witness the examination as well as the time the chaperone left. This not only provides a valuable time stamp denoting the period in which a chaperone is able to comment upon, but also creates a record of the duration of the examination. If a chaperone has been declined by a patient, this should also be documented in the aforementioned chaperone section.

III. MISCARRIAGE & ECTOPIC PREGNANCY

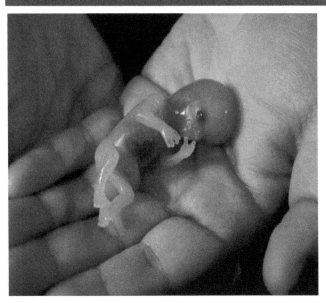

DEFINITIONS

- **Miscarriage** is the loss of a pregnancy before 23 completed weeks.
  - o **Early miscarriage** is more precisely defined as pregnancy loss in the first 12 weeks.
  - o **Late miscarriage** as pregnancy loss thereafter.
- **Ectopic pregnancy** occurs where a fertilized ovum is implanted in any tissue other than the uterine endometrium.
- **Antepartum haemorrhage (APH)** is defined as vaginal bleeding occurring from the 24th week of pregnancy and prior to the birth of the baby.
- **Postpartum haemorrhage (PPH)** is often defined as the loss of more than 500 ml or 1,000 ml of blood within the first 24 hours following childbirth.
- **Rhesus D antigen** is found on the surface of RBC and is capable of inducing intense antigenic reactions. Individuals without the antigen are determined rhesus negative and are homozygous recessive.

0-12 WEEKS	12-23 WEEKS	24 WEEKS-PREDELIVERY	24HRS TO 12 WEEKS POST DELIVERY
EARLY MISCARRIAGE	LATE MISCARRIAGE	APH	PPH

1. MISCARRIAGE

- Since 1997 the RCOG has encouraged the use of the term miscarriage rather than abortion.
- Miscarriage is subdivided as follows:
  - o **Threatened miscarriage:** bleeding or cramping in a continuing pregnancy. The cervical os is closed. An ultrasound scan is required to confirm foetal heart activity.

- o **Complete miscarriage:** all the foetal material has passed and the uterus is empty. The cervical os will be closed and where there has not previously been an US scan, one should be performed together with serum hCG to confirm pregnancy failure.
- o **Incomplete miscarriage:** there is retained products of conception within the uterus and the os remains open. The patient is at risk of haemorrhage and infection.
- o **Early embryonic/foetal demise** (previously known as missed/anembryonic pregnancy/blighted ovum): a non-viable pregnancy at 12 weeks where the products of conception have not been passed.
- o **Miscarriage with infection** (previously referred to as septic): this is secondary to either a spontaneous miscarriage or induced termination. Presentation is with fever and foul-smelling discharge.

CAUSATIVE FACTORS

- o Chromosomal abnormalities
- o Increasing maternal age
- o Smoking
- o Alcohol
- o Uterine abnormalities
- o Maternal infection
- o Co-morbidity

PRESENTATION

- o **Vaginal bleeding:** ranging from occasional spotting to significant haemorrhage or cervical shock.
- o **Abdominal pain**

Further reading:
Nice Guidelines CG126
https://www.nice.org.uk/guidance/ng126/chapter/Recommendations#early-pregnancy-assessment-services

2. ECTOPIC PREGNANCY [390]

OVERVIEW

- Ectopic pregnancy = fertilized ovum which implants outside the lining of the uterus

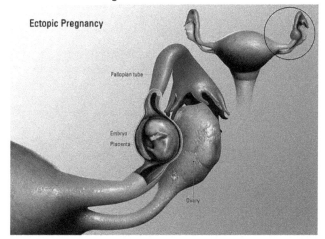

Ectopic Pregnancy

RISK FACTORS FOR ECTOPIC PREGNANCY

o *History of previous IUCD*
o *Maternal age of 35-44 years*
o *Previous ectopic pregnancy*
o *Previous pelvic or abdominal surgery*
o *Pelvic Inflammatory Disease (PID)*
o *Several induced abortions*
o *Conceiving after having a tubal ligation or while an IUD is in place*
o *Smoking*
o *Endometriosis*
o *Undergoing fertility treatments or using fertility medications*

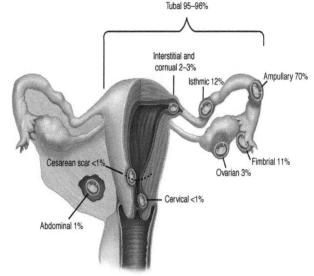

CORNUAL IMPLANTATION

o Patients with cornual implantation may rupture after 12 weeks with catastrophic blood loss. These patients sometimes present with symptoms of **gastroenteritis.**
o No single sign or combination of signs is diagnostic.
o Half of identified ectopics are in women with no known risk factors

CLINICAL FEATURES

- **History**
  o PV bleeding
  o Abdominal/Pelvic pain
  o 6-8 weeks LMP
  o Shoulder tip pain (large amount of bleeding)
  o Lightheadedness
  o Postural symptoms
- **Examination**
  o Adnexal tenderness and masses
  o State of cervix and material passing through it
  o Fetal heart (almost never heard in ectopic)

INVESTIGATIONS

- Beta-HCG (should almost double every 2 days)
- Bloods to rule out other causes of abdominal pain, Rh status
- MSU
- Transvaginal Ultrasound
  o If bHCG is > 1200 and there is no intra-uterine pregnancy = probable ectopic
  o An awareness of the limitations of US is as follows:
    - Cardioactivity needs to be seen to confirm intra-uterine pregnancy
    - Cardioactivity can be seen at gestational age **6-6.5 weeks.**
    - Cardioactivity does not exclude ectopic pregnancy in patients undergoing fertility treatment who are at risk of a **heterotopic pregnancy.**
    - Absence of an intrauterine pregnancy translates to a risk of ectopic of about 36%.

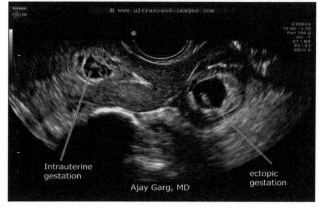

---

[390] *Nice Guidelines CG126, Ectopic pregnancy and miscarriage: diagnosis and initial management [NICE CG126]*

IV. ANTEPARTUM HAEMORRHAGE

INTRODUCTION

- Antepartum haemorrhage (APH) is defined as bleeding from or in to the genital tract, occurring from 24+0 weeks of pregnancy and prior to the birth of the baby.
- Obstetric haemorrhage remains one of the major causes of maternal death in developing countries and is the cause of up to 50% of the estimated 500 000 maternal deaths that occur globally each year.
- In the UK, deaths from obstetric haemorrhage are uncommon. In the 2006-08 report of the UK Confidential Enquiries into Maternal Deaths, haemorrhage was the sixth highest direct cause of maternal death (9 direct deaths; 3.9 deaths/million maternities) a decline from the 14 that occurred in the previous triennium (6.6 deaths/million maternities)[391].
- The most important causes of APH are placenta praevia and placental abruption, although these are not the most common. APH complicates 3-5% of pregnancies and is a leading cause of perinatal and maternal mortality worldwide. Up to one-fifth of very preterm babies are born in association with APH, and the known association of APH with cerebral palsy can be explained by preterm delivery

1. PLACENTA PRAEVIA

- Placenta praevia occurs when the placenta is implanted wholly or in part into the lower segment of the uterus.
- If the cervical os is completely covered it is considered a **major praevia (complete)** and if not, then it is considered a **minor praevia (marginal).**
- **Presentation:**
  o **Painless haemorrhage** or **foetal malpresentation** in late pregnancy are classical signs.
  o Abdominal pain can also occur

- **MANAGEMENT:**
  o Antenatal screening at 20 weeks enables detection and expectant management
  o Women who have had a bleed will be managed as in patients from 34 weeks.
  o Asymptomatic women may be managed as outpatients with close monitoring.
  o It is rare to have an undiagnosed placenta praevia present to the ED.

2. PLACENTAL ABRUPTION

- Placental abruption is the complete or partial premature separation of a normally implanted placenta from the uterus causing haemorrhage into the basalis decidua.

RISK FACTORS[392]

o Increased maternal age, Smoking, Use of cocaine,
o Hypertension, Multiple pregnancy, High parity,
o Prolonged rupture of membranes and trauma are all associated.
- The primary cause for abruption remains unknown except in cases of trauma.
- **Clinical:**
  o **Fundal tenderness** is associated with vaginal bleeding.
  o **Bleeding** may be concealed in up to 20%.
  o **Foetal distress** is indicative of abruption
  o **Foetal death** is common where separation is more than 50%.
  o **DIC** occurs in 10%, which can cause **long-term renal failure**

3. VASA PRAEVIA

- Vasa praevia is a condition in which the foetal blood vessels run freely and unsupported through the membranes, over the cervix across the internal os beneath the presenting part, unprotected by placenta or umbilical cord.

- **RISK FACTORS:**
  o Placenta praevia,
  o Multilobed placenta,
  o Velamentous insertion of the umbilical cord,
  o Multiple pregnancies
  o IVF pregnancies
- The foetal blood vessels may be ruptured at amniotomy, spontaneous rupture of membranes or during cervical dilatation.

- **Clinical:**
  o **Painless PV bleeding** and **foetal heart activity abnormalities** are common.
  o Pulsating vessels on vaginal examination are indicative; however, PV examination is normally contraindicated because of the possibility of placenta praevia.

[391] Lewis, G, editor. The Confidential Enquiry into Maternal and Child Health (CEMACH). Saving Mothers' Lives: reviewing maternal deaths to make motherhood safer, 2003-2005. The Seventh Report on Confidential Enquiries into Maternal Deaths in the United Kingdom. London: CEMACH; 2007.

[392] RCOG gtg63, Antepartum haemorroage [RCOG Online]

V. FETO-MATERNAL HAEMORRHAGE (FMH)

- Transplacental or fetomaternal haemorrhage (FMH) may occur during pregnancy or at delivery and lead to immunisation to the D antigen if the mother is D negative and the baby D positive. This can result in haemolytic disease of the fetus and newborn (HDN) in subsequent pregnancies.
- It is most common in the third trimester, during childbirth and following events associated with FMH.
- It is important to assess the volume of FMH to determine the dose of anti-D immunoglobulin required by a D negative woman to prevent sensitisation[393].
- Can occur in the absence of an observed potentially sensitising event
- **Potentially Sensitising Events in Pregnancy after 20 weeks of gestation:**
  o Amniocentesis, cordocentesis
  o Antepartum haemorrhage/ PV bleeding in pregnancy
  o External cephalic version, Fall, abdominal trauma
  o Intrauterine death and still birth
  o In-utero therapeutic interventions (transfusion, surgery)
  o Miscarriage, Therapeutic termination of pregnancy
- **Sensitisation:**
  o It has no effect on the mother and usually no adverse effect on the fetus in the primary pregnancy during which it occurs.
  o It is dependent on the volume of foetal blood entering the maternal circulation and the volume of the mother's immune response.
  o It is greatest with the first pregnancy (with the same father) and reduced with subsequent pregnancies
- Once occurred, **is irreversible.**
- **The immune response is:**
  o Usually not detected in the first pregnancy
  o Faster and greater in subsequent pregnancies
  o Causes **foetal anaemia** which in utero leads to **heart failure, hydrops foetalis** and **IUD**.
  o Neonatally, **haemolytic disease of the newborn** ensues causing **kernicterus**

CLINICAL ASSESSMENT

- A multidisciplinary approach to assessment and intervention of the shocked pregnant women is required.
- **History**
  o When possible take a full history.
  o Establish why the patient has attended the ED.

o Pertinent questions include LMP, parity, gravity and outcome of previous pregnancies not resulting in a live birth, paternity of previous pregnancies, rhesus status, sexual history, contraceptive history, fertility treatment, and pelvic surgery.
- **Ask about:**
  o Bleeding amount, colour and consistency and any previous bleeding in this or previous pregnancies
  o Scans in this pregnancy
  o Trauma
  o Pain location, nature and radiation
- **Establish if the patient is shocked:**
  o RR, Sats, HR, BP, CRT, Urine Output
- **Essential investigations**
  o **Urine+/-serum hCG**
  o **FBC, U&E, Clotting studies, G&S +/- Cross match** (at least 4 units if bleeding is heavy), **Blood grouping**
  o If gestation greater than 20/40, **Consider Kleihauer** (a blood test used to measure the amount of foetal hemoglobin transferred from a fetus to a mother's bloodstream), this determines the need for additional anti-D.
  o Consider **ECG**
  o Not required by: Individuals who are already sensitised are identified though an **indirect Coombs test**.

CLINICAL EXAMINATION

o Look for evidence of abdominal trauma
o Estimate PV loss as appropriate to the history
o **Do not** perform a vaginal examination in women presenting with PV bleeding after the 24th week as this can precipitate catastrophic haemorrhage in undiagnosed placenta praevia.
o The need for speculum examination should be considered on a case-by-case basis and should only be performed by a clinician competent in the technique.
  o **Use of Doppler and US**
    ▪ The foetal heart is audible with a Doppler probe from 10 weeks.
    ▪ Ongoing foetal monitoring should be by CTG.
    ▪ In the case of abdominal trauma, this should be prolonged monitoring, directed by local guidelines.
    ▪ Increasing availability of US in EDs should enable a rapid scan to be performed by a competent clinician.

---

[393] *Guidelines for the Estimation of Fetomaternal Haemorrhage Working Party of the British Committee for Standards in Haematology, Transfusion Taskforce. [Online]*

ED MANAGEMENT OF BLEEDING IN PREGNANCY

o **ABC DEFG**
o Oxygen ± airway management as appropriate
o IV access (2 wide bore cannulae) and volume replacement with crystalloid or colloid and blood
o **Left uterine displacement** can increase cardiac output by 30%
o Correction of coagulopathy
o Consider central venous catheterisation both for monitoring and access
o **Catheterisation.**
o **Analgesia**
• **Suspected ectopic pregnancy:** definitive management by the gynaecology team.
• **Suspected cervical shock:** remove products of conception from the os with the aid of a speculum and sponge forceps.
• **Continued haemorrhage:** consider administration of **ergometrine** and **oxytocin**.

• **Delivery of the baby:** in severe APH where foetal heart activity is detected, caesarean delivery of the baby should proceed. Where no foetal activity is identified vaginal delivery is advocated.
• **Administration of anti-D** to rhesus-negative women may not always be required.
   o In these circumstances, the dose to administer is:
      ▪ **Before 20 weeks:** 250 IU IMI to the Deltoid muscle
      ▪ **After 20 weeks:** 500 IU IMI to the Deltoid muscle
   o After 20 weeks gestation a **Kleihauer test** should be performed to establish the size of the FMH and additional anti-D given as required. This would not be done in the ED.
   o As anti-D immunoglobulin **is a blood product** there will be a small number of patients with particular religious beliefs to whom this treatment is unacceptable.
   o There is no passive immunisation and no alternative treatment.

VI. HYPEREMESIS GRAVIDARUM

• Vomiting is a normal feature of early pregnancy and occurs commonly between 7 and 12 weeks.
• Hyperemesis gravidarum is the presence of intractable, severe nausea and vomiting that results in fluid and electrolyte disturbance, marked ketonuria, nutritional deficiency and weight loss.
• It affects less than 1% of pregnancies.

RISK FACTORS FOR HYPEREMESIS GRAVIDARUM

o First pregnancy
o Multiple pregnancy
o Trophoblastic disease
o Obesity
o Prior or family history of hyperemesis gravidarum

POTENTIAL COMPLICATIONS OF HYPEREMESIS GRAVIDARUM

o Central pontine myelinosis
o Coagulopathy
o Mallory-Weiss tear
o Hypoglycaemia
o Pneumomediastinum
o Rhabdomyolysis
o Wernicke's encephalopathy
o Renal failure

ED MANAGEMENT OF HYPEREMESIS GRAVIDARUM

o Mild cases of nausea and vomiting in early pregnancy can often be controlled by dietary measures or non-pharmacological measures such as eating ginger and P6 wrist acupressure.
o In severe cases that are causing heavy ketonuria and marked dehydration admission to hospital is usually required for rehydration with intravenous fluids.
o **The NICE Clinical Knowledge Summary**[394] (NICE CKS) on nausea and vomiting in pregnancy recommends that if an anti-emetic is required **oral Promethazine** or **oral Cyclizine** should be used first-line.
o The situation should then be re-assessed after 24 hours.
o If the response to treatment is inadequate then a second-line drug such as **Metoclopramide, Prochlorperazine or Ondansetron** should be used.
o **Metoclopramide** should not be used in patients under the age of 20 due to the increased risk of extra-pyramidal side effects.
o **Proton pump inhibitors** (e.g. omeprazole) and **histamine H2-receptor antagonists** (e.g. ranitidine) are a useful adjunct in women that also have significant dyspepsia.

---

[394] https://cks.nice.org.uk/nauseavomiting-in-pregnancy

VII. POST PARTUM HAEMORRHAGE

INTRODUCTION

- Primary postpartum haemorrhage (PPH) is the most common form of major obstetric haemorrhage.
- The traditional definition of primary PPH is the loss of 500 ml or more of blood from the genital tract within 24 hours of the birth of a baby[395]. PPH can be minor (500-1000 ml) or major (more than 1000 ml).
- Major can be further subdivided into moderate (1001-2000 ml) and severe (more than 2000 ml).
- In women with lower body mass (e.g. less than 60 kg), a lower level of blood loss may be clinically significant[396].
- The recommendations in this guideline apply to women experiencing a primary PPH of 500 ml or more.
- Secondary PPH is defined as abnormal or excessive bleeding from the birth canal between 24 hours and 12 weeks postnatally.

RISK FACTORS

Thrombin	Pre-eclampsia Placenta abruption Pyrexia in labour Bleeding disorders: Haemophilia, anticoagulation, Von Willebrand
Tissue	Retained placenta Placenta accrete Retained products of conception
Tone	Placenta praevia Previous PPH Overdistension of the uterus: Multiple pregnancy, polyhydramnios, macrosomia
Trauma	Caesarean section Episiotomy Macrosomia
Other	Asian ethnicity Anaemia Induction BMI >35 Prolonged labour Age

CAUSES OF POSTPARTUM HAEMORRHAGE: "Four Ts"

FOUR TS	CAUSE
Tone	Atonic uterus
Trauma	Lacerations, Episiotomy, Hematomas, Inversion, Rupture
Tissue	Retained Placenta or products of conception, Invasive Placenta
Thrombin	Coagulopathies

PRIMARY POSTPARTUM HAEMORRHAGE

○ Primary PPH tends to be more severe than secondary PPH and is an obstetric emergency so call seniors immediately.

○ **ACTIVE MANAGEMENT**

- **Uterotonics** such as **oxytocin** reduces the risk of PPH by 60% when given prophylactically. (Syntocinon = synthetic oxytocin and is contra-indicated in patients with hypertension). Carbetocin is used to prevent PPH in caesarean delivery
- Early clamping of the umbilical cord
- Controlled traction of the placenta

⊥ *In a homebirth setting or where uterotropics are not available, **Misoprostol** (synthetic Prostaglandin E1) may be given to encourage uterine contraction.*

INVESTIGATIONS:

○ FBC
○ Blood cultures
○ Midstream Urine
○ High vaginal swab
○ Ultrasound can also be used to detect retained products of conception
- Long and complicated labour increase the risk of translocation of flora.
- **Group B Streptococcus (gram +ve) organisms** often cause **endometritis.**
- Endometritis is often polymicrobial and if endometritis is suspected then broad-spectrum antibiotics are required.
  ○ In a primary care setting, **amoxicillin or co-amoxiclav** is indicated
  ○ In a secondary care setting, **ampicillin or clindamycin and metronidazole** is recommended (RCOG, 2009).
  ○ **Gentamycin** is recommended in more severe cases.

395 Mousa HA, Blum J, Abou El Senoun G, Shakur H, Alfirevic Z. Treatment for primary postpartum haemorrhage. Cochrane Database Syst Rev 2014;(2):CD003249.

396 Knight M, Tuffnell D, Kenyon S, Shakespeare J, Gray R, Kurinczuk JJ, editors, on behalf of MBRRACE-UK. Saving Lives, Improving Mothers' Care - Surveillance of maternal deaths in the UK 2011-13 and lessons learned to inform maternity care from the UK and Ireland Confidential Enquiries into Maternal Deaths and Morbidity 2009–13. Oxford: National Perinatal Epidemiology Unit, University of Oxford; 2015.

ED MANAGEMENT OF PPH[397]

1. PRIMARY PPH

Resuscitation

- **Measures for minor PPH**
  - Measures for minor PPH (blood loss 500-1000 ml) without clinical shock:
    - Intravenous access (one 14-gauge cannula)
    - Urgent venepuncture (20 ml) for:-group and screen-full blood count-coagulation screen, including fibrinogen
    - Pulse, respiratory rate and blood pressure recording every 15 minutes
    - Commence warmed crystalloid infusion.

- **Measures for major PPH**
  - Full protocol for major PPH (blood loss greater than 1000 ml) and continuing to bleed or clinical shock:
    - A and B-assess airway and breathing
    - C-evaluate circulation
    - Position the patient flat
    - Keep the woman warm using appropriate available measures
    - Transfuse blood as soon as possible, if clinically required
    - Until blood is available, infuse up to 3.5 l of warmed clear fluids, initially 2 l of warmed isotonic crystalloid.
    - Further fluid resuscitation can continue with additional isotonic crystalloid or colloid (succinylated gelatin).
    - Hydroxyethyl starch should not be used.
    - The best equipment available should be used to achieverapid warmed infusion of fluids
    - Special blood filters should not be used, as they slow infusions.

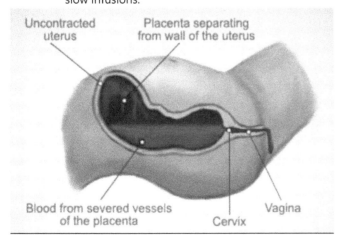

Uncontracted uterus

Placenta separating from wall of the uterus

Blood from severed vessels of the placenta

Cervix

Vagina

- **Blood transfusion**
  - There are no firm criteria for initiating red cell transfusion.
  - The decision to provide blood transfusion should be based on both clinical and haematological assessment. [New 2016]

2. SECONDARY PPH

- Secondary PPH occurs between **24h and 12 weeks** after delivery.
- Bleeding is less severe than in primary PPH.
- The cause is often **uterine atony** or **retained products of conception.**
- Secondary PPH commonly presents to primary care where a full obstetric and haematological history should be obtained.

RECOMMENDATIONS RCOG GREEN-TOP GUIDELINE NO. 52[398]

- In women presenting with secondary PPH, an assessment of vaginal microbiology should be performed (high vaginal and endocervical swabs) and appropriate use of antimicrobial therapy should be initiated when endometritis is suspected. [New 2016]
- A pelvic ultrasound may help to exclude the presence of retained products of conception, although the diagnosis of retained products is unreliable. [New 2016]
- Surgical evacuation of retained placental tissue should be undertaken or supervised by an experienced clinician.

COMPLICATIONS OF PPH

- *Sequelae of hypovolaemia (shock, renal failure)*
- *DIC*
- *Sepsis*
- *Transfusion or anaesthetic reaction*
- *Fluid overload (pulmonary oedema)*
- *DVT, VTE*
- *Anaemia (normocytic normochromic)*
- ***Sheehan syndrome*** *(postpartum hypopituitarism from pituitary necrosis) which can present as failure to lactate.*

[397] Mavrides E, Allard S, Chandraharan E, Collins P, Green L, Hunt BJ, Riris S, Thomson AJ on behalf of the Royal College of Obstetricians and Gynaecologists. Prevention and management of postpartum haemorrhage. BJOG 2016;124:e106–e149.

[398] RCOG, Postpartum Haemorrhage, Prevention and Management (Green-top Guideline No. 52) [Online]

VIII. SVT AND PREGNANCY

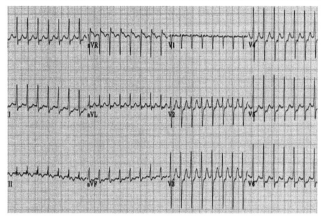

- Arrhythmias can cause cardiovascular complications in pregnancy. Palpitations are a common symptom in pregnancy, and electrocardiography (ECG) or ambulatory ECG monitoring can be conducted to determine correlation of the symptoms with arrhythmias.
- The differential diagnosis for supraventricular tachycardia (SVT) in pregnant patients is similar to that for non-pregnant patients, and includes atrioventricular nodal reentrant tachycardia (AVNRT), atrioventricular reentrant tachycardia (AVRT), atrial fibrillation (AF) or flutter, and atrial tachycardia (AT).
- Increase in circulating plasma volume and hyperdynamic circulation in pregnancy can predispose to SVT.
- SVT can occur in pregnant patients with structurally normal hearts or with structural heart diseases such as valvular heart disease, hypertrophic cardiomyopathy, or congenital heart disease.
- **Workup** of SVT in pregnancy should include a comprehensive history and physical examination.
- Attention must be paid to duration and frequency of episodes; concomitant cardiac symptoms such as chest pain, dyspnea, orthopnea, and syncope; past medical history of cardiac and non-cardiac disorders; and social history such as alcohol, drug, and caffeine intake.
- **Physical examination** will aid in detection of heart failure or structural heart disease. The ECG in tachycardia and sinus rhythm aids in the diagnosis of the specific etiology of the SVT.
- Attention must be paid to the presence of manifest pre-excitation and chamber enlargement on ECG.
- **Echocardiography** is an essential and safe tool to identify patients with structural heart disease in pregnancy.
- Laboratory studies should include evaluation for **anemia, electrolyte disorders, and thyroid function testing.**

ED MANAGEMENT OF SVT IN PREGNANCY

- Hemodynamically unstable patients with SVT should undergo **DC cardioversion**. The risk of fetal arrhythmia from cardioversion is minimal but present, and fetal monitoring should be performed.
- **For stable patients** with AVNRT or AVRT, vagal maneuvers such as **Valsalva maneuver** or carotid sinus massage are first-line therapy.
- **Intravenous adenosine** is unlikely to be harmful to the fetus due to its short half-life, and is an appropriate second choice.
- **AV nodal blocking** agents can be used as a third-line option. Among AV nodal blocking agents, **digoxin** is considered safe in pregnancy, followed by **calcium channel blockers** such as verapamil.
- **Beta blockers** other than atenolol can be used in the second or third trimester after appropriate counseling regarding intra-uterine growth restriction.
- **The use of atenolol** should be avoided in pregnancy. AV nodal blocking agents can also be used to prevent recurrent AVNRT and AVRT.
- Rate control of AF can be achieved by AV nodal blocking agents. Antiarrhythmic agents, including **flecainide and sotalol,** can be used in pregnancy as part of rhythm control strategy.
- Patients with valvular atrial fibrillation or non-valvular AF with high CHADS$_2$VASc scores are at risk for stroke, and anticoagulation, usually with heparin, must be continued in pregnancy and discontinued at the time of delivery.
- Electrical cardioversion is in general not recommended due to recurrence of tachycardia. Approximately 30% of atrial tachycardias may be terminated by adenosine.
- Catheter ablation should be considered in drug-resistant and poorly tolerated cases[399]. Catheter ablation can be considered in advanced centers for patients with frequent and symptomatic recurrences.
- Management of supraventricular tachycardia in pregnancy can be a challenging process due to drug-related toxicities to the mother and the fetus, and difficulty with ablation procedures due to risks of fluoroscopy. Addressing arrhythmias with potentially curative procedures such as ablation should be considered in women of childbearing age who are planning a pregnancy to prevent the quandary of arrhythmia management in the pregnant patient.

[399] European Society of Cardiology, ESC Guidelines on the management of cardiovascular diseases during pregnancy [European heart journal]

IX. PREGNANCY AND TRAUMA

- Manage pregnant trauma patients in accordance with the Advanced Trauma Life Support (ATLS) guidelines[400].
- 80% of women who survive haemorrhagic shock experience foetal death.
- **Additional issues:**
  - Anatomical and Physiological changes of pregnancy,
  - Pregnancy specific complications and Foetal issues.

ANATOMICAL AND PHYSIOLOGICAL CHANGES IN PREGNANCY

SYSTEMS	Changes in pregnancy
Cardiovascular system	
Plasma volume	Increased by up to 50%
Heart rate	Increased 15-20 beats per minute (bpm)
Cardiac output	Increased by 30 to 50% Significantly reduced by pressure of gravid uterus on IVC
Uterine blood flow	10% of cardiac output at term
Systemic vascular resistance	Decreased
Arterial blood pressure (BP)	Decreased by 10-15 mmHg
Venous return	Decreased by pressure of gravid uterus on IVC
Coagulation	Increased concentrations of most clotting factors
Respiratory system	
Respiratory rate	Increased
Oxygen consumption	Increased by 20 to 33%
Functional residual capacity	Decreased by 25%
Arterial pCO2	Decreased
Laryngeal oedema	Increased
Mucosal congestion	Increased
Airway size	Decreased
Upper airway blood supply	Increased
Other changes	
Gastric motility	Decreased
Gastro-oesophageal sphincters	Relaxed
Weight	Increased neck and mammary fat levels
Pelvic vasculature	Hypertrophied
Bowel	Superior displacement
Bladder	Anterior and superior displacement by uterus
Renal blood flow	Increased by 40%23. Serum urea, nitrogen, creatinine reduced

ED MANAGEMENT[401]

Airway and C-Spine

- **Increased risk of airway management difficulties due to:**
  - Weight gain
  - Respiratory tract mucosal oedema
  - Hyperaemia and hypersecretion of upper airway
  - Decreased functional residual capacity
  - Reduced respiratory system compliance o Increased airway resistance
  - Increased oxygen requirements
- Consider airway to be difficult and have most experienced provider secure and maintain airway
- Increased risk of failed or difficult intubation5–consider:
  - Early intubation
  - Use of a short handle laryngoscope
  - Smaller endotracheal tube (ETT)
  - Use of laryngeal mask airway if unable to intubate
- Increased risk of aspiration due to delayed gastric emptying in pregnancy
  - Ensure early gastric decompression with nasogastric or orogastric tube
- Apply cervical spine collar

Breathing and ventilation

- Increased risk of rapid desaturation
  - Provide oxygen supplementation to maintain maternal oxygen saturation greater than 95% to ensure adequate fetal oxygenation
- If safe to do so, raise the head of the bed to reduce weight of uterus on the diaphragm and facilitate breathing
- If a chest tube is indicated, insert 1-2 intercostal spaces higher than usual to avoid potential abdominal injury due to raised diaphragm
- Increased risk of aspiration1

Circulation and haemorrhage control

- Control obvious external haemorrhage
- Position with left lateral tilt 15-30 degrees (right side up) or perform manual left uterine (abdominal) displacement [refer to Appendix G: Positioning to relieve aortocaval compression]
- If seriously injured, insert two large bore intravenous (IV) lines
- Avoid femoral lines due to compression by gravid uterus
- If unable to achieve IV access, consider intraosseous lines
- Assess response–maintain an awareness of pregnancy related physiological parameters
- Aim to avoid large volumes of crystalloids (greater than 1 L) which may lead to pulmonary oedema due to the relatively low oncotic pressure in pregnancy
- Perform a thorough search for occult bleeding as maternal blood flow is maintained at expense of fetus
- If haemodynamically unstable, Focused Abdominal Sonography for Trauma (FAST) is useful to identify presence of free fluid in intraabdominal and intrathoracic cavities

Disability

- Rapid neurological evaluation utilising the Glasgow Coma Scale and assess for neurological deficits distally

Exposure

- Head to toe examination as for non-pregnant trauma patients
  - Expose and thoroughly examine all body parts
  - Prevent hypothermia

---

[400]Amercian College of Surgeons. Adv anced trauma lif e support: student course manual. 9th edition ed 2013.

[401] Maternity and Neonatal Clinical Guideline, Trauma in pregnancy, [Queensland Clinical Guidelines]

X. ABNORMAL VAGINAL BLEEDING

INTRODUCTION

- Abnormal uterine bleeding (formerly, **Dysfunctional Uterine Bleeding [DUB]**) is irregular uterine bleeding that occurs in the absence of recognizable pelvic pathology, general medical disease, or pregnancy.
- Heavy menstrual bleeding (HMB) is a prevalent condition that affects 20-30% of women of a reproductive age[402].
- It reflects a disruption in the normal cyclic pattern of ovulatory hormonal stimulation to the endometrial lining. The bleeding is unpredictable in many ways. It may be excessively heavy or light and may be prolonged, frequent, or random. There is a large differential diagnosis in women with abnormal vaginal bleeding.
- A careful menstrual history should be taken, including any history of post-coital or inter-menstrual bleeding. A pregnancy test must always be performed, regardless of whether the patient has missed a period or not.

VAGINAL BLEEDING TERMINOLOGY

- **Dysmenorrhea:** Painful cramps during menstruation.
- **Primary dysmenorrhea** is caused by menstruation itself.
- **Secondary dysmenorrhea** is triggered by another condition, such as endometriosis or uterine fibroids.
- **Amenorrhea:** Absence of menstruation.
- **Primary amenorrhea** is considered when a girl does not begin to menstruate by the age of 16.
- **Secondary amenorrhea** occurs when periods that were previously regular stop for at least 3 months.
- **Oligomenorrhea:** Menstrual bleeding with intervals of greater than 35 days.
- **Polymenorrhea**: Menstrual bleeding with intervals of less than 21 days.
- **Menorrhagia:** Menstrual bleeding with excessive flow or duration. Intervals are regular.
- **Metrorrhagia:** Irregular menstrual bleeding.
- **Menometrorrhagia:** Menstrual bleeding with excessive flow or duration. Intervals are irregular.
- **Intermenstrual bleeding:** Variable amounts of bleeding between normal regular menstrual periods.
- **Heavy menstrual bleeding** is both menorrhagia and menometrorrhagia, and refers to the menstrual blood loss of higher than 80 ml per month.

1. MENORRHAGIA

- Menorrhagia is excessive menstrual blood loss. The differential includes:
  - **Dysfunctional uterine bleeding**—heavy or irregular periods without obvious pelvic pathology. Often seen around menarche due to hormonal imbalance. Symptomatic relief with NSAIDs (e.g. mefenamic acid) are the mainstay of treatment.
  - **Fibroids, Endometriosis, Pelvic inflammatory disease, IUCD, Polyps.**
  - **Hypothyroidism.**

2. POST-MENOPAUSAL BLEEDING

- Post-menopausal bleeding is one of the most common presentations to a gynaecology clinic.
- The differential includes:
  - Atrophic vaginitis/ Fibroids/ Endometrial polyps.
  - Endometrial hyperplasia
  - Endometrial carcinoma/ Cervical carcinoma/ Vaginal carcinoma.
  - Bleeding from non-gynaecological sites, e.g. Urethra, Bladder, or Lower GI tract.
- An abdominal examination, speculum, and bimanual vaginal examination should be performed to look for evidence of tenderness or masses.
- Patients should be referred to gynaecology as an out-patient for further investigation.

3. VAGINAL BLEEDING UNRELATED TO MENSTRUATION OR PREGNANCY

- **Trauma, IUCD insertion.**
- **Post-gynaecological operations.**
- **Cervical erosions**—occur when the stratified squamous epithelium is replaced by columnar epithelium. The cervix appears red and the patient may experience post-coital or inter-menstrual bleeding.
- **Cervical polyp.**
- **Cervical cancer**—90% are squamous carcinoma.
- **Endometrial cancer/ Fibroids.**
- **Genital ulcers/ PID.**
- **Bleeding diathesis**, e.g. thrombocytopenia, haemophilia.
- **Anti-coagulant medication**.
- **Oral contraceptive problems**—breakthrough bleeding due to endometrial hyperplasia.

ED MANAGEMENT:

- Most patients with vaginal bleeding can be managed as outpatients with GP or gynaecology follow up.
- Patients with evidence of severe bleeding or hypovolaemia should be resuscitated and admitted.
- Patients with suspected genital tract malignancy should be referred urgently for gynaecology follow up.

---

402 RCOG, Advice for Heavy Menstrual Bleeding (HMB) Services and Commissioners [RCOG pdf]

XI. PREECLAMPSIA & ECLAMPSIA

1. DEFINITION

o **Preeclampsia** refers to the new onset of **hypertension** and **either proteinuria or end-organ dysfunction or both** after 20 weeks of gestation in a previously normotensive woman.

o **Eclampsia** refers to the development of **grand mal seizures** in a woman with preeclampsia, in the absence of other neurologic conditions that could account for the seizure.

2. Criteria of Pre-eclampsia

o SBP ≥140 mmHg or DBP ≥90 mmHg on 2 occasions at least 4 hours apart after 20 weeks of gestation in a previously normotensive patient

o If SBP ≥160 mmHg or DBP ≥110 mmHg, confirmation within minutes is sufficient **and**

o Proteinuria ≥0.3 grams in a 24-hour urine specimen or protein (mg/dL)/creatinine (mg/dL) ratio ≥0.3

o Dipstick ≥1+ proteinuria if a quantitative measurement is unavailable

• In patients with **new-onset hypertension without proteinuria**, the new onset of any of the following is diagnostic of preeclampsia:
   o Platelet count **<100,000/microliter**
   o Serum creatinine **>1.1 mg/dL** or doubling of serum creatinine in the absence of other renal disease
   o Liver transaminases **at least twice** the normal concentrations
   o Pulmonary oedema
   o Cerebral or visual symptoms

• **Severity of preeclampsia is based on BP measurement alone:**
   o **Mild:** SBP=140 to 149 mmHg and/or DBP=90 to 99 mmHg.
   o **Moderate:** SBP=150 to 159 mmHg and/or DBP=100 to 109 mmHg.
   o **Severe:** SBP is ≥160 mmHg and/or DBP ≥110 mmHg.

3. RISK FACTORS FOR THE DEVELOPMENT OF PRE-ECLAMPSIA

• *First pregnancy*
• *Age 40 years or older*
• *Pregnancy interval of more than 10 years*
• *Body mass index (bmi) of 35 kg/m² or more at first visit*
• *Family history of pre-eclampsia*
• *Multi-fetal pregnancy. [2010, amended 2019]*

4. FEATURES OF SEVERE PRE-ECLAMPSIA

Symptoms include[403]:
• *Severe headache*
• *Problems with vision, such as blurring or flashing before the eyes*
• *Severe pain just below the ribs*
• *Vomiting*
• *Sudden swelling of the face, hands or feet.*

5. COMPLICATIONS OF PRE-ECLAMPSIA

o *Eclampsia*
o *HELLP syndrome*
o *Disseminated intravascular coagulation*
o *Renal failure*
o *ARDS: Adult Respiratory Distress Syndrome*
o *Rupture of liver*
o *Stroke*
o *Cerebral haemorrhage*
o *Cortical blindness*
o *Pulmonary oedema*

6. INVESTIGATIONS FOR PRE-ECLAMPSIA

o **FBC**: risk of thrombocytopenia and haemoconcentration. Blood film should be checked because the patient may develop microangiopathic haemolytic anaemia.

o **Clotting screen**: should be checked if the patient is thrombocytopenic.

o **Renal function**: risk of renal failure.

o **LFTS**: elevated transaminases in HELLP syndrome.

o **Urinary dipstick**: ≥2 + protein indicates significant proteinuria and the need for 24-hour urine collection.

o Foetal monitoring via **ultrasound** and **cardiotocography**

7. ED MANAGEMENT OF PRE-ECLAMPSIA

o Upper abdominal pain in pregnancy may indicate pre-eclampsia

o **All women who present with upper abdominal pain and tenderness in pregnancy (usually after 20 weeks' gestation):**
   ▪ **Measure BP:** If > 140/90 mmHg seek advice from the obstetric unit in which the woman is booked
   ▪ **Test for proteinuria:** If proteinuria (i.e., more than a trace) is present in an MSU and especially if hypertension is detected refer immediately for admission to the maternity unit. (**Don't take "No" for an answer!!!**)

---

[403] *NICE Clinical Guideline, Hypertension in pregnancy: diagnosis and management ,NICE guideline [NG133]*

- o Once admitted, blood should be analysed for, among other things, **thrombocytopaenia** and **hepatic dysfunction**.
- o If you remain concerned about the epigastric pain and tenderness in the absence of hypertension or proteinuria review the following day.
- o Inform the on-call Obstetrics early, Move the patient to resuscitation room with full monitoring.
- o Consider positioning the patient left lateral.
- o Control hypertension with **IV labetalol or hydralazine.**
  - **Hydralazine:** Initial 5-10mg slow bolus; then repeat boluses or infusion 50-100µg/min
  - **Labetalol:** Initial 20-50mg slow bolus; then infusion 2mg/min, titrated as required
- o Careful fluid management is required.
- o Fluid overload is a significant cause of maternal death due to pulmonary oedema.
- o Limit fluids to approximately **1ml/kg/hr.**
- o Urine output should be monitored.
- o **Magnesium** should be considered in women with **severe pre-eclampsia** (systolic BP ≥170 mmHg or diastolic BP ≥110 mmHg plus significant proteinuria >1g/L).
- o **Delivery** is the definitive treatment for pre-eclampsia.
- o However, 44% of eclampsia occurs post-partum.

8. ED MANAGEMENT OF ECLAMPSIA
ABC approach
- o Airway and breathing adequacy should be assessed.
- o High-flow supplemental oxygen should be given.
- o Ventilation should be assisted if inadequate.
- o **Intubation** should be considered early due to the increased risks of aspiration and ventilatory inadequacy in pregnancy.
- o **Magnesium** is the therapy of choice to control seizures. A loading dose of **4 g IV should be given over 5–10 minutes followed by maintenance of 1 g/hour for 24 hours.**
- o A further **bolus of 2 g** can be given if the patient has recurrent seizures.
- **Management of HTN in Preeclampsia/Eclampsia**
  - o **Hydralazine:** Initial 5-10mg slow bolus; then repeat boluses or infusion 50-100µg/min
  - o **Labetalol:** Initial 20-50mg slow bolus; then infusion 2mg/min, titrated as required
  - o **Nicardipine:** Infusion of 2.5-5mg/hr; Increase to a maximum of 15mg/hr

+ *Nitroprusside should be avoided in pregnancy because of its potential toxicity to the foetus.*

MAGNESIUM SULPHATE

- **INDICATIONS**
  - o **Eclampsia**- Magnesium Sulphate rarely required to stop fit – usually self-limiting
  - o **Severe pre-eclampsia** where the decision to deliver has been made and where there is one other of the following criteria:
    - Hypertension with diastolic BP ≥ 110 mm Hg or systolic BP 170 mm Hg on two occasions and proteinuria ≥ 3+
    - Hypertension with diastolic BP ≥ 100mg Hg or systolic BP ≥ 150 mm Hg on two occasions and proteinuria ≥ 2+ (0.3 g/day) and at least two of the signs of imminent eclampsia.

- **CONTRA-INDICATIONS**
  - o Neuromuscular disease: Myasthenia gravis
  - o Renal failure,
  - o Cardiac disease

- **MgSO$_4$**
  - o **Loading dose: 4 grams I.V. over 5 mins**
  - o **Maintenance infusion**: **1g/hr for at least 24 hours** after the last seizure.
  - o Recurrent seizures should be treated by a further **bolus of 2g**

  - o **Side effects:**
    - Nausea, vomiting and flushing (use Maxolon)
    - Respiratory arrest
    - Renal failure
    - Hyporeflexia

  - o **Magnesium toxicity**
    - **Antidote**: **Calcium Gluconate 1 gram over 10 mins**
    - **Monitor**: reflexes, resps (>16/min), SpO$_2$, ECG for first hour

- **Recurrent seizures after MgSO4**
  - o Treat with a further bolus of 2g
  - o RSI with **Thiopentone/ventilation**
  - o Treat hypertension (MgSO$_4$ may reduce BP otherwise, give **Hydralazine**)

XII. HELLP SYNDROME

1. OVERVIEW

o HELLP syndrome, named for 3 features of the disease (**H**emolysis, **E**levated **L**iver enzyme levels, and **L**ow **P**latelet levels), is a life-threatening condition that can potentially complicate pregnancy[404].

o The cause of HELLP syndrome is currently unknown, although theories as described in Pathophysiology have been proposed.

2. RISK FACTORS FOR HELLP SYNDROME

o Maternal age older than 34 years

o Multiparity

o White race or European descent

o History of poor pregnancy

3. CLINICAL FEATURES

- **History**
  o No 'typical' clinical symptoms
  o Epigastric or RUQ pain,
  o Weight gain (oedema)
- **Examination**
  o Hypertension, Tender RUQ, Oedema
  o Polyuria from nephrogenic Diabetes Insipidus

4. INVESTIGATIONS

o Microangiopathic haemolytic anaemia (MAHA)

o Elevated LFT's – bilirubin, AST, ALT, LDH

o Low platelets, Normal PT, APTT & Coagulation screen

o Haemolysis on blood film

o Haptoglobins: low

5. COMPLICATIONS OF HELLP SYNDROME

o **Haemorrhage**
  - Abruption placentae, Severe PPH, DIC
  - Subcapsular liver haematoma
  - Intracerebral or brainstem haemorrhage

o **Infarction**
  - Liver infarct
  - Cerebral infarct

o **Pregnancy**
  - Overlap with preeclampsia
  - Preterm delivery
  - IUFD

o **Other**
  - Visual impairment due to retinopathy
  - Pulmonary oedema
  - Acute kidney injury

6. DIFFERENTIAL DIAGNOSIS

o Pre-eclampsia / Eclampsia

o Acute fatty liver of pregnancy/ Acute hepatitis

o Haemolytic-uremic syndrome (HUS)

o Thrombotic Thrombocytopenic Purpura (TTP/rare in pregnancy)

o Immune Thrombocytopenic Purpura (ITP)

o DIC (e.g. from PPH or amniotic fluid embolism)

o Other causes of haemolysis (e.g. AIHA, sepsis)

o Other causes of acute abdomen

7. ED MANAGEMENT OF HELLP SYNDROME

- **Resuscitation**
  o Prepare for major haemorrhage
  o Major life threats are hepatic haemorrhage, subcapsular hematoma, liver rupture, and multi-organ failure.

- **Specific treatment**
  o **Delivery** is indicated if the HELLP syndrome occurs after the 34th gestational week or the foetal and/or maternal conditions deteriorate.
  o **Seek and treat complications** (APO, DIC, MODS)
  o **Anti-hypertensives** to keep BP below 155/105 mmHg (Labetalol or Hydralazine or Nifedipine)
  o **MgSO4 IV** for eclamptic seizure prophylaxis
  o **Corticosteroids (IV) for Lung maturity**
    - No clear benefit for HELLP per se
    - Given for foetal lung maturity from 24 to 34 weeks: either 2 doses of 12 mg betamethasone 24 hours apart or 6 mg dexamethasone 12 hours apart before delivery.
  o **Liver haemorrhage**
    - Manage conservatively where possible
    - Correct coagulopathy
    - Surgery includes drainage of the hematoma, packing, oversewing of lacerations, or partial hepatectomy
    - Consider arterial embolisation
  o **Exchange transfusion**
    - Considered in situations of progressive elevation of bilirubin or falling Hb or PLTs and ongoing deterioration in maternal condition.

- **Supportive care and monitoring**
  o Consider invasive monitoring

- **Disposition**
  o OT or HDU/ ICU setting
  o Consider transfer to a liver transplant center

---

[404] *Intravascular hemolysis, thrombocytopenia and other hematologic abnormalities associated with severe toxemia of pregnancy. PRITCHARD JA, WEISMAN R Jr, RATNOFF OD, VOSBURGH GJ N Engl J Med. 1954 Jan 21; 250(3):89-98.*

XIII. EMERGENCY CONTRACEPTION

- Women requesting emergency contraception have 3 choices:

1. LEVONELLE 1.5mg

- o This is levonorgestrel and is licensed up to **72 hours** after UPSI (Unprotected Sexual Intercourse).
- o If vomiting occurs **within 2 hours of ingestion**, another tablet should be given.
- o It works mainly by inhibiting ovulation.

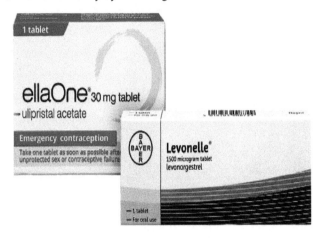

2. ULIPRISTAL ACETATE

- o This is the newest treatment available and is licensed up to **120 hours after UPSI**.
- o If vomiting occurs within **3 hours of ingestion** another tablet should be given.
- o It also works mainly by inhibiting ovulation.
- o It should be avoided in patients taking **enzyme-inducing drugs**, severe hepatic impairment or severe asthma that requires oral steroids.
- o Levonelle and ulipristal are less effective in women with higher BMIs.
- **Missed regular Oral contraception Pill**: If one pill has been missed (48-72 hours since last pill in current packet or 24-48 hours late starting first pill in new packet) then the following contraceptive cover is required:
  - o The missed pilled should be taken as soon as possible
  - o The remaining pills should be continued at the usual time
  - o Emergency contraception is not usually required but may need to be considered if pills have been missed earlier in the packet or in the last week of the previous packet.

3. COPPER IUD

- o This can be fitted up to **5 days after UPSI or ovulation**, whichever is longer.
- o Failure rate is less than 1 in a 1000, making it 10-20 times more effective than oral emergency contraceptive options.

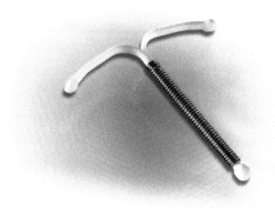

4. THE FRASER GUIDELINES (GILLICK COMPETENCE)

- Lord Fraser stated that a Doctor could proceed to give advice and treatment:
  - o **"Provided he is satisfied in the following criteria:**
    - That the girl (although under the age of 16 years of age) will understand his advice;
    - That he cannot persuade her to inform her parents or to allow him to inform the parents that she is seeking contraceptive advice;
    - That she is very likely to continue having sexual intercourse with or without contraceptive treatment;
    - That unless she receives contraceptive advice or treatment her physical or mental health or both are likely to suffer;
    - That her best interests require him to give her contraceptive advice, treatment or both without the parental consent." **(Gillick v West Norfolk, 1985)**

Further reading:

1. https://www.fsrh.org/standards-and-guidance/documents/ceu-clinical-guidance-emergency-contraception-march-2017/

2. https://www.nice.org.uk/guidance/qs129

34. Psychiatric Emergencies
I. MENTAL HEALTH ACT

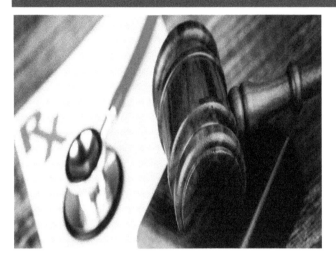

INTRODUCTION

- The Act sets out five principles that are designed to regulate decisions made under the legislation (any three will score a mark each):
  - A person must be assumed to have capacity unless it is established that he or she lacks capacity
  - A person is not to be treated as unable to make a decision unless all practicable steps have been taken to help him or her
  - A person is not to be treated as unable to make a decision just because he or she makes an unwise decision.
  - All decisions must be made in the incapacitated person's best interests
  - Decisions made must be least restrictive of the individual's fundamental rights or freedoms.
- The most important parts are **2, 3, 4, 5 & 135 and 136**[405].

SECTION 2

- **Section 2** aka an **Assessment Order**– allows a patient to be *sectioned* **for up to 28 days**.
- Must be **signed by 2 doctors and an ASW (ASW – approved social worker)**.
- These professionals must agree that the patient is mentally unwell, and they require a **full assessment** in a **psychiatric** setting.

- The patient must have been examined by the two doctors within 5 days of each other.
- The two doctors cannot be employed by the same organisation. One of the doctors has to have previously known the patient.
- It allows patients to be treated against their will, as they are seen to be mentally unstable.
- **Cannot be renewed**
- Commonly the doctors involved are the **patient's GP, and a psychiatrist**.
- Type of mental disorder that the patient is thought to be suffering from does not have to be disclosed.
- Treatment can be given against the patient's will – as this is considered part of the assessment process.

SECTION 3

- **Section 3** aka **treatment orders** – same as section 2, but **for 6 months.**
- The ASW must seek the consent of the nearest relative, and the patient cannot be detained if this relative objects.
- **Can be renewed** for 6 months or even sometimes for a year. The doctor has to state the category of mental illness the patient is thought to be suffering from (e.g. mental illness, psychosis, mental impairment)
- The majority of 'sectionings' are treatment orders
- **Treatment can be given** – but after 3 months, either:
  - The patient has to consent to treatment.
  - A third doctor has to review the patient and give their consent for treatment to be given
- To be discharged from sections 2 & 3, the patient has to be discharged by one of:
  - The RMO (registered medical officer)
  - Hospital managers
- The nearest relative can ask for discharge; however, in practice it is unlikely that patients will be discharged before the sectioning is over.
- **Appeal** – patient may appeal to mental health review tribunal
- **Section 2 appeal** – must be made within **14 days**
- **Section 3 appeal** – must been made within **6 months**

---

405 *NHS, Mental Health Act [Online]*

SECTION 4

- Requires support of one medical practitioner and allows **Emergency detainment for 72 hours for assessment.**
- The application can be made by an approved mental health practitioner or the nearest relative.
- **Renewal of section 4 is not possible** but it may be converted within 3 days of admission to a **section 2** by means of a second medical recommendation.

SECTION 5

SECTION 5(2)
- A Section 5(2) is known as the **Doctor's holding power**.
- The doctor in charge of the patient's care must write a report explaining the detainment and why informal treatment is inappropriate.
- A s5(2) can be used both in a mental health hospital and a general hospital.
- Under a s5(2), patient can be held for up to 72 hours.
- This is not renewable. Patient must be assessed as quickly as possible by an Approved Mental Health Professional (AMHP) and doctors for possible admission under the Mental Health Act.
- Under sections 5(2) and 5(4), patient can **refuse treatment** and **must give consent** for any treatment that is given to him/her.
- *Unless the patient:*
  - *Does not have the capacity to make a decision about treatment and the treatment is in the patient's best interests.*
  - *Needs treatment in an emergency to prevent serious harm to himself or others.*

B. SECTION 5 (4)
- A section 5(4) is known as the **Nurse's Holding Power**.
- This power can only be used:
  - *To prevent patient from leaving hospital for his/her own health or safety or for the protection of others*
  - *When it is not possible to get a Doctor, who can section the patient under s5(2)*
- Under s5(4), patient can be held up to 6 hours.
- This is not renewable.
- The holding power ends as soon as a doctor arrives.
- The doctor may transfer the patient onto a s5(2) or you may continue as a voluntary patient.
- If the patient needs to be detained under a section 2 or 3, an assessment by an Approved Mental Health Professional (AMHP) and doctors must be arranged as quickly as possible.

SECTION 135

- A police constable may enter the patient's premises and remove a person to a **'place of safety' for up to 72 hours.** Can use force if need be.
- Can only be used if a social worker has obtained a warrant. **Cannot treat against the patient's will**.

SECTION 136

- Section 136 of the MHA allows a police officer to remove someone who appears to be suffering from a mental health disorder to a place of safety.
- This allows detainment for **72 hours** and allows the patient to be assessed by a medical practitioner.
- Convert to s2 or s3 if admission is required.

IN EMERGENCIES, WHO DECIDES THAT SOMEONE SHOULD BE DETAINED? [406]

- An emergency is when someone seems to be at serious risk of harming themselves or others.
- Police have powers to enter a patient's home, if need be by force, under a Section 135 warrant.
- The patient may then be taken to a place of safety for an assessment by an approved mental health professional and a doctor. The patient can be kept there until the assessment is completed, for up to 24 hours.
- If the police find the patient in a public place and he/she appear to have a mental disorder and is in need of immediate care or control, they can take him/her to a place of safety (usually a hospital or sometimes the police station) and detain him/her there under Section 136.
- The patient will then be assessed by an approved mental health professional and a doctor.
- The patient can be kept there until the assessment is completed, for up to 24 hours.
- If the patient is already in hospital, certain nurses can stop him/her leaving under Section 5(4) until the doctor in charge of his/her care or treatment, or their nominated deputy, can make a decision about whether to detain him/her there under Section 5(2).
- Section 5(4) gives nurses the ability to detain someone in hospital for up to 6 hours.
- Section 5(2) gives doctors the ability to detain someone in hospital for up to 72 hours, during which time you should receive an assessment that decides if further detention under the Mental Health Act is necessary.

---

406 NHS, Mental Health Act [Online]

II. DELIBERATE SELF-HARM

A. GUIDELINE FOR ED STAFF

- **GENERAL PRINCIPLES**
  - o Patients who harm themselves have high rates of mental disorder, life stress and have an increased risk of further self-harm and suicide.
  - o **All** patients presenting to the ED following self-harm should have a brief mental health assessment by ED staff and should be referred to a trained mental health professional for assessment at the earliest possible opportunity.

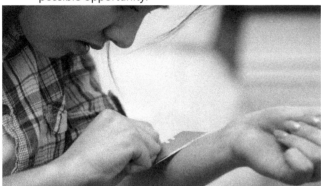

- **IMMEDIATE TRIAGE**
  - o Patients should be triaged on arrival with the mental health triage scale in addition to the standard triage.
  - o Staff should be aware of ongoing availability of means of repetition (e.g. tablets, weapon on person) and deal with this risk accordingly.

FACTORS ASSOCIATED WITH SELF HARM	
Demographics	Social isolation
	Lower social class
	Age >45
	Male
	Unemployment
	Single/divorced
	History of violence/criminal convictions
Features in the past medical history	Chronic alcohol and/or drug misuse
	Physical illness
	Previous self-harm
	Psychiatric disorder
	Personality disorder
	History of abuse
Psychological characteristics	Depression
	Hopelessness
	Continued suicidal intent

- **ED DOCTOR ASSESSMENT**
  - o In addition to necessary medical assessment and management, the ED Doctor should also consider the following:
    - Is the patient physically fit to wait?
    - Is there obvious severe emotional distress?
    - Is the person actively suicidal?
    - Is the person likely to wait for medical treatment and further mental health assessment?
    - Does the patient have mental capacity?

- **WHEN A PATIENT FOLLOWING SELF-HARM REFUSES TREATMENT**
  - o Remember that the **MHA cannot be used in the ED to give treatment** (medical or psychiatric) against a person's wishes.
  - o Consider whether or not the patient has the capacity to refuse treatment.
  - o If not, consider whether there is a situation of such urgent necessity that you proceed to treat the patient in their 'best interests' (i.e. under the common law).
  - o Do a brief mental health assessment.
  - o Consider whether there are grounds to apply for **involuntary admission** (under the MHA) to a psychiatric unit for treatment of a mental disorder.
  - o Seek the advice of a senior colleague and/or contact Psychiatric team.

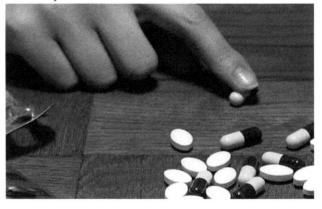

- **WHEN A PATIENT FOLLOWING SELF-HARM ABSCONDS FROM THE ED**
  - o Telephone the patient and ask him/her to come back for assessment / treatment.
  - o Contact the patient's next-of-kin.
  - o Contact security to search the hospital area.
  - o Consider contacting the Police.
  - o Complete an incident form and Inform the relevant clinical team and Document it.

- **REFERRAL BY ED STAFF TO PSYCHIATRY**
  - o All patients following self-harm should be referred to Psychiatry.
  - o Please inform the liaison psychiatry team of cases of **suicide** who die in the ED or in the community but are brought to ED by the emergency services.
- **REFERRAL TO SOCIAL WORK**
  - o All patients <18 yrs following self-harm should be referred to the Social Work in addition to Psychiatry.
  - o All cases of adult presentation where Child Protection/Welfare concerns are identified.
  - o All cases of adult self-harm presentation where Domestic / Elder Abuse is identified

B. ASSESSING SUICIDE RISK

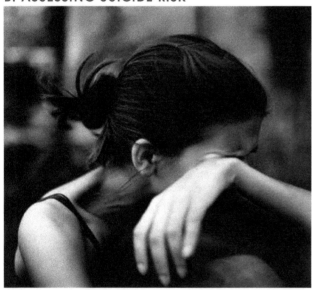

- There are many different risk assessment tools in use. Probably, the most commonly used is the **SAD PERSONS scale**.
- The accuracy of these scales in predicting future self-harm and suicide is poor.
- The advice from NICE is that a standardised risk assessment scale should only be used to aid identification of those at high risk of repetition of self-harm or suicide, and not to identify those patients who are supposedly 'low risk' who are then not offered services.

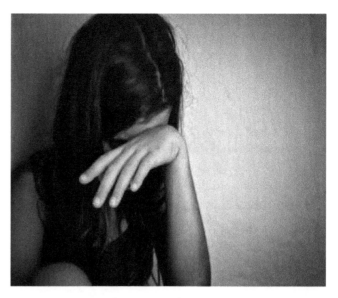

- Components of the modified **SAD PERSONS scale (DROS=2)** [407]

SAD PERSONS SCORE	
Sex (Male)	1 point
Age (15-25 or >59 years)	1 point
Depression/hopelessness	2 points
Previous attempt/psychiatric care	1 point
ETOH/Drug abuse	1 point
Rational thinking loss	2 points
Separated/divorced/single	1 point
Organised or serious attempt	2 points
No social support	1 point
Stated future intent	2 points

- This score is then mapped onto a risk assessment scale as follows:
  - o **0–5:** may be safe to discharge (depending upon circumstances).
  - o **6–8:** probably requires psychiatric consultation.
  - o **>8:** probably requires hospital admission

---

[407] Hockberger et al. Assessment of suicide potential by nonpsychiatrists using the SAD PERSONS score. J Emerg Med 6 (1988), pp. 99-107

35. Rashes:Life-threatening
I. TRANSFUSION REACTIONS

INTRODUCTION

- Acute transfusion reactions present as adverse signs or symptoms **during or within 24 hours** of a blood transfusion[408]. The most frequent reactions are fever, chills, pruritus, or urticaria, which typically resolve promptly without specific treatment or complications.
- Other signs occurring in temporal relationship with a blood transfusion, such as severe shortness of breath, red urine, high fever, or loss of consciousness may be the first indication of a more severe potentially fatal reaction[409].
- **The onset of red urine** during or shortly after a blood transfusion may represent **hemoglobinuria** (indicating an acute hemolytic reaction) or **hematuria** (indicating bleeding in the lower urinary tract). If freshly collected urine from a patient with hematuria is centrifuged, red blood cells settle at the bottom of the tube, leaving a clear yellow urine supernatant. If the red color is due to hemoglobinuria, the urine sample remains clear red after centrifugation.
- Transfusion reactions require immediate recognition, laboratory investigation, and clinical management. If a transfusion reaction is suspected during blood administration, **the safest practice is to stop the transfusion and keep the intravenous line open with 0.9% sodium chloride (normal saline).**

SUSPECTED REACTION WORKUP

- Indicated when possible reaction is suspected by a combination of signs/symptoms:
  - **Inflammatory:**
    - Fever/chills
    - Skin changes
    - Pain at infusion site
  - **Circulatory:**
    - Blood pressure changes
    - Shock
    - Hemoglobinemia/uria

[408] Frazier SK, Higgins J, Bugajski A, Jones AR, Brown MR. Adverse Reactions to Transfusion of Blood Products and Best Practices for Prevention. Crit Care Nurs Clin North Am. 2017 Sep. 29 (3):271-290.

[409] Fastman BR, Kaplan HS. Errors in transfusion medicine: have we learned our lesson?. Mt Sinai J Med. 2011 Nov-Dec. 78(6):854-64.

- **Pulmonary:**
  - Dyspnea, orthopnea, wheezing
  - Full respiratory failure
- **Coagulation:**
  - Unexplained increase in bleeding
  - DIC
- **Psychological:**
  - Sense of unease or impending "doom"!

CLASSIFICATION OF REACTIONS

- Below is an approach to screening transfusion reactions based on the presence or absence of fever and the timing of the reaction:
  - **Acute** = during or < 24 hrs after transfusion,
  - **Delayed** = > 24 hrs after transfusion)

Presenting With Fever	
Acute	**Delayed**
• Acute Hemolytic	• Delayed Hemolytic
• Febrile Non-hemolytic	• TA-GVHD
• Transfusion-related Sepsis	
• Transfusion-related acute lung injury (TRALI)	

Presenting Without Fever	
Acute	**Delayed**
• Allergic Hypotensive	• Delayed Serologic
• Tx-associated Dyspnea	• Post-transfusion Purpura
• TACO	• Iron Overload

A. ACUTE REACTIONS PRESENTING WITH FEVER
1. ACUTE HEMOLYTIC TRANSFUSION REACTIONS (AHTRS)

- Clerical errors (both in transfusion service and at bedside) are most common cause
- RBC destruction may be intravascular or extravascular

SIGNS/SYMPTOMS

- **Timing**
  - Severe reactions may occur early in transfusion (first 15 minutes)
  - Milder reactions may present later, but usually before end of transfusion

- **Specific signs/symptoms:**
  - Fever and chills- Most common (> 80%)
  - Back or infusion site pain
  - Hypotension/shock
  - Hemoglobinuria (may be first indication of hemolysis in anesthetized patients)
  - DIC/increased bleeding (also important in anesthetized patients)
  - Sense of "impending doom"

LAB FINDINGS

- Hemoglobinemia (pink or red serum/plasma); lasts several hours in those with adequate renal function
- Hemoglobinuria (typically clears by the end of one day)
- Positive DAT (unless all donor cells destroyed); may be "mixed field"
- Elevated indirect and direct bilirubin
- Lab findings of DIC (D-dimers, decreased fibrinogen,)
- RBC abnormalities
  - Schistocytes: Intravascular hemolysis
  - Spherocytes: Extravascular hemolysis

TREATMENT

- Hydration and diuresis are critical early components for hypotension treatment and renal function preservation
  - Maintain urine output > 1 mL/Kg/hr with saline +/- furosemide
  - Low-dose dopamine use is controversial (may not preserve function)
- Consider DIC; some use heparin during hypercoagulable phase of DIC
- Consider early exchange transfusion, esp. for high-volume incompatible transfusion

PREVENTION POSSIBILITIES

- Training and careful attention to phlebotomy, labeling, issue, and administration
- Some require two separate ABO/Rh types before transfusion
- Advanced methods (RFID, bar codes, etc) will likely be helpful in future

2. FEBRILE NONHEMOLYTIC TRANSFUSION REACTIONS (FNHTRS)

- Historically most frequently reported reaction
- Unexplained increase in temperature of 1°C
- Cause: Increased pyrogenic substances

SIGNS/SYMPTOMS

- Transient fever and chills (+/- rigors?) during or up to 2 hours after transfusion
- Symptoms tend to occur later in transfusion; if very early, be suspicious of transfusion-related sepsis

- Note that chills may be first; fever may be delayed up to one hour or more after transfusion in up to 10% of cases
- Variant versions in premedicated or head injury patients may never have fever

DIFFERENTIAL DIAGNOSIS:

- Acute HTR
- Transfusion-related sepsis

LAB FINDINGS

- None; negative hemolysis workup (diagnosis of exclusion)

TREATMENT

- Antipyretics (acetaminophen)
- Meperidine (Demerol) for more severe chills; use with caution!

PREVENTION

- Paracetamol premedication may prevent fever, but is not reliable
- Preventing FNH during RBC and platelet transfusions

3. TRANSFUSION-RELATED SEPSIS

Septic Transfusion Reaction, Bacterial Contamination

- Bacterial contamination is the number one infectious risk from transfusion, much more common than viruses
- Some sources: As many as 1 in 3000 platelet units are contaminated (many fewer reactions, however)
- Most contaminated products that cause reactions are closer to their expiration date than their collection date (gives bacteria time to proliferate and enter log phase)
- Organisms identified depend on product:
  - **Red cells**
    - **Gram-negative rods** (endotoxin-makers that like growing in cold temperatures): Yersinia enterocolitica (most common historically), E. coli, Enterobacter/Pantoea sp, Serratia marcescens and S. liquifaciens, Pseudomonas species
    - **Gram-positive cocci** (much less commonly): Staph. Epidermidis, Propionibacteria, Staph aureus
  - **Platelets**
    - Vast majority are gram-positive cocci (skin contaminants including those listed above); majority result in only mild reactions (if at all)
    - Gram negative rods can also contaminate and are much more likely to cause fatalities than gram-positives (reported examples include Serratia, E. coli, and Klebsiella species)
  - **Plasma products**
    - Uncommonly contaminated
    - Few reports involving water bath contamination with Pseudomonas species

SIGNS/SYMPTOMS

- Earlier symptoms seen in more severe reactions and more often with RBC transfusions (may occur within the first few minutes of transfusion)
- Rapid onset high fever (often greater than 2°C)
- Rigors (true shaking chills with rigidity)
- Abdominal cramping, nausea/vomiting
- Hypotension/shock
- DIC

DIFFERENTIAL DIAGNOSIS

- Acute HTR (always!); Severe septic reactions,
- Anaphylactic transfusion reaction: Can also be dramatic and very early in the transfusion. Usually NOT febrile.
- Febrile nonhemolytic transfusion reaction (FNHTR): Milder septic reactions and many PLT contaminations can overlap with FNHTR significantly (as a result, many culture units as part of FNHTR workup protocol)
- Sepsis from non-transfusion source (infected lines and/or fluids, coincidental presentation)

LAB FINDINGS

- Discolored RBC product (+/-); contaminated RBCs may turn DARK or purple
- May have hemoglobinemia/uria (non-immune)
- DAT negative (unless coincidental)
- Gram stain positive in only half to 2/3 of proven cases!
- Culture is proof positive (when same organism is cultured from both unit and recipient; even better if from the donor as well!)

TREATMENT

- Immediate IV antibiotics; treat presumptively with broad spectrum coverage, then adjust as necessary
- Pressure/respiratory/general support as needed
- Don't forget: Quarantine all other products from the same donation if a reaction suspicious for sepsis occurs! Notify blood collection agencies promptly!

PREVENTION

- Careful donor history
- Proper phlebotomy technique; use of diversion pouches (mandatory now), strict attention to possible site contaminants
- Leukocyte reduction filters may decrease risk (decrease in Yersinia concentration)
- Routine detection of platelet contamination required by AABB Standard
- Despite detection methods, false negatives occur, and pathogen reduction may be the ultimate answer

4. TRANSFUSION-RELATED ACUTE LUNG INJURY (TRALI)

- a. Currently the number one cause of transfusion-related fatality in the US!
- it is a new acute lung injury within 6 hours of a transfusion; ALI defined[410]:
  - Hypoxemia with PaO2/FiO2 < 300 mm Hg (or O2 sat <90%) and bilateral CXR infiltrates
  - Lack of other risk factors for pulmonary edema
  - No pre-existing acute lung injury
- Usually also with fever, chills, transient hypertension then hypotension
- Platelets/plasma transfusions most often, but also with RBCs/whole blood

DIFFERENTIAL DIAGNOSIS

- **ARDS:** TRALI may look exactly like ARDS, but TRALI usually resolves in 24-48 hours.
- **Transfusion-associated circulatory overload (TACO):** May be identical clinically, complete with a "wet" chest x-ray, but TRALI is usually associated with fever (unlike TACO) and does not respond to diuretics
- Anaphylactic reactions (generally afebrile)
- Acute pulmonary and myocardial disorders

DIAGNOSIS

- Difficult, as it is often confused for something else
- Typical early findings: bilateral CXR infiltrates, oxygen saturation less than 90%, no evidence of volume overload (no jugular venous distention, normal wedge pressure, normal BNP levels)
- Lab findings may include demonstration of anti-HLA and/or anti-neutrophil antibodies, and possibly increased biologic response modifiers in the bag.
- Remember, this is a clinical and radiographic diagnosis; confirming the presence of donor antibodies may take days or weeks!

TREATMENT

- Treat with respiratory support (oxygen, maybe intubation).
- Mortality reported between 5 and 25% 2) 80% recover quickly

PREVENTION

- Current AABB mandate for transfusion centers to reduce TRALI risk
- Implicated donors (with antibodies found) should be deferred from donation

---

[410] *National Heart, Lung, and Blood Institute (NHLBI) Working Group and Canadian Consensus Conference Panel*

- Use of all (or mostly) male plasma has been shown to decrease the risk of TRALI (females have more anti-HLA and anti-neutrophil antibodies because of pregnancy).
- Some centers have begun testing parous female PLT donors for anti-HLA +/- neutrophil antibodies and deferring those who have antibodies
- Strategies only address antibody-formers and ignore two hit model

B. ACUTE REACTIONS PRESENTING WITHOUT FEVER

1. ALLERGIC REACTIONS

a. Mild allergic (urticarial, cutaneous) transfusion reactions

- Very commonly reported reaction (1-3%) 2)
- Usually localized hives, but may have more severe swelling around eyes and lips (angioedema), mild respiratory symptoms, and laryngeal edema (see moderate reactions below)
- Type I (IgE-mediated) hypersensitivity to transfused plasma proteins (not usually a specific, identifiable allergen)
- Mast cell secretion of histamine and resultant cytokines and other mediators of allergic reactions

PREVENTION AND TREATMENT OPTIONS

- Diphenhydramine (Benadryl) IV 25-50 mg as treatment, may use PO form (same dose) as pre-transfusion prophylaxis
- Washed products work too (not usually done)
- May restart transfusion after hives clear.

b. Moderate allergic (anaphylactoid) transfusion reactions

- Some allergic reactions fall between the two classic categories
- May present with upper/lower airway obstruction +/- cutaneous manifestations
  - Upper airway: Stridor, hoarseness, "lump" in throat
  - Lower airway: Wheezing, chest tightness, dyspnea
- Some of these patients may respond to IV diphenhydramine and not require epinephrine, while others will need epinephrine

c. Severe allergic (anaphylactic) transfusion reactions

- Opposite end of hypersensitivity reaction spectrum
- Uncommon (1:20,000 to 50,000 transfusions)
- **Presentation**
  - Anaphylactic shock very early in the transfusion
  - Acute hypotension, lower airway obstruction, abdominal distress, systemic crash
  - Virtually all of these patients have skin findings (urticaria, angioedema, generalized pruritis)

DIFFERENTIAL DIAGNOSIS

- Acute HTR: Typically febrile
- Septic transfusion reaction: High fevers and lack of skin findings in septic reactions may be only ways to distinguish early; If unclear, give epinephrine anyway
- Acute hypotensive reactions: These reactions have hypotension only, without respiratory or skin findings

TREATMENT

- Epinephrine immediately (0.2-0.5 ml of 1:1000 IM/SQ)
- SQ or IM preferred, but may give IV if already crashed.

2. ACUTE HYPOTENSIVE REACTIONS

- Reactions that are similar to severe allergic reactions but ONLY have severe hypotension (no skin symptoms, no GI complaints, no respiratory issues)
- **CDC definition**[411]:
  - Over 30 mm Hg drop in systolic BP with diastolic < 80 mm Hg
  - Occurs less than 15 minutes after the start of transfusion
  - Resolves within 10 minutes after transfusion stopped
- Classically associated with two situations:
  - Patients taking angiotensin-converting enzyme inhibitors (ACEi)
  - Patients receiving blood through negatively charged filters

DIAGNOSIS

- Clearly a diagnosis of exclusion
- Rule out:
  - Acute HTR by workup and lack of fever
  - Severe allergic reaction by lack of skin and respiratory findings (as well as transient nature of process)
  - Septic reaction by lack of high fever and other clinical findings (GI complaints, transient nature of process)

MANAGEMENT

- STOP the transfusion! (short half life of bradykinin leads to rapid resolution)
- Give fluids, consider epinephrine if not resolved promptly

PREVENTION

- No routine prophylactic measures necessary
- Avoid bedside leukoreduction filters (not really a problem in most places, as most leukocyte reduction is done in blood centers or transfusion services)
- Stop ACEi before therapeutic apheresis procedures

---

[411] *National Healthcare Safety Network Bioviligance Component Hemovigilance Module Surveillance Protocol [Online]*

3. TRANSFUSION-ASSOCIATED DYSPNEA (TAD)

- Acute respiratory distress occurring within 24 hours of cessation of transfusion AND Allergic reaction, TACO, and TRALI definitions are not applicable.

4. TRANSFUSION-ASSOCIATED CIRCULATORY OVERLOAD (TACO)

- New onset or exacerbation of 3 or more of the following within 6 hours of cessation of transfusion[412]:
  o Acute respiratory distress (dyspnea, orthopnea, cough)
  o Elevated brain natriuretic peptide (BNP)
  o Elevated central venous pressure (CVP)
  o Evidence of left heart failure
  o Evidence of positive fluid balance
  o Radiographic evidence of pulmonary edema
- Proposed diagnostic criteria include some of the above signs/symptoms PLUS:
  o Hypoxemia
  o Bilateral CXR infiltrates
  o Reaction occurring within 6 hours of transfusion
- Patients most at risk (though any patient may get TACO if transfused rapidly):
  o Patients with pre-existing CHF
  o Very old (>85% occur in patients over age 60) and very young (to a lesser extent)
  o Renal failure
  o Chronic anemias (e.g., sickle cell, thallasemias), due to compensation for anemia with increased plasma volume

DIFFERENTIAL DIAGNOSIS:

- TRALI
- Allergic/anaphylactic reactions
- Coincidental cardiac or pulmonary issues unrelated to transfusion

TREATMENT

- Stop the transfusion, evaluate, sit patient up
- Give supplemental oxygen
- Diuretics to decrease blood volume
- In severe cases, therapeutic phlebotomy may be indicated

PREVENTION IN AT-RISK PATIENTS

- Control infusion rates (1 mL/Kg/hour).
- Split units into aliquots when possible.
- Consider lower volume units (using CPD-RBCs rather than AS-RBCs, for example) or volume reduction of certain products.

5. ACUTE PAIN REACTIONS

- Sudden onset pain in trunk/extremities
- No predictable risk factors, no way to prevent
- Lab workup is negative, and symptoms resolve shortly after transfusion
- May require narcotics to relieve pain

C. DELAYED REACTIONS PRESENTING WITH FEVER
1. DELAYED HEMOLYTIC TRANSFUSION REACTIONS (DHTRS)

- Positive direct antiglobulin test (DAT) for antibodies developed between 24 hours and 28 days after cessation of transfusion AND EITHER Positive elution test with alloantibody present on the transfused red blood cells OR Newly-identified red blood cell alloantibody in recipient serum AND EITHER Inadequate rise of post-transfusion hemoglobin level or rapid fall in hemoglobin back to pre-transfusion levels OR Otherwise unexplained appearance of spherocytes[413]

SIGNS/SYMPTOMS

- Often completely asymptomatic
- Fever and anemia of unknown origin
- Mild jaundice/scleral icterus may be seen

LAB FINDINGS

- Icteric serum
- DAT positive (classically "mixed field")
- Anemia
- Newly identified red cell antibody
- Spherocytes on peripheral smear
- Elevated LDH and indirect (and often direct) bilirubin, decreased haptoglobin (even if hemolysis is extravascular)

TREATMENT

- As for AHTR if severe and intravascular
- Often no treatment necessary

2. TRANSFUSION-ASSOCIATED GRAFT-VS-HOST DISEASE (TA-GVHD)

- A clinical syndrome occurring from 2 days to 6 weeks after cessation of transfusion characterized by:
  o Characteristic rash: erythematous, maculopapular eruption centrally that spreads to extremities and may, in severe cases, progress to generalized erythroderma and hemorrhagic bullous formation.
  o Diarrhea
  o Fever

---

[412] *National Healthcare Safety Network Biovigilance Component Hemovigilance Module Surveillance Protocol [Online]*

[413] *National Healthcare Safety Network Biovigilance Component Hemovigilance Module Surveillance Protocol [Online]*

- ○ Hepatomegaly
- ○ Liver dysfunction (i.e., elevated ALT, AST, Alkaline phosphatase, and bilirubin)
- ○ Marrow aplasia
- ○ Pancytopenia
- ○ AND Characteristic histological appearance of skin or liver biopsy.

D. DELAYED REACTIONS PRESENTING WITHOUT FEVER
1. DELAYED SEROLOGIC TRANSFUSION REACTION (DSTR)
- Absence of clinical signs of hemolysis
- AND Demonstration of new, clinically-significant antibodies against red blood cells BY EITHER Positive direct antiglobulin test (DAT)
- OR Positive antibody screen with newly identified RBC alloantibody[414]
- A new antibody in a recently transfused patient, without evidence of hemolysis

2. POST-TRANSFUSION PURPURA (PTP)
- Alloantibodies in the patient directed against HPA or other platelet specific antigen detected at or after development of thrombocytopenia
- AND Thrombocytopenia (i.e., decrease in platelets to less than 20% of pre-transfusion count).
- Caused by antibody vs common PLT antigen
  - ○ Anti-HPA-1A (PLA1; present in 98%) most common culprit (70-80% of cases)
  - ○ HPA-1A negative patients are exposed through pregnancy or transfusion.
  - ○ Transfusion after antibody is formed leads to devastating destruction of platelets.
  - ○ HPA-1A-positive transfused platelets and HPA-1a-negative patient platelets are both destroyed, which is weird, right?
- Most likely because antibody has autoantibody activity Passive adsorption of Ag/Ab complexes or soluble PLT Ags also suggested.

DIFFERENTIAL DIAGNOSIS
- TTP, ITP, DIC, HIT all can share features
- Even more difficult in patients already thrombocytopenic

TREATMENT
- IVIG reverses the process and normalizes platelet count in about 3-5 days

- ○ Due to this, plasma exchange is uncommon today (only if IVIG doesn't work)
- ○ Mortality historically 10% without treatment; now near 0% with treatment.
- Platelet transfusion should be avoided if possible (ineffective, may worsen?)
- Future platelet transfusions should be negative for target antigen

3. IRON OVERLOAD
- Each unit of RBCs: 200-250 mg iron (generally, 1 mg iron per 1 mL RBCs)
- Lifetime load of ~50-100 transfusions in 70 Kg person = risk for overload.
  - ○ Hepatic, cardiac, endocrine organ, RE system deposition is especially damaging
  - ○ May present with hepatic or cardiac failure, diabetes, thyroid abnormalities
  - ○ Big risk in chronically transfused patients
- Exchange transfusions reduce risk
- Iron chelators (deferoxamine, deferiprone, deferasirox) may remove iron from hepatic stores and from RE system

---

[414] *National Healthcare Safety Network Biovigilance Component Hemovigilance Module Surveillance Protocol [Online]*

II. LIFE-THREATENING SKIN RASHES

INTRODUCTION

- **Rash** is a nonspecific term that refers to any visible inflammation of the skin.
- Most rashes are not dangerous and are self-limited.
- **Life-threatening skin rashes** are rare, but when they do occur, medical assistance is absolutely necessary. Potentially life-threatening disorders that have a skin rash as a primary sign are
  1. Erythroderma
  2. Pemphigus Vulgaris (PV),
  3. Toxic Epidermal Necrolysis (TEN), also known as Stevens-Johnson syndrome (SJS) or Erythema Multiforme Major (EM),
  4. Drug Rash with Eosinophilia and Systemic Symptoms (DRESS) Syndrome,
  5. Toxic Shock Syndrome (TSS),
  6. Meningococcemia,
  7. Rocky Mountain spotted fever, and
  8. Necrotizing fasciitis.

1. ERYTHRODERMAS

- Erythroderma is a rare condition. The annual incidence has been estimated to be approximately 1 per 100,000 in the adult population[415].
- Erythroderma is the term used to describe intense and usually widespread reddening of the skin due to inflammatory skin disease. It often precedes or is associated with exfoliation (skin peeling off in scales or layers), when it may also be known as exfoliative dermatitis (ED). Idiopathic erythroderma is sometimes called the **'red man syndrome'**.

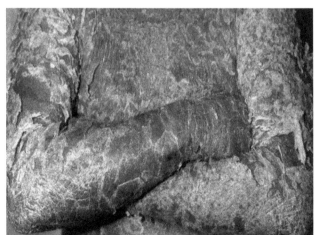

Erythrodermic Psoriasis

ETIOLOGY

The most common skin conditions to cause erythroderma are:

- **Drug eruption** – with numerous diverse drugs implicated.
- **Dermatitis** especially atopic dermatitis
- **Psoriasis,** especially after withdrawal of systemic steroids or other treatment
- **Pityriasis rubra pilaris**

Other skin diseases that less frequently because erythroderma include:

- Other forms of dermatitis: contact dermatitis (allergic or irritant), stasis dermatitis (venous eczema) and in babies, seborrheic dermatitis or staphylococcal scalded skin syndrome
- Blistering diseases including pemphigus and bullous pemphigoid
- Sezary syndrome (the erythrodermic form of cutaneous T-cell lymphoma)
- Several very rare congenital ichthyotic conditions

Erythroderma may also be a symptom or sign of a systemic disease. These may include:

- Haematological malignancies, eg lymphoma, leukaemia
- Internal malignancies, eg carcinoma of rectum, lung, fallopian tubes, colon
- Graft-versus-host disease
- HIV infection

CLINICAL FEATURES

- History is the most important aid in diagnosing exfoliative dermatitis (ED)[416].
- Patients may have a history of the primary disease (eg, psoriasis, atopic dermatitis). Elicit a comprehensive drug history, including over-the-counter drugs.
- Disease usually evolves rapidly when it results from drug allergens, lymphoma, leukemia, or staphylococcal scalded skin syndrome.
- Disease evolution is more gradual when it results from psoriasis, atopic dermatitis, or the spread of primary disease.
- Pruritus is a prominent and frequent symptom. Malaise, fever, and chills may occur.

Generalised erythema and oedema affects 90% or more of the skin surface.

- The skin feels warm to the touch.
- Itch is usually troublesome, and is sometimes intolerable.
- Rubbing and scratching leads to lichenification.
- Eyelid swelling may result in ectropion.
- Scaling begins 2-6 days after the onset of erythema, as fine flakes or large sheets.

415 Sigurdsson V, Steegmans PH, van Vloten WA. The incidence of erythroderma: a survey among all dermatologists in The Netherlands. J Am Acad Dermatol 2001; 45:675.

416 Yuan XY, Guo JY, Dang YP, Qiao L, Liu W. Erythroderma: A clinical-etiological study of 82 cases. Eur J Dermatol. 2010 May-Jun. 20(3):373-7.

- Thick scaling may develop on scalp with varying degrees of hair loss including complete baldness.
- Palms and soles may develop yellowish, diffuse keratoderma.
- Nails become dull, ridged, and thickened or develop onycholysis and may shed (onychomadesis).
- Lymph nodes become swollen (generalised dermatopathic lymphadenopathy).

COMPLICATIONS OF ERYTHRODERMA

- Complications in exfoliative dermatitis (ED) depend on underlying disease.
- Secondary infection, dehydration, electrolyte imbalance, temperature dysregulation, and high-output cardiac failure are potential complications in all cases.

DIAGNOSIS

- FBC may show anaemia, white cell count abnormalities, and eosinophilia. Marked eosinophilia should raise suspicions for lymphoma.
- >20% circulating Sézary cells suggests Sézary syndrome
- C-reactive protein may or may not be elevated.
- Proteins may reveal hypoalbuminaemia and abnormal liver function.
- Polyclonal gamma globulins are common, and raised immunoglobulin E (IgE) is typical of idiopathic erythroderma.
- Skin biopsies from several sites may be taken if the cause is unknown. They tend to show nonspecific inflammation on histopathology. Diagnostic features may be present however.
- Direct immunofluorescence is of benefit if an autoimmune blistering disease or connective tissue disease is considered.

TREATMENT FOR ERYTHRODERMA

- Erythroderma is potentially serious, even life-threatening, and most patients require hospitalisation for monitoring and to restore fluid and electrolyte balance, circulatory status and body temperature.

The following general measures apply:

- Discontinue all unnecessary medications
- Monitor fluid balance and body temperature
- Maintain skin moisture with wet wraps, other types of wet dressings, emollients and mild topical steroids
- Antibiotics are prescribed for bacterial infection
- Antihistamines may reduce severe itch and can provide some sedation
- Traditionally, topical corticosteroids under moist occlusion and phototherapy have been used to manage psoriatic erythroderma[417].

PREVENTION

- In most cases, erythroderma cannot be prevented.
- People with known drug allergy should be made aware that they should avoid the drug forever, and if their reaction was severe, wear a drug alert bracelet.
- All medical records should be updated if there is an adverse reaction to a medication, and referred to whenever starting a new drug.
- Patients with severe skin diseases should be informed if they are at known risk of erythroderma.
- They should be educated about the risks of discontinuing their medication.

PROGNOSIS

- Prognosis of erythroderma depends on the underlying disease process. If the cause can be removed or corrected, prognosis is generally good.

2. TOXIC SHOCK SYNDROME

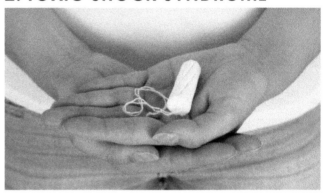

- Toxic Shock Syndrome is a rare multisystem disease with many widespread symptoms. It is caused by a toxin that is produced and secreted by the bacterium Staphylococcus aureus[418].
- The symptoms of Toxic Shock Syndrome may include a sudden high fever, nausea, vomiting, diarrhea, abnormally low blood pressure (hypotension), and a characteristic skin rash that resemble a bad sunburn.
- Subsequent reports identified an association with tampon use by menstruating women[419]. Other cases may occur in association with postoperative wound infections, nasal packing, or other factors.

Criteria for the diagnosis of TSS include:

- Temperature above 38.9°c,
- Hypotension,
- Esquamating rash,
- Involvement of at least three organ systems, and
- Exclusion of clinical mimics such as RMSF, leptospirosis, and measles.

417 Lee WK, Kim GW, Cho HH, Kim WJ, Mun JH, Song M, et al. Erythrodermic psoriasis treated with golimumab: a case report. Ann Dermatol. 2015 Aug. 27(4):446-9.

418 Rare diseases, Toxic Shock Syndrome [Online]

419 Davis JP, Chesney PJ, Wand PJ. Toxic-shock syndrome: epidemiologic features, recurrence, risk factors, and prevention. N Engl J Med. 1980 Dec 18. 303(25):1429-35.

ETIOLOGY

- Risk factors for the development of STSS are tampon use, vaginal colonization with toxin-producing *S aureus*, and lack of serum antibody to the staphylococcal toxin[420]. STSS also has occurred following use of nasal tampons for procedures of the ears, nose, and throat.
- The portal of entry for streptococci is unknown in almost one half of the cases.
- Procedures such as suction lipectomy, hysterectomy, vaginal delivery, and bone pinning have been identified as the portal of entry in many cases. Most commonly, infection begins at a site of minor local trauma, which may be nonpenetrating. Viral infections, such as varicella and influenza, also have provided a portal of entry.

RISK FACTORS OF TSS

- Menstrual tampons, (relatively rare) as most adults have developed protective antibodies to the exotoxin TSST-1.
- Previous TSS
- Localised or systemic infections.
- Recent childbirth, miscarriage or abortion.
- The use of birth control devices such as the diaphragm or contraceptive sponges.
- Foreign bodies, including nasal packing to stop nosebleeds and wound packing after surgery.
- Wound infection after surgery

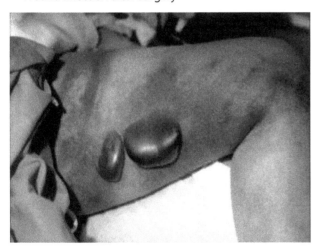

SIGNS AND SYMPTOMS

- The streptococcal TSS is identical to staphylococcal TSS (STSS), except that the blood cultures usually are positive for staphylococci in STSS. They share similar signs and symptoms.
- Fever, diffuse rash, low blood pressure, and multiple organ involvement are seen as the hallmarks of these diseases.

- Shedding of the skin in large sheets, especially of the palms and soles, is usually seen 1-2 weeks after the onset of illness.
- Individuals may experience symptoms and signs differently.

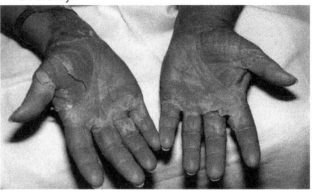

- Centres for Disease Control and Prevention (CDC) have clinical criteria for toxic shock syndrome and STSS.

CDC CRITERIA FOR TSS & STSS

CDC case definition for toxic shock syndrome requires presence of the following 5 clinical criteria:

1. Temperature ≥ 38.9 °C
2. Low BP (including fainting or dizziness on standing)
3. Widespread red flat rash
4. Shedding of skin, especially on palms and soles, 1-2 weeks after onset of illness
5. Abnormalities in 3 or more of the following organ systems:
   - **Gastrointestinal:** Vomiting or diarrhoea
   - **Muscular:** Severe muscle pain
   - **Hepatic:** Decreased liver function
   - **Renal:** Raised urea or creatinine levels
   - **Hematologic:** Bruising due to low blood platelet count
   - **CNS:** Disorientation or confusion
   - **Mucous membranes:** Red eyes, mouth and vagina due to increased blood flow to these areas.

CDC case definition for STSS requires isolation of group A streptococci and hypotension with 2 or more of the following clinical criteria:

1. Renal impairment: decreased urine output
2. Coagulopathy: bleeding problems
3. Liver problems
4. Rash that may shed, especially on palms and soles, 1-2 weeks after onset of illness
5. Difficulty breathing
6. Soft tissue necrosis including necrotising fasciitis, myositis and gangrene

---

[420] Park JS, Kim JS, Yi J, Kim EC. [Production and characterization of anti-staphylococcal toxic shock syndrome toxin-1 monoclonal antibody]. Korean J Lab Med. 2008 Dec. 28(6):449-56.

DIAGNOSIS

In addition to meeting CDC criteria for toxic shock syndrome and STSS, other diagnostic tests may include:

- Bacterial swabs from infected site of origin
- Blood cultures
- Blood tests: FBC, Renal and Liver Function, Creatine Kinase, Coagulation
- Urine tests: Urinalysis

- ❖ *Toxic shock syndrome diagnosis is confirmed if all 5 CDC clinical criteria are fulfilled.*
- ❖ *A probable case fulfils 4 of the 5 criteria.*

TREATMENT

Management of toxic shock syndrome and STSS is similar. The treatment starts with:

- Removing the source of infection ie tampons, vaginal sponges, or nasal packing
- Draining and cleaning the site of wound.

Treatment requires **hospitalisation** and **IV antibiotics** active against the causative organisms are given to eradicate the focus of the infection.

Flucloxacillin, nafcillin, oxacillin, linezolid and first-generation cephalosporin are the usual choices.

Vancomycin can be used as first line and in patients sensitive to penicillin.

For STSS, **Penicillin plus Clindamycin** is the most effective combination treatment.

Otherwise, treatment is largely supportive and may include:

- **Intravenous fluids** to treat shock and prevent organ damage
- **Cardiac medications** for patients with very low blood pressure
- **Dialysis** in patients who develop renal failure
- Administration of **blood products**
- **Infusions of intravenous immunoglobulin** in severe resistant cases
- **Oxygen and mechanical ventilation** to assist with breathing

PREVENTION OF TSS & STSS

- Women who have had toxic shock syndrome should avoid using tampons during menstruation as reinfection may occur.
- If worn, they should be changed ever 4-8 hours.
- The use of diaphragms and vaginal sponges may also increase the risk of toxic shock syndrome.
- Prompt and thorough wound care will help to avoid toxic shock syndrome and STSS.

3. STEVENS–JOHNSON SYNDROME & TOXIC EPIDERMAL NECROLYSIS

- Stevens-Johnson syndrome (SJS) and toxic epidermal necrolysis (TEN) are now believed to be variants of the same condition, distinct from erythema multiforme.
- The mucous membranes of the eyes, mouth, and/or genitals are also commonly affected[421].
- SJS and TEN previously were thought to be separate conditions, but they are now considered part of a disease spectrum. SJS is at the less severe end of the spectrum, and TEN is at the more severe end[422].

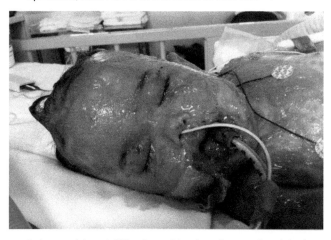

- It is considered SJS when skin detachment involves less than 10% of the body surface, and TEN when skin detachment involves more than 30% of the body surface.
- People with skin detachment involving 10-30% of the body surface are said to have "SJS/TEN overlap."
- All forms of SJS/TEN are a medical emergency that can be life-threatening.

More than 200 medications have been reported in association with SJS/TEN.

- It is more often seen with drugs with long half-lives compared to even a chemically similar related drug with a short half-life.
- The medications are usually systemic (taken by mouth or injection) but TEN has been reported after topical use.
- No drug is implicated in about 20% of cases
- SJS/TEN has rarely been associated with vaccination and infections such as mycoplasma and cytomegalovirus.
- Infections are generally associated mucosal involvement and less severe cutaneous disease than when drugs are the cause.

---

421 *High WA, Roujeau J-C. Stevens-Johnson syndrome and toxic epidermal necrolysis: Pathogenesis, clinical manifestations, and diagnosis. UpToDate. Waltham, MA: UpToDate; August 16, 2018;*

422 *Stevens-Johnson syndrome/toxic epidermal necrolysis. Genetics Home Reference (GHR). July 2015;*

The drugs that most commonly cause SJS/TEN are:

❖ Sulfonamides: cotrimoxazole;
❖ Beta-lactam: penicillins, cephalosporins
❖ Anticonvulsants: lamotrigine, carbamazepine, phenytoin, phenobarbitone
❖ Allopurinol
❖ Paracetamol
❖ Nevirapine (non-nucleoside reverse-transcriptase inhibitor)
❖ Nonsteroidal anti-inflammatory drugs (NSAIDs) (oxicam type mainly)

CLINICAL FEATURES OF SJS/TEN?

- SJS/TEN usually develops within the first week of antibiotic therapy but up to 2 months after starting an anticonvulsant. For most drugs the onset is within a few days up to 1 month.
- Before the rash appears, there is usually a prodromal illness of several days duration resembling an upper respiratory tract infection or 'flu-like illness. Symptoms may include:
  o Fever > 39 °C
  o Sore throat, difficulty swallowing
  o Runny nose and cough
  o Sore red eyes, conjunctivitis
  o General aches and pains.
- There is then an abrupt onset of a **tender/painful red skin rash** starting on the trunk and extending rapidly over hours to days onto the face and limbs (but rarely affecting scalp, palms or soles). The maximum extent is usually reached by 4 days.

The skin lesions may be:

- Macules – flat, red and diffuse (measles-like spots) or purple (purpuric) spots
- Diffuse erythema
- Targetoid – as in erythema multiforme
- Blisters – flaccid (ie not tense).

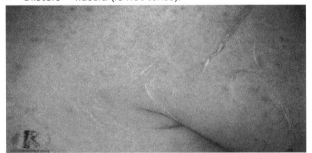

- The blisters then merge to form sheets of skin detachment, exposing red, oozing dermis.
- **The Nikolsky sign** is positive in areas of skin redness. This means that blisters and erosions appear when the skin is rubbed gently.

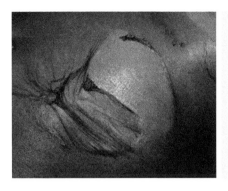

Nikolsky's sign is dislodgement of the epidermis with the appearance of a moist, glistening defect after pushing, rubbing, or rotating normal skin near bullous lesions

Mucosal involvement is prominent and severe, although not forming actual blisters.

At least 2 mucosal surfaces are affected including:

- **Eyes** (conjunctivitis, less often corneal ulceration, anterior uveitis, panophthalmitis) – red, sore, sticky, photosensitive eyes
- **Lips/mouth** (cheilitis, stomatitis) – red crusted lips, painful mouth ulcers
- **Pharynx, oesophagus** – causing difficulty eating
- **Genital area and urinary tract** – erosions, ulcers, urinary retention
- **Upper respiratory tract** (trachea and bronchi) – cough and respiratory distress
- **Gastrointestinal tract** – diarrhoea.

The patient is very ill, extremely anxious and in considerable pain. In addition to skin/mucosal involvement, other organs may be affected including liver, kidneys, lungs, bone marrow and joints.

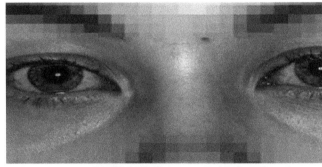

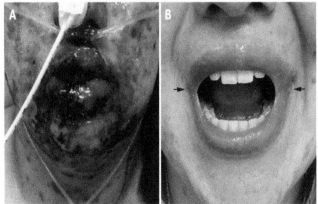

COMPLICATIONS OF SJS/TEN

SJS/TEN can be fatal due to complications in the acute phase. The mortality rate is up to 10% for SJS and at least 30% for TEN. During the acute phase, potentially fatal complications include:

- Dehydration and acute malnutrition
- Infection of skin, mucous membranes, pneumonia, septicaemia.
- Acute respiratory distress syndrome
- Gastrointestinal ulceration, perforation and intussusceptions
- Shock and multiple organ failure including kidney failure
- Thromboembolism and DIC.

DIAGNOSIS

SJS/TEN is suspected clinically and classified based on the skin surface area detached at maximum extent.

SJS

- Skin detachment < 10% of body surface area (BSA)
- Widespread erythematous or purpuric macules or flat atypical targets

Overlap SJS/TEN

- Detachment between 10% and 30% of BSA
- Widespread purpuric macules or flat atypical targets

TEN with spots

- Detachment > 30% of BSA
- Widespread purpuric macules or flat atypical targets

TEN without spots

- Detachment of > 10% of BSA
- Large epidermal sheets and no purpuric macules

The category cannot always be defined with certainty on initial presentation. The diagnosis may therefore change during the first few days in hospital.

INVESTIGATIONS IN SJS/TEN

1. If the test is available, elevated levels of **serum granulysin** taken in the first few days of a drug eruption may be predictive of SJS/TEN.
2. **Skin biopsy** is usually required to confirm the clinical diagnosis and to exclude staphylococcal scalded skin syndrome (SSSS) and other generalised rashes with blisters.
3. **The direct immunofluoresence test** on the skin biopsy is negative, indicating the disease is not due to deposition of antibodies in the skin.
4. **Blood tests** do not help to make the diagnosis but are essential to make sure fluid and vital nutrients have been replaced, to identify complications and to assess prognostic factors.

Abnormalities may include:

- **Anaemia** occurs in virtually all cases.
- **Leucopenia**, especially lymphopenia is very common
- **Neutropenia** if present, is a bad prognostic sign.
- **Eosinophilia** and atypical lymphocytosis do not occur.
- **Mildly raised liver enzymes** are common (30%) and approximately 10% develop overt hepatitis.
- **Mild proteinuria** occurs in about 50%. Some changes in kidney function occur in the majority.

SCORTEN

- SCORTEN is an illness severity score that has been developed to predict mortality in SJS and TEN cases.
- One point is scored for each of seven criteria present at the time of admission.

DIFFERENTIAL DIAGNOSIS OF SJS/TEN

- Histopathologic examination is necessary in differentiating these disorders from other severe bullous skin diseases, including the following[423].
  - Staphylococcal scalded skin syndrome
  - Toxic shock syndrome
  - Phototoxic skin reactions
  - Drug reaction with eosinophilia
  - Acute generalized exanthematous pustulosis
  - Paraneoplastic pemphigus
- **Other differentials:**
  - Acute Conjunctivitis (Pink Eye)
  - Chemical Burns
  - Exfoliative Dermatitis
  - Hypersensitivity Vasculitis
  - Pemphigus Vulgaris
  - Pseudoporphyria

TREATMENT FOR SJS/TEN

- Determined by the severity of the syndrome

Resuscitate

- **A** - may need to be intubated c/o mucosal involvement
- **B** - protective lung ventilation (can develop pulmonary complications: secretions, sloughing of bronchial epithelim, BOOP)
- **C** - fluid resuscitation similar to burn patient, large volumes proportional to BSA involved, will have a hyperdynamic circulation with vasodilatory shock (managed with careful fluids and inotropic support), monitor end-organ function -> urine output >1mL/kg/hr
- **D** - multimodal analgesia required -> may have to intubated and ventilated for analgesia
- **E** - keep warm and isolated if possible, to decrease risk of superinfection, humified environment, warm OT

---

[423] *Bachot N, Roujeau JC. Differential diagnosis of severe cutaneous drug eruptions. Am J Clin Dermatol. 2003. 4(8):561-72.*

Specific treatment
- Stop offending agent
- Identify and treat underlying disease and secondary infection (antibiotics)
- Burns dressings
- Antibiotics for documented invasive superinfection
- Avoid antibiotics that may exacerbate conditions (silver sulphadizine -> sulpha based)
- IgG and steroids - controversial (EuroSCAR study)
- Consider plasma exchange

General treatment
- Careful management of fluid-balance and electrolyte abnormalities required
- Nutrition
- Thromboprophylaxis

Disposition
- Management in a burns unit if large TBSA involvement
- Keep family informed
- Consult dermatology and plastic surgery early and involve burns nurse

LONG-TERM SEQUELAE INCLUDE
- Pigment change
- Skin scarring, especially at sites of pressure or infection
- Loss of nails with permanent scarring (pterygium) and failure to regrow
- Scarred genitalia – phimosis and vaginal adhesions
- Joint contractures
- Lung disease – bronchiolitis, bronchiectasis, obstructive disorders.
- Blindness

4. STAPHYLOCOCCAL SCALDED SKIN SYNDROME
OVERVIEW
- Staphylococcal scalded skin syndrome (SSSS) is a rare illness characterised by red blistering skin that looks like a burn or scald, hence its name staphylococcal scalded skin syndrome. SSSS is caused by the release of two exotoxins (**epidermolytic toxins A and B**) from toxigenic strains of the bacteria **Staphylococcus aureus**. SSSS has also been called **Ritter disease or Lyell disease** when it appears in newborns or young infants
- Primarily affects infants and young children (98% of patients are < 6 years of age).
- It is usually preceded by a mucocutaneous staphylococcal infection, such as **pharyngitis or bullous impetigo**, though this preceding infection may go unnoticed by patients and other caregivers.

- Following systemic dissemination of toxins from the local infection, SSSS itself typically begins with skin tenderness, erythema, and fever.
- This is followed a day or two later by flaccid blisters and sloughing off of the superficial layer of skin to reveal moist, red tissue underneath, giving the area a "scalded"-looking appearance.
- **Mucous membranes are spared.** A presumptive diagnosis of SSSS is based on clinical findings. **Biopsy** is only performed in unclear cases and shows separation of the epidermis at the granular layer.
- Treatment involves the administration of antibiotics and potential intensive care monitoring.
- The prognosis is generally good, and blisters heal without significant scarring.

ETIOLOGY
- **Pathogen**: **Staphylococcus aureus** strains that produce **exfoliative toxins**
- **Route of infection**: dissemination of toxins from a local infection:
  o Following a staphylococcal infection elsewhere (e.g., skin, mouth, nose, throat, GI tract, or umbilicus). The initial infection may also be completely undetected.
  o **Following bullous impetigo:** SSSS belongs to the spectrum of diseases mediated by specific staphylococcal toxins, which also includes bullous impetigo, toxic shock syndrome (TSS), and *Staphylococcus aureus* food poisoning. Unlike TSS, SSSS does not have systemic manifestations (e.g., liver, kidney, bone marrow, and CNS involvement)!

CLINICAL FEATURES
Initially
- Fever, malaise, and irritability
- Skin tenderness
- Diffuse or localized erythema, often beginning periorally
After 24–48 hours
- Flaccid, easily ruptured blisters that break to reveal moist, red skin beneath (i.e., with a "scalded" appearance) → **widespread sloughing of epidermal skin**
- **Nikolsky's sign**
- **No mucosal involvement**
- **Cracking**, and **crusting** is common
- Signs of shock (hypotension, tachycardia)

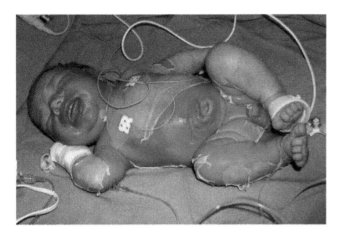

DIAGNOSTICS

- The presumptive diagnosis of SSSS is made based on clinical findings.
- **Cultures** (e.g., blood or nasopharynx) are usually taken for confirming the diagnosis, and a **biopsy** may be performed to exclude suspected differential diagnoses, but is usually not required.
- **History**: localized staphylococcal infection (e.g., pharyngitis, bullous impetigo)
- **Laboratory tests**: for confirming the diagnosis
  - ↑ WBCs
  - ↑ ESR
  - Cultures of potential sites of preceding infection (blood, urine, abnormal skin, nasopharynx, umbilicus, or any other suspected focus)
- **Biopsy**: indicated in unclear cases, especially when TEN or SJS are suspected
  - Intraepidermal fissure and blister formation at the granular layer
  - Lack of inflammatory cell infiltrate

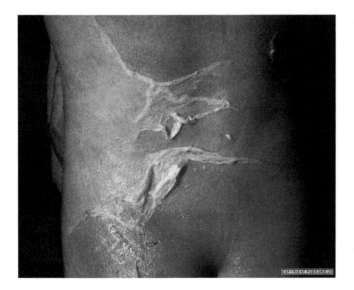

DIFFERENTIAL DIAGNOSES

Stevens-Johnson syndrome (SJS) or toxic epidermal necrolysis (TEN)

Differential diagnoses of severe exfoliative skin conditions			
	SSSS	**SJS**	**TEN**
Age of typical patient	**Children < 6 years**	Adults	Adults
Etiology	Infectious : *S. aureus* exfoliative toxins	Adverse drug reaction	Adverse drug reaction
Clinical features	Sloughing of skin, Nikolsky's sign Perioral erythema and crusting but **no mucous membrane involvement**	Sloughing of skin, Nikolsky's sign Mucous membrane involvement Typically < 10% of total body surface area	Sloughing of skin, Nikolsky's sign ≥ 2 mucous membranes involved > 30% of total body surface area
Biopsy	**Intraepidermal blistering** Lack of inflammatory infiltrate	Degeneration and blistering of **stratum basale of epidermis** → subepidermal blisters Eosinophils and mononuclear infiltrate in the papillary dermis	Eosinophilic **full-thickness epidermal necrosis** Cell-poor infiltrate, sparse, and with lymphocytes

The differential diagnoses listed here are not exhaustive.

TREATMENT

- In settings where adequate skin care can be provided outside of an intensive care unit or burn unit, most children do not require admission to an intensive care unit[424].
- A typical hospital stay for children lasts three to eight days[425]. In contrast, most adults with SSSS are seriously ill, and comorbidities or complications may warrant admission to an intensive care unit.
- **IV antibiotics**
  - Penicillinase-resistant penicillins are the drug of choice: **Nafcillin, Oxacillin**

---

[424] Neubauer HC, Hall M, Wallace SS, et al. Variation in Diagnostic Test Use and Associated Outcomes in Staphylococcal Scalded Skin Syndrome at Children's Hospitals. Hosp Pediatr 2018; 8:530.

[425] Staiman A, Hsu DY, Silverberg JI. Epidemiology of staphylococcal scalded skin syndrome in U.S. children. Br J Dermatol 2018; 178:704.

○ In areas with high **community-acquired MRSA** prevalence (or in patients who do not respond to treatment): **Vancomycin**

- **Supportive care:**
  ○ Fluid rehydration as indicated
  ○ Supportive skin care: emollients, covering denuded areas
  ○ NSAIDs as indicated for pain and fever
  ○ Steroids are contraindicated, as the etiology of SSSS is infectious! (They are, however, indicated in SJS and TEN.)

COMPLICATIONS

- The complications faced by SSSS patients are similar to those of patients with burns, as both have a compromised skin barrier:
  ○ Fluid and electrolyte imbalances
  ○ Thermal dysregulation
  ○ Secondary infections (e.g., pneumonia, sepsis)

PROGNOSIS

- **Mortality rate**
  ○ Children: < 5%
  ○ Adults: > 60%
- Blisters heal without scarring, as skin cleavage is intraepidermal

5. ROCKY MOUNTAIN SPOTTED FEVER

- Rocky Mountain spotted fever (RMSF) is a potentially lethal, but curable tick-borne disease, which was first described in Idaho in the 19th century. In 1906, Howard Ricketts demonstrated that RMSF was an infectious disease transmitted by ticks[426]. The clinical spectrum of human infection ranges from mild to fulminant disease[427].
- RMSF is a tickborne disease caused by *Rickettsia rickettsii*. After an incubation period of as little as two days, fever, headache, malaise, conjunctival suffusion, and myalgia usually develop.
- In most patients, a rash appears within the following week, initially on the wrists and ankles and later on the palms and soles, before spreading centripetally to include the arms, legs, face, and trunk.
- The differential diagnosis includes meningococcemia, infective endocarditis, measles, secondary syphilis, and other rickettsial diseases.

---

[426] *David H. Walker. Rickettsia rickettsii and other spotted fever group rickettsiae. In: Principles and Practice of Infectious Diseases, Gerald Mandell, John Bennett, Raphael Dolin (Eds).*

[427] *Thorner AR, Walker DH, Petri WA Jr. Rocky mountain spotted fever. Clin Infect Dis 1998; 27:1353.*

- The rash is at first erythematous and maculopapular. Progression to a petechial rash is often noted and, in severe cases of RMSF, purpura and hemorrhagic necrosis can occur.
- Associated thrombocytopenia can make the diagnosis of RMSF difficult to distinguish from meningococcemia.
- However, several clinical clues favor the diagnosis of RMSF, including a history of tick bite or visits to areas where RMSF-associated ticks are present, occurrence of the rash a median of three to four days following the onset of fever, relative leukopenia, and elevated aminotransferases.

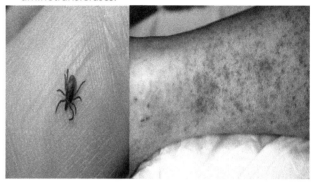

CLINICAL FEATURES RMSF

Symptoms generally appear **within 14 days** of a tick bite. However, the tick bite is painless and frequently goes unnoticed. The classic symptoms are **fever, severe headache, and a rash**. Fever and headache generally precede the rash by 2-5 days. **Myalgias** are also common. Other symptoms that may be present include:

- **Gastrointestinal** involvement producing abdominal pain, nausea, and vomiting.
- **Central nervous system** involvement which may cause confusion, lethargy, seizures, blindness, deafness, or coma.
- Any organ may become involved including the lungs, heart, kidneys, and liver.

More severe illness is experienced when treatment is delayed. The case-fatality rate of RMSF is 1-4%. Patients aged younger than 5 years or older than 70 years are at highest risk of death.

SKIN MANIFESTATIONS OF RMSF

Although the majority of patients with RMSF have a rash, in 4-26%, the rash is absent.

- The rash initially appears as **red macules** (flat spots). The macules are 1-5mm in size and may be itchy.
- Within days the lesions progress to become **papules** (small lumps), **petechiae** (small red or purple spots due to bleeding into the skin), and **ecchymoses** (bruises).

- The rash may become **haemorrhagic** (bloody) in around 50% of cases; or **necrotic** (blackened skin due to death of tissue) in 4%. These complications typically occur on the legs, scrotum, or vulva.
- The rash typically appears on days 3-5 of the illness, but this can be highly variable. The rash typically begins on the ankles and wrists, then spreads to the palms and soles (in around 50% of patients).
- The rash then spreads up the limbs, to the trunk.
- The face usually remains rash-free, but may become affected later in the course of the illness.
- As the patient recovers, the skin may be tender and may shed off in powdery scales. In severe cases, there may be sloughing of the skin, particularly the skin of the extremities and external genitals. This may resemble disseminated intravascular coagulation.
- Areas of petechiae may result in tiny scars. In rare cases, severe necrosis and gangrene may require amputation.

DIAGNOSIS OF RMSF

- Early treatment reduces mortality, so the diagnosis of RMSF is often made based on clinical observations before the results of laboratory tests are available.
- Serology is the mainstay to confirm diagnosis of rickettsial diseases. These are blood tests that detect the **presence of antibodies to rickettsial antigens.**
- The **indirect fluorescent antibody test** is the most reliable, with antibodies typically appearing 10-14 days after infection.
- Organisms may be seen by direct immunofluorescence of skin biopsies, but false-negatives are common.
- So, if clinical suspicion is high, treatment should commence even if the test is negative.

TREATMENT OF RMSF

- **Tetracyclines** are the preferred treatment for RMSF.
- **Doxycycline** should be used for children of any age, including those less than 9 years old (the risk of stained teeth is outweighed by the improved efficacy of doxycycline in treating this potentially life-threatening disease).
- **Chloramphenicol** is an alternative drug and can be used to treat pregnant women.
- Treatment should be continued until there has been no fever present for at least 2 or 3 days.

PREVENTION OF RMSF

- Avoid areas such as forests or fields where ticks are found.
- Use DEET insect repellents on the skin, and permethrin on the clothes.

- Wear long-sleeved clothing that fits tightly around the wrists, waist, and ankles.
- Check twice daily for attached ticks and remove immediately. While wearing protective gloves, gently grasp the tick with tweezers as close as possible to the skin and slowly, gently pull it away.

6. PEMPHIGUS VULGARIS

- Pemphigus vulgaris is a rare autoimmune disease that is characterised by blisters and erosions on the skin and mucous membranes, most commonly inside the mouth. It is the most common subtype of pemphigus, accounting for 70% of all pemphigus cases worldwide.
- The other two main subtypes of pemphigus are **pemphigus foliaceus** and **paraneoplastic pemphigus.**

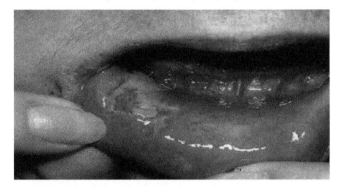

ETIOLOGY OF PEMPHIGUS VULGARIS

- Pemphigus vulgaris is an autoimmune blistering disease, which basically means that an individual's immune system starts reacting against his or her own tissue.
- In pemphigus vulgaris immunoglobulin type G (IgG) autoantibodies bind to a protein called desmoglein 3, which is found in desmosomes in the keratinocytes near the bottom of the epidermis. The result is the keratinocytes separate from each other, and are replaced by fluid, the blister.
- Pemphigus vulgaris affects people of all races, age and sex. It appears most commonly between the ages of 50-60 years, and is more common in Jews and Indians presumably for genetic reasons.

SIGNS AND SYMPTOMS OF PV

- Most patients first present with lesions on the mucous membranes such as the mouth and genitals. Several months' later blisters on the skin may develop or in some cases mucosal lesions are the only manifestation of the disease.
- The most common mucosal area affected is the inside of the mouth but others include the conjunctiva, oesophagus, labia, vagina, cervix, penis, urethra and anus.

Common features of oral mucosal pemphigus include:

- 50-70% of patients get oral lesions
- Blistering superficial and often appears as erosions
- Widespread involvement in the mouth
- Painful and slow to heal
- May spread to the larynx causing hoarseness when talking
- May make it difficult to eat or drink

DIAGNOSIS

- Diagnosis generally requires a **skin biopsy:** Pemphigus is confirmed by **direct immunofluorescence** staining of the skin biopsy sections to reveal antibodies.
- In most cases, circulating antibodies can be detected by a blood test (**indirect immunofluorescence test**). The level of antibodies fluctuates and may reflect the effectiveness of treatment.

TREATMENT OF PEMPHIGUS VULGARIS

- The goal of treatment in pemphigus is to induce complete remission while minimizing treatment-related adverse effects. The paucity of large, high-quality prospective trials that compare the therapeutic options for this disease as well as the variability in study protocols, outcome measures, and results have made definitive conclusions on the best approach to treatment difficult[428]. Adherence to the definitions for patient assessment outlined by a 2008 consensus of experts may facilitate systematic interpretation of published literature in the future[429].
- The primary aim of treatment is to decrease blister formation, prevent infections and promote healing of blisters and erosions.
- **Oral corticosteroids** are the mainstay of medical treatment for controlling the disease. Since their use, many deaths from pemphigus vulgaris have been prevented (mortality rate dropped from 99% to 5-15%).
- They are not a cure for the disease but improve the patient's quality of life by reducing disease activity.
- Unfortunately, higher doses of corticosteroids may result in serious side effects and risks. Other immune suppressive drugs are used to minimise steroid use.
- These include:
  - Azathioprine
  - Cyclophosphamide
  - Dapsone
  - Tetracyclines
  - Nicotinamide
  - Plasmapheresis
  - Gold
  - Mycophenolate mofetil
  - Intravenous immunoglobulin
  - The TNFα inhibitor, infliximab
  - Anti-CD20 monoclonal antibody (rituximab)
- At optimal therapy patients may still continue to experience mild disease activity.
- Appropriate wound care is particularly important, as this should promote healing of blisters and erosions.
- Patients should minimize activities that may traumatise the skin and mucous membranes during active phases of the disease.
- These include activities such as contact sports and eating or drinking food that may irritate or damage the inside of the mouth (spicy, acidic, hard and crunchy foods).
- There is future hope that future treatment for pemphigus will be more specific with fewer side effects. Investigators have engineered specific chimeric autoantibody receptor T-cells to eliminate Desmoglein-3-specific B cells in mice.

Differentiate Pemphigus from pemphigoid rash? (1)
- **Bullous Pemphigoid-** rash is the commonest autoimmune rash- associated with tense blisters.
- **Pemphigus Vulgaris** - Flaccid rash- no intact blisters found

Pemphigus Vulgaris	Bullous Pemphigoid
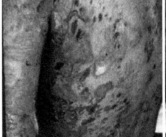	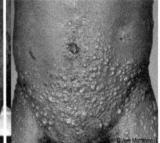

• Younger	• Older
• Mucous membrane involvement	• Rare mucous membrane involvement
• IgG through Epidermis	• IgG & C3 on basement membrane
• Monomorphic	• Polymorphic
• Rupture easily	• Tense and firm
• Fluid filled blister	• Often haemorrhagic
• Nikolsky positive	• Nikolsky negative
• Poor prognosis	• Prognosis favorable

---

[428] Martin LK, Werth VP, Villanueva EV, Murrell DF. A systematic review of randomized controlled trials for pemphigus vulgaris and pemphigus foliaceus. J Am Acad Dermatol 2011; 64:903.

[429] Murrell DF, Dick S, Ahmed AR, et al. Consensus statement on definitions of disease, end points, and therapeutic response for pemphigus. J Am Acad Dermatol 2008; 58:1043.

7. BULLOUS PEMPHIGOID

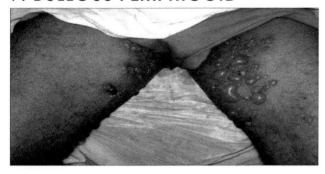

INTRODUCTION

- Bullous pemphigoid and mucous membrane pemphigoid (MMP) are autoimmune blistering diseases that most commonly arise in older adults.
- These disorders are characterized by subepithelial blister formation and the deposition of immunoglobulins and complement within the epidermal and/or mucosal basement membrane zone.

CLINICAL FEATURES

- A prodromal phase lasting weeks to months may precede the development of cutaneous bullae in patients with bullous pemphigoid[430].
- The prodromal phase may present with pruritic[431] eczematous, papular, or urticaria-like skin lesions.
- Some patients with bullous pemphigoid never develop blistering. Bullous pemphigoid may present with several distinct clinical presentations, as follows:
- **Generalized bullous form:** The most common presentation; tense bullae arise on any part of the skin surface, with a predilection for the flexural areas of the skin
- **Vesicular form:** Less common than the generalized bullous type; manifests as groups of small, tense blisters, often on an urticarial or erythematous base
- **Vegetative form:** Very uncommon, with vegetating plaques in intertriginous areas of the skin, such as the axillae, neck, groin, and inframammary areas
- **Generalized erythroderma form:** This rare presentation can resemble psoriasis, generalized atopic dermatitis, or other skin conditions characterized by an exfoliative erythroderma
- **Urticarial form:** Some patients with bullous pemphigoid initially present with persistent urticarial lesions that subsequently convert to bullous eruptions; in some patients, urticarial lesions are the sole manifestations of the disease

- **Nodular form:** This rare form, termed pemphigoid nodularis, has clinical features that resemble prurigo nodularis, with blisters arising on normal-appearing or nodular lesional skin
- **Acral form:** In childhood-onset bullous pemphigoid associated with vaccination, the bullous lesions predominantly affect the palms, soles, and face
- **Infant form:** In infants affected by bullous pemphigoid, the blisters tend to occur frequently on the palms, soles, and face, affecting the genital areas rarely; 60% of these infant patients have generalized blisters

DIAGNOSIS

- To establish a diagnosis of bullous pemphigoid, the following tests should be performed:
  - **Histopathologic analysis:** From the edge of a blister; the histopathologic examination demonstrates a subepidermal blister; the inflammatory infiltrate is typically polymorphous, with an eosinophil predominance; mast cells and basophils may be prominent early in the disease course
  - **Direct immunofluorescence (DIF) studies:** Performed on normal-appearing, perilesional skin (see the image below.
  - **Indirect immunofluorescence (IDIF) studies:** Performed on the patient's serum, if the DIF result is positive

DIFFERENTIAL DIAGNOSIS

- Pemphigus vulgaris
- Bullous impetigo
- Bullous insect bite
- Epidermolysis bullosa
- Drug eruptions which may be bullous in nature
- Erythema multiforme
- Urtricaria
- Dermatitis herpetiformis

MANAGEMENT

- The most commonly used medications for bullous pemphigoid are anti-inflammatory agents (eg, corticosteroids, tetracyclines, dapsone) and immunosuppressants (eg, azathioprine, methotrexate, mycophenolate mofetil, cyclophosphamide).
- Most patients affected with bullous pemphigoid require therapy for 6-60 months, after which many patients experience long-term remission of the disease. However, some patients have long-standing disease requiring treatment for years.

---

430 Schmidt E, della Torre R, Borradori L. Clinical features and practical diagnosis of bullous pemphigoid. Dermatol Clin 2011; 29:427.

431 Kasperkiewicz M, Zillikens D, Schmidt E. Pemphigoid diseases: pathogenesis, diagnosis, and treatment. Autoimmunity 2012; 45:55.

36. Research

Moussa Issa Bookstore

Your Official Moussa Issa Book Store

FRCEM FINAL CRITICAL APPRAISAL "Made Easy"

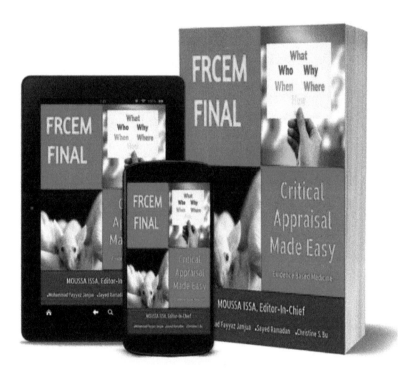

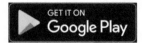
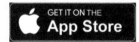

37. Sexual Assault

I. SEXUAL ASSAULT AND / OR RAPE IN ED

INTRODUCTION
- In England and Wales, under the Sexual Offences Act 2003 the definition of **rape** is the non-consensual penetration of vagina, mouth or anus by a penis[432].
- **Sexual assault by penetration** is the non-consensual, intentional insertion of an object or part of the body other than the penis into the vagina or anus. The Act also treats any sexual intercourse with a child under the age of 13 as rape and defines the age of consent as 16.

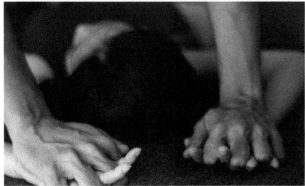

CONSEQUENCES OF SEXUAL ASSAULT
- Rape may result in physical injuries, sexually transmitted infections including HIV and Hepatitis B, unwanted pregnancy and psychological symptoms, which may culminate in post-traumatic stress disorder and affect immediate family or partners.
- These can range from sleeping difficulties, poor appetite, flashbacks, feelings of numbness, anger, shame and denial, avoidance behaviour, depression, suicidality, self-harm, relationship and sexual difficulties.

ASSESSMENT
- Patients who have been sexually assaulted may present to the ED after the assault. Whilst the ED can manage some aspects of their care, it is best practise to encourage patients to go to a **Sexual Assault Referral Centre (SARC.)**
- A SARC is a one-stop location where victims of sexual assault can receive a forensic examination, emergency contraception and post exposure prophylaxis, psychological counselling, legal advice and other support, all in one place from professionally trained staff.

- They bring together all of the different legal and medical agencies and departments, which helps both the victims and those investigating the crimes.
- Victims can choose to be dealt with anonymously if they do not wish any involvement form the police. A SARC cannot deal with acute injuries.

WHAT SHOULD OCCUR IN AN ED
- Patients who present to the Emergency Department should be assessed for physical injuries that may require treatment. Treatment of associated immediate life-threatening injuries takes priority over forensic examination.
- If a victim is unwilling to attend a SARC, Emergency Department staff should respect that decision and be able to manage emergency contraception and sexually transmitted infection risks. Assessment should be conducted in a non-judgemental, confidential and supportive manner. Do not attempt any form of pelvic examination unless there is significant bleeding, as this may disrupt any forensic evidence that may be taken at a later date.
- There are very few occasions when the collection of evidence should be considered in the Emergency Department e.g. if the victim has physical injuries requiring ongoing management. In such cases the forensic samples should be taken by an appropriately trained forensic physician.

EVALUATION FOR ACUTE TRAUMATIC INJURIES
○ **ANOGENITAL INJURIES**

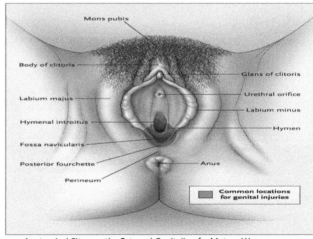

Anatomical Sites on the External Genitalia of a Mature Woman.

---

432 *RCEM, Management of Adult Patients who attend Emergency Departments after Sexual Assault and / or Rape [RCEM Website]*

- Anogenital injuries are not always seen after sexual assault, and clinicians should understand that the absence of such injuries does not equate with no assault.
- Common locations for genital injuries include[433].
  - Tears or abrasions of the posterior fourchette
  - Abrasion or bruising of the labia minora and fossa navicularis
  - Ecchymosis or tears of the hymen.
- The rate of detection of genital injuries varies according to the age of the victim (more common in the young and elderly), virginal status, degree of resistance, time from the assault to examination (more common if the victim is examined within 24 hours), and number of assailants or assaults. Despite the relatively low frequency of obvious injuries, the documentation of such injuries increases the chances of a successful prosecution.

PRE-TRANSFUSION BLOOD SAMPLE

- There is no requirement for pre-transfusion blood samples, unless this is performed as part of an assessment for exposure to blood borne viruses. If the police request a pre-transfusion blood sample, this service should be provided by a suitably trained doctor, usually a forensic medical examiner, who can quality assure the chain of evidence.

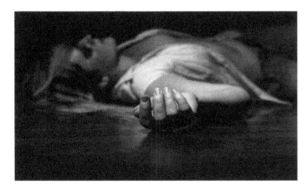

ROLE OF THE EMERGENCY PHYSICIAN

- The emergency physician must appreciate that their response to disclosure may have an important impact on their patient. The emergency physician should be sensitive and sympathetic. **The absence of injuries does not exclude sexual assault.** Take a careful history of the assault including time and location of the assault, characteristics of the assailant(s), physical violence, sexual acts (vaginal, oral, anal; Penile/digital penetration).
- Particular effort should be made to take accurate and contemporaneous notes. Any forensic medical examination should only be performed by a clinician with suitable specialist training, ideally in a forensically secure environment to avoid DNA contamination.

---

[433] *RCEM, Management of Adult Patients who attend Emergency Departments after Sexual Assault and / or Rape [RCEM Website]*

- The medical assessment should ideally be performed by the most senior or appropriately trained doctor in the emergency department.
- Patients should be offered a choice of gender of the doctor where possible.
- Examine everywhere where including inside the mouth looking for bruising, abrasions, and lacerations and any patterns such as fingertip marks.
- Look and treat for any bite marks.
- Document examination findings clearly as you may be asked to produce a statement later or go to court if the victim decides to press charges at a later date.
- **Consider the possibility of pregnancy:** Emergency contraception should be offered to the victim.
- Consider the possibility of exposure to **sexually transmitted infection.** Victims may need further referral to Social Services, Victim Support, a Community Safety Unit or other organizations which can offer them support after the assault. Any concerns about child welfare or vulnerable adults should lead to the activation of local safeguarding procedures.

2. EXPOSURE TO BLOOD BORNE VIRUSES

Baseline blood tests should be taken for **Hepatitis B, Hepatitis C and HIV in the ED**.

HEPATITIS B:

- If the perpetrator is not known to be Hepatitis B negative, then **accelerated Hepatitis B vaccination should be considered.**
- This usually involves a dose of Hepatitis B vaccine at the time of presentation and two further doses from the patient's General Practitioner at one and two months after the exposure.
- **Hepatitis B Immunoglobulin** can be provided in high risk situations at the time of presentation and provides passive immunisation for up to 7 days after an exposure. Follow up blood tests should be organised through the Genito-urinary medicine clinic or GP three months after exposure.

HIV:

- The decision to offer Post Exposure Prophylaxis after Sexual Exposure (PEPSE) is not always straightforward.
- PEPSE should be considered where:
  - The assailant is known to be HIV positive,
  - Has risk factors,
  - Anal rape,
  - Multiple assailants or
  - There is bleeding.
- PEPSE may be effective at reducing HIV transmission if it is administered **within 72 hours**, but is more effective when administered earlier.

3. EXPOSURE TO BACTERIAL INFECTIONS

- Transmission of sexually transmitted infections is more likely where there are multiple assailants, biting, defloration, wounds, or anal intercourse.
- Transmission is also likely when the assailant is a man who has sex with men, or injects illegal drugs.
- Prophylactic antibiotics should be offered.
- Local protocols vary but a common regime is **Cefixime 400mg + Azithromycin 1g + Metronidazole 2g as single oral stat doses**. This may reduce the need for follow up in some cases.
- For pregnant or breastfeeding women **Cefixime 400mg + Azithromycin 1g is regarded as safe** , but these cases can be discussed with the relevant on-call specialty, either infectious diseases or Genitor-urinary medicine.
- **Genito-urinary medicine follow-up** should be offered as the initial assessment may be too early for most sexually transmitted infections to be evident.
- Please refer to the British Association for Sexual Health and HIC guidelines for more detail.

PREVENTION OF STIs

Infection	Recommended treatment
Gonorrhoea	Ceftriaxone 250mg IM or Cefixime 400mg orally in a single dose; Azithromycin 2g po in a single dose in patients with penicillin allergy
Chlamydia	Azithromycin 1g orally in a single dose or Doxycycline 100mg po BD x 7 days
Trichomoniasis	Metronidazole 2g po in a single dose
Hepatitis B	Hep B vaccine if not already immunised, with 1st dose given in ED
HIV	Tenofovir + Emtricitabine (Truvada)1-tab po OD x 28 days
Tetanus	Tetanus booster
Pregnancy	Levonorgestrel 1.5mg po in a single dose within 72 hours of UPSI

Drug Therapies for the Prevention of Sexually Transmitted Infections and Pregnancy after Sexual Assault.
All patients should be offered prophylaxis in the ED for STIs.

4. PREGNANCY PREVENTION

- The risk of pregnancy after rape is approximately 5%.
- Progestin-only emergency contraception (1.5 mg of levonorgestrel), which is administered as a one-time dose within 120 hours after unprotected intercourse, has been shown to be 98.5% effective in preventing pregnancy. Since efficacy decreases with increasing time since unprotected intercourse, the drug should be **taken within 72 hours** after an assault.

- Although this medication should not be given if the person is already pregnant, it does not cause abortion, and there is no evidence that it causes harm to a pregnancy. Side effects include nausea, fatigue, abdominal pain, and vaginal bleeding.

PSYCHOSOCIAL CARE

- The victim often knows the perpetrator which may lead to psychosocial problems. Emergency physicians should be able to identify and support patients who develop **post-traumatic stress disorder and depression** by referring them to SARCs or the patient's GP. Appropriate written information about relevant services should be available in the Emergency Department.

INFORMATION SHARING WITH OUTSIDE AGENCIES

- Emergency physicians should assume that clinical information is confidential. Patients should be offered police involvement, but any decision not to involve the police should be respected. In exceptional circumstances, information can be shared with the police and statutory agencies such as social services.

These circumstances include:

- Where the victim is a child. Any sexual assault of a child should trigger **local safeguarding procedures**.
- Where **there are concerns about the welfare of children** of the victim.
- Where the **victim lacks capacity** and is unlikely to regain capacity.
- Where **guns or knives have been used** by the perpetrator.

FOLLOW-UP AND MANDATORY REPORTING

- Rape victims should be referred for both medical follow-up (testing for pregnancy, HIV, and hepatitis) and psychiatric support. The patient should be encouraged to follow up with her primary care doctor.
- Rape crisis centers can provide ongoing support, limited free confidential counseling, and legal services.

CONCLUSIONS AND RECOMMENDATIONS

A patient presenting for care after sexual assault, such as the woman described in the vignette, should:

- First be evaluated for acute traumatic physical injuries.
- Then be offered **prophylaxis for STIs and pregnancy**
- **toxicologic testing if indicated be offered forensic-evidence collection**
- Offer to call the police if the victim decides to report the assault.
- Finally, safe plans for discharge, including planned follow-up for medical care and psychological support, are critical.

II. MANAGEMENT OF DOMESTIC ABUSE

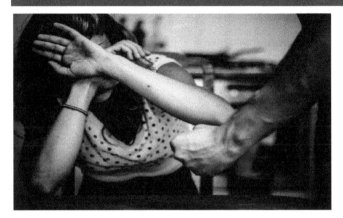

DEFINITION

- The Department of Health has provided a widely accepted definition of domestic abuse.
- **'Domestic violence refers** to a wide range of physical, sexual, emotional and financial abuse between partners / ex-partners – whether or not they are co-habiting.'[434]
- Both men and women can suffer abuse, though more women suffer abuse and this tends to be more severe.
- The terms 'Domestic abuse' and 'Domestic Violence' are used interchangeably.
- Though emergency physicians tend to focus on physical assault as the most obvious manifestation of abuse, the majority of abused patients report greater morbidity from the sexual and emotional abuse.

HEALTH CONSEQUENCES OF DOMESTIC ABUSE

- There are significant and strong associations between domestic abuse and many illnesses, notably psychiatric complaints; **depression, self-harm and drug and alcohol misuse**. Other strong associations exist with termination of pregnancy, sexually transmitted diseases and medically unexplained symptoms.

RECOGNITION OF DOMESTIC ABUSE

- Domestic abuse is frequently not disclosed, it is estimated that a woman will suffer 20 assaults before disclosure. Opportunities for confidential disclosure should be considered. Posters in the waiting room and leaflets in the women's toilets may encourage disclosure and should be encouraged.
- Most women will not disclose abuse unless directly asked. Simple, direct questions such as **'We know violence at home is a problem for many people, is there someone who is hurting you at home?'** are usually acceptable and effective.

- There is insufficient evidence of benefit to advocate screening all women for domestic abuse, but clinicians should be prepared to ask if there is any clinical suspicion. Men can also suffer domestic abuse.

THE ROLE OF THE ED CLINICIAN

- Up to 12% of emergency department attendances are suffering domestic abuse and 30% of domestic abuse commences during pregnancy. Emergency department staff are often in a good position to identify cases.

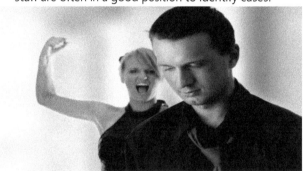

WHAT TO DO WHEN A PATIENT DISCLOSES DOMESTIC ABUSE[435]

- The patient should be believed.
- Enquiry about the extent and severity of the abuse should be made in a non-judgemental manner. An assessment should be made of the victim's immediate safety. Specific inquiry should identify whether there are any children living with the victim or perpetrator.
- Injuries, if present, should be photographed. If an Independent Domestic Violence Advocate (IDVA) is available immediately then they will make adequate records, but if not, as much information as possible should be recorded at the time of disclosure.
- Contact with the police and outside agencies should be offered from the safety of the emergency department.
- Information about local shelters and support agencies should available in written form and handed to the patient. Failure to involve outside help is common and may frustrate medical and nursing staff, who may believe that there has to be immediate action to be effective. This is not true, victims leave an abusive relationship when they feel ready, not when clinical staff feel they should. The risks to children growing up in an abusive household are greatly increased.
- Any concerns about child welfare should lead to the prompt activation of local child safeguarding procedures.

---

434 RCEM, *Management of Domestic Abuse [RCEM Website]*

435 RCEM, *Management of Domestic Abuse [RCEM Website]*

38. Sexually Transmitted Disease

1. PELVIC INFLAMMATORY DISEASE

BACKGROUND

- Pelvic inflammatory disease (PID) is usually the result of infection ascending from the endocervix causing endometritis, salpingitis, parametritis, oophoritis, tuboovarian abscess and/or pelvic peritonitis.
- Neisseria gonorrhoeae and Chlamydia trachomatis have been identified as causative agents[436], Mycoplasma genitalium is a likely cause[437] and anaerobes are also implicated. Microorganisms from the vaginal flora including streptococci, staphylococci, Escherichia coli and Haemophilus influenzae can be associated with upper genital tract inflammation.
- Mixed infections are common
- Laparoscopic studies have shown that in 30-40% of cases, PID is polymicrobial.

CAUSES OF PID

- **Sexually transmitted (90%):** Chlamydia, Gonorrhoea, Mycoplasma genitalium.
- **Non-sexually transmitted (10%, often post-surgical instrumentation):** *E. Coli*, Group B Strep, Bacteriodes, Gardenella.

CLINICAL FEATURES OF PID

- Lower abdominal pain and tenderness.
- Abnormal vaginal or cervical discharge.
- Fever (>38°C).
- Abnormal vaginal bleeding (intermenstrual, post-coital, or 'breakthrough').
- Deep dyspareunia.
- Cervical excitation.
- Adnexal tenderness mass.

INVESTIGATIONS IN PID

- Endocervical swabs for *Chlamydia* and *Gonorrhoea.*
- Urinary pregnancy test

- Bloods: ESR, CRP, and WCC are supportive but not specific.
- Transvaginal ultrasound may demonstrate inflamed or dilated Fallopian tubes or an abscess.

ED MANAGEMENT OF PID

- **Outpatient:**
  - Ceftriaxone 500mg IM/IV as single dose, then
  - Doxycycline 100mg PO BD + Metronidazole 400mg PO TDS
- **Inpatient management** is indicated in the following circumstances:
  - Clinically severe disease
  - Tubo-ovarian abscess
  - Intolerance or lack of response to oral therapy
  - Surgical emergency not excluded.
- Inpatient antibiotic therapy is:
  - IV Ceftriaxone 1g IV OD and
  - Doxycycline 100mg PO BD + Metronidazole 400mg PO TDS.
- **Surgical drainage** may be required for tubo-ovarian abscesses.
- Consideration should be given to **removing an IUCD** in patients presenting with PID, especially if symptoms have not resolved within 72 hours.
- **Sexual partners** from the previous 6 months should be contacted and offered screening via the genitourinary medicine clinic.

COMPLICATIONS OF PID

- Ectopic pregnancy
- Acute appendicitis
- Endometriosis
- Irritable bowel syndrome
- Complications of an ovarian cyst, i.e. Rupture, torsion
- functional pain (pain of unknown physical origin)

---

[436] Bevan CD, et al. Clinical, laparoscopic and microbiological findings in acute salpingitis: report on a United Kingdom cohort. Br J Obstet Gynaecol 1995; 102: 407–414.

[437] Lis R, Rowhani-Rahbar A and Manhart LE. Mycoplasma genitalium infection and female reproductive tract disease: a meta-analysis. Clin Infect Dis 2015; 61: 418–426.

2. VAGINAL CANDIDIASIS

- Vulvovaginal candidiasis may be caused by *Candida albicans* (80-92%) or non-*albicans* species of yeast such as *C. glabrata*. The symptoms caused by the different species are indistinguishable[438].
- Risk factors for its development include:
  - Diabetes mellitus
  - Recent antibiotic treatment
  - Pregnancy
  - Immunosuppression

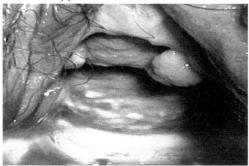

- Patients typically present with a **white 'cheesy' discharge, vaginal itching, dyspareunia and dysuria**.
- Examination will reveal **vulval erythema, oedema, satellite lesions** and sometimes associated **fissuring**.
- Treatment is with topical antifungals, such as **Clotrimazole and Miconazole**, is usually adequate.
- More severe cases sometimes require **Oral Fluconazole or Itraconazole.**

3. TRICHOMONAS VAGINALIS

- Infection is most commonly seen in sexually active females between the ages of 18 and 35 years.
- It is usually, but not always, acquired through sexual transmission.

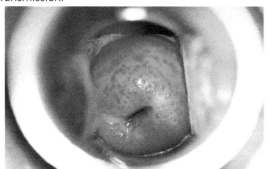

- It typically presents with a profuse, offensive, **thin vaginal discharge**. The colour is usually **yellow or green**.
- It is often associated with vulval itching and soreness, dysuria, dyspareunia and abdominal pain.

- On examination, there will be **vulval and cervical erythema** and some patients will have a **'strawberry cervix'** where the ectocervix resembles the surface of a strawberry. The vaginal pH will be > 4.5 in Trichomonas vaginalis infection.
- **Trichomonas vaginalis infection is associated with:**
  - Pelvic inflammatory disease
  - Increased risk of HIV infection
  - Preterm delivery and other pregnancy complications
- Treatment is with **Metronidazole or Tinidazole**[439].

4. PRIMARY SYPHILIS

- Syphilis is caused by infection with the spirochete bacterium *Treponema pallidum subspecies pallidum.*
- Approximately one-third of sexual contacts of infectious syphilis will develop the disease.
- Transmission is by direct contact with an infectious lesion or by vertical transmission during pregnancy (T. pallidum crosses the placenta)[440].
- Site of bacterial entry is typically genital in heterosexual patients, but 32-36% of transmissions among men who have sex with men (MSM) may be at extragenital (anal, rectal, oral) sites through oral-anal or genital-anal contact. The typical incubation period is 2-3 weeks but can be as long as 3 months.
- A primary lesion develops at the site of contact, initially as a **small painless nodule** that subsequently ulcerates and forms **a large painless ulcer.**

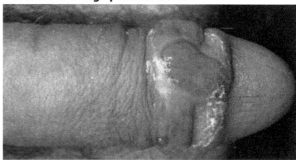

- The margins are typically indurated and red and there is often a clear serous discharge.
- Painless regional lymphadenopathy is also usually present.
- The treatment of choice for primary syphilis is long-acting procaine **Benzylpenicillin 600 mg daily by IMI for 10-12 days**.
- For CNS disease, secondary and tertiary syphilis, the treatment regime is for 14 days.

---

438 *British Association for Sexual Health and HIV, The 2007 United Kingdom national guideline on the management of vulvovaginal candidiasis [Online]*

439 *BASHH Guidelines, Trichomonas vaginalis [Bashh Website]*
440 *BASHH Guidelines, Syphilis [Bashh Website]*

5. CHANCROID

- A sexually transmitted infection caused by the fastidious Gram-negative bacteria **Haemophilus ducreyi.**
- It is spread by direct sexual contact.
- H. ducreyi, the microbial causative agent of chancroid, is a Gram-negative facultative anaerobic coccobacillus and is placed in the family Pasteurellacae[441].
- Chancroid is relatively rare in the UK but is endemic in Africa, Asia and South America.
- HIV is an important co-factor, with a 60% association in Africa.
- The disease is characterized by the development of **painful ulcers on the genitalia**. In women the most common site of ulcer development is the labia majora.
- **'Kissing ulcers'** can develop where ulcers are situated in opposing surfaces of the labia.
- Painful lymphadenopathy occurs in 30-60% of patients and these can further develop into abscesses (buboes).

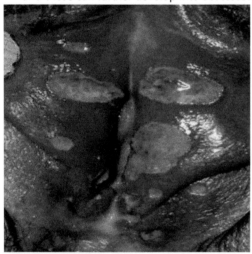

ED MANAGEMENT

- The CDC recommends a single oral dose of **1 gram of azithromycin** or a **single IM dose of ceftriaxone** for the treatment of chancroid.
- **A 7-day course of oral Erythromycin** is an acceptable alternative.
- H. ducreyi is resistant to penicillins, tetracyclines, trimethoprim, ciprofloxacin, aminoglycosides and sulfonamides.

- **POTENTIAL COMPLICATIONS INCLUDE:**
  - Extensive adenitis
  - Large inguinal abscesses and/or sinuses
  - Phimosis
  - Superinfection with *Fusarium spp.* or *Bacteroides spp.*

6. BACTERIAL VAGINOSIS

- Bacterial vaginosis (BV) is the commonest cause of abnormal discharge in women of childbearing age.
- The reported prevalence has varied from 5% in a group of asymptomatic college students to as high as 50% of women in rural Uganda. A prevalence of 12% was found in pregnant women attending an antenatal clinic in the United Kingdom, and of 30% in women undergoing termination of pregnancy. Lactobacilli are the dominant bacteria in the healthy vagina[442].
- Anaerobic organisms, such as ***Gardnerella vaginalis, Mobiluncus* spp. and *Bacteriodes spp.*** proliferate and replace lactobacilli. *Gardnerella vaginalis* is the most commonly implicated bacteria.
- The commonest presenting symptom of BV is an **unpleasant, fishy-smelling discharge**.
- It is often worse after intercourse but there is not usually any accompanying vaginal soreness or irritation.
- Diagnosis can be made on the basis of **Amsel's criteria**, with any 3 of the following being required:
  - Thin, white or yellow, homogenous discharge
  - **Clue cells** (epithelial vaginal cells with a distinctive stippled appearance)
  - Vaginal pH > 4.5 (can be as high as 7.0)
  - **Positive 'whiff test'** (fishy odor released on addition of 10% potassium hydroxide to vaginal fluid)
- Treatment is with **Metronidazole or Clindamycin.**

7. CHLAMYDIA

AETIOLOGY

- Genital chlamydial infection is caused by the obligate intracellular bacterium ***C. trachomatis.***
- Chlamydia is the most commonly reported curable bacterial STI in the UK. The highest prevalence rates are in 15-24-year olds. Chlamydia infection has a high frequency of transmission, with concordance rates of up to 75% of partners being reported[443].

CLINICAL FEATURES

1. Women
Symptoms:
- In the majority, infection is asymptomatic
- Increased vaginal discharge
- Post-coital and intermenstrual bleeding
- Dysuria, Lower abdominal pain, Deep dyspareunia

Signs:
- Mucopurulent cervicitis with or without contact bleeding
- Pelvic tenderness, Cervical motion tenderness

---

441 BASHH Guidelines, chancroid [Bashh Website]

442 BASHH Guidelines, Bacterial vaginosis [Bashh Website]

443 BASHH Guidelines, chlamydia [Bashh Website]

2. Men
Symptoms (may be so mild as to be unnoticed):
- Urethral discharge
- Dysuria

Signs: Urethral discharge

3. Extra-genital infections:
- **Rectal infection:**
  - Rectal infection is usually asymptomatic, but anal discharge and anorectal discomfort may occur
  - **Pharyngeal infections:** Usually asymptomatic
- **Conjunctival infections**
  - Usually sexually acquired - the usual presentation is of unilateral low-grade irritation; however, the condition may be bilateral

COMPLICATIONS[444]
- **Women**
  - PID, Endometritis, Salpingitis
  - Tubal infertility
  - Ectopic pregnancy
  - Sexually acquired reactive arthritis (SARA) (<1%)
  - Perihepatitis
- **Men**
  - Sexually aquired reactive arthritis
  - Epididymo-orchitis.

DIAGNOSIS
- Nucleic Acid Amplification **Test** (**NAAT**)
- Vulvo-vaginal swabs (VVS)
- Endocervical swabs
- First-catch urine
- Urethral swabs
- **Extra-genital sampling:**
  - Rectal swabs
  - Pharyngeal swabs

MANAGEMENT OF CHLAMYDIA
1. Uncomplicated urogenital infection and pharyngeal infection:
- Doxycycline 100mg bd for 7 days (contraindicated in pregnancy) or
- Azithromycin 1g orally in a single dose

2. Alternative regimens:
if either of the above treatment is contraindicated:
- Erythromycin 500mg bd for 10-14 days or
- Ofloxacin 200mg bd or 400mg od for 7 days

3. Pregnancy and breast feeding
Doxycyline and ofloxacin are contraindicated in pregnancy
- Azithromycin 1g as a single dose or
- Erythromycin 500mg QID for 7 days or

- Erythromycin 500mg BD for 14 days or
- Amoxicillin 500mg TDS for 7 days

4. Management of sexual partners:
- All sexual partners should be offered, and encouraged to take up, full STI screening, including HIV testing and if indicated, hepatitis B screening and vaccination.

8. GONORRHOEA
ETIOLOGY
- Gonorrhoea is caused by the Gram-negative diplococcus *Neisseria gonorrhoeae*.
- The primary sites of infection are the columnar epithelium-lined mucous membranes of the urethra, endocervix, rectum, pharynx and conjunctiva.
- Transmission is by direct inoculation of infected secretions from one mucous membrane to another.
- Secondary infection to other anatomical sites, through systemic or transluminal spread, can also occur[445].

CLINICAL FEATURES
Symptoms
Men
- Urethral discharge and/or dysuria within 2-5 days
- Urethral infection can be asymptomatic
- Rectal infection is usually asymptomatic but may cause anal discharge or perianal/anal pain or discomfort
- Pharyngeal infection is usually asymptomatic

Women
- Infection at the endocervix is frequently asymptomatic
- Increased or altered vaginal discharge is the most common symptom
- Lower abdominal pain may be present
- Urethral infection may cause dysuria but not frequency
- Gonorrhoea is a rare cause of intermenstrual bleeding or menorrhagia
- Rectal infection is usually asymptomatic
- Pharyngeal infection is usually asymptomatic

Signs
Men
- Mucopurulent or purulent urethral discharge
- Rarely, epididymal tenderness/swelling or balanitis may be present

Women
- Mucopurulent endocervical discharge and easily induced endocervical bleeding
- Pelvic/lower abdominal tenderness
- Commonly, no abnormal findings are present on examination

---

444 *BASHH Guidelines, chlamydia [Bashh Website]*

445 *BASHH Guidelines, Gonorrhoea [Bashh Website]*

COMPLICATIONS

- Transluminal spread my result in epididymo-orchitis or prostatitis in men and pelvic inflammatory disease (PID) in women.
- Disseminated gonoccoccal infection may occur following haematogenous dissemination causing skin lesions, arthralgia, arthritis and tenosynovitis.

DIAGNOSIS

- Microscopy of Gram-stained genital specimens allows direct visualization of N. gonorrhoeae as monomorphic Gram-negative diplococci within polymorphonuclear leukocytes.
- Nucleic Acid Amplification **Test (NAAT)**
- Culture

MANAGEMENT OF GONORRHOEA[446]

1. General advice

- Detailed explanation of condition, long term implications for health of themselves and partner(s), reinforced with clear and accurate written information.
- Patients should be advised to abstain from sexual intercourse until they and their partner(s) have completed treatment; if azithromycin is used, this will be 7 days after treatment was given
- Screening for other STIs

2. Treatment for uncomplicated anogenital infection

- Ceftriaxone 500 mg I.M. as a single dose with azithromycin 1 g oral as a single dose.
- Azithromycin is recommended as co-treatment irrespective of the results of chlamydia testing, to delay the onset of cephalosporin resistance.

3. Alternative regimens (all in combination with azithromycin 1g single dose)

- Cefixime 400 mg oral as a single dose. Only advisable if an I.M. injection is contraindicated or refused by the patient
- Spectinomycin 2 g I.M. as a single dose
- Cefotaxime 500 mg I.M. as a single dose or Cefoxitin 2 g I.M. as a single dose plus Probenecid 1 g oral
- **Quinolones** cannot be recommended due to high prevalence of resistance. When an infection is known to be quinolone sensitive, ciprofloxacin 500 mg orally as a single dose or ofloxacin 400 mg orally as a single dose have proven efficacy
- **High-dose azithromycin 2g** as a single dose has shown acceptable efficacy in clinical trials, but was associated with high gastrointestinal intolerance. Single dose 1g azithromycin is not recommended (II, C)

---

446 *BASHH Guidelines, Gonorrhoea [Bashh Website]*

9. VARICELLA ZOSTER & PREGNANCY

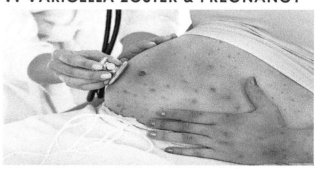

- Varicella can cause serious complications in pregnant women. The risk of the foetus being affected is around 1% if the mother develops varicella in the first 28 weeks of pregnancy. The result is **foetal varicella syndrome (FVS),** which is characterised by *eye defects, limb hypoplasia, skin scarring and neurological abnormalities.*
- Any pregnant woman who has not had chickenpox or who is found to be seronegative for **VZV IgG** should be advised to minimize any contact with chickenpox and shingles and to seek medical help immediately if exposed. If a pregnant woman is exposed, the first course of action is to perform a blood test and check for **VZV immunity**. If she is not immune and the history of the exposure is significant, she should be given **VZV immunoglobulin** as soon as possible.
- It is effective **up to 10 days after being exposed**.
- A pregnant woman that develops chickenpox should seek medical help urgently. There is an increased maternal risk of **Pneumonia, Encephalitis** and **Hepatitis** as well as the 1% risk of developing **FVS**.
- **Acyclovir** should be used with caution before 20 weeks gestation, but is recommended after 20 weeks if the woman presents within 24 hours of the onset of the rash.

MATERNAL INFECTION	POTENTIAL CONSEQUENCES
< 20 weeks of gestation	Spontaneous abortion Foetal varicella syndrome
Any stage	Foetal death Herpes zoster 1st year of life
Near term	Congenital; Disseminated varicella Varicella Pneumonia (can be fatal)

39. Shocked Patient

I. ED APPROACH TO A SHOCKED PATIENT

DEFINITION

○ Shock is a pathophysiologic state in which the oxygen supply to body tissues inadequately meets metabolic demands, resulting in dysfunction of end-organs.

○ Effects of shock are reversible in the early stages, and a delay in diagnosis and/or timely initiation of treatment can lead to irreversible changes, including multiorgan failure (MOF) and death[447].

○ Shock may arise by impaired delivery of oxygen to tissues, impaired utilization of oxygen by tissues, increased oxygen consumption by tissues, or a combination of these processes[448].

○ While circulatory failure and hypotension is the most common and readily identified clinical presentation of shock, the manifestations of shock exist along a continuum of illness severity, thus a patient with initially normal vital signs may still be in shock.

CAUSES OF SHOCK	
Hypovolaemic	○ Haemorrhage
	○ Gastroenteritis, stomal losses
	○ Intussusception, volvulus
	○ Burns
	○ Peritonitis
Distributive	○ Septicaemia
	○ Anaphylaxis
	○ Vasodilating drugs
	○ Spinal cord injury
Cardiogenic	○ Arrhythmias
	○ Heart failure (cardiomyopathy, myocarditis)
	○ Valvular disease
	○ Myocardial contusion
Obstructive	○ Tension/haemopneumothorax
	○ Flail chest
	○ Cardiac tamponade
	○ Pulmonary embolism
	○ Congenital cardiac (coarctation, hypoplastic left heart, aortic stenosis)
Dissociative	○ Profound anaemia
	○ Carbon monoxide poisoning
	○ Methaemoglobinaemia

CLINICAL ASSESSMENT

○ Clinical features and symptoms can vary according to the type and stage of shock.

○ The most common clinical features/labs which are suggestive of shock include hypotension, tachycardia, tachypnea, obtundation or abnormal mental status, cold, clammy extremities, mottled skin, oliguria, metabolic acidosis, and hyperlactatemia[449].

○ **Patients with hypovolemic shock** can have general features as mentioned above as well as evidence of orthostatic hypotension, pallor, flattened jugular venous pulsations, may have sequelae of chronic liver disease (in case of variceal bleeding).

○ **Patients with septic shock** may present with symptoms suggestive of the source of infection (example-skin manifestations of primary infection such as erysipelas, cellulitis, necrotizing soft-tissue infections), and cutaneous manifestations of infective endocarditis.

○ **Patients with anaphylactic shock** can have hypotension, flushing, urticaria, tachypnea, hoarseness of voice, oral and facial edema, hives, wheeze, inspiratory stridor, and history of exposure to common allergens such as medications or food items the patient is allergic to or insect stings.

○ **Tension pneumothorax** should be suspected in a patient with undifferentiated shock who has tachypnea, unilateral pleuritic chest pain, absent or diminished breath sounds, tracheal deviation to the normal side, distended neck veins and also has pertinent risk factors for tension pneumothorax such as recent trauma, mechanical ventilation, underlying cystic lung disease).

○ **In a patient with undifferentiated shock,** diagnostic clues to pericardial tamponade as the etiology include dyspnea, the Beck triad (elevated jugular venous pressure, muffled heart sounds, hypotension), pulses paradoxus, and known risk factors such as trauma, the recent history of pericardial effusion, and thoracic procedures[450].

○ **Cardiogenic shock** should be considered as the etiology if the patient with undifferentiated shock had chest pain suggestive of cardiac origin, narrow pulse pressure, elevated jugular venous pulsations or lung crackles, and significant arrhythmias on telemetry or ECG.

---

447 *Haseer Koya H, Paul M. Shock. [Updated 2020 Jul 26]. In: StatPearls [Internet]. Treasure Island (FL): StatPearls Publishing; 2020 Jan-. [Online]*

448 *Benjamin J. Sandefur, Approach to shock [CDEM Online]*

449 *Kraut JA, Madias NE. Lactic acidosis. N. Engl. J. Med. 2015 Mar 12;372(11):1078-9. [PubMed]*

450 *Haseer Koya H, Paul M. Shock. [Updated 2020 Jul 26]. In: StatPearls [Internet]. Treasure Island (FL): StatPearls Publishing; 2020 Jan-. [Online]*

CLASSIFICATION OF SHOCK

Class of shock	Class I	Class II	Class III	Class IV
Volume Blood loss (ml)	Up to 750	750-1500	1500-2000	>2000
Volume of blood loss (%)	0-15%	15-30%	30-40%	>40%
Heart Rate	<100	>100	>120	>140
Blood Pressure	Normal	Normal	Decrease	Decrease
Pulse Pressure	Normal or increase	Decrease	Decrease	Decrease
Respiratory Rate	14-20	20-30	30-40	>35
Urine output (ml/h)	>30	20-30	5-15	Negligible
Mental State	Slightly anxious	Mildly anxious	Anxious, confused	Confused, lethargic
Initial fluid replacement	Crystalloid	Crystalloid	Crystalloid & blood	Crystalloid & blood

- o Note also **a reduction in pulse pressure occurs before a reduction in systolic BP** as the diastolic increases in response to vasoconstriction.
- o The Mean Arterial Pressure (MAP) is a better representation of organ perfusion than the systolic. A MAP of 65mmHg is considered to be sufficient for organ perfusion in a healthy adult[451].

MAP = (systolic + 2 x diastolic) / 3.

$$MAP = \frac{SP + 2DP}{3}$$

- **Other history and examination findings:**
  (Reproduced from RCEM Learning website[452])

FINDING	POSSIBLE CAUSE
Pain radiating to testicle	o Abdominal aortic or iliac aneurysm
Chest pain radiating to back	o Thoracic aortic dissection
Onset with food	o Anaphylaxis
History of active rheumatoid arthritis	o Addisonian crisis
Muffled heart sounds	o Cardiac tamponade
Priapism	o Neurogenic shock
Unequal radial pulses	o Thoracic aortic dissection
Distended neck veins	o Tension pneumothorax
Sweet smelling breath	o Diabetic ketoacidosis

INVESTIGATION STRATEGIES

- FBC with differential, U&E, LFT, glucose
- Blood gas & Lactate
- Coagulation studies
- Pregnancy test (blood or urine)
- Calcium
- Urinalysis
- ECG
- Chest radiograph
- If a particular etiology of shock is suspected, further studies may be indicated:
  - o Hemorrhagic etiology – type and screen
  - o Infectious etiology – blood and urine cultures; CSF studies; focused CT or ultrasound
  - o Cardiogenic – cardiac enzymes (ACS, myocarditis); echocardiogram (heart failure or structural etiology)
  - o Obstructive – CT (PE); echocardiogram (pericardial tamponade)

ED MANAGEMENT OF A SHOCKED PATIENT

- Timely empiric treatment for the shock patient is crucial to minimize morbidity and mortality.
- Critical findings involving the airway, breathing, and circulation (i.e. "the ABCs") should be emergently addressed.
- Ensuring proper oxygenation is critical for all of the etiologies of shock, and arterial oxygen saturation should be maximized.

GENERAL MANAGEMENT:

- **MOVER: M**onitor, **O**xygen, **V**ital Signs, **E**CG, **R**esus
  - o **A**: Patent airway
  - o **B:** Maximise oxygen delivery
    - Consider early **intubation and ventilation** in many shocked patients.
  - o **C:** 2 large bore IV Cannula;
    - Get blood: **ABG, FBC, U&E, LFT, CRP, Blood Cultures, Cross match, tryptase**...
    - **IV fluid** (crystalloids) bolus: Small volumes (e.g. 250ml) given quickly (over 5-10 min).
    - Consider **intubation** once fluid resuscitation **exceeds 40-60 ml/kg.**
    - **Judicious transfusion:** reasonable target: **7-9 g/dl** in otherwise healthy patients.
  - o **D: Inotropes**: indicated in some conditions
    - **There is no role for steroid use** in the initial resuscitation and treatment of a shocked patient. (except in case of **adrenal insufficiency (Addisonian crisis).**

---

451 Jonathan M Jones, Shock [RCEMlearning Online]

452 Jonathan M Jones, Shock [RCEMlearning Online]

II. SEPSIS

INTRODUCTION

- **Sepsis** is characterised by a life-threatening organ dysfunction due to a dysregulated host response to infection.'
- **Septic shock:** 'sepsis with persistent hypotension requiring vasopressors to maintain MAP ≥65mm Hg and having a serum lactate >2mmol/L despite adequate volume resuscitation'.
- Modified SIRS criteria, adapted from the Surviving Sepsis campaign[453]:

Temperature >38.3°C or <36.0 °C	New confusion/drowsiness
Pulse >90/min	WBC >12 or < 4.0×10^9 /L
RR >20/min	Blood glucose >7.7 mmol/L (not if diabetic)

- The 2016 taskforce identified **'life-threatening organ dysfunction'** by 'an increase [from baseline] in the Sequential [Sepsis-related] Organ Failure Assessment **(SOFA) score of 2 points or more'.**
- Patients with an increase of 2 or more in the SOFA score have an estimated in hospital mortality of 10% due to sepsis and a 2-fold to 25-fold increased risk of death compared with patients with a SOFA score of <2.
- As a result, the task force recommended that patients with sepsis meeting this definition be observed in a location with a 'greater level of monitoring' than a routine inpatient floor environment.

THE 'QUICKSOFA' (QSOFA) SCORE

- qSOFA, or 'quick-SOFA', is a tool proposed by the Sepsis-3 Task Force to aid in the identification of patients with infection who have a high risk of death.
- 'SOFA' is derived from the Sequential (or Sepsis-related) Organ Failure Assessment (SOFA) score, which is described below[454]:

Respiratory rate of 22/min or greater

Altered mentation (GCS of less than 15)

Systolic blood pressure of 100 mm hg or less

- The quickSOFA score does not define sepsis, but is an indicator of increased risk for clinical deterioration.

- The key benefits of the qSOFA score are that **it is simple to measure** and does not require laboratory testing; thus it can be performed rapidly and repeatedly.
- For patients identified with organ dysfunction, the group emphasizes adherence to the **3-hour and 6-hour bundles.**

ED MANAGEMENT OF SEPSIS

- In July 2016, NICE issued NG51[455], which dealt with the identification and management of sepsis in the community and in hospitals, but did not include Critical Care management of sepsis

3-HOUR & 6-HOUR SEPSIS BUNDLES
Within 3 hours of presentation:
o   Measure lactate level
o   Obtain blood cultures prior to administration of antibiotics
o   Administer broad spectrum antibiotics
o   Administer 30 ml/kg crystalloid for hypotension or lactate ≥ 4mmol/L

Within 6 hours of presentation:
o   Apply vasopressors (for hypotension that does not respond to initial fluid resuscitation) to maintain a mean arterial pressure (MAP) ≥ 65mmHg
o   In the event of persistent hypotension after initial fluid administration (MAP < 65Hg) or if initial lactate was ≥4 mmol/L, re-assess volume status and tissue perfusion and document findings according to note below.
o   Re-measure lactate if initial lactate elevated.

Note:
- Document Reassesment of Volume Status and Tissue Perfusion with:
- **Either:**
  o   Repeated focused exam (after initial fluid resuscitation) by licensed independent practitioner including vital signs, cardiopulmonary, capillary refill, pulse and skin findings

- **Or two of the following:**
  o   Measure CVP
  o   Measure $ScvO_2$
  o   Bedside cardiovascular ultrasound
  o   Dynamic assessment of fluid responsiveness with passive leg raise or fluid challenge

[453] The sepsis manual 4th edition 2017 – 2018.pdf Edited by Dr Ron Daniels and Professor Tim Nutbeam

[454] The sepsis manual 4th edition 2017 - 2018 Edited by Dr Ron Daniels and Professor Tim Nutbeam

[455] NICE guideline [NG51], Sepsis: recognition, diagnosis and early management [NICE CG51]

The relationship of lactate level in sepsis to mortality[456]:

Lactate	Mortality
<2	15%
2-4	25%
>2	38%

NICE NG 31 GUIDELINES[457]

1. **Arrange for immediate review** by the senior clinical decision maker to assess the person and think about alternative diagnoses to sepsis
2. Carry out a **venous blood test** for the following:
   ○ ABG, Blood culture, FBC, U&ES, CRP, Clotting screen
3. **Give a broad-spectrum antimicrobial** within 1 hour:
   • Take **blood cultures** before antibiotics are given.
   • If meningococcal disease is suspected (fever and purpuric rash) give **IV ceftriaxone**.
   • **For children younger than 3 months**, give an additional antibiotic active **against listeria** (for example, **ampicillin or amoxicillin**).
   • Treat neonates presenting in hospital with suspected sepsis in their first 72 hours with **intravenous benzylpenicillin and gentamicin**.
   • Treat neonates who are more than 40 weeks with **ceftriaxone 50 mg/kg** unless already receiving an intravenous calcium infusion at the time.
4. Discuss with a consultant
5. **Give intravenous fluid bolus** within 1 hour of identifying that they meet any high risk:
   • Use crystalloids that contain sodium in the range 130-154 mmol/litre with a bolus of **500 ml over less than 15 minutes.**
   • If children and young people up to 16 years, give a bolus of 20 ml/kg over less than 10 minutes.
   • If neonates need intravenous fluid resuscitation, use glucose-free crystalloids that contain sodium in the range 130-154 mmol/litre, with a **bolus of 10–20 ml/kg over less than 10 minutes.**
   • Reassess the patient after completion of the intravenous fluid bolus, and **if no improvement give a second bolus**. If there is no improvement after a second bolus **alert a consultant to attend**.
   • Do not use starch-based solutions or hydroxyethyl starches for fluid resuscitation for people with sepsis.
   • Consider human albumin solution 4-5% for fluid resuscitation only in patients with sepsis and shock.

7. **Using oxygen in people with suspected sepsis:**
   • Give oxygen to achieve a target saturation of **94–98% for adult patients or 88–92% for those at risk of hypercapnic respiratory failure.**
   • Oxygen should be given to children with suspected sepsis who have signs of shock or oxygen saturation (SpO2) of less than 92% when breathing air.
   • Treatment with oxygen should also be considered for children with an SpO2 of greater than 92%, as clinically indicated.
8. **Refer to critical care** for review of management including need for **central venous access and initiation of inotropes or vasopressors**.
9. **Monitor continuously:**
   • A minimum of once every 30 min depending on setting.
   • Monitor the mental state
   • Alert a consultant to attend in person if patient fails to respond within 1 hour of initial antibiotic and/or intravenous fluid resuscitation.

   Failure to respond is indicated by any of:
   ○ Systolic blood pressure persistently below 90 mmhg
   ○ Reduced level of consciousness despite resuscitation
   ○ Respiratory rate over 25 breaths per minute or a new need for mechanical ventilation
   ○ Lactate not reduced by more than 20% of initial value within 1 hour.
10. **Investigations**
   • Consider **urine analysis and chest X-ray** to identify the source of infection in all
   • Consider **imaging of the abdomen and pelvis** if no likely source of infection is identified after clinical examination and initial tests.
   • **Do not perform a lumbar puncture** without consultant instruction if any of the following contraindications are present:
   ○ Signs suggesting raised intracranial pressure or reduced or fluctuating level of consciousness (GCS <9 or a drop of 3 points or more)
   ○ Relative bradycardia and hypertension
   ○ Focal neurological signs
   ○ Abnormal posture or posturing
   ○ Unequal, dilated or poorly responsive pupils
   ○ Papilloedema, Abnormal 'doll's eye' movements
   ○ Shock
   ○ Extensive or spreading purpura
   ○ After convulsions until stabilised

456 Trzeciak S, Dellinger RP, Chansky ME, Arnold RC, Schorr C, Milcarek B, et al. Intensive Care Med 2007, 33(6):970-7

457 NICE guideline [NG51], Sepsis: recognition, diagnosis and early management [NICE CG51]

40. Cardio-Respiratory Arrest
I. ADVANCED CARDIAC LIFE SUPPORT

o   Routine cricoid pressure not recommended
o   Use continuous capnography if intubated
o   Emphasis on high quality CPR
o   **Atropine** no longer used in PEA/Asystole
o   **Adenosine** is recommended in stable, undifferentiated, regular monomorphic wide complex tachycardia
o   Trial of chronotropic drugs before pacing suggested for unstable bradycardia

Adapted from Resuscitation council UK[458]

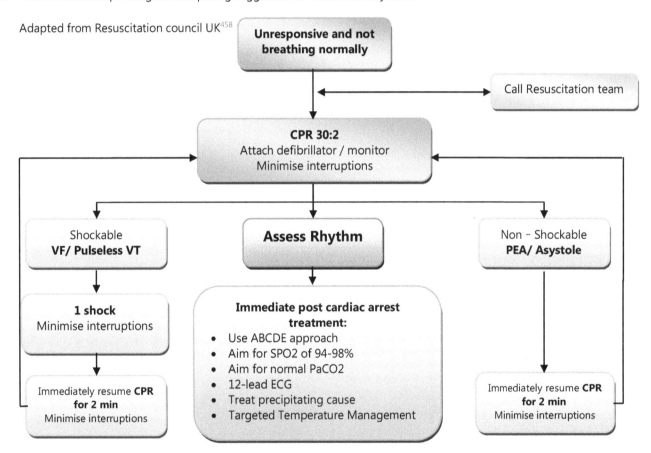

During CPR:	Treat Reversible causes:	Consider:
• Ensure high quality Chest compressions • Minimise interruptions to compressions • Give Oxygen • Use Waveform capnography • Continuous compressions when advanced airway in place • Vascular access (IV/ IO) • Give Adrenaline every 3-5 min • Give Amiodarone after 3 shocks	• Hypoxia • Hypovolaemia • Hypo/ Hyperkalaemia/Metabolic • Hypothermia • Thrombosis: Coronary/pulmonary • Tension pneumothorax • Tamponade- cardiac • Toxins	• Ultrasound imaging • Mechanical chest compressions to facilitate transfer/ treatment • Coronary angiography and percutaneous coronary intervention • Extracorporeal CPR

---

458 *Jasmeet Soar,Charles Deakin, Andrew Lockey, Jerry Nolan, Gavin Perkins, Guidelines: Adult advanced life support [Resuscitation Council UK]*

REVERSIBLE CAUSES

The "Hs"

- o **H**ypoxia
- o **H**ypovolaemia
- o **H**ypokalaemia/**H**yperkalaemia,
- o **H**ypothermia
- o **H**ydrogen: Acidaemia
- o Other metabolic disorders:
  - o **H**ypoglycaemia, **H**ypocalcaemia,

The "Ts"

- o **T**hrombosis: coronary or pulmonary
- o **T**ension pneumothorax
- o **T**amponade – cardiac
- o **T**oxins

- **HYPOXIA**:
  - o Adequate ventilation with the maximal possible inspired oxygen during CPR.
  - o Adequate chest rise and bilateral breath sounds.
  - o Check that the tracheal tube is not misplaced in a bronchus or the oesophagus.

- **HYPOVOLAEMIA:**
  - o Usually due to severe haemorrhage >>> **Stop the haemorrhage.** Restore intravascular volume with fluid and blood products.

- **Hyperkalaemia, Hypokalaemia, Hypocalcaemia, Acidaemia and Other Metabolic Disorders:**
  - o Detected by biochemical tests or suggested by the patient's medical history (e.g. renal failure).
  - o Give **IV calcium chloride** in the presence of hyperkalaemia, hypocalcaemia and calcium channel-blocker overdose.

- **HYPOTHERMIA**:
  - o Should be suspected based on the history such as cardiac arrest associated with drowning.
  - o Rewarm the patient up to 34⁰C

- **CORONARY THROMBOSIS**:
  - o Associated with an **acute coronary syndrome** or **ischaemic heart disease** is the most common cause of sudden cardiac arrest.
  - o An ACS is usually diagnosed and treated after ROSC is achieved.
  - o If an ACS is suspected, and ROSC has not been achieved, consider **urgent coronary angiography** when feasible and, if required, **percutaneous coronary intervention.**
  - o **Mechanical chest compression** devices and **extracorporeal CPR** can help facilitate this.

- **Pulmonary Embolism**:
  - o If PE is thought to be the cause of cardiac arrest consider giving a **fibrinolytic drug** immediately.
  - o Following fibrinolysis during CPR for acute pulmonary embolism, survival and good neurological outcome have been reported, even in cases requiring in excess of 60 min of CPR.
  - o If a fibrinolytic drug is given in these circumstances, consider performing CPR for **at least 60–90 min** before termination of resuscitation attempts.
  - o In some settings extracorporeal CPR, and/or surgical or mechanical thrombectomy can also be used to treat pulmonary embolism.

- **TENSION PNEUMOTHORAX:**
  - o Can be the primary cause of PEA and may be associated with trauma.
  - o The diagnosis is made clinically or by ultrasound.
  - o **Decompress rapidly** by thoracostomy or needle thoracocentesis, and then insert a chest drain.

- **CARDIAC TAMPONADE:**
  - o Usually difficult to diagnose because the typical signs of distended neck veins and hypotension are usually obscured by the arrest itself.
  - o Cardiac arrest after penetrating chest trauma is highly suggestive of tamponade and is an indication for **resuscitative thoracotomy**.
  - o The use of ultrasound will make the diagnosis of cardiac tamponade much more reliable.

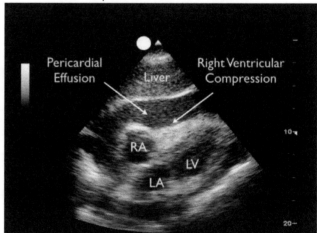

- **TOXINS:**
  - o In the absence of a specific history, the accidental or deliberate ingestion of therapeutic or toxic substances may be revealed only by laboratory investigations.
  - o Where available, the **appropriate antidotes** should be used, but most often treatment is supportive and standard ALS protocols should be followed.

USE OF ULTRASOUND IMAGING DURING ADVANCED LIFE SUPPORT

- Absence of cardiac motion on sonography during resuscitation of patients in cardiac arrest is highly predictive of death although sensitivity and specificity has not been reported.

WAVEFORM CAPNOGRAPHY DURING ADVANCED LIFE SUPPORT

- **Advantages:**
  - o **Ensuring tracheal tube placement in the trachea**: although it will not distinguish between bronchial and tracheal placement.
  - o **Monitoring ventilation rate during CPR**: avoiding hyperventilation.
  - o **Monitoring the quality of chest compressions** during CPR.
  - o **Identifying ROSC during CPR**: An increase in end-tidal CO_2 during CPR can indicate ROSC and prevent unnecessary and potentially harmful dosing of adrenaline in a patient with ROSC.
  - o **Prognostication during CPR:** The Resuscitation Council (UK) recommends that a specific end-tidal CO_2 value at any time during CPR should not be used alone to stop CPR efforts.
  - o End-tidal CO_2 values should be considered only as part of a multi-modal approach to decision-making for prognostication during CPR.

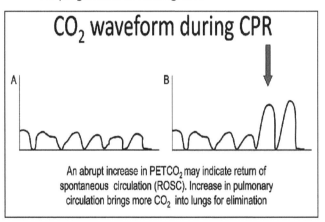

An abrupt increase in $PETCO_2$ may indicate return of spontaneous circulation (ROSC). Increase in pulmonary circulation brings more CO_2 into lungs for elimination

DEFIBRILLATION (MANUAL DEFIBRILLATORS)

- Continue chest compressions during defibrillator charging,
- Interruption in chest compressions of no more than 5 seconds.
- Immediately resume chest compressions following defibrillation.
- Deliver the first shock with an energy of **at least 150 J.**

- If an initial shock has been unsuccessful it is worth attempting the second and subsequent shocks with a higher energy level if the defibrillator is capable of delivering a higher energy but, based on current evidence, both fixed and escalating strategies are acceptable.
- If VF/pVT recurs during a cardiac arrest (refibrillation) give subsequent shocks with a higher energy level if the defibrillator is capable of delivering a higher energy.

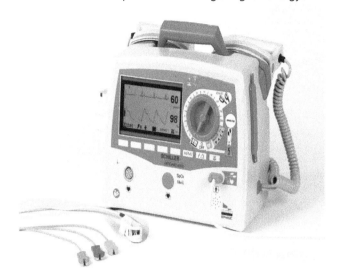

AIRWAY MANAGEMENT AND VENTILATION[459]

- The options for airway management and ventilation during CPR vary according to patient factors, the phase of the resuscitation attempt (during CPR, after ROSC), and the skills of rescuers.
- They include:
  - o No airway and No ventilation (compression-only CPR),
  - o Compression-only CPR with the airway held open (with or without oxygen),
  - o Mouth-To-Mouth breaths, Mouth-To-Mask, Bag-Mask Ventilation with simple airway adjuncts,
  - o Supraglottic Airways (SGAs),
  - o Tracheal Intubation (inserted with the aid of direct laryngoscopy or videolaryngoscopy, or via a SGA).
- Anyone attempting tracheal intubation must be well trained and equipped with waveform capnography.
- In the absence of these, use **bag-mask ventilation** and/or an **SGA** until appropriately experienced and equipped personnel are present.

---

459 Jasmeet Soar,Charles Deakin, Andrew Lockey, Jerry Nolan, Gavin Perkins, Guidelines: Adult advanced life support [Resuscitation Council UK]

II. POST CARDIAC ARREST: CARE OF THE ROSC PATIENT

1. TARGETED TEMPERATURE MANAGEMENT (TTM) [460]

- TTM which was previously called **therapeutic hypothermia** is the only intervention that has been shown to improve neurological outcomes after cardiac arrest. Induced hypothermia should occur soon after ROSC (return of spontaneous circulation).
- The decision point for the use of therapeutic hypothermia is whether or not the patient can follow commands. (Lack of meaningful response to verbal commands). One of the most common methods used for inducing therapeutic hypothermia is a rapid infusion of ice-cold **(4° C),** isotonic, non-glucose-containing fluid to a volume of **30 ml/kg.**
- The optimum temperature for therapeutic hypothermia is **32-36 ° C** (89.6 to 96.8 ° F).
- A single target temperature, within this range, should be selected, achieved, and maintained for **at least 24 hours**.
- During induced TTM, the patient's core temperature should be monitored with any one of the following: oesophageal thermometer, a bladder catheter in the nonanuric patients, or a pulmonary artery catheter if one is already in place. Axillary and oral temperatures are inadequate for monitoring core temperatures.

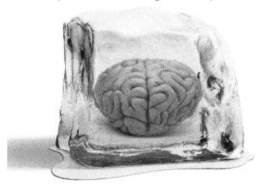

2. VENTILATION OPTIMIZATION

- During the post-cardiac arrest phase, inspired oxygen should be titrated to maintain an arterial oxygen saturation of ≥ 94%. This reduces the risk of oxygen toxicity.
- Excessive ventilation should also be avoided because of the potential for reduced cerebral blood flow related to a decrease in PaCO2 levels.

- Also, excessive ventilation should be avoided because of the risk of high intrathoracic pressures which can lead to adverse hemodynamic effects during the post-arrest phase.
- Quantitative waveform capnography can be used to regulate and titrate ventilation rates during the post-arrest phase. Avoid excessive ventilations.
- Ventilation should start at 10/min and should be titrated according to the target **PETCO2 of 35-40 mmHg.**

3. HEMODYNAMIC OPTIMIZATION

- Hypotension, a systolic blood pressure < **90 mmHg** should be treated and the administration of **fluids and vasoactive medications** can be used to optimize the patient's hemodynamic status.
- While the optimal blood pressure during the post-cardiac arrest phase is not known, the primary objective is adequate systemic perfusion, and a **Mean Arterial Pressure of ≥ 65 mmHg** should accomplish this.
- A systolic blood pressure greater than 90 mmHg and a mean arterial pressure greater than 65 mmHg should be maintained during the post-cardiac arrest phase.
- The goal of post-cardiac arrest care should be to return the patient to a level of functioning equivalent to their prearrest condition.

4. IV INFUSIONS FOR THE CONTROL OF POST-ARREST HYPOTENSION

- **IV Fluid Bolus**: Give 1-2 L of normal saline or LR
- **Epinephrine** 0.1-0.5 mcg/kg/min
- **Dopamine** 5-10 mcg/kg/min
- **Norepinephrine** 0.1-0.5 mcg/kg/min).

5. OTHER CONSIDERATIONS

- Moderate glycemic control measures should be implemented to maintain glucose levels from **8-10 mmol/L**, and since there is an increased risk for hypoglycaemia in the post-arrest phase these more moderate levels should be maintained rather than normal levels of 4.4-6.1 mg/dl.
- Every effort should be made to provide coronary reperfusion (PCI), and interventions should be directed with this goal in mind.
- PCI has been shown to be safe and effective in both the alert and comatose patient, and hypothermia does not contraindicate PCI.

[460] Jasmeet Soar, Charles Deakin, Andrew Lockey, Jerry Nolan, Gavin Perkins, Guidelines: Adult advanced life support [Resuscitation Council UK]

ADULT IMMEDIATE POST-CARDIAC CARE ALGORITHM-2015 Update[461]

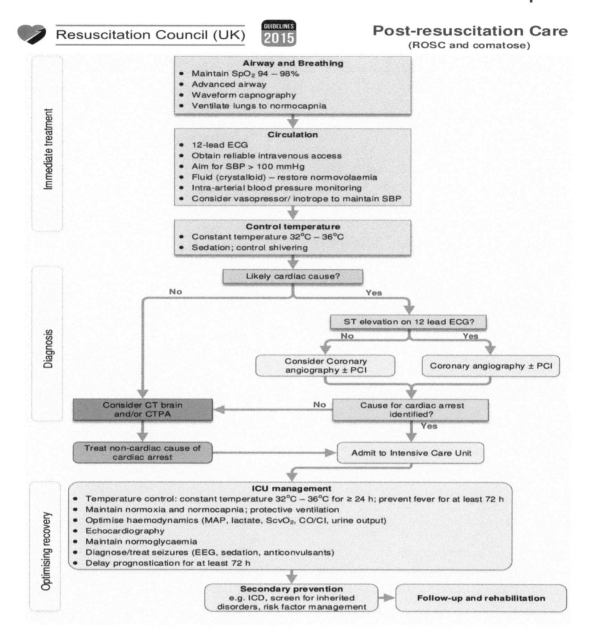

DRUGS FOR CARDIAC ARREST

1. ADRENALINE	2. AMIODARONE	PAEDS ANTI-ARYHYTHMICS
o Adult: Adrenaline **1 mg IV/IO** o Give **as soon as possible in PEA/ asystole**. o Give **after the 3rd shock in VF/ pVT**. o **Repeat every 3–5 min** (alternate cycles).	o Adult: Amiodarone dose **300 mg IV/IO bolus after the 3rd shock in VF/VT.** o A further **150 mg** may be given for refractory VF/VT (5th shock) o Followed by a **900mg infusion over 24 h.** o **If Amiodarone not available, give Lidocaine 1mg/kg IV**	• **Amiodarone** 5mg/kg -in paediatrics • **Lignocaine** 1mg/kg - paediatrics • **Magnesium** 0.1-0.2mmol/kg - paediatrics • **Atropine** 1-3mg or 20mcg/kg - removed from adult PEA/asystole guidelines, still paediatrics • **NaHCO3:** 1mmol/kg - paediatrics

[461] Jasmeet Soar,Charles Deakin, Andrew Lockey, Jerry Nolan, Gavin Perkins, Guidelines: Adult advanced life support [Resuscitation Council UK]

III. RESUSCITATION IN SPECIAL CIRCUMSTANCES

1. OPIOID OVERDOSE

- In known opioid overdose associated with respiratory depression, respiratory arrest, or to help diagnose suspected opioid overdose, the usual initial adult dosage of **Naloxone Hydrochloride is 400–2000 mcg IV, given at 2–3 min intervals and titrated to response.**
- Naloxone may be given for cardiac arrest associated with opioid overdose, but its benefit is uncertain.
- **If no response is observed after a total of 10 mg IV Naloxone,** consider a non-opioid related drug or other process. If the IV route is not available, naloxone may be given by IM, IO, SC or intranasal routes.
- Additional doses may be necessary if the patient's level of consciousness falls, or if the patient's respiratory rate decreases again, because the half-life of naloxone can be shorter than the opioid causing the respiratory depression. Only give as much as is necessary to achieve an adequate respiratory rate, as an excessive dose, particularly in chronic opioid users, can cause **agitation and occasionally seizures**.

2. CARDIAC ARREST IN PREGNANCY

- **Causes of cardiac arrest in pregnancy:**
  - Haemorrhage,
  - Embolism (thomboembolic and amniotic fluid),
  - Hypertensive disorders of pregnancy,
  - Abortion
  - Genital tract sepsis

- **Differential diagnosis for chest pain/cardiac arrest in pregnancy:**
  - Pulmonary embolism
  - Aortic dissection
  - ACS
  - Spontaneous Coronary Artery Dissection **(SCAD)** (21% of AMI post partum)
  - Arrhythmia including Long QTc

- **Approach of cardiac arrest in pregnancy**
  - Use the **ABCDE approach** and follow ALS algorithm
  - **Identify and treat the underlying cause** (e.g. rapid recognition and treatment of sepsis, including early intravenous antibiotics).
  - Place the patient in the **left lateral position** or **manually displace the uterus to the left.**
  - Give **high-flow oxygen**, guided by pulse oximetry and aim to correct hypoxaemia.
  - Establish **IV access and give a fluid bolus** (250 mL) if there is hypotension or hypovolaemia.
  - Seek **expert help early**: Obstetric, anaesthetic and neonatal specialists should be involved early in the resuscitation.
  - **Defibrillation** energy levels are as recommended for standard defibrillation. If left lateral tilt and large breasts make it difficult to place an apical defibrillator electrode, use **an antero-posterior or bi-axillary electrode position**.
  - If resuscitation attempts fail to achieve ROSC, consider an **immediate caesarean section to deliver the foetus**.

3. TRAUMATIC CARDIAC ARREST

- **REVERSIBLE CAUSES OF TRAUMATIC CARDIAC ARREST**
  - **H**ypovolaemia,
  - **H**ypoxia (Oxygenation)
  - **T**ension pneumothorax
  - **T**amponade – cardiac
- Patients with traumatic cardiac arrest commonly have one or more injuries resulting in severe hypovolaemia, critical hypoxaemia, tamponade or tension pneumothorax, either in isolation or concurrently.
- Each of these conditions needs to be addressed simultaneously by the prehospital team and active management commenced.

A. HYPOVOLAEMIA & FLUID REPLACEMENT
  - Immediately control active external haemorrhage by applying **direct pressure** to bleeding wounds.
  - Then **volume re-expansion** should follow.
  - **Splint fractures** of the pelvis and long bones and if there is a suspicion of a pelvic fracture, apply a **pelvic binder** to reduce the pelvis to an anatomical position taking care to minimise patient movement.
  - **Reduce long bone fractures** to an anatomical position and apply splints.
  - **Tranexamic Acid**
    - Give adult trauma patients with suspected haemorrhage a prehospital dose of **Tranexamic acid 1g IV/IO over 10 min.**

B. HYPOXAEMIA

o Initial attention should be paid to high quality, basic airway management **with cervical spine control**, using airway adjuncts if required.

o Attention to basic airway management is vital in the unconscious trauma patient who is at risk of airway compromise.

o Secure a definitive airway by insertion of a **cuffed tracheal tube** as early as possible.

C. TENSION PNEUMOTHORAX

o Manage any open pneumothorax or sucking chest with a **dressing** that enables air to be released from the pleural cavity.

o **Bilateral needle chest decompression** is rapid and within the skill set of most EMS personnel and should be performed immediately.

o Tracheal intubation, positive pressure ventilation and formal chest decompression will effectively treat tension pneumothorax in patients with traumatic cardiac arrest.

o **Simple thoracostomy** is straightforward and used in several prehospital physician services.

4. ASTHMA

- If IV or IO access cannot be established rapidly, give **IM adrenaline** if cardiorespiratory arrest has occurred recently.

- When the appropriate skills are available **intubate** the trachea to enable ventilation of stiff lungs and avoid gastric insufflation.

- **Identify and treat tension pneumothorax** with needle decompression or thoracostomy as appropriate.

- Cardiac arrest associated with asthma results from respiratory exhaustion, respiratory acidosis and impaired venous return caused by high intrathoracic pressures.

- It may also be precipitated by a tension pneumothorax that is, on rare occasions, bilateral.

- If there is a history of a severe asthma attack leading to cardiac arrest, **adrenaline 0.5 mg IM can be given early**, if IV access is not immediately available.

5. HYPOXIA

- Cardiac arrest caused by pure hypoxaemia is uncommon.

- It is seen more commonly as a consequence of asphyxia, which accounts for most of the non-cardiac causes of cardiac arrest.

- **Causes of asphyxial cardiac arrest:**

  o **Airway obstruction:** soft tissues (coma), laryngospasm, aspiration

o Anaemia
o Asthma
o Avalanche burial
o Central hypoventilation - brain or spinal cord injury
o Chronic obstructive pulmonary disease
o Drowning
o Hanging,
o High altitude
o Impaired alveolar ventilation from neuromuscular disease Pneumonia
o Tension pneumothorax
o Trauma,
o Traumatic asphyxia or compression asphyxia (e.g. crowd crush)

- **Treatment**
  o Effective ventilation with supplementary oxygen

6. HYPERKALAEMIA

- Hyperkalaemia is the most common electrolyte disorder associated with life threatening arrhythmias and cardiac arrest. It is defined as $K_{(S)} > 5.0$ mmol/l.

Mild	*5.0-5.9 mmol/l*
Moderate	*6.0-6.4 mmol/l*
Severe	*> 6.5 mmol/l*

- Mild hyperkalaemia is common and often well tolerated in patients with chronic renal failure.

- **$K_{(S)} > 10$ mmol/l is usually fatal.**

CLASSIC CAUSES OF HYPERKALAEMIA

Drugs	Renal & Metabolic
▪ Angiotensin converting enzyme inhibitors (ACEI) ▪ Angiotensin receptor blockers (ARB) ▪ Non-steroidal anti-inflammatory (NSAIDs) ▪ Beta blockers ▪ Suxamethonium ▪ K⁺ supplementation ▪ K⁺ sparing diuretics	▪ Acute and Chronic Renal Failure ▪ Type 4 Renal Tubular Acidosis ▪ Metabolic acidosis ▪ Diet ▪ Fasting caused by a relative lack of insulin

Endocrine disorders	Others
▪ Addison's disease ▪ Hyporeninaemia ▪ Insulin deficiency	▪ Tumour lysis ▪ Rhabdomyolysis ▪ Massive transfusion ▪ Massive haemolysis ▪ Haemolysis (in laboratory tube) ▪ Thrombocytosis ▪ Leukocytosis ▪ Venepuncture technique (e.g. prolonged tourniquet application)

- **CLINICAL MANIFESTATIONS**
  - o Patients with hyperkalaemia frequently appear well.
  - o The following symptoms usually occur in severe cases but are very non-specific:
    - Flaccid paralysis
    - Paraesthesia
    - Respiratory difficulties
    - Signs such as depressed deep tendon reflexes
    - Arrhythmias: VT, VF, PEA...
- **Bradycardia** is also common in hyperkalaemia and causes a dilemma in that calcium salt administration can worsen the situation. The response to atropine is also poor.

ECG IN HYPERKALAEMIA

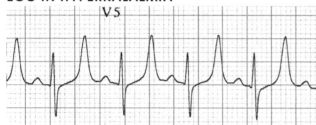

- o **Serum potassium > 5.5 mEq/L** is associated with **repolarization abnormalities**:
  - Peaked T waves (usually the earliest sign of hyperkalaemia)

- o **Serum potassium > 6.5 mEq/L** is associated with **progressive paralysis of the atria**:
  - P wave widens and flattens
  - PR segment lengthens
  - P waves eventually disappear

- o **Serum potassium > 7.0 mEq/L** is associated with **conduction abnormalities** and **bradycardia**:
  - Prolonged QRS interval with bizarre QRS morphology
    - High-grade AV block with slow junctional and ventricular escape rhythms
    - Any kind of conduction block (bundle branch blocks, fascicular blocks)
    - Sinus bradycardia or slow AF
    - Development of a sine wave appearance (a pre-terminal rhythm)

- o **Serum potassium level of > 9.0 mEq/L** causes **cardiac arrest** due to:
  - Asystole
  - Ventricular fibrillation
  - PEA with bizarre, wide complex rhythm

ED MANAGEMENT OF HYPERKALAEMIA

- o Treatment of hyperkalaemia involves stabilizing the myocardium to prevent arrhythmias, shifting potassium back into the intracellular space and removing excess potassium from the body.

Mechanism	Drug/ Method	Dose	Onset (min)
Stabilizing membranes	**Calcium chloride**	10ml 10% IV	1-30
Shift K⁺	**Insulin/ Glucose**	10U in 100ml of DW 10%	15-30
	Salbutamol	0.5mg IV 20mg Nebs	15-30
	Na⁺ Bicarbonate	1mmol/kg IV	15-30
Remove excess K⁺	**Calcium resonium**	15-30g PO/PR	Variable
	Dialysis	Most immediate and reliable method of K⁺ removal. Can lower K⁺ by 1mmol/L in 1st hr and another 1mmol/L over the next 2 hrs.	

INDICATIONS FOR DIALYSIS

- o The main indications for dialysis in patients with hyperkalaemia are:
  - Severe life-threatening hyperkalaemia with or without ECG changes or arrhythmia;
  - Hyperkalaemia resistant to medical treatment;
  - End-stage renal disease;
  - Oliguric acute kidney injury (<400 mL/day urine output);
  - Marked tissue breakdown (e.g. rhabdomyolysis).

7. HYPOKALAEMIA

- Hypokalaemia is defined as **K(S) < 3.5 mmol/l,** symptoms are more likely with increasing severity.

Mild	3.0-3.5 mmol/l
Moderate	2.5-3.0 mmol/l
Severe	< 2.0 mmol/l

- **Causes:**
  - o The most common cause of hypokalaemia **is potassium depletion**.
  - o In critically ill patients the most common cause is **abnormal losses** which occur in stool and urine (from metabolic alkalosis and chloride depletion).

- o **Other causes of hypokalaemia are:**
  - ▪ **Gastrointestinal loss** (e.g. Diarrhoea, vomiting, ileostomy, intestinal fistula);
  - ▪ **Drugs** (e.g. Diuretics, laxatives, steroids);
  - ▪ **Renal losses** (e.g. Renal tubular disorders, diabetes insipidus, dialysis);
  - ▪ **Endocrine disorders** (e.g. Cushing's/Conn's syndromes, hyperaldosteronism);
  - ▪ **Transcellular shift**: Insulin/Glucose, Theophylline, Caffeine, Hyperthyroidism
  - ▪ **Metabolic alkalosis**;
  - ▪ Magnesium depletion & Poor dietary intake.

ECG FEATURES OF HYPOKALAEMIA ARE:

- o ***U*** *waves Prominent;*
- o ***T*** *wave flattening;*
- o ***ST*** *segment depression*
- o ***PR*** *interval prolonged*
- o ***P*** *wave slightly peaked*

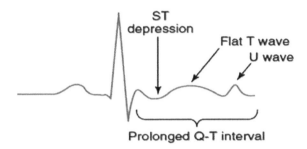

ED MANAGEMENT OF HYPOKALAEMIA

1. MILD/MODERATE HYPOKALAEMIA

- • Dietary supplementation and monitoring may suffice.
- • Gradual Potassium administration.
- • **Magnesium supplementation** facilitates more rapid correction of hypokalaemia.

2. SEVERE HYPOKALAEMIA

- • In severe hypokalaemia, intravenous replacement must be used.
- • This must be rigorously controlled using infusion pumps according to local protocols.
- • The maximal rate of correction is **20 mmol/h K⁺.**
- • **Magnesium 5 ml of 50% over 30 minutes** should commence soon after.
- • Never bolus inject potassium and always ensure adequate mixing of the solution occurs before the infusion is started.

3. CARDIAC ARREST

- • Cardiac arrest due to hypokalaemia may require **20mmol KCl IV over 2-3 minutes, repeated until potassium is > 4.0 mmol/l.**

8. HYPOTHERMIA

INTRODUCTION

- o **Accidental hypothermia:** An involuntary drop in core body temperature to <35°C (95°F) [462]
- o **Primary hypothermia:** Simple environmental exposure, when heat production in an otherwise healthy person is overcome by the stress of excessive cold
- o **Secondary hypothermia:** Impaired thermoregulation, much more common in urban ED
- o Can occur in ill persons with a wide variety of medical conditions, even in a warm environment.

AETIOLOGY/CAUSES		
General:	**Drugs:**	**Trauma:**
Young and old	Ethanol	Multiple trauma
Systemic illness	Sedatives (BDZ,	Minor trauma,
Sepsis	TCAs, opioids OD)	Immobility: NOF
Malnutrition	Phenothiazines	Major burns
	(impaired	
Environmental:	shivering)	**Endocrine:**
Cold, wet, windy		Hypoglycaemia
conditions	**Neurological:**	and diabetes
Cold water	CVA	Hypothyroidism
immersion	Paraplegia	Hypoadrenalism
Exhaustion	Parkinson's disease	
Marathon runners		

PREDISPOSING FACTORS

- • Extremes of age (elderly, infants)
- • Ethanol use
- • Lack of shelter (homeless persons)
- • Exposure (winter sports)
- • Underlying illness

CLINICAL ASSESSMENT:

- • In determining whether hypothermia is playing a significant role in your patient's presentation consider:
  - o Where they were found
  - o The ambient temperature and weather conditions
  - o The patient's clothing
  - o The patient's age
  - o Co-morbid conditions and state of nutrition
  - o Alcohol and drug use
- • **Sinus bradycardia** develops followed by A-Fib..
- • **Below 32°C,** ventricular arrhythmias including ventricular fibrillation (VF) may occur. Finally, asystole results.
- • Note that malignant arrhythmias are unlikely to be hypothermia-induced at temperatures above 32°C-consider alternative causes such as acute coronary syndrome (ACS).

---

[462] *Salman Ahsan, Hypothermia [Core EM]*

ECG IN HYPOTHERMIA[463]

- Most common abnormality is prolongation of PR/QRS/QT intervals
- Most common dysrhythmia is atrial fibrillation
- Shivering produces mechanical artifact in baseline
- Osborn wave: A deflection occurring at the junction of the QRS and ST segment is invariably present in patients with temperatures <86°F (<30°C)
- Size of J-point deflection related to temperature decrease
- Not prognostically significant
- Cardiac arrest due to VT, VF or asystole

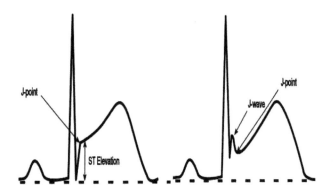

Classic Early Repolarization Without a J-wave   Classic Early Repolarization With a J-wave

Stage	Core T°	Signs and symptoms
Mild	35-32°C	Alert Shivering Hypertension Tachycardia and Tachypnoea
Moderate	32-30°C	Reduced LOC Shivering diminishes Loss of fine motor control Cyanosis
	30-28°C	Shivering stops Fixed dilated pupils
Severe	28-25°C	Unconscious Shivering has stopped rigid muscles Appears Dead Potential arrhythmias
	25-20°C	Cardiac arrest
Profound	<20°C	No detectable vital signs

MANAGEMENT OF HYPOTHERMIA IN THE ED

- **General Approach**
  - **ABC approach** including **D**on't **E**ver **F**orget **G**lucose
  - Removal of wet, cold clothes is the cornerstone of management
  - Prevention of further heat loss;
  - Initiation of re-warming appropriate to the degree of hypothermia
    - The patient must be placed on a cardiac monitor,
    - Intravenous access established
    - Active re-warming measures initiated.
  - Treatment of complications and other medical factors (such as alcohol intoxication, central nervous system disease, trauma and infection should be considered and treated concurrently).

- Salman Ahsan[464] has published a summary of steps regarding the ED management of Hypothermic patients:

ABCs APPROACH

- **Airway:** Do not delay intubation when it is indicated.
  - The advantages of adequate oxygenation and protection from aspiration outweigh the minimal risk of triggering VF by performing tracheal intubation.

- **Breathing:**
  - Do not correct blood gas for temperature as blood gas machine automatically rewarms blood, interpret as if patient normothermic to guide ventilation management, whether spontaneously breathing or mechanically ventilated.

- **Circulation:**
  - When hypotension occurs in a patient with hypothermia, it may be a result of the presence of bradycardia and volume depletion; however, hypotension may be a predictor of infection, particularly when associated with a slow rewarming rate (Vassallo, 2015)

- **Rewarming as management of circulation**
  - Passive external: Involves covering the patient with blankets and protecting the patient from further heat loss
    - Uses the patient's own endogenous heat production for rewarming and is most successful in healthy patients with mild to moderate hypothermia whose capacity for endogenous heat production is intact.

  - **Active External:** Bair hugger or other forced air surface rewarming device

---

463 Vassallo 1999, PMID: 10569384)

464 Salman Ahsan, Hypothermia [Core EM]

- Hypothetical concern for suppressing shivering mechanism and peripheral vasodilation causing hypotension and worsening demand on cold myocardium
- Has not been replicated in animal studies. Remains controversial even though there is no evidence to support these concerns (Golden 1981)
- Recent literature supports forced air surface rewarming has a safe and effective method with no arrhythmia or aftedrop detected.

o **Minimally invasive active internal rewarming**
  - **IV fluids:** Normal Saline should be given to expand intravascular volume. Urine output is an important indicator of organ perfusion and the adequacy of intravascular volume in hypothermic patients, although the initial cold diuresis may lead to underestimation of fluid needs.
  - **Cold diuresis:** Occurs when increases in central blood volume result in inhibition of the release of antidiuretic hormone, results in large volume dilute urine (Vassallo 2015, Hamlet 1983)
  - Warmed saline has not been shown to speed rewarming but is theorized to prevent further iatrogenic heat loss, thus preferable but not essential to resuscitation
  - Warm humidified oxygen, delivered by face mask or endotracheal tube.

o **Invasive internal circulation management:** Central rewarming devices (Zoll, Alsius), thoracic/peritoneal/bladder lavage, extracorporeal membrane oxygenation (ECMO) or cardiopulmonary bypass (CPB)
  - **Central rewarming devices**
  - Newer generation devices that have both a triple lumen function and a large volume infuser with a temperature control system
  - Newer generation devices may reverse trauma associated coagulopathy.
  - If a central venous catheter is considered necessary, it should not be allowed to touch the endocardium .
  - Body cavity lavage: Form of active internal rewarming, suggested use for cardiac instability (VT/VF, cardiac arrest if ECMO/CPB or transfer to center with ECMO/CPB are not available)
  - Thoracic lavage
  - Peritoneal lavage with warmed dialysate
  - ECMO or cardiopulmonary bypass should be considered for patients with severe hypothermia and subsequent cardiac instability.

HYPOTHERMIC CARDIAC ARREST

- **DEFIBRILLATION AND PACING**
  o *Defibrillation is less effective in hypothermia.*
  o For ventricular fibrillation/ventricular tachycardia (VF/VT) defibrillation may be tried up to three times but is then not tried **until the temperature reaches 30^0C.**
  o *Pacing is generally ineffective.* Do not try it unless bradycardia persists when normothermia is reached.
  o Sinus bradycardia may be a physiological response and is not treated specifically.

- **VENTILATION**
  o Normocapnia will be achieved at lower minute volumes than normal and hyperventilation risks cerebral hypoxia through reduction of cerebral blood flow.
  o Aim for a normal CO_2 on ABG (**not** corrected for the patient's temperature).

- **INTUBATION**
  o In a patient with a perfusing rhythm, intubation (or other rough handling of the patient) may precipitate VF, although the evidence for this is mainly animal-based and it is rare.

- **RESUSCITATION DRUGS**
  o Drugs are often ineffective and will undergo reduced metabolism; so these are **withheld below 30^0C then given with twice the time interval between doses** until either normothermia is approached or circulation restored.
  o So, adrenaline would be given about **every 8-10 minutes** once the core temperature is above 30^0 C.

- **CHEST COMPRESSIONS**
  o Hypothermia causes muscular stiffness: chest compressions may be harder work than normal.
  o Make sure that the individual performing chest compressions is swapped frequently.

"Nobody is dead until warm and dead"

Further Reading:
European Resuscitation Council Guidelines for Resuscitation 2015: Section 4. Cardiac arrest in special circumstance [Online]

41. Allergic Reactions
I. ANAPHYLAXIS

- **DEFINITION**
- Anaphylaxis is a severe, life-threatening, generalised or systemic hypersensitivity reaction. It is characterised by rapidly developing life-threatening airway and/or breathing and/or circulation problems usually associated with skin and mucosal changes. Anaphylaxis can be triggered by a very broad range of triggers, but those most commonly identified include food, drugs and venom.
- The relative importance of these varies very considerably with age, with food being particularly important in children and medicinal products being much more common triggers in older people[465].

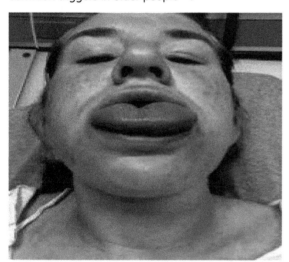

- **Anaphylaxis is likely when all three of the following criteria are met:**
  - o *Acute onset of illness and sudden progression*
  - o *Skin and/ or mucosal changes, e.g. flushing, urticaria, angioedema*
  - o *Life threatening Airway and/ or Breathing and/ or Circulation problems*
- *Skin or mucosal changes alone are not a sign of an anaphylactic reaction.*
- *Skin or mucosal changes can be subtle or absent in up to 20% of reactions, e.g. some patients can have only a decrease in blood pressure, i.e. a circulation problem.*

465 *Emergency treatment of anaphylactic reactions: Guidelines for healthcare providers [Resuscitation Council UK]*

- **PATHOPHYSIOLOGY**
  - o Anaphylaxis can be caused by an either allergic or non-allergic mechanism. The clinical presentation and management is the same regardless of whether the reaction has an allergic or nonallergic mechanism. Allergic anaphylaxis is an example of **immediate type 1 hypersensitivity.**
  - o The response is caused by the binding of an antigen to an antigen-specific antibody leading to mediating mast cell activation. Histamine and other mediators, including leukotrienes, tumour necrosis factor and various cytokines, are released from mast cells and basophils following exposure to this antigen.
  - o This causes bronchial smooth muscle tone to increase (causing wheeze and shortness of breath), decreased vascular tone and increased capillary permeability (leading to hypotension and an urticarial rash). The response is usually **uniphasic**, although a **biphasic response** occurs in approximately 20% of individuals.

- **COMMON AGENTS CAUSING ANAPHYLAXIS INCLUDE:**
  - o **Drugs:**
    - **Antibiotics**: Penicillin is the most common cause of drug induced anaphylaxis,
    - **Aspirin and NSAIDs:** second most common cause of drug induced anaphylaxis.
    - **Angiotensin Converting Enzyme Inhibitors**
  - o **Food:** e.g. peanuts, egg and seafood (food is the most common cause of anaphylaxis in children). The clinical cross-reactivity with other foods in the same group is unpredictable.
  - o **Insect stings**: bees and wasps
  - o **Hereditary C1 esterase inhibitor deficiency:** usually inherited as an autosomal dominant, but also occurs with lymphoma and certain connective tissue disorders.
  - o **Idiopathic**

- **LESS COMMONLY:**
  - o Physical triggers, e.g. exercise, cold
  - o Biological fluids, e.g. transfusions, semen
  - o Latex

- **SIGNS AND SYMPTOMS**
  - **Skin and mucosal**: urticaria, erythema, pruritus
  - **Airway problems:** lip and tongue swelling/ angioedema, nasal congestion, sneezing, tightness of throat/ hoarse voice/ stridor
  - **Breathing problems**: tachypnoea, bronchospasm/ wheeze, increased mucous secretions, exhaustion, confusion, cyanosis, respiratory arrest.
  - **Circulation problems:** hypotension, tachycardia, arrhythmia, myocardial ischemia, cardiac arrest.
  - **Neurological problems:** confusion, agitation, loss of consciousness.
  - **Gastrointestinal:** stomach cramps, nausea, vomiting, diarrhoea
  - **Other:** feeling of impending doom

- **INVESTIGATION**
  - **Mast cell tryptase** is released during the anaphylactic reaction and may be measured in the blood.
  - It reaches its peak blood concentration approximately **1-2 hours** after the reaction.
  - This is useful to aid later diagnosis and treatment and can help in the diagnosis in uncertain cases.
  - The half-life of tryptase is short (approximately 2 hours), and concentrations may be back to normal **within 6-8 hours**, so timing of any blood samples is very important.
  - **Three timed samples:**
    - **Initial** sample **as soon as feasible** after resuscitation has started – do not delay resuscitation to take sample.
    - **Second** sample **at 1-2 hours after** the start of the symptoms.
    - **Third** sample either at **24 hours or in convalescence** (for example in a follow up allergy clinic). This provides baseline tryptase levels - some individuals have an elevated baseline level.

- **TREATMENT OF ANAPHYLAXIS** (see algorithm below)
  - **Epinephrine** is the most important drug in the treatment of anaphylaxis.
  - **Oxygen and fluid resuscitation**
  - **Antihistamines:**
  - **H1 blockers** help to overcome the histamine-induced vasodilatation.
  - **Corticosteroids** are slow acting drugs that take between six and eight hours to reduce the immune-mediated reaction. They may be useful in preventing, or reducing the severity of, a biphasic response.

- **FURTHER MANAGEMENT**
  - Most patients who have suffered an anaphylactic reaction will need admission and observation **for 6 hours.**
  - Patients with the following may need observation for **up to 24 hours:**
    - *Previous history of biphasic reactions or known asthmatics*
    - *Possibility of continuing absorption of allergen (fully eaten peanut butter sandwich)*
    - *Poor access to emergency care*
    - *Presentation in the evening or at night*
    - *Severe reactions with slow onset caused by idiopathic anaphylaxis.*
  - **Biphasic reactions** are not easy to predict. Patients who have suffered an anaphylactic reaction are likely to suffer future episodes and follow-up should be arranged.
  - **Outpatient follow-up** is useful to help identify the allergen and provide training in the use of **an epipen**.
  - Patients should be given an **epipen** and instructions as to how to use it.
  - There is no benefit from providing an additional course of steroids.

URTICARIA (HIVES)

- Histamine mediated **localised oedema of the dermis**.
- It is at one end of the allergic reaction spectrum with anaphylactic shock at the other end.
- Exposure to an allergenic protein produces IgE mediated mast cell degranulation and histamine release.
- This produces vascular dilation and transudation of fluid from the affected vessels.
- Unlike in allergic angioedema and anaphylaxis, this vascular dilatation is limited to the dermis.

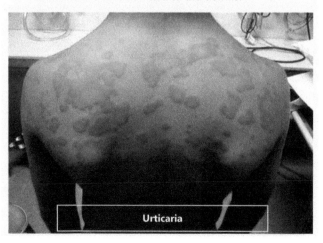

Urticaria

ANAPHYLAXIS ALGORITHM

Anaphylactic Reaction?

⇓

Airway. Breathing, Circulation, Disability, Exposure?

⇓

Diagnosis- look for:
- Acute onset of illness
- Life-threatening Airway and/or Breathing and/or circulation problems
- And usually skin changes

⇓

Adapted from Resuscitation council UK[466]

- **Call for help**
- Lie the patient flat
- Raise patient's legs

⇓

ADRENALINE[2]

⇓

When skills and equipment available:
- Establish Airway
- High flow oxygen
- IV fluid challenge
- Chlorphenamine
- Hydrocortisone

Monitor:
- Pulse oximetry
- ECG
- Blood Pressure

⇓

1. **Life-threatening problems:**
   - **Airway**: intraoral swelling, hoarseness, stridor, swollen tongue
   - **Breathing**: rapid breathing, wheeze, fatigue, cyanosis, SPO2 <92%, confusion
   - **Circulation**: pale, clammy, low BP, faintness, drowsy/ coma

2. **Adrenaline** (give IM unless experienced with IV adrenaline)
IM dose of 1:1000 Adrenaline (repeat after 5min if no better)

- Adult   :   500 mcg IM (0.5 ml)
- Child > 12 years   :   500 mcg IM (0.5 ml)
- Child 6-12 years   :   300 mcg IM (0.3 ml)
- Child < 6 years   :   150 mcg IM (0.15 ml)

Adrenaline IV only if experienced specialists
Titrate: Adults 50 mcg, Children 1mcg/Kg

3. **IV Fluid challenge:**
- Adult: 500-1000 ml
- Child: crystalloid 20ml/Kg

Stop IV colloid if this might be the cause of anaphylaxis

Age	4. Chlorphenamine (IM/ slow IV)	5. Hydrocortisone (IM/ slow IV)
Adult	• 10 mg	• 200 mg
Child > 12 years	• 5 mg	• 100 mg
Child 6-12 years	• 2.5 mg	• 50 mg
Child < 6 years	• 250mcg/Kg	• 25 mg

[466] *Emergency treatment of anaphylactic reactions: Guidelines for healthcare providers [Resuscitation Council UK]*

II. ANGIOEDEMA

OVERVIEW

- Angioedema is a relatively common presentation in the emergency department (ED). Diagnosis of the specific type of angioedema is essential for appropriate treatment; however, many ED physicians may not know how to distinguish different types of angioedema or how to effectively treat less common presentations[467].
- Angioedema may be life-threatening, depending on the underlying cause and the body location affected
- Airway involvement is usually the immediate life-threat
- The possibility of anaphylaxis must be considered

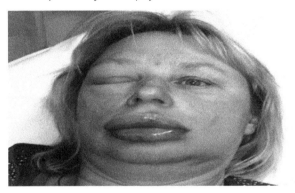

CAUSE

- **Hereditary angioedema (HAE) (type 1 and type 2)**
  - C1 esterase inhibitor deficiency (functionally abnormal C1E-INH leads to bradykinin over-production)
  - Affects 1/50,000 people, 50% present with recurrent episodes of angioedema by age 10 years
  - Type 1 has low antigen and functional levels of C1E-INH
  - Type 2 has normal antigen levels but low functional levels of C1E-INH
  - HAE without C1E-INH deficiency has also been described
- **Acquired**
  - **Medications**
    - **ACE Inhibitors (ACEI)**
      - Up to 1% incidence
      - Angioedema is a class effect and is not dose dependent – symptoms can occur any time from a few hours up to 10 years after the initial dose (winters et al, 2013)
      - More common in african americans and patients on immunosuppressants

- Note that angioedema can occur in patients switched to an angiotensin receptor blocker
    - **NSAIDS**
      - Usually localised to the face +/- uritcaria
    - **Opiates**
    - **Dextrans**
  - **Acquired C1 esterase inhibitor deficiency**
    - Due to an underlying lymphoproliferative disorder and/or an antibody directed against C1E-INH
  - **Food**
  - **Latex**
  - **Local trauma**
  - *Hymenoptera* envenomations and other insect stings
- **Idiopathic** (most cases are thought to be histamine-mediated)

PATHOGENESIS

Angioedema may be histamine-mediated or non-histamine mediated:

- **Histamine-mediated angioedema** may co-exist with urticaria and is mast-cell mediated
  - E.g. anaphylaxis, allergies, some drug reactions
- **Non-histaminergic (bradykinin-mediated) angioedema** tends to be more severe, more prolonged and less responsive to adrenaline
  - Another cause of bradykinin-mediated angioedema is associated with ACEis. Angiotensin-converting enzyme is one of the two enzymes that degrade bradykinin; ACEis can cause accumulation of bradykinin that results in angioedema (ACEi-induced angioedema)[468].

CLINICAL FEATURES

- Abrupt onset of non-pitting, non-pruritic swelling
  - Well demarcated
  - Usually asymmetric
  - Located in non-dependent areas
  - Transient (up to 7 days duration)
- Angioedema may be isolated or co-exist with urticaria
- Areas affected
  - Asymmetric swelling of the lips and face
  - Tongue, the floor of the mouth, neck, and eyelids
  - May affect extremities, genitalia or viscera (e.g. Intensitines)
- Features of significant airway involvement:

[467] Lombardi C, Crivellaro M, Dama A, Senna G, Gargioni S, Passalacqua G Chest. 2005 Aug; 128(2):976-9.

[468] Kaplan AP, Joseph K, Silverberg M J Allergy Clin Immunol. 2002 Feb; 109(2):195-209.

- o Dyspnea, dysphagia, dysphonia, odynophagia, stridor, hoarseness, and drooling
  - o Can progress to complete airway obstruction and death
- Features of gastrointestinal involvement:
  - o Abdominal pain, nausea, vomiting, altered bowel habit
  - o May mimic an acute surgical abdomen
- Previous episodes
- Identify triggers
  - o Exposures (may not be new, e.g. 40% of ACEI-related angioedema occurs months to years after initiation)
  - o HAE patients may have prodroma symptoms
    - ▪ E.g. erythema marginatum, an erythematous serpentine but nonpruritic and non-raised rash (do not confuse with urticaria)
  - o Family history

INVESTIGATIONS

- There are no point-of-care tests that can guide management in the emergency situation, but investigations may help guide long-term management.

Bedside

- Fibreoptic laryngoscopy (significant airway swelling can occur in rare cases even in the absence of clinical features suggesting significant airway involvement)

Laboratory

- Identify underlying cause
  - o **C1 esterase inhibitor (C1E-INH) assays** (low/ abnormal in HAE)
  - o **C4 levels** (low in HAE attacks, usually normal between attacks)
  - o **Serial Tryptase Levels** (may be elevated in anaphylaxis/ mast cell-mediated angioedema)

Imaging

- CT abdomen may show evidence of angioedema in patients presenting with abdominal pain:
  - o May involve GI and GU tracts
  - o Angioedema of the visceral organs is often accompanied by adjacent fluid
  - o involvement may be multifocal or asymmetric (not always be diffuse or concentric)
- CT neck primarily has a role in excluding conditions that may mimic angioedema (e.g. soft tissue infection)
  - o Glossomegaly is common
  - o Shows the extent of airway involvement

MANAGEMENT
Resuscitation

- Airway obstruction is the potential life-threat in most patients with angioedema
  - o If stable and cooperative, awake fiberoptic intubation (AFOI) with anaesthetist and ENT involvement is preferred
    - ▪ Be aware that failed attempts at intubation may worsen airway compromise
  - o If unstable with hypoxia and progressive airway obstruction, then laryngoscopy with a **'double setup'** emergency surgical airway should be attempted
- Hypovolaemic shock may also occur due to vasodilation and increased vascular permeability
  - o Fluid resuscitation
  - o Vasopressors

Specific therapy

- **FFP**
- **Therapies for HAE attacks**
  - o These include:
    - ▪ **Icatibant** – a bradykinin 2 receptor inhibitor
    - ▪ **Ecallantide** – a kallikrein inhibitor (kallikrein is the enzyme that produces bradykinin from high-molecular-weight kininogen (HMWK))
    - ▪ **C1E-INH concentrate** – C1 esterase inhibitor blocks the pathways that produce (the C1-INH concentrate may be plasma-derived or recombinant)
- Role of adrenaline, steroids and antihistamines
  - o Unlikely to be effective for ACEI-related angioedema
  - o Should be administered if the underlying cause of angioedema is uncertain (i.e. anaphylaxis is possible)

DISPOSITION

- All angioedema patients with potential airway involvement should be observed in a high visibility area until marked resolution has occurred
- This often requires admission to an HDU/ICU
- Admission to hospital, rather than in ED, is preferred in the following situations (Winters et al, 2013):
  - o Previous history of angioedema
  - o Tongue edema
  - o Pharyngeal edema (palate, uvula)
  - o Laryngeal edema (true vocal cords, false vocal cords, arytenoids, aryepiglottic folds, epiglottis; the term upper airway oedema is probably more useful)
  - o Lack of improvement during the ED course
- Patients with isolated angioedema of the face or lips and be usually be observed in ED for 4 to 8 hours for progression of symptoms, then discharged

42. Visual loss - Atraumatic

I. TRANSIENT VISUAL LOSS

INTRODUCTION

- Transient loss of vision is an ophthalmological symptom which instills apprehension in both the minds of the patient and the ophthalmologist. The patient is usually worried about a permanent loss of vision and the physician about a serious underlying condition.

ETIOLOGY

- The term Transient loss of vision can be used for episodes of reversible visual loss lasting less than 24 hours. It can be monocular or binocular.
- **Transient monocular loss of vision** is caused most commonly by a lesion anterior to the chiasm, at the level of the eyes or optic nerve, whereas **binocular loss of vision** could be of chiasmal or retro chiasmal origin or it could be due to the bilateral involvement of the eyes or optic nerve.

Common causes:
- **Monocular transient loss of vision include:**
  - **Amaurosis fugax",**
  - Thromboembolic or stenotic vascular diseases,
  - Vasospasm,
  - Retinal migraine,
  - Closed angle glaucoma,
  - Papilledema, etc.
- **Bilateral transient loss of vision may be caused by:**
  - Occipital epilepsy, Complex migraines,
  - Papilloedema, Hypoperfusion, etc.

TREATMENT / MANAGEMENT

It is very important to distinguish whether the episode of TVL is due to high-risk cause or a low-risk cause.
- **Management of TVL due to embolism** is directed to the underlying cause. In patients with a cardiac source, treatment is anticoagulation and proper management of the underlying cardiac cause.
- **Internal carotid artery stenosis** may be managed with antiplatelet therapy, management of systemic risk factors, carotid endarterectomy or stenting if indicated.
- **Giant cell arteritis** is managed with corticosteroid therapy. **Retinal vasospasm** could be treated with Aspirin or Calcium channel blockers.
- **A retinal migraine** is controlled by conventional migraine treatments.
- **Angle-closure glaucoma** is also treated as per standard therapies for the condition.

1. AMAUROSIS FUGAX

INTRODUCTION

- In amaurosis fugax, the loss of vision is usually unilateral, painless and transient[469]. In most cases, the vision loss may vary from a few seconds to a few minutes.

ETIOLOGY

- Amaurosis fugax is a result of an **occlusion or stenosis** of the internal carotid artery circulation.

EPIDEMIOLOGY

- Amaurosis fugax usually occurs in patients over the age of 50 who have other vascular risk factors which include hypertension, hypercholesterolemia, smoking, previous episodes of transient ischemic attacks (TIAs), and claudication.
- The risk of hemispheric stroke in patients with amaurosis fugax is estimated to be 2% per year and 3% per year for those presenting with retinal emboli.

HISTOPATHOLOGY

- During the retinal examination, one may see the cholesterol plaque lodged within a retinal vessel.
- It is known as a **Hollenhorst plaque**, and the cholesterol particle appears refractile yellow and bright.

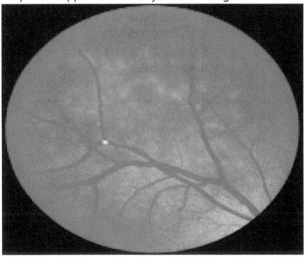

TREATMENT / MANAGEMENT

- Treatment is first aimed at controlling and treating the underlying vascular risk factors, such as hypertension, diabetes, and hyperlipidemia.
- Refer patient to Medical team for further evaluation and management.

469 Bernstein EF. Amaurosis fugax, Springer-Verlag, New York 1987. p.286.

II. CENTRAL RETINAL ARTERY OCCLUSION

INTRODUCTION

- Central retinal artery occlusion (CRAO) is an ocular emergency. Patients typically present with profound, acute, painless monocular visual loss—with 80% of affected individuals having a final visual acuity of counting fingers or worse.
- CRAO is the ocular analogue of a cerebral stroke—and, as such, the clinical approach and management are relatively similar to the management of stroke, in which clinicians treat the acute event, identify the site of vascular occlusion, and try to prevent further occurrences.
- The incidence of CRAO is approximately 1 to 2 in 100,000,[470] with a male predominance and mean age of 60-65 years.

RISK FACTORS

- The major risk factors for CRAO can be divided into nonarteritic and arteritic.
- **Nonarteritic.** More than 90% of CRAOs are nonarteritic in origin. Ipsilateral carotid artery atherosclerosis is the most common cause of retinal artery occlusion with a prevalence as high as 70% reported among patients with CRAO or branch retinal artery occlusion[471]. Other causes of nonarteritic retinal artery occlusion include cardiogenic embolism, hematological conditions (sickle cell disease, hypercoagulable states, leukemia, lymphoma, etc.), and other vascular diseases, such as carotid artery dissection, moyamoya disease, and Fabry disease.
- **Arteritic.** CRAO of arteritic etiology is mostly caused by giant cell arteritis, although other vasculitic disorders such as Susac syndrome, systemic lupus erythematosus, polyarteritis nodosa, and granulomatosis with polyangiitis have also been associated with retinal artery occlusion.

SIGNS AND SYMPTOMS

- Patients with CRAO usually present with sudden and profound unilateral loss of vision.
- In a study of 260 eyes with CRAO, 74% had presenting visual acuity of counting fingers or worse, while the remainder showed some degree of macular sparing that perfused the fovea with resultant better visual acuity[472].

- On examination, a relative afferent pupillary defect occurs regardless of the visual acuity or macular sparing.
- **Classic ophthalmoscopic signs** include retinal edema (ischemic retinal whitening), **cherry red spot** (due to underlying normal choroidal circulation), retinal arteriolar attenuation, and, in the acute phase, segmentation of blood in retinal arterioles (also known as box-carring).
- A retinal embolus may be visible in up to 40% of patients[473].
- The embolic material can be a shiny cholesterol plaque, gray-white platelet plaque, or white calcium plaque.
- Associated signs and symptoms may point toward a specific etiology such as headache and scalp tenderness in giant cell arteritis, or contralateral sensory or motor deficits in carotid artery disease.

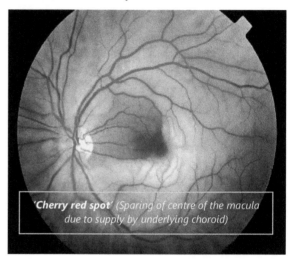

'Cherry red spot' *(Sparing of centre of the macula due to supply by underlying choroid)*

EVALUATION

- Urgent ESR and CRP to exclude GCA.
- TIA and vasculitis work up as per amaurosis fugax

TREATMENT

Treatment is unproven but includes:

- Immediate ocular massage
- anterior chamber paracentesis
- IOP reduction with acetazolamide (e.g. 500mg IV) or Timolol (0.5% topical drops bd)
- Breathe into a paper bag (respiratory acidosis induces retinal vasodilation)

---

[470] Rumelt S et al. Am J Ophthalmol. 1999;128(6):733-738.

[471] Babikian V et al. Cerebrovasc Dis. 2001;12:108-113.

[472] Hayreh SS, Zimmerman MB. Am J Ophthalmol. 2005;140(3):376.e1-e18.

[473] Sharma S et al. Arch Ophthalmol. 1998;116(12):1602.

III. CENTRAL RETINAL VEIN OCCLUSION

INTRODUCTION

- Sudden painless loss of vision, in a patient with risk factors and a '**blood and thunder**' retinal appearance (**Stormy sunset appearance).**
- Retinal vein occlusion (RVO) is a common cause of vision loss in older individuals, and the second most common retinal vascular disease after diabetic retinopathy[474].
- There are two distinct types, classified according to the site of occlusion: in central RVO (CRVO), the occlusion is at or proximal to the lamina cribrosa of the optic nerve, where the central retinal vein exits the eye[475].
- CRVO is further divided into the categories of perfused (nonischemic) and nonperfused (ischemic), each of which has implications for prognosis and treatment

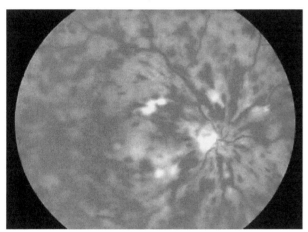

Stormy sunset' appearance

RISK FACTORS

- Glaucoma
- Old age
- Hypertension
- Diabetes mellitus
- Hypercoagulable state
- Atherosclerosis (vein is compressed by adjacent artery)
- Retrobulbar compressive lesions (e.g. Thyroid disease, orbital tumour)
- Vasculitis

SYMPTOMS AND SIGNS

- **History**
  - Sudden and painless loss of vision
  - Assess for risk factors/ underlying causes
- **Examination**

---

[474] Cugati S, Wang JJ. Retinal vein occlusion and vascular mortality: pooled data Analysis of 2 population-based cohorts. Ophthalmology 114, 520–524.

[475] Mitchell P, Smith W, Chang A. Prevalence and associations of retinal vein occlusion in Australia. The Blue Mountains Eye Study. Arch. Ophthalmol. 114, 1243–1247.

- **Visual acuity** – variable depending on severity and duration since onset
- **A Marcus-Gunn pupil** may be present if ischemic CRVO (Relative Afferent Pupillary Defect = RAPD)
- **Red reflex** – may be abnormal
- **Fundoscopy** – large areas of haemorrhage:
  - **Non-Ischemic CRVO**: dilated tortuous veins, retinal haemorrhages, cotton wool spots, retinal oedema, disc swelling.
  - **Ischemic CRVO** (more severe): classic '**blood and thunder**' appearance (**Stormy sunset appearance)** from widespread haemorrhages that obscure most fundal details.

MANAGEMENT

- **Refer to an ophthalmologist**: photocoagulation may be performed if there is neovascularisation.
- **Refer to a physician** for ongoing work-up and treatment of underlying causes
- **Screen for risk factors** (cardiovascular disease, diabetes, vasculitis, etc)
- **Consider low-dose aspirin** (unproven)

IV. VITREOUS HAEMORRHAGE & RETINAL TEARS

- The vitreous body represents 80% of the eye and is 99% water and 1% hyaluronic acid/collagen.
- It fills the space between the lens and the retina.
- It is adherent to the retina in three places: anteriorly at the border of the retina, at the macula, and at the optic nerve.
- With increasing age, the vitreous may liquefy and the collagen fibres clump together, causing the vitreous to collapse.
- The pockets left by the collapsed vitreous after often seen as 'floaters'.
- Vitreous haemorrhage can occur due to rupture of abnormal blood vessels or due to stress on normal vessels.

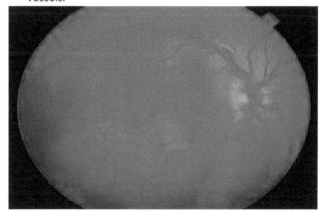

RISK FACTORS

- The population at risk for vitreous hemorrhage will have the demographic and clinical characteristics according to its common causes. For example, poorly controlled diabetics with end-organ damage such as proliferative diabetic retinopathy are at high risk.
- People younger than 40 with vitreous hemorrhage often have a history of recent ocular trauma whereas older, non-diabetic populations with vitreous hemorrhage often suffered an acute PVD and/or retinal tear.
- Although anticoagulants and antiplatelet agents do not likely cause spontaneous vitreous hemorrhage, they may enhance bleeding from pathology[476].
- Notably, however, the Early Treatment of Diabetic Retinopathy Study did not show increased risk of vitreous hemorrhage among aspirin users[477]. Patients with systemic coagulation disorders and blood dyscrasias such as leukemia and thrombocytopenia may have an increased risk of vitreous hemorrhage, but these cases are rare.

CLINICAL FEATURES

- Early or mild haemorrhage may present as floaters, cobwebs, haze, shadows, or a red hue. In large bleeds, visual acuity may be severely reduced.
- Loss of red reflex.
- Retina is difficult to visualise on fundoscopy.

ED MANAGEMENT

- Sit the patient head up to allow blood to collect inferiorly.
- Refer to ophthalmology.
- Urgent assessment is required to assess for an associated retinal tear.

V. RETINAL DETACHMENT

- This is the separation of the sensory retina from the underlying pigmented retinal epithelium.
- **Findings:**
  - **Ultrasound:** The detached retina is visible as a free floating echogenic membrane separated from the globe posteriorly. It moves with eye movement and is attached at the optic disc.
  - **Ophthalmoscopy**: The detached retina appears corrugated and partially opaque.
  - **Funduscopy:** the detached portion will appear out of focus.

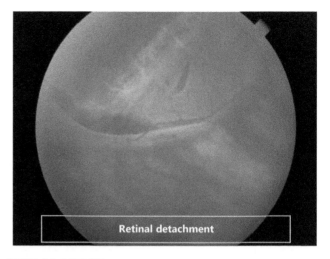

Retinal detachment

RISK FACTORS

- Lattice degeneration
- Peripheral retinal breaks
- Pathologic myopia
- Previous intraocular surgery
- Trauma
- Previous retinal detachment
- Family history
- **Lattice degeneration** is considered the most important peripheral retinal degeneration process that predisposes to a rhegmatogenous retinal detachment[478].
- Other peripheral lesions having slight increased risk of retinal detachment include Ora bays, meridional folds and complexes, and cystic retinal tufts.

CLINICAL FEATURES

- **History**
  - **Painless loss of vision** (central, peripheral or both)
  - Recent history of increased numbers of **flashes** (due to traction on the retina) and **floaters** (due to haemorrhage and debris in the vitreous).
  - Presence of a **dark shadow or curtain** moving over the visual field of the affected eye.

- **Examination**
  - **Visual acuity**: reduced if the macula is involved.
  - **Red reflex**: abnormal; a mobile detached retina may be visible.
  - **Visual fields**: reduced.
  - **Pupils:** a mild relative afferent pupillary defect (RAPD) may be present depending the size of the retinal detachment
  - **Ophthalmoscopy:** The detached retina appears corrugated and partially opaque.
  - **Funduscopy:** the detached portion will appear out of focus.

476 Witmer MT, Cohen SM. Oral anticoagulation and the risk of vitreous hemorrhage and retinal tears in eyes with acute posterior vitreous detachment. Retina. 2013 Mar;33(3):621-6.

477 Early Treatment Diabetic Retinopathy Study design and baseline patient characteristics. ETDRS report number 7. Ophthalmology. 1991 May;98(5Suppl):741-56.

478 Lewis H. Peripheral Retinal Degenerations and the Risk of Retinal Detachment. Am J Ophthalmol 2003; 136:155–160.

INVESTIGATION

o **Direct funduscopy** in the Emergency Department cannot rule out retinal detachment
o **Ultrasound** is a useful investigation for diagnosing retinal detachment in the ED.

MANAGEMENT

o Urgent ophthalmologist opinion.
o Minimise activity: bed rest with toilet privileges.
o Treatment of underlying cause (especially if exudative).
o Surgical options include laser photocoagulation, cryotherapy, pneumatic retinopexy, vitrectomy, and scleral buckle.
o Close follow up is required.

VI. POSTERIOR VITREOUS DETACHMENT

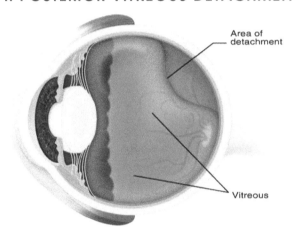

- Occurs when the vitreous membrane separates from the retina.

RISK FACTORS

o Increasing Age
o Diabetes Mellitus
o Eye Trauma
o Myopia
o Recent Cataract Surgery

CLINICAL FEATURES

o **Flashes** of light (photopsia)
o Increased numbers of **floaters**
o **A ring floaters** to the temporal side of central vision
o A feeling of heaviness in the eye

- **Weiss' ring** (an irregular ring of translucent floating material in the vitreous)
- There is a small associated risk of retinal detachment in the 6-12 weeks following a posterior vitreous detachment.
- Retinal detachment can be distinguished from posterior vitreous detachment by the presence of:

o A dense shadow in the periphery that spreads centrally
o A 'curtain drawing across the eye'
o Straight lines suddenly appearing curved (**positive Amsler grid test)**
o Central visual loss and decreased visual acuity

DIFFERENTIAL DIAGNOSIS

- Retinal detachment
- Asteroid hyalosis/Synchysis scintillans
- Vitreous syneresis
- Vitreous inflammation (infectious and non infectious)
- Vitreous haemorrhage
- Vitreous amyloidosis
- Ocular large cell lymphoma

VII. OPTIC NEURITIS

- optic neuritis is a demyelinating inflammation of the optic nerve.
- It affects the optic nerve peripheral to the **optic chiasm.**
- The commonest cause is **Multiple Sclerosis (MS).**
- It usually presents with **sudden onset loss of vision**, which can be partial or complete, and painful eye movements. It can be the first presentation of multiple sclerosis or occur as part of a relapse.

- **OTHER CAUSES INCLUDE:**
  o **Infections** e.g. Herpes zoster, Lyme disease
  o **Autoimmune disorders** e.g. SLE, Neurosarcoidosis
  o **Poisoning** e.g. Methanol
  o **Diabetes mellitus**
  o **Vitamin B12 deficiency**
- Any sudden increase (i.e. over a 24-48-hour period) in symptoms of MS should be urgently assessed by a neurologist with expertise in the management of the condition.
- Daily IV Methylprednisolone 500mg infusion/4hr X 5/7 treatment should be considered, and if initiated, should be done so at the earliest opportunity.

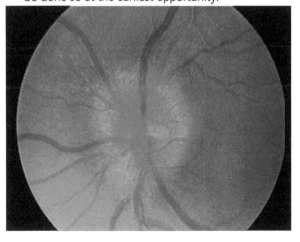

VIII. TEMPORAL ARTERITIS

- Temporal arteritis, also known as **Giant Cell Arteritis (GCA),** is a type of chronic vasculitis characterized by granulomatous inflammation in the walls of medium and large arteries.
- It usually affects people over 50 years of age.

CLINICAL FEATURES

- Headache
- Scalp tenderness
- Jaw claudication
- Amaurosis fugax or sudden blindness (typically unilateral).
- Some patients also present with systemic features such as fever, fatigue, anorexia, weight loss, and depression.
- It is associated with polymyalgia rheumatica (PMR) in 50% of cases (bilateral upper arm stiffness, aching, and tenderness; pelvic girdle pain).
- Visual loss occurs early in the course of disease and, once established, it rarely improves.
- Early treatment with **high-dose corticosteroids (40-60 mg prednisolone daily)** is imperative to prevent further visual loss and other ischaemic complications.
- An urgent referral for specialist evaluation (same day ophthalmology assessment for those with visual symptoms) and **temporal artery biopsy should** also be organised.

IX. RETINITIS PIGMENTOSA

- Retinitis pigmentosa is a group of inherited disorders characterized by:
- Night blindness (nyctalopia)
- Loss of peripheral vision (tunnel vision)
- Altered colour vision
- Pigmentary retinopathy

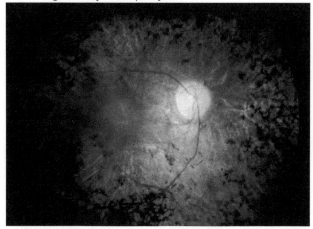

A fundoscopic examination revealing **bony spicule-shaped pigment deposits** in the periphery with preservation of the macula is characteristic of retinitis pigmentosa.

- Retinitis pigmentosa can be passed on by all forms of inheritance, but 50% of patients have no known affected relatives.
- There is often also an association with rare systemic disorders including:
- Laurence-Moon-Biedl-Bardet syndrome
- Abetalipoproteinaemia
- Refsum's disease
- Kearns-Sayre syndrome
- Usher's disease
- Freidreich's ataxia
- These patients should be referred on for genetic counselling and an ophthalmology assessment.

X. DIABETIC MACULOPATHY

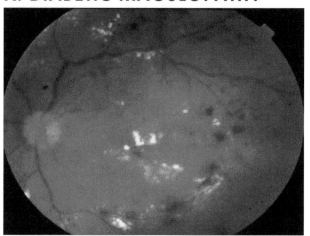

Above fundoscopic images are consistent with that of diabetic maculopathy and patient should be referred for an ophthalmology opinion with 4 weeks.

- The following are the recommended referral criteria for diabetic retinopathy:
- **Referral for an opinion within 4 weeks if:**
- There is an unexplained drop in visual acuity
- There are hard exudates within 1 disc diameter of the fovea
- Macular oedema is present
- There are unexplained retinal findings
- Pre-proliferative or severe retinopathy is present
- **Referral to ophthalmology specialist within 1 week if:**
- There is new vessel formation
- There is evidence of pre-retinal and/or vitreous haemorrhage
- Rubeosis iridis is present

- **Emergency referral to ophthalmology specialist on the same day if:**
- There is sudden loss of vision
- There is evidence of retinal detachment

XI. OCULAR NERVES PALSY

Nerve	Presentation & Causes
CN 3	• Inability to move the eye superiorly, inferiorly and medially • Ptosis • Pupil fixed and dilated (mydriasis) • The eye rest, sits in the **"down and out"** position due to preservation of the superior oblique (moving the eye downwards) and lateral rectus (moving the eye outwards). **Causes:** • Aneurysm of PCA • Tumour • Trauma • Microvascular disease: DM, HTN • Infection: Herpes zoster

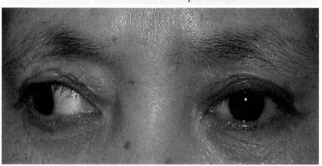

Nerve	Presentation & Causes
CN 4	• Failure of depression when the eye is in the adducted position (i.e. inability to look down towards the nose) • May manifest as vertical diplopia when reading/ going down stairs. • Patient classically have a compensatory head tilt **Causes:** • Trauma • Vascular disease: DM, HTN • Demyelinating disorders: Multiple sclerosis • Idiopathic • Congenital

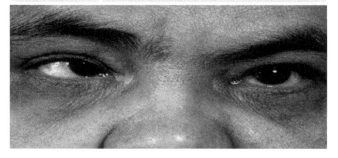

Nerve	Presentation & Causes
CN 6	• Failure of abduction • Manifests as horizontal diplopia, that is worse when looking towards affected side **Common Causes:** • Trauma • Vascular disease: DM, HTN • Idiopathic **Less common causes:** • Raised ICP, Tumour, Aneurysm, • Thrombosis of cavernous sinus, • MS, Post-viral syndrome in children

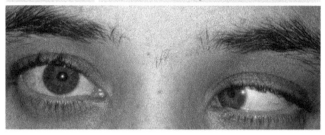

Ocular muscles innervation: **LR6 (SO4) Rest 3**

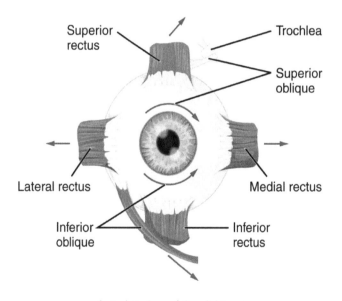

Anterior view of the right eye

❖ **The superior rectus** moves the eye up and in.

❖ **The inferior oblique** pulls the eye up and out

❖ **The inferior rectus** pulls the eye down and in.

❖ **The superior oblique** pulls the eye down and out.

❖ **The lateral rectus** is responsible for moving the eye out

❖ **The medial rectus** is responsible for moving the eye in.

43. Red Eye

I. ATRAUMATIC RED EYE

1. CONJUNCTIVITIS

- Conjunctivitis is the most common ocular condition diagnosed at emergency departments (ED), although it is generally not an emergent condition. Bacterial conjunctivitis is an infection of the eye's mucous membrane, the conjunctiva, which extends from the back surface of the eyelids (palpebral and tarsal conjunctiva), into the fornices, and onto the globe (bulbar conjunctiva) until it fuses with the cornea at the limbus.

ETIOLOGY

- **Acute bacterial conjunctivitis** is primary due to Staphylococcus aureus, Streptococcus pneumoniae, and Haemophilus influenzae. Other pathogens responsible for acute disease are Pseudomonas aeruginosa, Moraxella lacunata, Streptococcus viridans, and Proteus mirabilis. These organisms may be spread from hand to eye contact or through adjacent mucosal tissues colonization such as nasal or sinus mucosa.
- **Hyperacute conjunctivitis** is primarily due to Neisseria gonorrhoeae, which is a sexually transmitted disease. Neisseria meningitidis is also in the differential and is important to consider as it can lead to potentially fatal meningeal or systemic infection.
- **Chronic conjuctivitis** is primarily due to Chlamydia trachomatis. However, chronically ill, debilitated, or hospital patients can become colonized with other virulent bacteria responsible for chronic conjunctivitis. Staphylococcus aureus and Moraxella lacunata may also cause chronic conjunctivitis in patients with associated blepharitis.

RISK FACTORS

- Poor hygenic habits
- Poor contact lens hygiene
- Contaminated cosmetics
- Crowded living or social conditions such elementary schools, military barracks etc
- Ocular diseases including dry eye, blepharitis, and anatomic abnormalities of the ocular surface and lids
- Recent ocular surgery, exposed sutures or ocular foreign bodies
- Chronic use of topical medications
- Immune compromise

PRIMARY PREVENTION

- Handwashing and good hygiene techniques

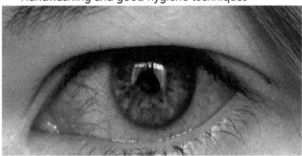

HISTORY

- Patients may complain of redness, discharge, crusting and sticking or gluing of the eyelids upon waking, blurry vision, light sensitivity, and irritation.

PHYSICAL EXAMINATION
Symptoms
- Red eye: Either unilateral, bilateral, or sequentially bilateral
- Discharge: Classically purulent, but may be thin or thick muco-purulent or watery
- Irritation, burning, stinging, discomfort
- Tearing
- Light sensitivity
- Intolerance to contact lens
- Fluctuating or decreased vision

Signs
- Bulbar conjunctival injection
- Palpebral conjunctival papillary reaction
- Muco-purulent or watery discharge
- Chemosis
- Lid erythema

DIAGNOSTIC PROCEDURES

- **Gram stain & Cultures:** Primarily used in cases of atypical conjunctivitis such as hyperacute or chronic/non-responding. Also important in neonatal.
- There has not been a role for these tests in routine cases due to the cost and high likelihood of success with either empiric treatment or observation
- **RPS Adeno Detector:** May be used to establish diagnosis of viral conjunctivitis instead of bacterial.
- Treatment of infective conjunctivitis with topical antibiotics is controversial.

- Antibiotics may lead to quicker clinical and microbiological remission compared with placebo, at least in the first 2-5 days of therapy. This may result in decreased transmission of the disease and lower incidences within the population[479].
- **Always prescribe topical antibiotics:**
  - Purulent / mucopurulent secretion and patient discomfort and ocular redness
  - Patients and staff in nursing homes, neonatal units, critical care units etc
  - Children going to nursery
  - Contact lens wearers
  - Patients with dry eyes or corneal epithelial disease
- **Usually prescribe topical antibiotics:**
  - Purulent / mucopurulent secretion and severe ocular redness
  - Patients with previously known external ocular disease
- **Delayed prescription or no antibiotic treatment:**
  - Patients who do not want immediate antibiotic treatment
  - Patients with moderate mucopurulent discharge and little or no discomfort
  - Co-operative and well informed patients

2. NON-TRAUMATIC SUBCONJUNCTIVAL HAEMORRHAGE

- Subconjunctival hemorrhage is a common eye disease that is caused by the rupture of a conjunctival vessel, resulting in a local extravasation of blood into the subconjunctival tissue and subconjunctival episcleral space. Spontaneous in 50-87% of cases; may be recurrent. Valsalva manoeuvre (e.g. coughing, straining, vomiting) producing rise in central venous pressure
- Due to the benign natural course of the disorder, therapy is normally not necessary; however, a subconjunctival hemorrhage frequently causes considerable alarm to the patient, therefore, most affected patients may have sought medical help[480].

3. KERATITIS & KERATOCONJUNCTIVITIS

- Keratoconjunctivitis refers to an inflammatory process that involves both the conjunctiva – conjunctivitis – and the superficial cornea – keratitis – which can occur in association with viral, bacterial, autoimmune, toxic, and allergic etiologies.

[479] Sheikh A, Hurwitz B. Antibiotics versus placebo for acute bacterial conjunctivitis. Cochrane Database Syst Rev 2006 Issue 2. Art No: CD001211. DOI: 10.1002/14651858.CD001211.pub2.

[480] Tarlan B1, Kiratli H. Subconjunctival hemorrhage: risk factors and potential indicators. Clin Ophthalmol. 2013; 7:1163–1170. 10.2147/OPTH.S35062 [PubMed]

ETIOLOGY

- **Infectious keratoconjunctivitis**:
  - Viral: accounting for the majority of all-comers suspected of an infectious etiology. HSV epithelial keratitis usually resolves spontaneously,
  - Bacterial: rare
- **Non-infectious keratoconjunctivitis**:
  - Allergic,
  - Toxic, or
  - immune-mediated: Collagen vascular diseases, like rheumatoid arthritis, granulomatosis with polyangiitis, polyarteritis nodosa, relapsing polychondritis, systemic lupus erythematosus, and others

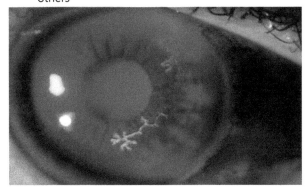

- Dual staining with Rose-Bengal and fluorescein stain is a very important clinical tool to make a diagnosis of HSV epithelial disease. Fluorescein stain makes the dendrites and geographical ulcers more evident by staining the base of ulcer, and Rose-Bengal stains the cells at the margin of the ulcer, which are loaded with viruses.
- Symptoms common to keratoconjunctivitis, regardless of etiology, include eye discomfort/irritation, pruritis, light sensitivity, minor blurring of vision (often intermittent), epiphora. Common signs include conjunctival injection, conjunctival chemosis, and eye discharge.
- Systemic conditions, including autoimmune conditions, atopy, and thyroid disease, should be discerned during the historical investigation.
- For HSV necrotizing stromal keratitis, treatment has to be given at the earliest to avoid corneal melt and subsequent perforation. The loading dose of antiviral both topical acyclovir (3%) and oral (acyclovir 400 mg 5 times daily) is given for the initial three days. Topical steroid is added on the third day.
- For bacterial keratitis, patients are started on fortified topical antibiotics empirically until culture reports are available. Fortified cefazolin 5% or vancomycin and fluoroquinolones or tobramycin or gentamicin give complete coverage against both gram-positive and gram-negative organisms.
- Refer all patients for ophthalmologist review

4. ACUTE ANGLE CLOSURE GLAUCOMA

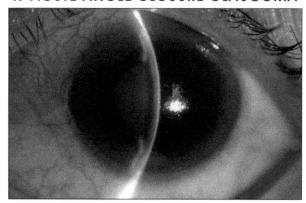

- AACG is defined as closure (or narrowing) of the anterior chamber angle, causing elevated intraocular pressure and eventual optic nerve damage.

RISK FACTORS
- Female gender (Female to male ratio 4:1)
- African or Asian ethnicity
- Hypermetropia (long-sightedness)
- Increasing age (anterior chamber becomes shallower)
- Family history of glaucoma
- Diabetes mellitus

CLINICAL
- Severe eye pain
- Loss of vision or decreased visual acuity
- Congestion and circumcorneal erythema
- Corneal oedema and cloudy
- A fixed semi-dilated ovoid pupil
- Nausea and vomiting
- Preceding episodes of blurred vision or haloes

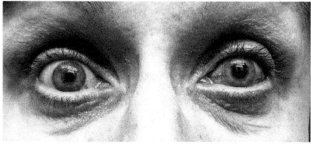

Acute Angle-Closure Glaucoma | NEJM

ED MANAGEMENT
- **Topical 2% Pilocarpine drops** to both eyes **every 15 minutes**
- **Topical 0.5% Timolol drops**
- IV Morphine titrated to pain
- IV anti-emetic e.g. Metoclopramide
- IV Acetazolamide 500mg
- Urgent referral to on-call ophthalmologists
- Definitive treatment is a **laser iridotomy or iridectomy**

5. EPISCLERITIS

- Episcleritis is defined as idiopathic inflammation of the episclera, which is the vascularized tissue between conjunctiva and sclera[481].
- Episcleritis risk factors include female gender (70%), age (fifth decade of life), and systemic autoimmune conditions.
- Redness is usually focal in the interpalpebral zone (the area visible when the eye is open).

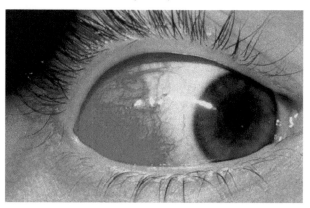

CLINICAL
- Pain: Mild irritation is possible; chronic or nodular episcleritis may have pain
- Photophobia: None
- Response to topical anesthetic: May improve irritation
- Response to phenylephrine: Resolution of episcleral redness after 10-15 minutes (key feature)
- Visual Acuity: Normal
- Pupils: Normal
- Anterior Chamber: Clear
- Fluorescein: No uptake

DIAGNOSIS
- The key feature in distinguishing between episcleritis and scleritis is **the patient's response to phenylephrine**.
- The vessels in episcleritis will constrict and the eye redness will improve; this is not true of scleritis.
- Additionally, the inflamed vessels of episcleritis will move with gentle pressure from a cotton-tipped applicator.
- Patients with episcleritis are treated with topical lubricants and oral non-steroidal anti-inflammatory drugs.
- Patients can follow up with primary care for continued management and for workup of any underlying cause.
- Patients should be given return precautions for symptoms of scleritis (worsening pain).

481 Gilani CJ, Yang A, Yonkers M, Boysen-Osborn M. Differentiating Urgent and Emergent Causes of Acute Red Eye for the Emergency Physician. West J Emerg Med. 2017;18(3):509-517. doi:10.5811/westjem.2016.12.31798

6. SCLERITIS

- Anterior scleritis is defined as scleral inflammation that is frequently associated with autoimmune systemic disease.
- Fifty percent of patients with anterior scleritis have associated autoimmune, systemic disease (rheumatoid arthritis, granulomatosis with polyangiitis, formerly known as Wegener's granulomatosis), while 4-10% have associated infectious processes.
- There are three forms of anterior scleritis: diffuse, nodular, and necrotizing, the latter of which usually causes the most severe pain and has the worst outcome.
- The sclera may have a typical blush in natural light as uveal tissue may be apparent through a thin and inflamed sclera.

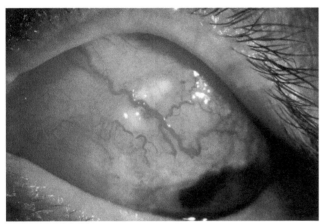

Necrotizing scleritis | Moran CORE

CLINICAL

- Pain: Gradual onset, severe, boring, and piercing eye pain. Pain is worse at night, with extraocular movements, and may radiate to the face[482]
- Photophobia: May be present
- Response to topical anesthetic: Should not improve pain
- Response to phenylephrine: Redness does not improve
- Visual Acuity: Normal or decreased, depending on extent of the disease
- Pupils: Normal
- Anterior Chamber: Clear
- Fluorescein: May show peripheral keratitis, which is more common in the necrotizing form.

MANAGEMENT

- Patients with anterior scleritis should be referred emergently to ophthalmology to initiate treatment and to prevent scleral melting.
- If there is excessive scleral thinning, patients are at risk for perforation and an eye shield should be placed.

7. ANTERIOR UVEITIS (IRITIS)

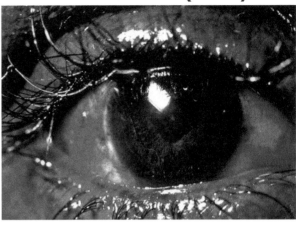

- A painful eye with perilimbal injection, photophobia and an irregular pupil are all indicative of anterior uveitis.
- The presence of keratitic precipitates, inflammatory cells and flare confirm the diagnosis. Anterior uveitis is defined as idiopathic inflammation of the uvea (iris, choroid, and/or ciliary body), causing redness and pain. Risk factors include systemic diseases (spondyloarthropathies), infectious processes (syphilis, tuberculosis, Lyme disease, toxoplasmosis, herpesviruses, cytomegalovirus), and certain drugs (rifabutin, cidofovir, sulfas, moxifloxacin). Patients present with pain, diffuse redness pronounced at the limbus (ciliary flush), consensual photophobia, tearing, and possibly decreased vision.
- Pain: Moderate to severe
- Photophobia: Consensual photophobia (key feature)
- Response to topical anesthetic: Should not improve pain
- Response to phenylephrine: Redness does not improve
- Visual Acuity: Normal or decreased
- Pupils: Constricted or irregular
- Anterior Chamber: Cells and flare present
- Fluorescein: May reveal dendrites if the underlying cause is HSV.

MANAGEMENT

- The treatment for anterior uveitis is topical steroids, although this should only be done in conjunction with ophthalmologic consultation, since topical steroids may worsen the prognosis for patients with HSV keratitis.
- Patients may also be treated with dilating drops to help to prevent scarring of the iris to the lens (synechiae). Patients must follow up with ophthalmology within 24 hours to control symptoms, limit inflammatory consequences, and to consider lab work for an underlying cause[483].

482 Gilani CJ, Yang A, Yonkers M, Boysen-Osborn M. Differentiating Urgent and Emergent Causes of Acute Red Eye for the Emergency Physician. West J Emerg Med. 2017;18(3):509-517. doi:10.5811/westjem.2016.12.31798

483 Gilani CJ, Yang A, Yonkers M, Boysen-Osborn M. Differentiating Urgent and Emergent Causes of Acute Red Eye for the Emergency Physician. West J Emerg Med. 2017;18(3):509-517. doi:10.5811/westjem.2016.12.31798

II. TRAUMATIC OCULAR INJURIES

1. GLOBE RUPTURE

- **Definition**: Full-thickness perforation or laceration of the ocular globe

- **Mechanism of injury**: Sharp objects or high-velocity blunt objects

- **Clinical features**
  - ○ Gross deformity of the eye (ocular rupture with fluid volume loss) or prolapsing uvea (full-thickness laceration)
  - ○ Afferent pupillary defect and impaired visual acuity
  - ○ All sequelae of ocular contusion are possible (see above).

- **Diagnosis**
  - ○ Careful investigation of the anterior and posterior segment of the eye (by slit lamp and fundoscopy, respectively)
  - ○ Fluorescein stain if inconclusive: corneal abrasions and foreign bodies
  - ○ Nonenhanced CT can be used if the eye cannot be directly visualized or to exclude the possibility of an intraocular foreign body.
  - ○ Culture of the vitreous if a foreign body or infection is suspected

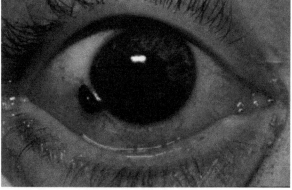

Penetrating Globe Injury

- **Treatment**
  - ○ Urgent stabilization and resuscitation
  - ○ Analgesia (e.g., IV morphine), antiemetics (e.g., IV ondansetron), and tetanus vaccine or booster
  - ○ Systemic antibiotic therapy for foreign bodies
  - ○ Urgent ophthalmologic consultation for surgical repair

- **Complications**
  - ○ Permanent vision loss
  - ○ Loss of eye

- ○ **Endophthalmitis**: inflammation of the tissues or fluid inside the eye (especially with retained intraocular foreign bodies), often presenting with deep ocular pain, a red eye, and reduced visual acuity
- ○ **Sympathetic ophthalmia**: bilateral granulomatous panuveitis after unilateral penetrating injury (and rarely after intraocular surgery) → bilateral blindness may occur

2. HYPHEMA

DEFINITION
- Blood in the anterior chamber of the eye occurring usually as a result of a ruptured iris root vessel, if secondary to trauma.

DIAGNOSIS
- Gross inspection of blood in anterior chamber
- Slit lamp exam à check anterior chamber for blood

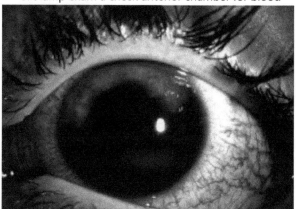

PEOPLE AT RISK
- Sickle cell disease
- Bleeding diatheses
- Anticoagulant or antiplatelet medications

MANAGEMENT
- Interventions aimed preventing secondary hemorrhage
  - ○ Elevate head of bed
  - ○ Dilate pupil
  - ○ Control intraocular pressure with topical beta-blockers, topical alpha-adrenergic agonists, or topical carbonic anhydrase inhibitors
- Although recommended, no solid evidence supports the use of cyclopegics, corticosteroids, bed rest, or patching to decrease secondary hemorrhage or affect visual acuity
- Limited studies supporting tranexamic acid and other antifibrinolytics to decrease secondary hemorrhage
- Consult ophthalmology

3. RETROBULBAR HEMATOMA/ ORBITAL COMPARTMENT SYNDROME

DEFINITION

Blood found behind the globe but within the orbit, mostly occurring secondary to trauma, which can lead to optic nerve and retinal ischemia and ultimately, vision loss.

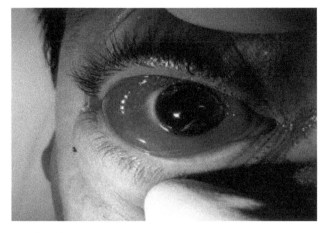

DIAGNOSIS

- **Physical findings:**
  o Proptosis
  o Decreased visual acuity
  o Afferent pupillary defect
  o Decreased extraocular movements
- Increased intraocular pressure (> 40 mmHg)
- CT scan (do not delay management for CT scan if orbital compartment syndrome highly suspected)

MANAGEMENT

- Consider lateral canthotomy if any of the following
  o Decreased visual acuity
  o Restricted extraocular movement
  o Afferent pupillary defect
  o Proptosis
  o Intraocular pressure > 40 mmHg
- **Expeditious performance of a lateral canthotomy is vision saving. Do not delay.**
- Consult ophthalmology emergently

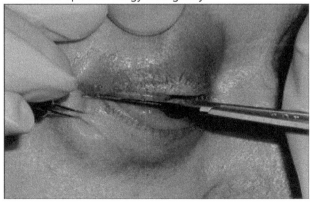

4. RETINAL DETACHMENT

- Retina separates from the underlying retinal pigment epithelium and choroid, either from accumulation of fluid between the two layers or vitreous traction on the retina.

DIAGNOSIS

- History (trauma followed by flashing lights/floaters/dark veil/curtains, or history of diabetes/sickle disease with the same complaints)
- Decreased peripheral or central visual acuity
- Direct fundoscopic exam à pale billowing parachute with a large retinal detachment
- Dilated indirect ophthalmoscopic evaluation by ophthalmologist
- **Ocular ultrasound** of retinal detachment seen as hyperechoic membrane is posterior part of eye, sensitivity ranges from 97%-100%, specificity 83%-100%.

MANAGEMENT

- Consult ophthalmology for surgical repair

5. CORNEAL FOREIGN BODY (INCLUDING RUST RING)

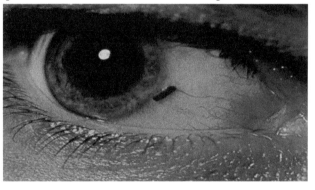

- Small metallic foreign bodies can come into contact with the eyes, most commonly when someone is drilling or grinding a metal surface. Special attention should be paid to the identification of a corneal rust ring. Iron in its neutral form is relatively insoluble in the corneal layers.
- However, over time a metallic foreign body's surface oxidises and diffuses into the stroma. A rust ring is then formed by the combination of oxidised iron and cellular infiltrate at the level of the superficial stroma.
- **A rust ring can lead to:**
  o Permanent corneal staining,
  o Chronic inflammation,
  o Corneal vascularisation,
  o Necrosis

Therefore, should be removed within a few days of it being identified.

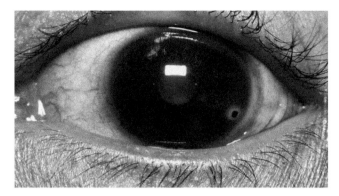

ANGLE GRINDING

o Patients will not always recall a foreign body having entered the eye so it is important to have a high index of suspicion and examine for a conjunctival or corneal foreign body if a patient presents with an uncomfortable red eye.

o Local anaesthetic may be needed both to examine the eye and to remove any foreign body – **Proxymetacaine** has been shown to be the optimal agent.

o If there is a history of a possible foreign body entering the eye and it cannot be seen then **the eyelid must be everted** to exclude a subtarsal foreign body, provided a penetrating injury is not suspected. If a subtarsal foreign body is present, it is easily removed using a cotton bud.

o Also, where the history is of a high velocity foreign body (e.g. metallic fragment from angle grinding or hammering a metal chisel) the possibility of a penetrating injury with intraocular foreign body must be considered.

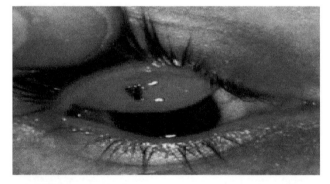

ED MANAGEMENT

o **Instillation of local anaesthetic**

o Small loose conjunctival foreign bodies can be **washed out with water or removed with a cotton bud.**

o If the foreign body is adherent or embedded in the cornea, a **needle may be used to lift it out of the cornea.** This must be done either using a slit lamp or loupes to ensure accuracy and minimal damage to the cornea.

o Once the foreign body has been removed any remaining epithelial defect can be treated as an abrasion.

o Rust rings can be removed either **by a needle** or **by ophthalmic burr.** It may be easier to remove rust rings 2-3 days after presentation as local necrosis will separate the rust ring from the corneal epithelium.

o If there is any doubt, these patients should be **referred to an ophthalmologist**

6. CHEMICAL EYE INJURIES

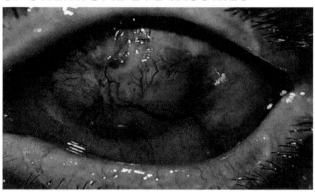

- **Definition**: chemical burn of the eye with acidic or alkaline compounds
- **Clinical features**
  o Intense pain
  o Visual impairment
  o Blepharospasm: involuntary eyelid closure
  o Erythematous conjunctiva or whitening of the conjunctiva
  o Photophobia
- **Treatment**
  o Immediate and thorough irrigation with copious sterile saline (preferred if available) or cold tap water
  o Continued irrigation in the emergency department (ED) with a plastic scleral lens (Morgan® lens) until the pH normalizes for acidic agents or for 2-3 hours for alkaline agents
  o Mechanical removal of solid particles that become acidic or alkaline when combined with water, e.g., dry lime
  o Antibiotic eye drops (e.g., tetracycline)
  o Ophthalmologic consultation
  o Topical glucocorticoids (prednisolone acetate 1%)
- **Complications**
  o Scarring, clouding, and/or ulceration of the cornea
  o Neovascularization of the cornea
  o Adhesion of the eyelid (palpebral conjunctiva) to the globe (bulbar conjunctiva)
  o Blindness

Patients should be advised to irrigate with a copious volume of water or saline for at least 15 minutes before arrival to the ED because immediate irrigation is the most important factor in preventing morbidity!

III. ABNORMAL PUPILLARY RESPONSES

I. ANISOCORIA

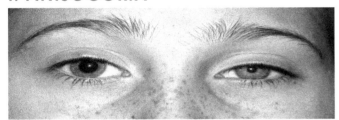

- Refers to the asymmetric sizes of pupils
- Physiologic anisocoria can is very common and a normal variant in up to 20% of the population. The variation should be no more than 1mm and both eyes should react to light normally.
- The goal of evaluation is to elucidate the physiologic mechanism of anisocoria[484]. By identifying certain mechanisms (eg, Horner syndrome, 3rd cranial nerve palsy), clinicians can diagnose the occasional serious occult disorder (eg, tumor, aneurysm) manifesting with anisocoria.
- Consider further workup such as imaging if anisocoria is suspected to be from a pathologic process.
- Treatment of anisocoria itself is unnecessary. Underlying disorders (eg, Horner syndrome) should be evaluated and treated as indicated.

RELATIVE AFFERENT PUPILLARY DEFECT (RAPD, Marcus Gunn Pupil)

- An RAPD is a defect in the direct response. It is due to **damage in optic nerve** or **severe retinal disease**.
- It is important to be able to differentiate whether a patient is complaining of decreased vision from an ocular problem such as cataract or from a defect of the optic nerve.
- If an optic nerve lesion is present the affected pupil will not constrict to light when light is shone in the that pupil during the swinging flashlight test. However, it will constrict if light is shone in the other eye (consensual response).
- **The swinging flashlight** test is helpful in separating these two etiologies as only patients with optic nerve damage will have a positive RAPD.
- Swing a light back and forth in front of the two pupils and compare the reaction to stimulation in both eyes.
- When light reaches a pupil there should be a normal direct and consensual response.

---

484 *Christopher J. Brady*, Anisocoria [Online]

- An RAPD is diagnosed by observing paradoxical dilatation when light is directly shone in the affected pupil after being shown in the healthy pupild to be from a pathologic process.

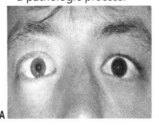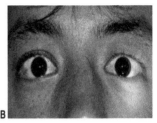

A   B

- This decrease in constriction or widening of the pupil is due to reduced stimulation of the visual pathway by the pupil on the affected side. By not being able to relay the intensity of the light as accurately as the healthy pupil and visual pathway, the diseased side causes the visual pathway to mistakenly respond to the decrease in stimulation as if the flashlight itself were less luminous.
- This explains the healthy eye is able to undergo both direct and consensual dilatation seen on the swinging flashlight test.
- **Some causes of a RAPD include:**
  1. Optic neuritis
  2. Ischemic optic disease or retinal disease
  3. Severe glaucoma causing trauma to optic nerve
  4. Direct optic nerve damage (trauma, radiation, tumor)
  5. Retinal detachment
  6. Very severe macular degeneration
  7. Retinal infection (CMV, herpes)

ADIE'S (TONIC) PUPIL

- Common in women in the 3rd/4th decade of life (but also can be present in men). Either no or sluggish response to light (both direct and consensual responses)
- Thought to be caused from denervation in the postganglionic parasympathetic nerve
- Associated with **Holmes-Adie syndrome** described with Adie's pupil and absent deep tendon reflexes
- Overall, this is a benign process (including Holmes-Adie syndrome)

ARGYLL ROBERTSON PUPIL

- This lesion is a hallmark of tertiary neurosyphillis
- Pupils will NOT constrict to light but they WILL constrict with accommodation. Pupils are small at baseline and usually both involved (although degree may be asymmetrical)

IV. EYE INFECTIONS

1. ORBITAL CELLULITIS

DISEASE ENTITY

- **Orbital or postseptal cellulitis** is an inflammation of the soft tissues of the eye socket behind the orbital septum, a thin tissue which divides the eyelid from the eye socket. Infection isolated anterior to the orbital septum is considered to be **preorbital or preseptal cellulitis.**
- Orbital cellulitis most commonly refers to an acute spread of infection into the eye socket from either the adjacent sinuses, skin or from spread through the blood.

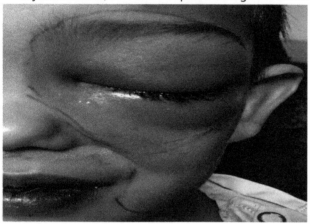

ETIOLOGY

Orbital cellulitis occurs in the following 3 situations[485]:

- Extension of an infection from the paranasal sinuses or other periorbital structures such as the face, globe, or lacrimal sac
- Direct inoculation of the orbit from trauma or surgery
- Hematogenous spread from bacteremia
- The orbital tissues are infiltrated by acute and chronic inflammatory cells and the infectious organisms may be identified on the tissue sections.
- The organisms are best identified by microbiologic culture.
  - Streptococcus species,
  - Staphylococcus aureus,
  - Haemophilus influenzae type B are the most common bacterial causes
  - Pseudomonas, Klebsiella, Eikenella, and Enterococcus are less common culprits.
  - Polymicrobial infections with aerobic and anaerobic bacteria are more common in patients aged 16 years or older.

RISK FACTORS

- Risk factors include recent upper respiratory illness, acute or chronic bacterial sinusitis, recent trauma, recent ocular or periocular infection, or systemic infection.

PRIMARY PREVENTION

- Identifying patients and effectively treating upper respiratory or sinus infections before they evolve into orbital cellulitis is an important aspect of preventing preseptal cellulitis from progressing to orbital cellulitis.
- Equally important in preventing orbital cellulitis is prompt and appropriate treatment of preseptal skin infections or even odentogenic infections before they spread into the orbit.

DIAGNOSIS

- The diagnosis of orbital cellulitis is based on clinical examination. The presence of below orbital signs confirm the diagnosis:
  - Proptosis,
  - Pain with eye movements,
  - Ophthalmoplegia,
  - Optic nerve involvement
  - Fever
  - Leukocytosis.

HISTORY

- A thorough history and physical examination are critical in establishing a diagnosis of orbital cellulitis. Patients with orbital cellulitis frequently complain of fever, malaise, and a history of recent sinusitis or upper respiratory tract infection. Questioning the patient about any recent facial trauma or surgery, dental work[486], or infection elsewhere in the body is important.
- Diverse conditions such as sickle cell orbitopathy, bisphosphonate use, and cosmetic fillers can cause orbital inflammation that can be mistaken for infection.

PHYSICAL EXAMINATION

- Proptosis and ophthalmoplegia are the cardinal signs of orbital cellulitis. The symptoms and signs of orbital cellulitis can advance at an alarming rate and eventually lead to prostration.
- Proptosis and ophthalmoplegia may be accompanied by the following:
  - Decreased vision, dyschromatopsia, and relative afferent pupillary defect

[485] Anari S, Karagama YG, Fulton B, et al. Neonatal disseminated methicillin-resistant Staphylococcus aureus presenting as orbital cellulitis. J Laryngol Otol. 2005 Jan. 119(1):64-7.

[486] Grimes D, Fan K, Huppa C. Case report: dental infection leading to orbital cellulitis. Dent Update. 2006 May. 33(4):217-8, 220.

- o Elevated intraocular pressure
- o Pain on eye movement
- o Conjunctival chemosis
- o Orbital pain and tenderness - Are present early
- o Dark red discoloration of the eyelids, chemosis, hyperemia of the conjunctiva, and resistance to retropulsion of the globe may be present
- o Purulent nasal discharge may be present
- Vision may be normal early, but it may become difficult to evaluate in very ill children with marked edema.
- The above signs may be accompanied by the following:
  - o Fever
  - o Headache
  - o Lid edema
  - o Rhinorrhoea
  - o Increasing malaise

DIAGNOSTIC PROCEDURES

- **Computed tomography (CT)of the orbit**
  - o CT scan is the imaging modality of choice for patients with orbital cellulitis.
  - o **MRI** may be helpful in defining orbital abscesses and in evaluating the possibility of cavernous sinus disease.

LABORATORY TEST

- Admission to the hospital is warranted in all cases of orbital cellulitis.
- An **FBC** with differential as well as **blood cultures** should be ordered.
- **Nasal, throat swabs**

GENERAL TREATMENT

- The management of orbital cellulitis requires **admission to the hospital** and initiation of **broad-spectrum I.V. antibiotics.**
- In infants with orbital cellulitis a **3rd generation cephalosporin** is usually initiated such as cefotaxime, ceftriaxone or ceftazidime along with a **Co-Amoxiclav.**
- In older children, since sinusitis is most commonly associated with aerobic and anaerobic organisms, **clindamycin** might be another option.
- **Metronidazole** is also being increasingly used in children.
- Refer to ophthalmology

COMPLICATIONS

- Optic neuropathy,
- Retinal vein occlusion,
- Severe exposure keratopathy,
- Cavernous sinus thrombosis,
- Meningitis
- Death.

2. PERIORBITAL CELLULITIS

Your patient is a child who is systemically well. He has developed redness and swelling around his left eye over the past few days (see image):

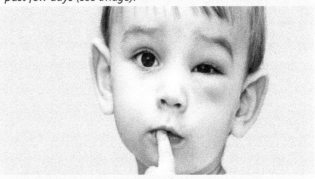

Q1. What is the likely diagnosis?
- Periorbital/ pre-septal cellulitis

Q2. What are the clinical features of this condition, and how is it distinguished from the fisherman's diagnosis?
- Periorbital (or preseptal) cellulitis is a soft-tissue infection of the eyelids that does not extend **past the orbital septum posteriorly**.
- It causes eyelid and periorbital oedema, redness, and discomfort.
- The ocular exam should be essentially normal:
  - o *Normal visual acuity*
  - o **FROEM** *without significant discomfort*
  - o *Absence of proptosis*
- Sometimes the clinical distinction is unclear and imaging is necessary (e.g. CT orbits and sinuses).

Q3. What organisms cause this condition in children <5 years of age?
- Much the same as for orbital cellulitis:
  - o Staphylococcus aureus
  - o Streptococcus pneumoniae
  - o Streptococcus anginosus/milleri group
  - o Haemophilus influenzae type b (Hib) **in the unvaccinated**

Q4. What is the antibiotic treatment of this condition?
- Systemically well children <5 years of age:
  - o **Amoxycillin+Clavulanate for 7 days or Cephalexin 12.5 mg/kg orally QID for 7 days**
- Older children or adults or children with an infected wound or stye, etc:
  - o **Flucloxacillin 500 mg orally, 6-hourly for 7 days**
  - o (cephalexin and clindamycin are options in the setting of penicillin hypersensitivity)
  - o If systemically unwell it is best to treat and investigate for orbital cellulitis.

44. Complex Older Patients
I. FALLS IN ELDERLY

1. RISK FACTORS FOR FALLS
- Older age (≥ 75 years)
- A history of previous falls, Fear
- Acute illness
- Chronic conditions, especially neuromuscular disorders
- Gait deficit, Balance deficit
- Visual impairment, Mobility impairment,
- Cognitive impairment, Hearing impairment
- Urinary incontinence
- Living alone
- Home hazards
- Multiple medications

2. COMMON CAUSES OF FALLS[487]

I	Inflammation of joints (or joint deformity)
H	Hypotension (orthostatic blood pressure changes)
A	Auditory and visual abnormalities
T	Tremor (Parkinson's disease or other causes of tremor)
E	Equilibrium (balance) problem
F	Foot problems
A	Arrhythmia, heart block or valvular disease
L	Leg-length discrepancy
L	Lack of conditioning (generalized weakness)
I	Illness
N	Nutrition (poor; weight loss)
G	Gait disturbance

3. DRUGS INCREASING THE RISK OF FALLS[488]
- Sedative-hypnotic and anxiolytic drugs (especially long-acting benzodiazepines)
- Tricyclic antidepressants
- Major tranquilizers (phenothiazines and butyrophenones)
- Antihypertensive drugs
- Cardiac medications
- Corticosteroids
- Nonsteroidal anti-inflammatory drugs
- Anticholinergic drugs
- Hypoglycaemic agents
- Any medication that is likely to affect balance

4. IDENTIFICATION OF PEOPLE WHO HAVE FALLEN
- The recommendation from the NICE guidance[489] on the assessment and prevention of falls in older people is that all older people in contact with healthcare professionals should be routinely asked whether they have fallen in the past year and asked about the frequency, context, and characteristics of the fall.
- Therefore, all older patients (aged 65 or older) presenting to the ED for any condition should be asked about falls. Older people who present to the ED following a fall or considered at risk of falling should be offered a **multifactorial risk assessment** (e.g. referred to a specialist falls service).

5. ASSESSMENT OF PEOPLE WHO HAVE FALLEN
History and examination[490]
- The history should ideally be obtained from the patient and, if available, a witness account of events should be sought. Pertinent points in the history include:
  - **Circumstances of events**
    - Is there a clear history of a simple trip or slip?
    - Is there history suggestive of a preceding illness (e.g. chest pain, palpitations, limb weakness, dizziness, etc.)?
  - **Loss of consciousness**
    - Is there any reported loss of consciousness or amnesia pre-or post-fall?
    - Does the patient have a history of falling or collapsing?
    - Does the patient feel dizzy on sudden changes in posture?
  - **Vision**: Does the patient require glasses? When was their last eyesight test? Do they have cataracts?
  - **Recent illnesses:** Has the patient had any recent illnesses that could have precipitated the 'fall' (e.g. urinary tract infection)?

487 Sloan JP. Mobility failure. In: Protocols in primary care geriatrics. 2d ed. New York: Springer, 1997:33–8.

488 Svensson ML, Rundgren A, Larsson M, Oden A, Sund V, Landahl S. Accidents in the institutionalized elderly: a risk analysis. Aging [Milano]. 1991;3:181–92.

489 Falls Assessment and prevention of falls in older people Issued: June 2013 NICE guidance number [online]

490 Falls Assessment and prevention of falls in older people Issued: June 2013 NICE guidance number [online]

- o **Past medical history**
  - ▪ Cardiac, Respiratory, Neurological, and Metabolic.
  - ▪ Have they previously sustained a fragility fracture?
- o **Drug history**
  - ▪ Are there medications that could have caused orthostatic hypotension or resulted in dizziness or poor balance (e.g. anti-hypertensives, antidepressants, antipsychotics, anticholinergics, opiates)?
  - ▪ Are there any recent medication changes?
- o **Social history**: What is the patient's social support? Do they have home hazards that are contributing to falls (e.g. loose-fitting rugs, poor lighting, stairs, upstairs bathroom...)?
- o **Alcohol history:** Is there a history of alcohol excess?

- In addition to the examination of any injuries the patient should have a full cardiovascular and neurological examination to screen for evidence of any underlying cause for the fall.

6. INVESTIGATIONS FOR PATIENTS WHO HAVE FALLEN

- Investigations should be guided by the particular presentation of the patient and any injuries sustained.
- In addition, the following investigations should be considered:
  - o Blood glucose/
  - o ECG.
  - o Postural blood pressures
  - o Urinalysis
  - o **Creatinine kinase** and **renal function** should be checked if the patient has had a prolonged period of immobility, to screen for **rhabdomyolysis.**

7. ED MANAGEMENT OF A PATIENT WHO HAS FALLEN

- ED management should focus on treating the consequences of a fall and identifying any potential underlying causes.
- Patients who have fallen should be offered referral on to a specialist falls service for a multifactorial assessment.
- Prior to discharge the patient and/or carers should be given written information about the assessment they are going to receive and how to prevent further falls.

8. COMPLICATIONS OF FALLS

- Falling, particularly falling repeatedly, increases risk of injury, hospitalization, and death, particularly in elderly people who are frail and have preexisting disease comorbidities (e.g., osteoporosis) and deficits in activities of daily living (e.g., incontinence).

- Longer-term complications can include *decreased physical function, fear of falling, and institutionalization*.
- Falls reportedly contribute to > 40% of nursing home admissions.
- Over 50% of falls among elderly people result in an injury.
- Although most injuries are not serious (e.g., contusions, abrasions), fall-related injuries account for about 5% of hospitalizations in patients ≥ 65.
- Although most falls do not result in serious injury, the consequences for an individual of falling or of not being able to get up after a fall can include:
  - o Fear of further falls and thus limitation of activities. This is one of the most important effects, as unchecked it can lead to isolation, further physical decline, depression and even institutionalization
  - o Head injury
  - o Soft tissue injury
  - o Fractures – wrist, hip, pelvis, rib and vertebral fractures are common
  - o About half of elderly people who fall cannot get up without help. Remaining on the floor for > 2 h after a fall increases risk of:
    - ▪ Dehydration,
    - ▪ Pressure ulcers,
    - ▪ Rhabdomyolysis,
    - ▪ Hypothermia
    - ▪ Pneumonia.
  - o 2-5 falls may lead to hospitalisation with its own complications

9. CRITICAL STEPS IN REDUCING THE RISK OF FALLS IN THE ELDERLY[491]

- o Home hazards assessment
- o Vision assessment and referral
- o Strength and balance training
- o Review medication
- o Provide opportunities for socialization and encouragement
- o Improve home supports
- o Modify restraints
- o Involve the family
- o Provide follow-up

---

[491] *Speechley M, Tinetti M. Falls and injuries in frail and vigorous community elderly persons. J Am Geriatr Soc. 1991;39:46–52.*

II. DELIRIUM

OVERVIEW

o The DSM-5 defines **delirium** as a disturbance from baseline in attention, awareness, and cognition, over a short period of time, with fluctuation in severity throughout the day.

o These changes must not be explained by another neurocognitive disorder, and there must be evidence that the condition is explained by another condition such as infection, substance intoxication (including antihistamines or sedatives), or withdrawal. **Inattention** is one of the hallmarks and pivotal features of delirium

o 3 subtypes: hyperactive, hypoactive and mixed

o Prevalence in the critically ill is about 80%

RISK-FACTORS OF DELIRIUM

RISK FACTORS	PRECIPITATING FACTORS
• Old age	• Immobility
• Severe illness	• Use of physical restraint
• Dementia	• Use of bladder catheter
• Physical frailty	• Iatrogenic events
• Admission with infection or dehydration	• Malnutrition
• Visual impairment	• Psychoactive medications
• Polypharmacy	• Intercurrent illness
• Surgery (e.g. NOF)	• Dehydration
• Alcohol excess	
• Renal impairment	

CAUSES OF DELIRIUM: "I WATCH DEATH" [492]

I	Infections	Pneumonia, Urinary, Skin/soft tissue, CNS
W	Withdrawal	Often unintentional, from alcohol, Sedatives, Barbiturates
A	Acute metabolic changes	Altered pH, hypo/hyper Na^+/ Ca^{2+}, Acute liver or renal failure
T	Trauma	Brain Injury, Subdural Hematoma
C	CNS pathology	Post-Ictal, Stroke, Tumour, Brain Mets
H	Hypoxia	CHF, Anaemia
D	Deficiencies	Thiamine, Niacin, B12
E	Endocrinopathies	Hypo-/Hyper-Cortisol, Hypoglycaemia
A	Acute vascular	Hypertensive encephalopathy, Septic Hypotension
T	Toxins and Drugs	Anticholinergics, Opioids, Benzodiazepines
H	Heavy metals	Lead, Manganese, Mercury

[492] *Delirium Differential Diagnosis – I WATCH DEATH, Family medicine reference* [Online]

LIFE-THREATENING CAUSES: "WHIP X 2"

• **W**ernicke's, **W**ithdrawal
• **H**ypertensive encephalopathy, **H**ypoglycaemia and metabolic/endocrine
• **I**nfection, **I**ntracranial disease
• **P**oisons, and **P**orphyria

ASSESSMENT

o **ASSESSMENT APPROACH**
  ▪ Focussed History, Examination and Investigations
  ▪ Assess for predisposing, Precipitating and Perpetuating factors (e.g. features of underlying illness).

MANAGEMENT OF DELIRIUM IN ED

o **EARLY RECOGNITION**
  ▪ Routine monitoring
  ▪ Seek and treat cause – especially life-threatening causes (**WHIP x 2**)

o **NON-PHARMACOLOGIC TREATMENT**
  ▪ Recurrent orientation of patients
  ▪ Early mobilisation and physiotherapy
  ▪ Early removal of catheters
  ▪ Day-night routine
  ▪ Sleep hygiene
  ▪ Involve family
  ▪ Noise control at night
  ▪ Correct vision and Hearing impairment

PHARMACOLOGIC TREATMENT

▪ **Decrease** analgesics, sedatives and anticholinergic drugs, e.g. protocolised sedation or daily interrupted sedation
▪ **Thiamine** (if suspect alcohol consumption or poor nutrition)
▪ **Atypical antipsychotics** (evidence suggests may reduce duration of delirium)
▪ **Dexmedetomidine** (less delirium than benzodiazepine infusions, and a recent meta-analysis also suggests less than propofol infusions too)
▪ **Lorazepam/ Midazolam and Haloperidol/ Triperidol** may be required for acute chemical restraint
▪ NOTE there are NO FDA approved drugs for the treatment of delirium
▪ No strong evidence for a pharmacological delirium protocol or any specific drugs in preventing delirium.
▪ **Rivastigmine** (cholinesterase inhibitor) should not be used (increased mortality in one study)

III. DEMENTIA

OVERVIEW

- Dementia is a disorder, characterised by progressive cognitive impairment that is associated with impairment in functional abilities and in many cases behavioural and psychological symptoms[493]. Dementia is a major cause of disability and dependency[494]. Despite this being a long-term condition, most people live well with dementia for much of this journey. The global prevalence of dementia is rising, primarily due to an ageing population [495], although the incidence appears to be decreasing in some countries (e.g. US and UK). Dementia usually presents in older age, with an exponential increase in incidence with age ≥65 years; overall approximately 80% of people with dementia are aged ≥75 years. Dementia has a major impact on patients and their families with significant societal and financial implications.

TYPES OF DEMENTIA

- There are many different types of dementia, the most common are Alzheimer's disease (AD), vascular dementia (VaD), dementia with Lewy bodies (DLB) and frontotemporal dementia (FTD); mixed dementia with more than one sub-type is also common.
- Other types of dementia include alcohol-related dementia and HIV-dementia.

Type of Dementia	Main characteristics
Alzheimer's disease (AD)	• Occurs in approx. 60 to 80% of patients with dementia. Insidious and irreversible memory decline is the most recognised feature, beginning with short-term deficits but other areas of cognition such as word-finding, visuoconstructional and executive abilities can also decline
Vascular dementia (VaD)	• Causes or contributes to 25 to 50% of patients with dementia. Due to cardiovascular or cerebrovascular disease; may occur following stroke. • Progressive or stepwise cognitive decline and prominent impairment of executive function

| Dementia with Lewy bodies (DLB) | • Occurs in approx. 15% of patients with dementia.
• Progressive cognitive decline accompanied by core features: visual hallucinations, fluctuating attention and cognition and motor features of parkinsonism. Up to 40% of patients with Parkinson's disease (PD) develop PD dementia (PDD).
• The main clinical distinction between DLB and PDD is temporal; in DLB the dementia presents before the parkinson symptoms, while in PDD, the dementia symptoms develop after the patient has PD for many years |
| Frontotemporal dementia (FTD) | • Most common early-onset dementia; onset usually in the 6th decade of life. Substantial genetic component.
• Group of heterogenous disorders characterised by prominent changes in social behaviour and personality or aphasia associated with progressive atrophy of the frontal and/or temporal lobes.
• May develop a concomitant motor syndrome such as parkinsonism |

CRITERIA FOR DIAGNOSIS OF DEMENTIA (DSM-5)

- Evidence of significant cognitive decline from a previous level of performance in one or more cognitive domains:
  - Learning and memory
  - Language
  - Executive function
  - Complex attention
  - Perceptual-motor
  - Social cognition
- The cognitive deficits interfere with independence in everyday activities. At a minimum, assistance should be required with complex instrumental activities of daily living, such as paying bills or managing medications
- The cognitive deficits do not occur exclusively in the context of a delirium
- The cognitive deficits are not better explained by another mental disorder (e.g. major depressive disorder, schizophrenia)

[493] Foley T, Swanwick G, Quality in Practice Committee – Dementia: Diagnosis and Management in General Practice published 2014, downloaded from www.icgp.ie on the 7th February 2019

[494] NICE guideline – Dementia: assessment, management and support for people living with dementia and their carers, Published June 2018 downloaded from www.nice.org.uk on the 7th February 2019

[495] Livingston G et al, Dementia prevention, intervention and care, Lancet 2017;390:2673-734

[496] UpToDate, Evaluation of cognitive impairment and dementia downloaded from www.uptodate.com on the 25th February 2019

ASSESSMENT OF DEMENTIA IN PRIMARY CARE

- Blood tests: Full blood count, thyroid function, renal and liver function, calcium, glucose and vitamin B12
- Chest X-ray and MSU if clinically indicated and ECG
- Cognitive assessment tools used in primary care include:
  - Mini-Mental State Examination (MMSE)
  - General Practitioner Assessment of Cognition
  - Mini-Cognitive Assessment Instrument (Mini-Cog)
  - Memory Impairment Screen (MIS)

MANAGEMENT

- The first step in the management of dementia is a timely diagnosis, and disclosure of the diagnosis in a sensitive way to the patient and their family/carer as appropriate[497]. Disclosure of the diagnosis has been shown to decrease depression and anxiety in patients and their family/carers. Patients and their family/carers should be informed of the dementia subtype, the HCPs involved in their care, medico-legal issues, local support groups and the effect of dementia on driving if appropriate. A patient-centred approach is recommended to enable the patient to stay living at home for as long as possible. If possible physicians may encourage patients to draw up advance directives containing future treatment and care preferences.
- People with dementia present with complex problems and experience symptoms in many domains including cognition, neuropsychiatric symptoms, ADL and they may also have co-morbidities; the patient's needs will change with time. Multidisciplinary input from HCPs include GPs, neurologists, geriatricians, pharmacists, public health nurses, physiotherapists, occupational therapists, speech and language therapists, social workers, dietitians and psychologists.

DELIRIUM VS. DEMENTIA

In a patient who presents to the ED with new cognitive complaints, the first consideration is whether this represents dementia, delirium, or delirium imposed upon underlying dementia. Delirium in ED patients is associated with an increase in mortality and inpatient length of stay.
Cognitive impairment and delirium are associated with a risk of repeat ED visits and increased length of stay.
Generally, a major difference between delirium and dementia is the rapidity of onset:

- Progression of symptoms is usually acute in delirium, rather than insidious and slowly progressive as in dementia. However, a stroke could also cause a rapid decline in cognition that could be defined as dementia.

- Additionally, delirium may cause disturbance in the level of consciousness, attention, and vital signs, whereas dementia should not. The DSM-5 defines **delirium** as a disturbance from baseline in attention, awareness, and cognition, over a short period of time, with fluctuation in severity throughout the day.
- These changes must not be explained by another neurocognitive disorder, and there must be evidence that the condition is explained by another condition such as infection, substance intoxication (including antihistamines or sedatives), or withdrawal. For any patient with a subacute or chronic complaint of cognitive difficulty, **depression** should be considered in the differential. **Acute psychosis** may be considered if the behavior change occurs abruptly, but is more likely in a patient with a preexisting psychiatric history.

COMPARISON OF CLINICAL PRESENTATION OF DEMENTIA, DELIRIUM, AND ACUTE PSYCHOSIS

Characteristic	Dementia	Delirium	Psychosis
Onset	Gradual (months to years)	Acute (days to weeks)	Acute (acute)
Psychomotor activity	Unchanged	Can have marked changes	Can have marked changes
Vital signs	Normal	Typically abnormal (fever, tachycardia, hypertension)	Typically normal
Level of consciousness	Normal	Altered and changing levels	Normal
Course	Gradual, progressive	Rapidly fluctuates	Stable
Hallucinations	Unusual (except with Lewy body dementia)	Visual or auditory	Primarily auditory
Cognitive functions			
Orientation	May be impaired	Usually impaired	May be impaired
Attention	Normal	Short, impaired	Disorganized
Concentration	May be impaired	Impaired	Impaired
Speech	May have difficulty with word finding	Pressured, slow, may be incoherent	Coherent

497 Hort J et al, EFNS-ENS guidelines on the diagnosis and management of Alzheimer's disease, European Journal of Neurology 2010;17:1236-1248

IV. ATYPICAL PRESENTATIONS IN OLDER PEOPLE

OVERVIEW/DEFINITION

Because illness in older adults is complicated by physical changes of aging and by multiple medical problems, it is essential to recognize more commonly seen atypical presentations of illness in older adults. For example, subtle changes like a decrease in function or a diminished appetite very often are the first signs of illness in an older adult.

RISK FACTORS

- Over age 85 in particular
- Multiple co-morbidities
- Multiple medications
- Cognitive or functional impairment

CONSEQUENCES (OF NOT IDENTIFYING)

- Increased morbidity and mortality
- Missed diagnosis
- Unnecessary use of Emergency Rooms

ASSESSMENT/SCREENING TOOLS

Three strategies to assess for atypical presentation of illness:

- Vague Presentation of Illness;
- Altered Presentation of Illness; and
- Non-presentation (under-reporting) of Illness.

1. VAGUE PRESENTATION OF ILLNESS

The Table below lists some non-specific symptoms, such as falls, confusion or other symptoms that may signify an impending acute illness in an older adult.

Non-specific Symptoms that may Represent Specific Illness:

- Confusion, Self-neglect
- Falling, Incontinence
- Apathy, Anorexia
- Dyspnea
- Fatigue

2. ALTERED PRESENTATION OF ILLNESS

- The presentation of a symptom or a group of symptoms in older adults may present a confusing picture to health care provides. The classic presentation of common illnesses in a general adult population such as chest pain during a myocardial infarction, burning with a urinary tract infection or sadness with depression does not hold true with older adults.
- For example, a change in mental status is one of the most frequently presenting symptoms at the onset of acute illness in older adults.

ALTERED PRESENTATION OF ILLNESS IN ELDERLY PERSONS

ILLNESS	ATYPICAL PRESENTATION
Infectious diseases	• Absence of fever • Sepsis without usual leukocytosis and fever • Falls, decreased appetite or fluid intake, confusion, change in functional status
"Silent" acute abdomen	• Absence of symptoms (silent presentation) • Mild discomfort and constipation • Some tachypnea and possibly vague respiratory symptoms
"Silent" malignancy	• Back pain secondary to metastases from slow growing breast masses • Silent masses of the bowel
"Silent" myocardial infarction	• Absence of chest pain • Vague symptoms of fatigue, nausea and a decrease in functional status. • Classic presentation: shortness of breath more common complaint than chest pain
Non-dyspneic pulmonary edema	• May not subjectively experience the classic symptoms such as paroxysmal nocturnal dyspnea or coughing • Typical onset is insidious with change in function, food or fluid intake, or confusion
Thyroid disease	• Hyperthyroidism presenting as "apathetic thyrotoxicosis," i.e. fatigue and a slowing down • Hypothyroidism, presenting with confusion and agitation
Depression	• Lack of sadness • Somatic complaints, such as appetite changes, vague GI symptoms, constipation, and sleep disturbances • Hyper activity • Sadness misinterpreted by provider as normal consequence of aging • Medical problems that mask depression
Medical illness that presents as depression	• Hypo- and hyper- thyroid disease that presents as diminished energy and apathy

"Hidden" Illness in Older Adults[498]

- Depression, Incontinence,
- Musculoskeletal stiffness, Falling,
- Alcoholism, Osteoporosis, Hearing loss
- Dementia, Dental Problems, Poor nutrition
- Sexual dysfunction, Osteoarthritis

---

[498] Ham, R., Sloane,D. & Warshaw,G. (2002). Primary Care Geriatrics: A Case Based Approach. pp 32-33.St Louis, MO:Mosby. Reprinted with permission from Elsevier.

V. FRAILTY SYNDROMES

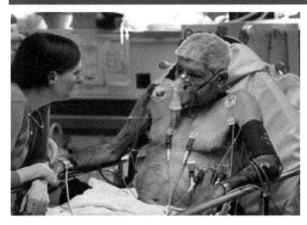

OVERVIEW

Frailty is a vitally important issue in the treatment of the elderly. It is something that most people who live to an advanced age will probably face.

Frailty can strongly affect how an elderly person will respond to medical treatment, as well as how long and how well they will live. Surprisingly, though common, it remains poorly understood.

Part of the problem is that it defies exact definition. Frailty is not really a disease but rather a combination of the natural aging process and a variety of medical problems.

Frailty may not be a disease, but there is no question that certain diseases and medical problems play a large role in it.

Recently, however, gerontologists have been putting a new focus on frailty, beginning with a more precise definition.

Gerontologists suggest that if someone has three or more of five factors, then that person should be considered frail.

These factors are:

1. Unintentional weight loss (10 pounds or more in a year)
2. General feeling of exhaustion
3. Weakness (as measured by grip strength)
4. Slow walking speed
5. Low levels of physical activity.

The frail faced an immediate future of falls, deteriorating mobility, disability, hospitalization and death. Frailty was also highly associated with cardiovascular disease, low education and poverty.

HOW A PERSON BECOMES FRAIL

The definition above, which is known as the Fried framework after its author, Dr. Linda Fried, has made it easier to identify frailty and to understand the complex interaction between physiological factors, external factors and aging that causes it. By the Fried definition, frailty is not a disease but rather a sort of intermediate state — between being functional and nonfunctional, and between being healthy and being sick.

Frailty may not be a disease, but there is no question that certain diseases and medical problems play a large role in it, which other researchers believe also need to be considered.

These include:

- Anorexia, or loss of appetite
- Sarcopenia, or loss of body mass
- Immobility or decreased physical activity
- Atherosclerosis
- Balance impairment
- Depression
- Cognitive impairment

ANOREXIA

It is well recognized that older persons often develop anorexia, loss of appetite, as a natural part of the aging process. Add this to eating problems caused by certain diseases and the result is chronic undernutrition and, eventually, fatigue, weakness, cachexia and micronutrient (vitamins and minerals) deficiencies. Hormone problems such as testosterone deficiency can aggravate anorexia.

SARCOPENIA

Sarcopenia is defined as an excessive loss of muscle associated with aging. While genetically predetermined to some extent, several factors can accelerate the process.

They include, among others, decreased physical activity, and testosterone and growth hormone deficiencies.

IMMOBILITY

Immobility can be caused by illnesses such as arthritis, which decreases the ability to move a joint, or by pain.

Illness can also cause fatigue.

Osteoporosis can set the stage for hip fracture which initiates a cycle of immobility whose endpoint is frailty.

ATHEROSCLEROSIS

Atherosclerosis produces frailty as less oxygen reaches the tissues and organs. It can also cause small strokes, which, in turn, can lead to cognitive impairment. In the legs, vascular disease caused by atherosclerosis can result in nutrient deprivation of the muscles, slowed walking speed and, ultimately, sarcopenia.

BALANCE IMPAIRMENT

Balance deteriorates naturally over a person's lifetime. Decreased balance can initiate a vicious cycle in which accidental falls lead to a fear of falling, which leads to decreased mobility, which makes frailty worse.

DEPRESSION

Depression can result in a reduction in mobility and a pervasive feeling of fatigue. Depression also produces a slowing of thought processes. Depressed people are more likely to develop major illnesses, such as myocardial infarction, and to have more difficult, slower recoveries. Depression is also a major cause of anorexia and weight loss in the elderly.

COGNITIVE IMPAIRMENT

Cognitive impairment can lead to a decline in mental processing time and reaction speed, resulting in a more frequent fall.

PRISMA 7 QUESTIONNAIRE

Which is a seven-item questionnaire to identify disability that has been used in earlier frailty studies and is also suitable for postal completion.

A score of > 3 is considered to identify frailty:

1. Are you more than 85 years?
2. Male?
3. In general, do you have any health problems that require you to limit your activities?
4. Do you need someone to help you on a regular basis?
5. In general, do you have any health problems that require you to stay at home?
6. In case of need can you count on someone close to you
7. Do you regularly use a stick, walker or wheelchair to get about?

Common problems in frailty which need to be addressed to reduce severity and improve outcomes:

- Falls
- Cognitive Impairment
- Continence
- Mobility
- Weight loss/nutrition
- Low mood
- Polypharmacy
- Physical inactivity
- Smoking
- Alcohol excess
- Vision problems
- Social isolation and loneliness

PREVENTING FRAILTY

- **F**ood: maintain intake
- **R**esistance: exercises
- **A**therosclerosis: prevent
- **I**solation: avoid (i.e., go out and do things)
- **L**imit pain
- **T**ai Chi or other balance exercises
- **Y**early check for testosterone deficiency

MANAGEMENT

Management strategies that may be of benefit:

- Early physiotherapy (e.g. early mobilisation) and occupational therapy input to establish usual functional baseline, provide walking aids and prevent unnecessary deterioration by prolonged bed rest.

- **Pharmacology**
  - Dose reduction is often appropriate in the frail elderly
  - Pharmacy involvement for medicines reconciliation to reduce drug interactions and iatrogenic harm

- **Early assessment and treatment of complications of acute illness that are common in patients with frailty:**
  - Delirium
  - Falls risk
  - Pressure sore risk
- Nutrition support
- Early discussion of end of life goals and appropriate limitation of invasive therapies to avoid unnecessary iatrogenic harm

PROGNOSIS

- Assessment of frailty and poor physiological reserve is becoming increasingly important as we become more cognisant of the poor long-term outcomes and costs associated with intensive care of the frail
  - Critically ill elderly frail patients, compared to similarly aged non-frail patients have worse outcomes (morbidity, mortality and institutionalisation)
  - Critically ill patients of all ages may share characteristics with frail elderly patients: "deficits associated with frailty, which typically take years to accumulate in the outpatient geriatric population, rapidly develop in a large proportion of critically ill patients independent of age and illness severity" (McDermid et al, 2009)

RECOMMENDATIONS

- Older people should be assessed for the possible presence of frailty during all encounters with health and social care professionals. Slow gait speed, the PRISMA questionnaire, the timed up-and-go test are recommended as reasonable assessments.
- The Edmonton Frail Scale is recommended in elective surgical settings.
- Provide training in frailty recognition to all health and social care staff who are likely to encounter older people.
- Do not offer routine population screening for frailty.

VI. ABUSE IN OLDER PEOPLE

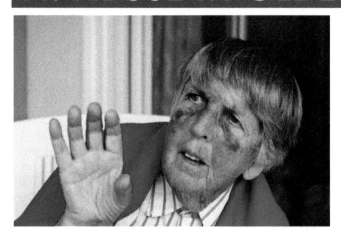

INTRODUCTION

- **Abuse and neglect** of the elderly refer to physical, emotional, sexual abuse, or abandonment of the aged by relatives or caregivers. Elder abuse refers to any form of maltreatment of an older dependent person.
- The abuser typically has a close relationship to the elderly person e.g. spouse, sibling, child or be a friend or care giver. Elder abuse is under recognised

RISK FACTORS

- **Relating to the older person:**
  - Cognitive impairment
  - Behavioural problems
  - Psychiatric illness or psychological problems
  - Functional dependence (requiring assistance with activities of daily living)
  - Poor physical health or frailty
  - Low income or wealth
  - Trauma or past abuse
  - Ethnicity (increased risk among non-whites for overall abuse, African Americans for financial abuse and Canadian Aboriginals for physical and sexual abuse)
- **Relating to the perpetrator:**
  - Caregiver burden or stress
  - Psychiatric illness or psychological problems
- **Relating to the relationship:**
  - Family disharmony with poor or conflictual relationships
- **Relating to the environment:**
  - Low social support
  - Living with others (except in financial abuse)

TYPES OF ELDER ABUSE

- **Categories**
  - Domestic (in the home of the elderly person or the carer)
  - Institutional (occurring in a residential facility such as a hostel or nursing home)
- **Forms of elder abuse**
  - Physical
  - Neglect, including abandonment
  - Financial or material
  - Psychological or emotional
  - Sexual (rare)

ASSESSMENT

Take a history from the suspected victim privately using tailored questions such as:

- Do you feel safe where you live? Who prepares your meals? Who pays your bills? If you want money to buy something, how do you get it? Who does your banking?
- How do you get on with your husband / Wife / Son / Daughter?
- Do you ever have disagreements? Tell me about what happens when you have a disagreement.
- Does your husband / wife / son / daughter ever get angry or upset with you? What happens when they get angry? Are you ever frightened when your husband / Wife / Son / Daughter gets angry?
- Do they ever hurt you?
- Look for features on history and examination of the different forms of abuse.

1. PHYSICAL ABUSE

- **Definition**
  - The use of physical force or violent acts that result in bodily injury, pain or impairment.
  - For example, striking, hitting, beating, pushing, shaking, slapping, kicking, pinching and burning
  - Also includes forced feeding and physical restraints.
- **Possible indicators include:**
  - Inappropriate delays between injuries and presentation for medical attention (e.g. lacerations healing by secondary intention or radiological evidence of healed fractures for which no medical attention was sought)
  - Disparity in histories given by the patient and the suspected abuser.
  - Implausible or vague explanations provided by either party (e.g. fractures that are not explained by the purported mechanism of injury)
  - Multiple physical injuries seen of variable ages
  - Multiple bruising, including black eyes, welts, lacerations and rope/belt marks
  - Skull fractures, Repeated falls / injuries

2. NEGLECT & ABANDONMENT

- **Definition**
  - The failure or refusal to fulfil any part of the person's obligations or duties of care to the elder.
  - **Neglect** means the failure to provide an elderly person with such life necessities as food, water, clothing, shelter, heating, personal hygiene, medicine, comfort, safety.
  - **Institutional neglect** is used when an aged care facility fails to provide adequate supervision and safety necessary for the wellbeing of the elder.
  - **Abandonment** is defined as the desertion of an elder person for any length of time deemed to be unsafe and inappropriate.

- **Possible indicators include:**
  - Dehydration, Malnutrition, Untreated injuries
  - Severe and untreated pressure sores
  - Poor personal hygiene
  - Frequent visits to the ED for exacerbation of chronic disease despite a plan for medical care and adequate resources
  - Presentation of a functionally impaired patient without his/her designated caregiver (patient with significant dementia who presents to the ED alone)
  - Lack or inappropriate use of medication,
  - Unkempt appearance, e.g. dirt, fleas, lice, soiled bedding, fecal, /urine smell, long uncut nails
  - Inappropriate delays between onset of illness and the seeking of medical help
  - Repeated Falls / Injuries
  - Prolonged periods of no visitation (without credible reason)
  - Unexplained banking withdrawals or unexplained loss of elder person's money, (financial abuse)
  - Abrupt changes in will or banking details
  - Lack of adequate heating, running water, or electricity

3. FINANCIAL OR MATERIAL ABUSE

- **Definition**
  - Deliberate misuse of a person's property or financial resources
  - Includes misuse, misappropriation of money, valuables or property, denial of right of access to or control of personal funds and interference in financial decisions.
- **Possible indicators include complaints or allegations that:**
  - The patient does not have appropriate access to their funds

  - The patient does not have access to spending money for personal items such as toiletries and clothing
  - An Enduring Power of Attorney is not being executed appropriately and, in the patient's, best interests
  - Funds or assets are being misappropriated

4. PSYCHOLOGICAL/ EMOTIONAL ABUSE

- **Definition**
  - Inflicting pain, distress and anxiety through verbal and non- verbal acts.
- **Possible indicators include:**
  - Agitation and distress in the presence of Carer
  - Extremely withdrawn, non-communicative and/or non-responsive
  - Scared, takes foetal position avoids eye contact
  - Helplessness and Hesitation to talk openly

5. SEXUAL ABUSE

- **Definition**
  - Non-consensual sexual acts with the older person
  - Also includes sexual acts with an older person incapable of giving consent
  - Includes examples such as any form of unwanted touching, explicit photographing, nudity, and acts of sexual contact such as rape and abuse
- **Possible indicators include the following:**
  - Contusions around the breasts or genital area
  - Venereal disease or other genital infections
  - Unexplained vaginal or anal bleeding

MANAGEMENT

General

- Attend to any life-threats and treat any specific medical issues

Management of potential abuse

- Document any concerns about elder abuse in the medical record
  - Carefully document why you are concerned that abuse may be occurring
  - Notes should be detailed and accurate particularly with respect to any physical injuries
  - Drawings are useful
- Determine competency as may influence management
- Legal requirement for mandatory reporting

DISPOSITION

- Issues of either home or institutional neglect / abandonment may be managed as an outpatient Hospital admission is mandated if there is genuine concern for the safety of a patient such that they are at high risk should they return home.

45. Unconscious Patient

I. COMA

OVERVIEW

- There are two main mechanisms to explain coma: The first is a diffuse insult to both cerebral hemispheres and the second a disruption of the ascending reticular activating system in the midbrain and pons, where signals are carried to the thalamus and cortex.
- The thalamus plays a crucial role in maintaining arousal. The thalamus and ascending reticular activating system can be damaged either by direct insult or by problems arising within the brainstem[499].

CAUSES OF COMA

Mnemonics "TIPS AEIOU" [500]

- o **T**rauma to head
- o **I**nsulin: too little or too much
- o **P**sychogenic
- o **S**troke
- o **A**cidosis/ **A**lcohol
- o **E**pilepsy
- o **I**nfection
- o **O**verdose
- o **U**raemia

DIFFERENTIAL DIAGNOSIS:

Traumatic	• Head Injury
Primary CNS or Structural	• Tumors: Primary, Metastatic • Hemorrhage: Spontaneous, Traumatic • Edema: HTN encephalopathy, Obstructive hydrocephalus, Tumor • Seizure: Post-ictal state • Dementia
Pharmacologic or Toxic	• Medication effects: antihypertensives, Steroids, Sedatives, Opiates, Sleep aids, Anticholinergics, Antiepileptics, • Polypharmacy • Alcohols: Ethanol (ETOH), Methanol/ethylene glycol • Illicit drugs: Withdrawal, Alcohol, Benzodiazepine, Opiates
Infectious	• Primary CNS: Meningitis, Encephalitis, Abscesses • Other site of infection: UTI, Pneumonia, Skin/decubitus ulcer, Intra-abdominal, Viral syndrome
Other	• Shock: Cardiogenic, Hypovolemic, Hemorrhagic, Distributive • Complicated migraine • Psychiatric disorder • Sundowning/ICU delirium

CLASSIC PRESENTATION

- Unfortunately, there is no classic presentation for a patient with AMS.
- The terms, "Altered mental status" and "altered level of consciousness" (ALOC) are common acronyms, but are vague nondescript terms.
- The same can be said about terms such as lethargy or obtundation. Both represent some level of decreased consciousness but are more subjective descriptors than true objective findings.
- The "AMS" label may be applied to a patient who is postictal or perhaps a patient who has dementia. Because the varied presentations that can range from global CNS depression to confusion to the other extreme, agitation, it is important to be clear with terminology on how we describe a patient's mental status.

1. BELL'S PHENOMENON

- o This is a normal reflex that is lost with decreasing consciousness.
- o When the eye closes, the eye rolls upwards and inwards. This reflex is lost with a reduced level of consciousness.
- o A patient with **an organic cause of coma** will have lost this reflex, so the eye will not move. The eyelids will close slowly and incompletely.
- o A patient with a **psychogenic cause of coma** will have an intact reflex, so the eye will roll upwards. Also, the eyelids will close at a normal speed and completely.

2. THE HAND DROP TEST.

- o With the patient lying supine, lift the patient's hand above the face and allow it to drop onto the face.

---

[499] Edlow J. Rabinstein A. Traub S. Wijdicks E. Diagnosis of reversible causes of coma. Lancet. 2014;384:206476.

[500] Rok Petrovčič, Hypoglycemia, International Emergency Medicine Education Project [Online]

---

o A patient with **psychogenic cause of coma** will guide the hand to fall away from the face, while a patient with an **organic cause of coma** will allow the hand to fall onto the face.

3. CORNEAL REFLEXES/ PUPILLARY RESPONSES
- **The pupillary light reflex**[501]. is an autonomic reflex that constricts the pupil in response to light, thereby adjusting the amount of light that reaches the retina.
- Pupillary constriction occurs via innervation of the iris sphincter muscle, which is controlled by the parasympathetic system
- **The dark reflex** dilates the pupil in response to dark[502]. It can also occur due to a generalized sympathetic response to physical stimuli and can be enhanced by psychosensory stimuli, such as by a sudden noise or by pinching the back of the neck, or a passive return of the pupil to its relaxed state.

ED MANAGEMENT OF COMA
- **Bed side test: Blood Glucose**
- **ABC DEFG** approach
- Treat **Hypoxia and Hypotension** to prevent further neurological damage: **15 l/min O2 via a well-fitting non-re-breath mask.**
- **Urgent ABG analysis** and calculation of the **anion gap.**
- **A serum lactate**: degree of tissue hypo-perfusion and is useful as a marker in sepsis
- In cases of non-traumatic coma, the attending doctor should consider specific treatment with **Naloxone, Flumazenil, Thiamine and Glucose.**
- **Flumazenil** and **Naloxone:** if overdose of benzodiazepines or opiates.
- Wernicke's encephalopathy is a rare cause of coma, however indiscriminate infusion of glucose in (thiamine deficient) alcoholics can precipitate further acute neurological damage.
- In consequence, all malnourished and alcoholic patients in coma should receive **100 mg thiamine slowly over 5 minutes prior to the administration of glucose.**
- **Surgical evacuation** of cerebellar haematomas is proven to improve outcome; surgical evacuation of intracerebral haematomas is not.Coma following cardiac arrest is not of itself an indication to withdraw therapy.
- All patients who present in coma with pyrexia should receive broad spectrum antibiotic therapy urgently.

PROGNOSIS & FOLLOW UP STRATEGIES
- Prognosis depends on a number of factors. In one systematic review the mortality rate varied from 25-87%[503]. Non-traumatic unconscious patients presenting with a stroke have the highest mortality, while those presenting with epilepsy and poisoning have the best prognosis.
- A Swedish study of coma patients presenting to the Emergency Department found initial inpatient mortality to be 27%, rising to 39% at 1 year. Patients with a lower GCS at presentation, 3-5, have a significantly higher mortality than those with a GCS of 7-10[504]. Reversible causes of coma are generally more likely when a CT scan of the brain is unremarkable and the patient has no focal neurology. Patients not responding to initial treatment and who remain comatose are likely to require critical care admission unless withdrawal of treatment and palliation of symptoms is more appropriate. Early communication with the next of kin, family or appropriate advocate is always necessary. When the prognosis is poor these discussions will include ceiling of care, consideration of future withdrawal of treatment and cardiopulmonary resuscitation.

1. LOCKED IN SYNDROME
- Locked-in syndrome is a rare neurological disorder in which there is complete paralysis of all voluntary muscles except for the ones that control the movements of the eyes. Individuals with locked-in syndrome are conscious and awake, but have no ability to produce movements (outside of eye movement) or to speak (aphonia). Cognitive function is usually unaffected. Communication is possible through eye movements or blinking.
- Locked-in syndrome is caused by damaged to the pons, a part of the brainstem that contains nerve fibers that relay information to other areas of the brain.

2. MALINGERING
- Malingering is falsification or profound exaggeration of illness (physical or mental) to gain external benefits such as avoiding work or responsibility, seeking drugs, avoiding trial (law), seeking attention, avoiding military services, leave from school, paid leave from a job, among others.

[501] Dragoi, Valentin. "Chapter 7: Ocular Motor System". Neuroscience Online: An Electronic Textbook for the Neurosciences. Department of Neurobiology and Anatomy, The University of Texas Medical School at Houston.

[502] Hunyor, AP. Reflexes and the Eye. Aust N Z J Ophthalmol. 1994;22(3):155-159. doi:10.1111/j.1442-9071.1994.tb01709.x

[503] Horsting M. Franken M. Meulenbelt J. van Klei W. de Lange D. The etiology and outcome of non-traumatic coma in critical care: a systematic review. BMC Anesthesiol. 2015;15:65.

[504] Sacco R. Van Gool R. Mohr JP. Hauser WA. Nontraumatic coma. Glasgow Coma Score and coma etiology as predictors of 2 week outcome. Arch Neurol. 1990;47:1181-4.

46. Vomiting & Nausea

I. INTRODUCTION

- **Nausea**, the unpleasant sensation of being about to vomit, can occur alone or can accompany **vomiting** (the forceful expulsion of gastric contents), dyspepsia, or other gastrointestinal symptoms.
- Nausea can occur without vomiting and, less commonly, vomiting occurs without nausea.
- Nausea is often more bothersome and disabling than vomiting.
- **Retching** differs from vomiting in the absence of expulsion of gastric content. In addition, patients may confuse vomiting with regurgitation, which is the return of Esophageal contents to the hypopharynx with little effort.

APPROACH TO MANAGEMENT

- Patients with acute vomiting, typically for hours to a few days, most often present to an emergency department, whereas patients with chronic symptoms are more often initially evaluated in outpatient office settings.
- Emergency department physicians should expeditiously exclude life-threatening disorders such as **bowel obstruction, mesenteric ischemia, acute pancreatitis, and myocardial infarction**.
- The etiology should be sought, taking into account whether the patient has acute nausea and vomiting or chronic symptoms (at least one month in duration).
- The consequences or complications of nausea and vomiting (eg, fluid **depletion, hypokalemia, and metabolic alkalosis**) should be identified and corrected.
- Targeted therapy should be provided, when possible (eg, surgery for bowel obstruction or malignancy).
- In other cases, the symptoms should be treated.

HISTORY AND PHYSICAL EXAMINATION

- An initial careful history and physical examination should be performed. In most cases, the cause of the nausea and vomiting can be determined from the history and physical examination and additional testing is not required. If additional testing is needed, it should be guided by the symptom duration, frequency, and severity, as well as the characteristics of vomiting episodes and associated symptoms.
- The following clinical features are especially important:
  - Drug use can cause nausea and vomiting, particularly opioids and cannabis
  - Abdominal pain with vomiting often indicates an organic etiology (eg, cholelithiasis)
  - Abdominal distension and tenderness suggest bowel obstruction.
  - Vomiting of food eaten several hours earlier and a succession splash detected on abdominal examination suggest gastric obstruction or gastroparesis.
  - Vomiting of blood or coffee ground-like material indicates upper gastrointestinal bleeding.
  - Heartburn with nausea often indicates gastroesophageal reflux disease (GERD), and GERD can present as chronic nausea without typical reflux symptoms
  - Early morning vomiting is characteristic of pregnancy
  - Feculent vomiting suggests intestinal obstruction or a gastrocolic fistula.
  - Vertigo and nystagmus are typical of vestibular neuritis and other causes of vertigo.
  - Bulimia is associated with dental enamel erosion, parotid gland enlargement, lanugo-like hair, and calluses on the dorsal surface of the hand
  - Headache may indicate migraine-associated vomiting. Neurogenic vomiting may be positional and is usually associated with other neurologic signs or symptoms.
- A similar illness suffered concurrently by people in personal contact with the patient or who had ingested food or liquid from the same source at about the same time suggests a common viral or bacterial pathogen.

SPECIFIC ACUTE DISORDERS

1. ACUTE GASTROENTERITIS

- Acute gastroenteritis is second only to the common cold as a cause of lost productivity. Bacterial, viral, and parasitic pathogens cause this illness which is characterized by diarrhea and/or vomiting.
- Vomiting is especially common with infections caused by **rotaviruses, enteric adenovirus, norovirus, and *Staphylococcus aureus.***
- Laboratory testing usually is unnecessary in adults with domestically acquired illness.
- Stool cultures had higher yields in patients with fever or diarrhea of more than two days' duration.

2. POSTOPERATIVE NAUSEA AND VOMITING

- About one-third of surgical patients have nausea, vomiting, or both after receiving general anesthesia.
- Most research has been directed toward prevention rather than therapy of established symptoms.
- Risk factors include female sex, non-smoker status, previous history of postoperative nausea and vomiting, and use of postoperative opioids.

3. VESTIBULAR NEURITIS

- This acute labyrinthine disorder is characterized by rapid onset of severe vertigo with nausea, vomiting and gait instability.

4. CHEMOTHERAPY-INDUCED NAUSEA AND VOMITING

- Nausea and vomiting are common side effects of cancer chemotherapy. Anticipatory antiemetic therapy is indicated when highly emetogenic chemotherapy regimens are given.

TREATMENT

1. Antiemetics and prokinetics

- **Prochlorperazine** is an antiemetic that often partially alleviates acute nausea and vomiting (eg, acute gastroenteritis), but is associated with risks of hypotension and extrapyramidal side effects. Prochlorperazine should usually be considered in such cases before trying serotonin receptor antagonists or prokinetic drugs.
- The dopamine receptor antagonist, **metoclopramide,** has combined antiemetic and prokinetic properties. However, it can be associated with extrapyramidal side effects. It can be given orally or intravenously. When given intravenously, using a slow infusion over 15 minutes is associated with a lower incidence of akathisia compared with bolus dosing, without a decrease in efficacy.
- Another dopamine antagonist, **domperidone**, penetrates the blood-brain barrier poorly. As a result, anxiety and dystonia are much less common than with metoclopramide.

2. Antidepressants

- In patients with chronic nausea and vomiting syndrome or cyclic vomiting syndrome, antinausea drugs are usually ineffective

3. Gastric electrical stimulation

- Gastric electrical stimulation via implanted electrodes has been applied to highly selected patients with gastroparesis that is refractory to conventional therapy.

II. BOERHAAVE'S SYNDROME

- Diagnosis of Boerhaave syndrome can be difficult, because often no classic symptoms are present and delays in presentation for medical care are common[505].
- Although Boerhaave syndrome classically presents as the **Mackler triad** of chest pain, vomiting, and subcutaneous emphysema due to esophageal rupture, these symptoms are not always present.
- In fact, approximately one third of all cases of Boerhaave syndrome are clinically atypical.

CLINICAL PRESENTATION

History

- The classic clinical presentation of Boerhaave syndrome usually consists of repeated episodes of retching and vomiting, typically in a middle-aged man with recent excessive dietary and alcohol intake.
- These repeated episodes of retching and vomiting are followed by a sudden onset of severe chest pain in the lower thorax and the upper abdomen.
- The pain may radiate to the back or to the left shoulder.
- Swallowing often aggravates the pain and may precipitate coughing because of the communication between the esophagus and the pleural cavity..
- Typically, hematemesis is not seen after esophageal rupture, which helps to distinguish it from the more common **Mallory-Weiss tear.**
- Shortness of breath is a common complaint and is due to pleuritic pain or pleural effusion.

Physical Examination

- Although the Mackler triad of vomiting, lower thoracic pain, and subcutaneous emphysema is the classic presentation of Boerhaave syndrome, this triad is actually rare, which may then lead to a delay in diagnosis[506].
- Patients' presentation may vary depending on the following:
  - o The location of the tear
  - o The cause of the injury
  - o The amount of time that has passed from the perforation to the intervention

INVESTIGATIONS

- **Laboratory findings**: are often nonspecific in patients with Boerhaave syndrome.
- Patients may present with leukocytosis and a left shift.

---

[505] *Turner AR, Turner SD. Boerhaave syndrome. StatPearls [Internet]. 2018 Jan.*

[506] *Garas G, Zarogoulidis P, Efthymiou A, et al. Spontaneous esophageal rupture as the underlying cause of pneumothorax: early recognition is crucial. J Thorac Dis. 2014 Dec. 6 (12):1655-8.*

- **Upright chest radiography**
  - The most common finding is a **unilateral effusion**, usually on the left.
  - Other findings may include:
    - Free air in the mediastinum or peritoneum,
    - Pneumothorax, hydropneumothorax,
    - Pneumomediastinum,
    - Subcutaneous emphysema, or
    - Mediastinal widening.
  - The **V-sign of Naclerio** has been described as a chest radiograph finding in as many as 20% of patients.
  - Overall, 10% of chest radiographs are normal.

- **Esophagography**
  - It typically shows extravasation of contrast material into the pleural cavity.

- **Computed tomography (CT) scanning**
  - It is helpful in patients too ill to tolerate esophagrams, and it localizes collections of fluid for surgical drainage.

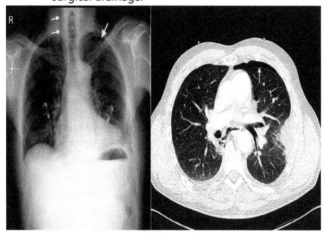

MANAGEMENT
- This is a highly **lethal condition** - it is essentially 100% fatal if left untreated.
- Overall mortality is about 30%.
- The cornerstones of management are:
  - **Aggressive resuscitation**
  - **Broad-spectrum antibiotics**
  - **Early referral for surgical intervention**

III. MALLORY-WEISS TEAR
- **INTRODUCTION**
  - Superficial longitudinal mucosal lacerations of the distal oesophagus or proximal stomach. Associated with forceful retching, alcoholism, and hiatal hernias.
  - Amount of blood loss is usually small and self-limited
  - Accounts for approximately 5% of all presentations of upper GI bleeds.

- **PRESENTATION**
  - **Symptoms**
    - Blood in vomit, Blood in stool, Dark stools
    - Epigastric pain, Back pain

- **PHYSICAL EXAM**
  - Upper GI bleed, Hemodynamic instability
  - Can occur with large bleeds
  - Signs include hypotension/tachycardia

- **EVALUATION**
  - Mallory-Weiss tears are diagnosed via direct visualization under **endoscopy**

- **DIFFERENTIAL**
  - Oesophageal varices, Boerhaave's syndrome, ulcerative diseases of the oesophagus (including reflux esophagitis or infectious esophagitis)

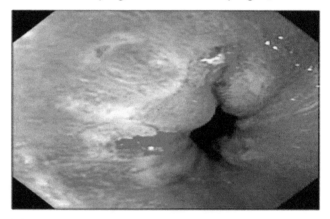

ED MANAGEMENT OF MALLORY WEISS TEAR
- **Medical management**
  - **Supportive therapy and observation**
    - Management of hemodynamic instability including
      - IV fluids
      - Blood transfusion if needed
      - Most bleeds resolve spontaneously
    - Refer to Surgery

- **PROGNOSIS**
  - Bleeding stops spontaneously in 80-90% of patients
  - Up to 10% of patients will experience hemodynamic instability
  - Recurrence of Mallory Weiss tears is rare

- **PREVENTION:** Avoid engaging in activities that lead to excessive coughing or vomiting (i.e. binge drinking).

- **COMPLICATIONS**
  - Hypovolemic shock,
  - Organ infarction,
  - Death if bleeding is not controlled

47. Weakness & Stroke
I. TRANSIENT ISCHAEMIC ATTACK

DEFINITION

- A transient ischaemic attack (TIA) is a transient episode of neurological dysfunction caused by focal brain, spinal cord, or retinal ischaemia, without acute infarction[507]. This replaced the former definition of focal neurological impairment lasting less than 24 hours.
- The majority of TIAs resolve within the first hour, and diagnostic imaging allows recognition that some events with rapid clinical resolution are associated with permanent cerebral infarction[508 509].
- The arbitrary definition of duration of symptoms for TIA should not deter aggressive therapy for a patient who presents with new neurological deficit.

ETIOLOGY

The TIA workup should focus on emergency/urgent risk stratification and management. Numerous potential underlying causes can be readily identified, including the following:

- Atherosclerosis of extracranial carotid and vertebral or intracranial arteries
- Embolic sources - Valvular disease, ventricular thrombus, or thrombus formation from atrial fibrillation, aortic arch disease, paradoxical embolism via a patent foramen ovale (PFO) or atrial-septal defect (ASD)
- Arterial dissection
- Arteritis - Inflammation of the arteries occurring primarily in elderly persons, especially women; noninfectious necrotizing vasculitis (primary cause); drugs; irradiation; local trauma; connective tissue diseases
- Sympathomimetic drugs (eg, cocaine)
- Mass lesions (eg, tumors or subdural hematomas) – These less frequently cause transient symptoms and more often result in progressive persistent symptoms
- Hypercoagulable states (eg, genetic or associated with cancer or infection)

SIGNS AND SYMPTOMS

- A TIA may last only minutes, and symptoms often resolve before the patient presents to a clinician. Thus, historical questions should be addressed not just to the patient but also to family members, witnesses, and emergency medical services (EMS) personnel regarding changes in any of the following[510]:
  o Behavior
  o Speech
  o Gait
  o Memory
  o Movement
- Initial vital signs should include the following[510]:
  o Temperature
  o Blood pressure, Heart rate and rhythm
  o Respiratory rate and pattern and Oxygen saturation
- The examiner should assess the patient's overall health and appearance, making an assessment of the following:
  o Attentiveness
  o Ability to interact with the examiner
  o Language and memory skills
  o Overall hydration status
  o Development
- The goals of the physical examination are to uncover any neurologic deficits, to evaluate for underlying cardiovascular risk factors, and to seek any potential thrombotic or embolic source of the event[510].
- Ideally, any neurologic deficits should be recorded with the aid of a formal and reproducible stroke scale, such as the National Institutes of Health Stroke Scale (NIHSS).
- A neurologic examination is the foundation of the TIA evaluation and should focus in particular on the neurovascular distribution suggested by the patient's symptoms. Subsets of the neurologic examination include the following:
  o Cranial nerve testing
  o Determination of somatic motor strength
  o Somatic sensory testing
  o Speech and language testing
  o Assessment of the cerebellar system (be sure to watch the patient walk)

[507] Easton JD, Saver JL, Albers GW, et al. Definition and evaluation of transient ischemic attack. Stroke. 2009;40:2276-2293.

[508] National Institute of Neurological Disorders and Stroke rt-PA Stroke Study Group. Tissue plasminogen activator for acute ischemic stroke. N Engl J Med. 1995 Dec 14;333(24):1581-7.

[509] Kidwell CS, Alger JR, Di Salle F, et al. Diffusion MRI in patients with transient ischemic attacks. Stroke. 1999 Jun;30(6):1174-80.

[510] Ashish Nanda, Transient Ischemic Attack [Medscape online]

TIA SYMPTOMS FOR DIAGNOSIS

Carotid Territory TIA should have:	Focal loss of function One of: - • unilateral sensory/motor disturbance • unilateral visual disturbance • monocular blindness (amarosis fugax) • total aphasia or dysphasia
Carotid Territory TIA should NOT have:	• Loss of consciousness • Confusion, • Dizziness • Generalised weakness • Urinary incontinence • Vertigo, • Diplopia, • Dysphagia • Tinnitus • Loss of balance • Amnesia • Drop attacks • Scintillating scotoma • Sensory symptoms in part of limb or face
Vertebral Territory TIA may have:	• Bilateral motor/sensory loss • Bilateral visual loss • Ataxia • Combination of vertigo, diplopia & dysarthria

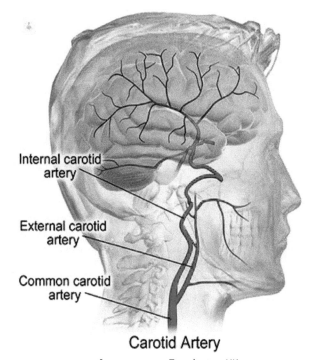

Internal carotid artery

External carotid artery

Common carotid artery

Carotid Artery
Image source -Top doctors UK

DIAGNOSIS

- Standard investigations should include:
  - o **Blood tests:** Plasma glucose FBC, U&E, Lipid profile, LFTs
  - o **ECG**
- NICE Clinical guidance[511] recommended that imaging of the brain should be performed within 24 hours of symptom onset, as follows:
  - o Magnetic resonance imaging (MRI) with diffusion-weighted imaging (preferred)
  - o Noncontrast computed tomography (CT; ordered if MRI is not available)
- The cerebral vasculature should be imaged urgently, preferably at the same time as the brain. Vascular imaging for TIA includes the following:
  - o Carotid Doppler ultrasonography of the neck
  - o CT angiography (CTA)
  - o Magnetic resonance angiography (MRA)

DIFFERENTIAL DIAGNOSIS

There are a number of conditions that can be mistaken for a TIA:

- o Hypoglycaemia
- o Ocular disorders
- o Peripheral vascular disease
- o Arteritis
- o CNS tumour
- o Subdural haematoma
- o Migraine
- o Partial seizure
- o Vestibular disorders
- o Presyncope/syncope
- o Neuropathy
- o Radiculopathy

ABCD² Score

- o One recent study used a combination of the California score and the ABCD score used in the UK to derive a score designed to predict two-day risk of stroke.
- o Individuals with an ABCD² score of 6 or 7 have an 8% risk of stroke within 2 days, whereas those with an
- o ABCD² score lower than 4 have a 1% risk of stroke within 2 days[512].
- o Some of these patients with lower scores may well have non-TIA events rather than true TIAs.

---

[511] *National Institute for Health and Clinical Excellence (NICE) Stroke Guidelines. Available at Accessed: September 22, 2010. [Nice Guideline]*

[512] *Johnston SC, Rothwell PM, Nguyen-Huynh MN, Giles MF, Elkins JS, Bernstein AL, et al. Validation and refinement of scores to predict very early stroke risk after transient ischaemic attack. Lancet. 2007 Jan 27. 369(9558):283-92.*

ABCD² Score
Adapted from emed.ie

Parameter	Feature	Score
Age	>60	1
Blood pressure	SBP > 140mmHg or DBP > 90mmHg	1
Clinical features	Unilateral weakness	2
	Speech impairment with no weakness	1
	Other	0
Duration of symptoms	>60 minutes	2
	10-59 minutes	1
	<10 minutes	0
Diabetes	Yes	1
0-3: low risk	**4-6: Moderate Risk**	**6-9: High Risk**

0 - 3	1%	Hospital observation may be unnecessary without another indication (e.g. new AF)
4 - 5	4.1%	Hospital admission justified in most situations
6 - 7	8.1%	Hospital admission recommended

- Patients with a **score of 4 or more** should receive:
  o Immediate aspirin (300mg),
  o Specialist assessment **within 24 hours of symptom onset** and Secondary prevention as soon as the diagnosis is confirmed.
- **Low-risk patients** should receive the same care **but within 7 days of symptom onset.**
- Other **high-risk patients** are:
  o Those with new onset atrial fibrillation (AF)
  o Patients already on warfarin.
  o Those who have had more than one TIA in a week.

MANAGEMENT
- The following should be done urgently in patients with TIA[513] :
  o Evaluation
  o Risk stratification (eg, with the ABCD score [)
  o Initiation of stroke prevention therapy
- Soluble Aspirin 300mg stat, then 75mg od (give PPI if h/o dyspepsia).
- Only use Clopidogrel in cases of aspirin hypersensitivity or severe dyspepsia from aspirin not resolved by PPI
- Urgent Referral to TIA clinic

- Consider admission if crescendo TIAs (>1 in 7 days), fluctuating neurological symptoms/signs, if there is significant headache or the patient is on anticoagulants.
- For patients with a recent (≤1 week) TIA, guidelines recommend a timely hospital referral with hospitalization for the following:
  o Crescendo TIAs
  o Duration of symptoms longer than 1 hour
  o Symptomatic internal carotid stenosis greater than 50%
  o Known cardiac source of embolus (eg, atrial fibrillation)
  o Known hypercoagulable state
  o Appropriate combination of the California score or ABCD score (category 4)

DISPOSAL
- Low risk: refer to local TIA service
- Moderate and high risk: immediate access to the available thrombolytic therapy

DRIVING ADVICE
- All patients suffering a TIA who are group 1 licensed drivers should be advised that current (as of August 2015) Driver and Vehicle Licensing Authority (DVLA) regulations state they would not be allowed to drive for 1 month following a TIA.
- Currently group 2 license holders are required to notify the DVLA and their license is revoked for 1 year. You should always check the DVLA regulations to provide the most up to date information for the patient (www.dvla.gov.uk).

NICE (1) state that[514] :
- *Do not offer CT brain scanning to people with a suspected TIA unless there is clinical suspicion of an alternative diagnosis that CT could detect*
- *After specialist assessment in the TIA clinic, consider MRI (including diffusionweighted and blood-sensitive sequences) to determine the territory of ischaemia, or to detect haemorrhage or alternative pathologies. If MRI is done, perform it on the same day as the assessment.*

---

513 White H, Boden-Albala B, Wang C, Elkind MS, Rundek T, Wright CB, et al. Ischemic stroke subtype incidence among whites, blacks, and Hispanics: the Northern Manhattan Study. Circulation. 2005 Mar 15. 111(10):1327-31. [Medline].

514 NICE (May 2019). Stroke and transient ischaemic attack in over 16s: diagnosis and initial management [NICE NG128]

II. ISCHEMIC STROKES

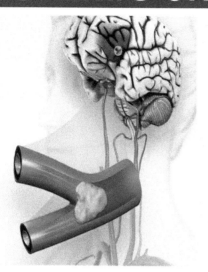

INTRODUCTION

- Ischemic stroke is characterized by the sudden loss of blood circulation to an area of the brain, resulting in a corresponding loss of neurologic function.
- Acute ischemic stroke is caused by thrombotic or embolic occlusion of a cerebral artery and is more common than hemorrhagic stroke.
- Approximately **85%** of strokes are caused by occlusion of one of the arteries supplying the brain (**ischemic stroke**) and approximately **15%** are caused by non-traumatic intracerebral haemorrhage (ICH).
- **Circulation Territories:** Refer to TIA

CLINICAL ASSESSMENT AND RISK STRATIFICATION

1. FAST SCORE

- This is a tool to raise the awareness of a possible stroke - recognising the signs of stroke or mini-stroke and calling ambulanace service is crucial[515].
- The quicker a patient arrives at a specialist stroke unit, the quicker they will receive appropriate treatment and the more likely they are to make a better recovery.
- The FAST test is outlined below.
  - **Facial weakness:** Can the person smile? Has their face fallen on one side?
  - **Arm weakness:** Can the person raise both arms and keep them there?
  - **Speech problems:** Can the person speak clearly and understand what you say? Is their speech slurred?
  - **Time:** If you see any one of these three signs, it's TIME to call the local emergency number.

---

515 *FAST tool for stroke and TIA, [GP Notebook]*

2. ROSIER SCORE

Rule Out Stroke In the Emergency Room[516]

Clinical history	Yes	No
• Loss of consciousness	-1	0
• Convulsive fit	-1	0
Neuro signs: Score +1 for each "FALS V"	**Yes**	**No**
• **F**ace weakness	1	0
• **A**rm weakness	1	0
• **L**eg weakness	1	0
• **S**peech disturbance	1	0
• **V**isual field defect	1	0

- If score > 0 (stroke is likely)
- If score </= 0 (stroke is unlikely but not completely excluded!)

INVESTIGATIONS

- The stages in the investigation of a stroke include:
  - Confirmation of the diagnosis
  - Establishing the site of the primary pathology
  - Identifying factors which may influence management

- NICE NG128[517] state that:
  - brain imaging should be performed immediately (ideally the next slot and definitely within 1 hour, whichever is sooner) for people with acute stroke if any of the following apply:
    - indications for thrombolysis or early anticoagulation treatment
    - on anticoagulant treatment
    - a known bleeding tendency
    - a depressed level of consciousness (Glasgow Coma Score below 13)
    - unexplained progressive or fluctuating symptoms
    - papilloedema, neck stiffness or fever
    - severe headache at onset of stroke symptom
  - for all people with acute stroke without indications for immediate brain imaging, scanning should be performed as soon as possible (within a maximum of 24 hours after onset of symptoms)
  - If thrombectomy might be indicated, perform imaging with CT contrast angiography following initial non-enhanced CT. Add CT perfusion imaging (or MR equivalent) if thrombectomy might be indicated beyond 6 hours of symptom onset.

---

516 *Pandora Spilman-Henham, Lightning Learning: ROSIER Score [EM3 nline]*

517 *NICE (May 2019). Stroke and transient ischaemic attack in over 16s: diagnosis and initial management [NICE NG128]*

o People with intracerebral haemorrhage should be monitored by specialists in neurosurgical or stroke care for deterioration in function and referred immediately for brain imaging when necessary.

3. OTHER TESTS

All patients		Selected patients:
o FBC	o ESR	• Toxicology screen
o U&E	o ECG	• Pregnancy test
o Lipid profile	o CXR	• LFTs
o Clotting profile		

ACLS SUSPECTED STROKE ALGORITHM

- Using the Suspected Stroke Algorithm for Managing Acute Ischemic Stroke. The ACLS Suspected Stroke Algorithm[518] emphasizes critical actions for out-of-hospital and in-hospital care and treatment.

National Institute of Neurological Disorders and Stroke Critical Time Goals
- Included in the algorithm are critical time goals set by the National Institute of Neurological Disorders (NINDS) for in-hospital assessment and management.
- These time goals are based on findings from large studies of stroke victims:
- Immediate general assessment by a stoke team, emergency physician, or other expert **within 10 minutes of arrival**, including the order for an urgent CT scan
- Neurologic assessment by stroke team and CT scan performed **within 25 minutes of arrival**
- Interpretation of CT scan **within 45 minutes of ED arrival**
- Initiation of fibrinolytic therapy, if appropriate, **within 1 hour of hospital arrival and 3 hours from onset of symptoms**.
- **rTpa** can be administered in "well screened" patients who are at low risk for bleeding for **up to 4.5 hours**.
- **Door-to-admission time of 3 hours in all patients**

TIME BENCHMARKS FOR POTENTIAL THROMBOLYSIS
o Door to CT scan completion: **25 minutes**
o Door to CT scan interpretation: **45 minutes**
o Door to treatment: **60 minutes**

GENERAL ASSESSMENT IN THE ED
NINDS time goal: 10 min
- Within 10 minutes of the patient's arrival in the ED, take the following actions:
  1. Assess ABC and evaluate vital signs.
  2. Give oxygen if patient is hypoxemic (less than 94% saturation).

3. Consider oxygen if patient is not hypoxemic.
4. Make sure that an IV has been established.
   a. Take blood samples for blood count, coagulation studies, and blood glucose.
   b. Check the patient's blood glucose and treat if indicated. Give dextrose if the patient is hypoglycemic. Give insulin if the patient's serum glucose is more than 300.
   c. Give thiamine if the patient is an alcoholic or malnourished.
5. Obtain a 12-lead ECG and assess for arrhythmias.
6. Assess the patient using a neurological screening assessment, such as the NIH Stroke Scale (NIHSS).
7. Order a CT brain scan without contrast and have it read quickly by a qualified specialist.
8. Refer to neurologist or stroke team

❖ *Do not delay the CT scan to obtain the ECG.*
❖ *The ECG is taken to identify a recent or ongoing acute MI or arrhythmia (such as atrial fibrillation) as a cause of embolic stroke.*
❖ *Life-threatening arrhythmias can happen with or follow a stroke.*

Early CT scan
- Ideally **within 1-hour ED arrival**, if any of indications for lysis or early anticoagulation:
o On warfarin;
o Known bleeding tendency;
o Depressed GCS <13;
o Unexplained progressive or fluctuating symptoms;
o Suspected meningitis;
o Severe headache at onset.
Otherwise **within 24 hours** (see later).

- **Antiplatelet treatment**:
  o **Aspirin 300 mg orally** (or via NGT / PR) **early and then daily** if stroke is non-haemorrhagic on CT or for TIA, ideally within first 24 hours. Continue for at least 2 weeks.
  o Addition of **dipyridamole 200 mg po bd** for TIAs and minor ischaemic stroke preferred, but note more side effects including headache!

THROMBOLYSIS:
o **The indications for considering thrombolysis are:**
  ▪ Aged ≥16 years with symptoms of acute stroke
  ▪ Clear time of onset
  ▪ Onset within last 4.5 hours*
  ▪ Measurable deficit on NIHSS
  ▪ Absence of haemorrhage or stroke mimic on baseline CT

---

518 *ACL training centre, ACLS Suspected Stroke Algorithm [Online]*

* proceed with caution between 3-4.5h window if age >80y, NIHSS>25 and/or early infarct change >one third of the MCA territory

- o **The recommended medication is:**
  - ▪ The recommended dose of **Alteplase** is 0.9 mg/kg (not to exceed 90 mg total dose), with 10% of the total dose administered as an initial intravenous bolus over 1 minute and the remainder infused over 60 minutes[519].

CONTRA-INDICATIONS FOR THROMBOLYSIS OF ACUTE ISCHAEMIC STROKE

- **Absolute Contra-indications include:**
  - o Systolic BP>185 and/or diastolic BP >110
  - o Symptoms and signs suggestive of a subarachnoid haemorrhage
  - o Any evidence of active bleeding
  - o History of any intracranial haemorrhage
  - o Arterial puncture at non-compressible site within 7 days
  - o Recent lumbar puncture within last 7 days
  - o Known or strongly suspected bacterial endocarditis
  - o Known or confirmed aortic dissection if suspected
  - o Major head trauma; brain or spinal surgery within last 3 months
  - o Platelet count <100 x10^9/l if high-level of clinical suspicion
  - o Heparin or NOAC∞ within last 48 hours; or INR >1.7 on warfarin

∞ direct thrombin inhibitors (e.g. dabigatran) or factor Xa inhibitors (e.g. rivaroxaban)

- **Relative Contra-indications include:**
  - o Pregnancy
  - o Stroke within last 3 months
  - o Major surgery or non-head trauma within last 2 weeks
  - o Brain tumour, cerebral aneurysm or AVM#
  - o Gastro-intestinal, urinary or gynaecological haemorrhage within last 21 days

\# may consider if underlying CNS lesions at low-risk of bleeding such as small unruptured aneurysms (

COMPLICATION

- The major complication of IV tPA is intracranial hemorrhage.

519 Alteplase, indication and usage FDA document page 3 [Online]

MANAGING HYPERTENSION IN tpa CANDIDATES

- For patients who are candidates for fibrinolytic therapy, you need to control their blood pressure to lower their risk of intracerebral hemorrhage following administration of tPA. See the general guidelines below.

NOT ELIGIBLE FOR FIBRINOLYTIC THERAPY

Blood pressure level, mm Hg	Treatment
Systolic ≤220 or Diastolic ≤120	**Observe patient** unless there is other end-organ involvement. **Treat the patient's other symptoms** of stroke (headache, pain, nausea, etc). Treat other acute complications of stroke, including hypoxia, increased intracranial pressure, seizures, or hypoglycemia.
Systolic > 220 or Diastolic 121 - 140	**Labetalol** 10 to 20 mg IV for 1-2 min—may repeat or double every 10 min to a maximum dose of 300 mg or **Nicardipine** 5 mg/hr IV infusion as initial dose; titrate to desired effect by increasing 2.5 mg/hr every 5 min to max of 15 mg/hr **Aim for a 10% to 15% reduction in blood pressure**
Diastolic > 140	**Nitroprusside** 0.5 µg/kg per min IV infusion as initial dose with continuous blood pressure monitoring. **Aim for a 10% to 15% reduction in blood pressure.**

STROKE PATIENTS ELIGIBLE FOR A FIBRINOLYTIC

PRETREATMENT	
SBP > 185 or DBP > 110	**Labetalol** 10 to 20 mg IV for 1-2 min—may repeat 1 time or nitropaste 1-2 inches
During or after TREATMENT	
Monitor blood pressure	**Check blood pressure** every 15 min for 2 hrs, then every 30 min for 6 hrs, and finally every hr for 16 hrs
Diastolic > 140	**Sodium nitroprusside** 0.5 µg/kg per minute IV infusion as initial dose and titrate to desired blood pressure
SBP > 230 or DBP 121 to 140	**Labetalol** 10 mg IV for 1-2 min—may repeat or double every 10 min to maximum dose of 300 mg or give initial labetalol dose and then start labetalol drip at 2 to 8 mg/min OR nicardipine 5 mg/hr IV infusion as initial dose and titrate to desired effect by increasing 2.5 mg/hr every 5 min to maximum of 15 mg/hr; if blood pressure is not controlled by nicardipine, consider sodium nitroprusside
SBP180 to 230 or DBP 105 to 120	**Labetalol** 10 mg IV for 1-2 min—may repeat or double every 10 to 20 min to a maximum dose of 300 mg or give initial labetalol dose, then start labetalol drip at 2 to 8 mg/min

III. FACIAL NERVE PALSY

1. BELL'S PALSY
INTRODUCTION

- Bell's palsy is an idiopathic, acute peripheral-nerve palsy involving the facial nerve, which supplies all the muscles of facial expression.
- The facial nerve also contains parasympathetic fibers to the lacrimal and salivary glands, as well as limited sensory fibers supplying taste to the anterior two thirds of the tongue[520]. The facial nerve also contains parasympathetic fibers to the lacrimal and salivary glands, as well as limited sensory fibers supplying taste to the anterior two thirds of the tongue
- The cause of Bell's palsy has long been debated but only recently has evidence started to accumulate for a viral origin. **Reactivation of latent herpes simplex or zoster virus**[521] is the most likely scenario. Left untreated, 85 percent of patients will show at least partial recovery within three weeks of onset

COMMON SEQUELAE OF BELL'S PALSY

o Irreversible damage to the facial nerve
o Abnormal regrowth of nerve fibers, resulting in involuntary contraction of certain muscles when trying to move others (synkinesis)
o Hearing loss
o Residual partial facial weakness
o Blindness of the affected eye due to excessive dryness and scratching of the cornea
o Loss of taste functions of the tongue (Ageusia)
o Crocodile tears syndrome: Spontaneous tearing in parallel with the normal salivation of eating.

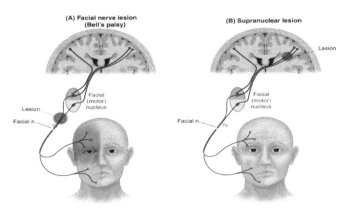

CLINICAL ASSESSMENT

- Patients with Bell's palsy typically complain of:
  o Weakness or complete paralysis of all the muscles on one side of the face.
  o The facial creases and nasolabial fold disappear,
  o The forehead unfurrows,
  o The corner of the mouth droops.
  o The eyelids will not close and the lower lid sags; on attempted closure, the eye rolls upward (Bell's phenomenon).
  o Eye irritation often results from lack of lubrication and constant exposure.
  o Tear production decreases; however, the eye may appear to tear excessively because of loss of lid control, which allows tears to spill freely from the eye.
  o Food and saliva can pool in the affected side of the mouth and may spill out from the corner.
  o Patients often complain of a feeling of numbness from the paralysis, but facial sensation is preserved.
- Patients with Bell's palsy usually progress from onset of symptoms to maximal weakness within three days and almost always within one week. A more insidious onset or progression over more than two weeks should prompt reconsideration of the diagnosis.

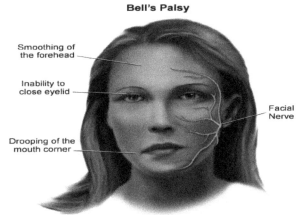

BELL'S PALSY VS STROKE

- **Differentiating Facial Weakness Caused by Bell's Palsy vs. Acute Stroke**[522]:
  o Ask yourself two questions when assessing a patient with an acute facial weakness:
    - Is the palsy an upper or lower motor neurone lesion?
    - Is the weakness a Bell's palsy another cause?

[520] Jeffrey D. Tiemstra, Nandini Khatkhat, Bell's Palsy: Diagnosis and Management [Online]

[521] Schirm J, Mulkens PS. Bell's palsy and herpes simplex virus. APMIS. 1997 Nov. 105(11):815-23.

[522] Michael T. Mullen, Caitlin Loomis , Differentiating Facial Weakness Caused by Bell's Palsy vs. Acute Stroke, JEMS, Issue 5 and Volume 39. [Online]

1. Is this an upper or lower motor neurone lesion?

1. Talk to the patient.

- Ask the patient when they first noticed the weakness and how quickly it developed.
- Although both Bell's palsy and acute stroke cause "acute" facial weakness, ischemic stroke is much more acute in onset, reaching maximum severity within seconds to minutes.
- Bell's palsy reaches maximum severity within hours to a few days. Patients often don't know the exact time of onset, but family members, co-workers, or other witnesses may have more information.
- It's crucial to determine the time they were last seen normal when assessing onset, rather than the time they first noticed the deficit.

2. Perform a brief neurologic exam.

- You want to determine if the facial weakness is caused by a peripheral or central lesion.
- **Mouth:**
  - **First, Look at the nasolabial fold**—the wrinkle between the corner of their nose and the corner of their mouth. Facial weakness or drooping can obscure this wrinkle, as the face is pulled down by gravity.
  - **Next, have the patient smile.** If the facial palsy is severe, they'll be unable to lift the side of their mouth. If the patient is able to smile symmetrically but has flattening of the nasolabial fold, this is still a sign of mild facial weakness. Mouth weakness will be present in both central and peripheral facial palsies.
- **Eyes:**
  - **First, inspect the eyes at rest.** Look at the palpebral fissure—the space between the eyelids—to determine if one eye is opened more widely than the other. This may be a subtle sign of eye closure weakness.
  - **Next, ask the patient to close their eyes tightly.** Normally, patients should be able to squeeze their eyes so tightly that the eyelashes are no longer visible. Asymmetry in eyelid closure is a sign of peripheral facial nerve palsy.
- **Forehead:**
  - Have the patient wrinkle their forehead, as if they're surprised.
    - In a central lesion, the forehead should lift symmetrically, due to bilateral cortical innervation of the frontalis muscle. However, in a peripheral lesion, the patient will be unable to wrinkle their forehead on one side, or have fewer wrinkles on that side.
    - Asymmetry in forehead wrinkles is a sign of peripheral facial nerve palsy.

3. Look for associated signs/symptoms.

- Key signs to look for include the following:
  - Weakness or numbness in the arm or leg
  - Slurred speech (dysarthria)
  - Double vision (diplopia)
  - Facial numbness
  - Difficulty swallowing (dysphagia)
  - Incoordination (ataxia
  - Vertigo
- *If the patient has any of these features present on exam, it's most likely a stroke, as the territory involved includes more than just the facial nerve. If the patient has a peripheral pattern of weakness and nothing else, it's most likely Bell's palsy.*

Patient A *shows a flattened nasolabial fold and inability to smile on the affected side with sparing of the forehead and eye closure muscles and resulting in a partial paralysis of the face which is caused by a **Stroke**.*

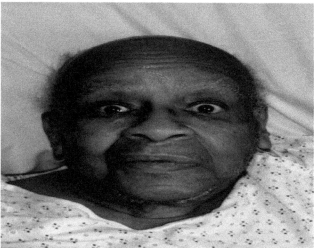

Patient B *shows flattening of the nasolabial fold, widened palpebral fissure, and absence of forehead winkles on the right. This lesion is what causes **Bell's palsy**.*

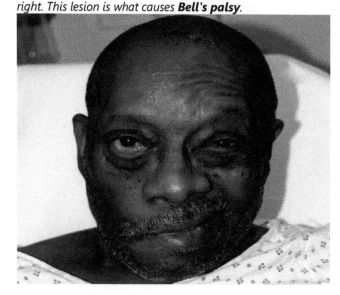

2. Is the weakness a Bell's palsy or another cause?

- Many conditions can produce isolated facial nerve palsy identical to Bell's palsy:
    o Cholesteatoma,
    o Salivary tumors
    o Guillain-Barré syndrome,
    o Lyme disease,
    o Otitis media,
    o Diabetes
    o Ramsay Hunt syndrome
    o Sarcoidosis,
    o HIV

INVESTIGATIONS

- Laboratory testing is not usually indicated. However, because diabetes mellitus is present in more than 10 percent of patients with Bell's palsy, fasting glucose or A1C testing may be performed in patients with additional risk factors (e.g., family history, obesity, older than 30 years) [523].

HOUSE-BRACKMANN CLASSIFICATION[524]

- *Grade I - Normal*
    o *Normal facial function in all areas*
- *Grade II - Slight Dysfunction*
    o *Gross: slight weakness noticeable on close inspection; may have very slight synkinesis*
    o *At rest: normal symmetry and tone*
    o *Motion: forehead - moderate to good function; eye - complete closure with minimum effort; mouth - slight asymmetry.*
- *Grade III - Moderate Dysfunction*
    o *Gross: obvious but not disfiguring difference between two sides; noticeable but not severe synkinesis, contracture, and/or hemi-facial spasm.*
    o *At rest: normal symmetry and tone*
    o *Motion: forehead - slight to moderate movement; eye - complete closure with effort; mouth - slightly weak with maximum effort.*
- *Grade IV - Moderate Severe Dysfunction*
    o *Gross: obvious weakness and/or disfiguring asymmetry*
    o *At rest: normal symmetry and tone*
    o *Motion: forehead - none; eye - incomplete closure; mouth - asymmetric with maximum effort.*
- *Grade V - Severe Dysfunction*
    o *Gross: only barely perceptible motion*
    o *At rest: asymmetry*
    o *Motion: forehead - none; eye - incomplete closure; mouth - slight movement*
- *Grade VI - Total Paralysis*
    o *No movement*

[523] *Jeffrey D. Tiemstra, Nandini Khatkhat, Bell's Palsy: Diagnosis and Management [Online]*

[524] *House, J.W., Brackmann, D.E. Facial nerve grading system. Otolaryngol. Head Neck Surg, [93] 146–147. 1985.*

ED MANAGEMENT OF BELL'S PALSY

- **Treatment directed at the facial nerve**
    o Prednisone is typically prescribed in a 10-day tapering course starting at 50-60 mg OD x10 days.
    o Antiviral drugs: The antiviral drugs used in trials were aciclovir (400 mg five times daily for five days) or valaciclovir (1000 mg/day for five days). There is currently no evidence to support the use of either antiviral drug on its own, and there is uncertainty regarding the benefit of adding them to corticosteroids.

- **Treatment of the consequences of facial muscle weakness.**
    o The incomplete closure of the eyelid may lead to exposure keratitis and corneal ulcers:
        - Topical ocular lubrication (with artificial tears during the day and lubricating ophthalmic ointment at night, or occasionally ointment day and night) is sufficient to prevent the complications of corneal exposure.
        - Occluding the eyelids by using tape or by applying a patch for 1 or 2 days may help to heal corneal erosions.
        - Ophthalmology referral.
    o Physical therapies including tailored facial exercises, acupuncture to affected muscles, massage, thermotherapy and electrical stimulation have been used to hasten recovery. However, there is no evidence for any significant benefit.

2. RAMSAY HUNT SYNDROME

- Ramsay Hunt described a syndromic occurrence of facial paralysis, herpetiform vesicular eruptions, and vestibulocochlear dysfunction[525]. It is believed to be caused by the reactivation of herpes zoster virus.
- Patients presenting with Ramsay Hunt syndrome generally have a greater risk of hearing loss than do patients with Bell palsy, and the course of disease is more painful. Moreover, a lower recovery rate is observed in these patients. Ramsay Hunt syndrome is commonly accompanied by associated symptoms such as **hearing loss and vestibular disturbance due** to involvement of structures adjacent to the facial nerve.
- Medical treatment is equivalent to that for Bell palsy; most often, a combination of steroids and antiviral agents is used[526]: Prednisolone 60mg once daily for 10 days and acyclovir 800mg five times a day for 7 days.

[525] *Hunt JR. On herpetiform inflammation of the geniculate ganglion: A new syndrome and its complications. Nerve Ment Dis. 1907. 34:73.*

[526] *Niparko JK. The acute facial palsies. Jackler RK, ed. Neurotology. St. Louis: Mosby; 1994. 1311.*

IV. GUILLAIN-BARRE SYNDROME

INTRODUCTION

- Guillain-Barré syndrome (GBS) can be described as a collection of clinical syndromes that manifests as an acute inflammatory polyradiculoneuropathy with resultant weakness and diminished reflexes.
- Although the classic description of GBS is that of a demyelinating neuropathy with ascending weakness, many clinical variants have been well documented in the medical literature.

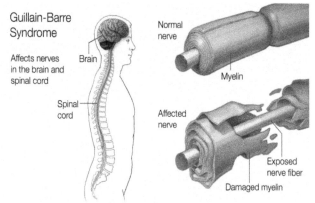

Guillain-Barre Syndrome
Affects nerves in the brain and spinal cord
Brain
Spinal cord
Normal nerve
Myelin
Affected nerve
Exposed nerve fiber
Damaged myelin

SIGNS AND SYMPTOMS

- The typical patient with GBS, which in most cases will manifest as acute inflammatory demyelinating polyradiculoneuropathy (AIDP), presents 2-4 weeks following a relatively benign respiratory or gastrointestinal illness with complaints of finger dysesthesias and proximal muscle weakness of the lower extremities.
- The weakness may progress over hours to days to involve the arms, truncal muscles, cranial nerves, and muscles of respiration.
- **Common complaints associated with cranial nerve involvement in GBS include the following:**
  - Facial droop (may mimic Bell palsy)
  - Diplopias
  - Dysarthria
  - Dysphagia
  - Ophthalmoplegia
  - Pupillary disturbances
- Most patients complain of paresthesias, numbness, or similar sensory changes. Paresthesias generally begin in the toes and fingertips, progressing upward but generally not extending beyond the wrists or ankles.
- Pain associated with GBS is most severe in the shoulder girdle, back, buttocks, and thighs and may occur with even the slightest movements. The pain is often described as aching or throbbing in nature.

- **Autonomic changes in GBS can include the following:**
  - Tachycardia
  - Bradycardia
  - Facial flushing
  - Paroxysmal hypertension
  - Orthostatic hypotension
  - Anhidrosis and/or diaphoresis
  - Urinary retention
- **Typical respiratory complaints in GBS include the following:**
  - Dyspnea on exertion
  - Shortness of breath
  - Difficulty swallowing
  - Slurred speech
- Ventilatory failure with required respiratory support occurs in up to one third of patients at some time during the course of their disease.

Features make the diagnosis of GBS doubtful:

- Sensory level (decrement or loss of sensation below a spinal cord root level as determined by neurologic examination).
- Marked, persistent asymmetry of weakness
- Bowel and bladder dysfunction at onset
- Severe and persistent bowel and bladder dysfunction
- Severe pulmonary dysfunction with little or no limb weakness at onset
- Severe sensory signs with little or no weakness at onset
- Fever at onset
- CSF pleocytosis with a WCC >50/mm³

ETIOLOGY

- EBVGuillain-Barre syndrome may be triggered by:
  - Most commonly, infection with **campylobacter,** a type of bacteria often found in undercooked poultry
  - Influenza virus
  - Cytomegalovirus
  - Epstein-Barr virus
  - Hepatitis A, B, C and E
  - Zika virus
  - HIV, the virus that causes AIDS
  - Mycoplasma pneumonia
  - Surgery
  - Trauma
  - Hodgkin's lymphoma
  - Influenza vaccinations or childhood vaccinations
  - COVID-19

COVID-19 & GBS

- *Evidence exists that coronavirus disease 2019 (COVID-19) is linked to the development of neurologic complications, including GBS[527].*
- *By April 20, 2020, one case of GBS in a patient with COVID-19 had been reported out of China and five such cases had been reported out of Italy. A report on the Italian cases said that GBS developed 5-10 days after COVID-19 had been diagnosed, with three of the patients having the demyelinating form of GBS, and the other two appearing to have an axonal variant.*

DIFFERENTIAL DIAGNOSIS

- Acute Life-threatening Causes of Weakness:
  - Myasthenia gravis
  - Guillain-Barre Syndrome
  - Botulism
  - Adrenal insufficiency/hypermagnesemia
  - Organophosphate poisoning
  - Carbon monoxide poisoning
  - Hypokalemia
  - Cerebrovascular accident
  - Seizure
  - Spinal cord compression
  - Encephalopathy
  - Sepsis
  - Intubation/RSI pearls

Guillain-Barré Syndrome

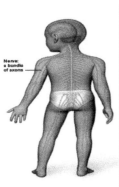
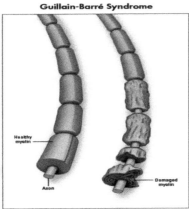

INVESTIGATION STRATEGIES

- LFTs, FBC, U&E, CRP, ESR, CPK, Glucose, CMP
- Lumbar puncture (LP)
- Stool culture: testing for C jejuni and others
- Serology
- Spinal MRI
- Chest x-ray
- Spirometry
- Nerve conduction studies
- Antiganglioside antibody

- HIV antibodies
- Borrelia burgdorferi serology
- CSF PCR, CSF cytology, CSF angiotensin-converting enzyme
- CSF VDRL, CSF West Nile PCR

MANAGEMENT
General measures

- The first priority in any patient arriving to the Emergency department should focus on ABCs and a quick review of life threatening causes of weakness.
- Weakness of the respiratory muscles can cause patients with GBS to require artificial ventilation in up to 25% of patients. Regular monitor of vital capacity: Lunf function every 4 hours
- Electrocardiogram and BP monitoring
- Early intubation is recommended for patients for airway protection
- Analgesia
- Consider DVT prophylaxis
- Eye care
- Meticulous nursing to avoid pressure sores
- Physiotherapy referral to prevent contractures
- Other potential indications would be inability to lift head or shoulders, inability cough, rapid onset of symptoms.
- Regarding RSI: succinylcholine should be avoided due to significant risk of hyperkalemia, which results due to the upregulation of muscle acetylcholine receptors.
- ICU admission for more severe patients

Medication Considerations

- Plasma exchange (PE) vs immunoglobulin (IVIG) therapy are the mainstay therapy and are more efficacious when started during the first 2 weeks of symptoms:
- IVIG (or rarely PE)- for those unable to walk, ideally to start within 4 weeks or onset of symptoms.
- IVIG: **0.4g/Kg for 5 days**
- PE: **total exchange of 5 plasma volumes in 4 weeks**
- If secondary deterioration Consider further doses of IVIG.

INTENSIVE CARE UNIT

- Admission to the intensive care unit (ICU) should be considered for all patients with labile dysautonomia, a forced vital capacity of less than 20 mL/kg, or severe bulbar palsy[528]. Any patients exhibiting clinical signs of respiratory compromise to any degree also should be admitted to an ICU[529].

[527] McNamara D. More Evidence Supports COVID-19/Guillain-Barre Link. Medscape Medical News. 2020 Apr 20.

[528] Walgaard C, Lingsma HF, Ruts L, Drenthen J, van Koningsveld R, Garssen MJ, et al. Prediction of respiratory insufficiency in Guillain-Barré syndrome. Ann Neurol. 2010 Jun. 67(6):781-7.

[529] Hughes RA, Rees JH. Clinical and epidemiologic features of Guillain-Barré syndrome. J Infect Dis. 1997 Dec. 176 Suppl 2:S92-8.

V. ACUTE DYSTONIC REACTIONS

DEFINITION

- Drug-induced acute dystonic reactions are a common presentation to the emergency department.
- They occur in 0.5% to 1% of patients given metoclopramide or prochlorperazine[530].
- Up to 33% of acutely psychotic patients will have some sort of drug-induced movement disorder within the first few days of treatment with a typical antipsychotic drug.
- Younger men are at higher risk of acute extra pyramidal symptoms.
- Although there are case reports of oculogyric crises from other classes of drugs, including H_2 antagonists, erythromycin and antihistamines, the majority of patients will have received an antiemetic or an antipsychotic drug.

RISK FACTORS

- Suggested risk factors for acute dystonic reactions include:
  - Male gender
  - Young age (children are particularly susceptible)
  - A previous episode of acute dystonia
  - Higher potency D2 receptor antagonists used in high doses
  - Family history of dystonia
  - Recent cocaine use

PATHOPHYSIOLOGY

- Acute dystonic reactions result from an imbalance of dopaminergic and cholinergic neurotransmission.
- The dominant mechanism n acute dystonia is thought to be nigrostriatal dopamine D2 receptor blockade, which leads to an excess of striatal cholinergic output.
- High potency D2 receptor antagonists, such as the butyrophenone haloperidol, are most likely to produce acute dystonic reactions.
- Higher dosages are often linked to acute dystonic reactions, but the relationship is unpredictable and reactions are generally idiosyncratic.

AETIOLOGY

- **Medications can cause this condition?**
  - **Antipyschotics** are the most important cause of acute dystonic reactions – all currently available antipsychotics (e.g. phenothiazines, butyrophenones and newer atypical agents) have the potential to cause acute dystonic reactions.
  - Acute dystonic reactions can also be caused by drugs other than antipsychotics. They include:
  - **Antiemetics** – e.g. metaclopramide, proclorperazine
  - **Antidepressants and serotonin receptor agonists** – e.g. SSRIs, buspirone, sumitriptan
  - **Antibiotics** – e.g. erythromycin
  - **Antimalarials** – e.g. chloroquine
  - **Anticonvulsants** – e.g. carbamazepine, vigabatrin
  - **H2 receptor antagonists** – e.g. ranitadine, cimetidine
  - **Recreational drugs** – e.g. cocaine

CLINICAL ASSESSMENT

Oculogyric crisis	• Spasm of the extraorbital muscles, causing upwards and outwards deviation of the eyes Blephorospasm
Torticollis	• Head held turned to one side
Opisthotonus	• Painful forced extension of the neck. • When severe the back is involved and the patient arches off the bed.
Macroglossia	• The tongue does not swell, but it protrudes and feels swollen
Buccolingual crisis	May be accompanied by: • Trismus, • Risus sardonicus, • Dysarthria • Grimacing • Dysphagia • Grimacing • Tongue protrusion or sensation of the tongue feeling swollen
Laryngospasm	• Uncommon but frightening, presents as **stridor**
Spasticity	• Trunk muscles and less commonly limbs can be affected

---

[530] *Bateman DN, Darling WM, Boys R, Rawlins MD. Extrapyramidal reactions to metoclopramide and prochlorperazine. QJM 1989;71:307-11.*

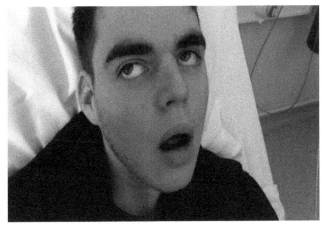

Oculogyric Crisis

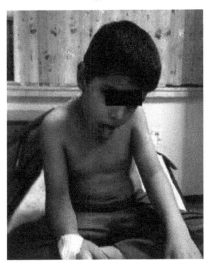

Bucolingual Crisis

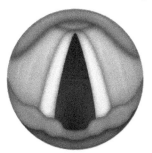 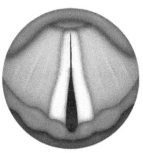

NORMAL VOCAL CORDS   LARYNGOSPASM

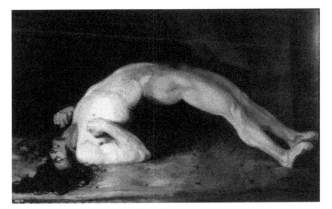

Opisthotonos

CONSEQUENCES OF ACUTE DYSTONIC EPISODES

Finally, patients may present with the consequences of acute dystonic episodes such as:

- Chipped teeth
- Temporomandibular joint (TMJ) dislocation
- Tongue lacerations
- Respiratory distress secondary to pharyngeal muscle involvement

DIFFERENTIAL DIAGNOSIS

The differential diagnosis for acute dystonias includes:

- Many conditions may resemble the different types of acute dystonic reaction. They include:
- **Neurological:**
  - Status epilepticus
  - Stroke
  - Stiff Man Syndrome
  - Other movement disorders
- **Toxicological:**
  - Strychnine
  - Serotonin toxicity
  - Anticholinergic syndrome
  - Other drug-induced movement disorders
- **Infectious:**
  - Meningitis
  - Tetanus
  - Oropharyngeal infections
- **Metabolic:**
  - Hypocalcaemia
  - Hypomagnesaemia
  - Metabolic or respiratory alkalosis
- **Psychiatric:**
  - Conversion disorder
  - Hyperventilation due to anxiety (carpopedal spasm)
- **Drug seeking behaviour:** there are reports of patients who misuse anticholinergics and present to the ED feigning a dystonic reaction to obtain their drug of abuse

INVESTIGATION STRATEGIES

- The diagnosis of acute dystonic reaction is a clinical one based on characteristic signs and symptoms in combination with of ingestion of above mentioned drugs. The diagnosis is confirmed by a rapid resolution of symptoms in response to treatment given.
- If there is any doubt, it is reasonable to treat as an acute dystonic reaction in the first instance, and investigate further if there is no response.

ED MANAGEMENT
Resuscitation:
- Attend to ABCs.
- On rare occasions acute dystonic reactions may be life-threatening:
  - Airway compromise e.g. Laryngeal dysphonia
  - Respiratory compromise e.g. Chest wall rigidity.
  - Administer oxygen, obtain iv access and assist ventilation as required.
- Treat with centrally acting anticholinergic: **Procyclidine 5-10mg IV bolus repeated in 20minutes** (max. dose 20mg)
- Dramatic resolution of symptoms occurs within 5 minutes and complete resolution usually within 15 minutes.
- **Diazepam 5-10mg IV bolus** repeated at regular intervals may help in cases of dystonic reactions not amenable to adequate doses of anticholinergic medication.
- If symptoms are not settling with the above standard treatment, other diagnoses should be considered.

- Diazepam may also be effective in such cases but has side effects of drowsiness and respiratory depression.
- Warn patients not to drive or perform tasks that require full alertness whilst on sedative medications.
- Patients can be discharge home when symptoms have resolved.
- Consider admitting patients that experienced airway or respiratory compromise to an observation ward for 24-48 hours.
- Advise the patient to return if they have a recurrence and to avoid taking the offending medication in the future.
- Patients requiring ongoing antipyschotic treatment may require long-term anticholinergic treatment (e.g. benztropine) to prevent symptoms, or an alternative antipsychotic agent (e.g. a newer atypical agent) may be tried.

Acute ystonic reaction | Curtesy life in the fast lane

DISPOSITION
- There are no criteria for admission and patients can be discharged once symptoms have settled[531].
- Advice patient that symptoms may recur with continued usage of the offending medication.
- This may be treated with procyclidine 5mg PO tds.

---

531 Nabil El Hindy, Dr Íomhar O' Sullivan. Acute Dystonic Reactions [Emed Website]

Further Reading
- Bateman DN, Darling WM, Boys R, Rawlins MD. Extrapyramidal reactions to metoclopramide and prochlorperazine. QJM 1989;71:307-11.
- Fauci AS, Braunwald E, Isselbacher KJ, Wilson JD, Martin JB, Kasper DL, et al. Harrison's Principles of Internal Medicine. 14th ed. New York: McGraw-Hill; 1998. p. 2361.
- Shy K, Rund DA. Psychotropic Medications. In Tintinalli JE, Ruiz E, Krome RL, editors. Emergency Medicine: A comprehensive study guide. 4th ed. New York: McGraw-Hill; 1996.
- Hope RA, Longmore JM, McManus SK, Wood-Allum CA. Oxford Handbook of Clinical Medicine. 4th ed. Oxford: Oxford University Press; 1998. p. 428.

VI. MYASTHENIA GRAVIS IN THE ED

OVERVIEW

- Myasthenia gravis is a potentially serious but treatable organ specific autoimmune disorder characterised by weakness and fatigability of the voluntary muscles that is caused by autoantibodies against the nicotinic acetylcholine receptor (AChR) on the postsynaptic membrane at the neuromuscular junction[532].
- A reduction in the number of ACh receptors results in a characteristic pattern of progressively reduced muscle strength with repeated use of the muscle and recovery of muscle strength following a period of rest.
- **The bulbar muscles** are affected most commonly and most severely, but most patients also develop some degree of fluctuating generalized weakness.

ETIOLOGY

- The most common cause of myasthenic crisis often is **infection,** although idiopathic causes are also common.
- Many other factors influence cholinergic transmission, including **drugs, temperature, and emotional state**.
- There are four classes based on the aetiology:
  - Acquired autoimmune.
  - Transient neonatal caused by the passive transfer of maternal anti-AChR antibodies
  - Drug induced: D-penicillamine is the prototype of drug induced myasthenia gravis. Clinical presentation may be identical to typical acquired autoimmune myasthenia gravis and the antibody to AChR may be found[533]. Disease tends to remit after cessation of the drug. Other drugs that can cause myasthenia-like weakness or that exacerbate weakness of myasthenia gravis include curare, aminoglycosides, quinine, procainamide, and calcium channel blockers.
  - Congenital myasthenic syndromes (AChR deficiency, slow channel syndrome, and fast channel syndrome) are distinct heritable disorders of postsynaptic neuromuscular transmission with characteristic age of onset, pathology, electrophysiology, and treatment.

PATIENT HISTORY

- Most patients who present to the ED have an established diagnosis of myasthenia gravis and are already taking appropriate medications. The activity of the disease fluctuates, and adjustments in medication dosages must be made accordingly.

- Noncompliance with medications, infection, and other physiologic stressors may result in a fulminant **exacerbation of the disease**.
- Thyroid disorders may be seen in as many as 10% of patients with myasthenia gravis, and symptoms of hyperthyroidism or hypothyroidism may be present.
- Rarely does a patient present with undiagnosed myasthenia gravis. However, if this situation does occur, typical complaints are of generalized weakness and reduced exercise tolerance that improves with rest.
- Patients with myasthenia gravis do not present with primary complaints of sleepiness or muscle pain.
- The patient may also complain of a specific weakness of certain muscle groups (eg, those used when climbing stairs). The distribution of muscle weakness follows a characteristic pattern; initially 85% of patients have involvement of the eyelids and extraocular muscles, resulting in **ptosis and/or diplopia.**
- The involvement of the facial muscles results in changes in expression and speech, whereas involvement of the pharyngeal muscles results in progressive difficulty with mastication and deglutition. In 15-20% of patients, myasthenia gravis affects the bulbar muscles alone. The other patients progress to generalized myasthenia gravis. Neck and proximal limb weakness may occur.
- Respiratory failure occurs in 1% of patients.

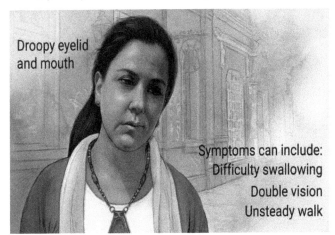

Droopy eyelid and mouth

Symptoms can include:
Difficulty swallowing
Double vision
Unsteady walk

PHYSICAL EXAMINATION
1. SEVERE EXACERBATIONS

- Severe exacerbations of myasthenia gravis may present dramatically and should be considered a true neurological emergency.
- **Findings can include the following:**
  - Facial muscles may be slack, and the face may be expressionless

532 ***Drachman D*** . *Myasthenia gravis.* In: Rose N, Mackay I, eds. *The autoimmune diseases.* 3rd Ed. San Diego: Academic Press, 1998:637–62

533 ***Penn AS***, *Low BW, Jaffe JL, et al. Drug-induced autoimmune myasthenia gravis. Ann N Y Acad Sci* 1998; **841**:433–49.

- The patient may be unable to support his or her head, which will fall onto the chest while the patient is seated
- Jaw is slack
- Voice has a nasal quality
- Body is limp
- Gag reflex is often absent, and such patients are at risk for aspiration of oral secretions.
- Respiratory distress
- The patient's ability to generate adequate ventilation and to clear bronchial secretions is of utmost concern with severe exacerbations of myasthenia gravis.
- Inability to cough leads to an accumulation of secretions; therefore, rales, rhonchi, and wheezes may be auscultated locally or diffusely.
- The patient may have evidence of pneumonia (ie, fever, cough, dyspnea, consolidation).
- The patient may appear anxious, with rapid and shallow breathing. Paradoxical chest movements due to diaphragmatic weakness may be present.

2. CHOLINERGIC CRISIS

- One of the confusing factors in treating patients with myasthenia gravis is that **insufficient medication (ie, myasthenic crisis)** and **excessive medication (ie, cholinergic crisis)** can present in similar ways.
- **Cholinergic crisis** results from an excess of cholinesterase inhibitors (ie, neostigmine, pyridostigmine, physostigmine) and resembles organophosphate poisoning. In this case, excessive ACh stimulation of striated muscle at nicotinic junctions produces **flaccid muscle paralysis** that is clinically indistinguishable from weakness due to myasthenia gravis.
- Despite muscle weakness, **deep tendon reflexes are preserved.**
- Both myasthenic crisis and cholinergic crisis may cause bronchospasm with wheezing, Bronchorrhoea, respiratory failure, diaphoresis, and cyanosis.
- **Miosis and the SLUDGE syndrome** (ie, salivation, lacrimation, urinary incontinence, diarrhea, gastrointestinal [GI] upset and hypermotility, emesis) also may mark cholinergic crisis. However, these findings are not inevitably present.

IMAGING TESTS

- **Chest radiography**: aspiration or other pneumonias,
- **CT scanning and MRI:** in detecting thymomas. E
- **Tensilon (Edrophonium) Challenge Test:** in distinguishing myasthenic crisis from cholinergic crisis, due to its rapid onset and short duration of action.

- **Ice Pack Test:** In a patient with myasthenia gravis who has ptosis, placing ice over an eyelid will lead to cooling of the lid, which leads to improvement of the ptosis. Lightly placing ice that is in a surgical glove or that is wrapped in a towel over the eyelid will cool it within 2 minutes. A positive test is clear resolution of the ptosis.
- **Additional Testing:** not available in ED
  - Standard electromyography,
  - Single-fiber electromyography,
  - Repetitive nerve stimulation,
  - Assays for ACh receptor antibody [ARA])
- **Patients with respiratory distress should have:**
  - Pulse oximetry,
  - ABG
  - Pulmonary function tests: peak expiratory flow, forced expiratory volume in 1 second [FEV1])

ED MANAGEMENT OF MYASTHENIA GRAVIS

- Patients with myasthenia gravis who are in respiratory distress may be experiencing a myasthenic crisis or a cholinergic crisis. Before these possibilities can be differentiated, ensuring **adequate ventilation and oxygenation** is important.
- Patients with myasthenic crisis can develop apnea very suddenly, and they must be observed closely.
- Evidence of respiratory failure may be noted through ABG determination, pulmonary function tests, or pulse oximetry.

1. Airway maneuvers

- Open the airway by suctioning secretions after positioning the jaw and tongue.
- Administer high-flow oxygen, and measure oxygen saturation by pulse oximetry.
- If respirations remain inadequate, ventilate by bag-valve mask while preparing to intubate.
- In the patient without an intact gag reflex, an oral airway may be placed.

2. Endotracheal intubation

- Rapid sequence intubation should be modified, because depolarizing paralytic agents (eg, **succinylcholine**) have less predictable results in patients with myasthenia gravis.
- **The relative lack of ACh receptors** makes these patients relatively **resistant to succinylcholine**; therefore, **higher doses must be used** to induce paralysis. Once paralysis is achieved, it may be prolonged.
- A rapid-onset, nondepolarizing agent (ie, **rocuronium, vecuronium**) is the preferred paralytic agent for these patients.

- Although nondepolarizing agents delay the onset of paralysis, compared with succinylcholine, these medications do not result in unwanted prolonged paralysis. Following paralysis, intubation is accomplished as usual. ABG sampling guides ventilator settings.

INVESTIGATION AND TREATMENT

- Once the airway is secured, investigation into the cause of the exacerbation of myasthenia gravis may proceed, with the most common reason for an exacerbation being **infection**, followed by **inadequate treatment with cholinesterase inhibitors**. However, up to 30% of patients will not have an identified cause of their exacerbation. Differentiation from cholinergic crisis can proceed as described above.
- In less severely ill patients, **oral pyridostigmine** can be administered until clinical improvement is seen. The patient should be closely observed and monitored during this trial.
- Other reasons for the exacerbation can then be investigated. Although patients with myasthenia gravis can develop any common infection that can result in decompensation, the most likely source of infection is pulmonary.
- **Cultures of blood, sputum**, and **urine** may be indicated on an individual basis.
- **Chest radiography** is important in detecting pneumonia.
- Appropriate **broad-spectrum antibiotics** are indicated for sepsis and pneumonia.
- It is important to consider that fluoroquinolones and antibiotics may adversely affect cholinergic transmission in patients with myasthenia gravis, and these antibiotics should be avoided if possible.
- Patients with myasthenia gravis are sensitive to high temperatures (core or ambient), and their muscle strength can improve when temperature is lowered with **cooling measures or antipyretics.**

INPATIENT CARE

- Patients who present to the ED with myasthenic or cholinergic crisis will often require admission to an intensive care unit; while patients with increasing muscle weakness of a less severe degree require admission to a monitored setting, because their course is unpredictable.
- Patients with complications of the disease or treatment are admitted to a level of care corresponding to the nature and severity of the complication.
- Patients with pneumonia should be admitted because they often are taking immunosuppressant medications and are at a high risk for aspiration pneumonia.

PLASMAPHERESIS

- It has been found to be an effective short-term treatment of acute exacerbations of myasthenia gravis.
- Plasmapheresis removes circulating antibodies, including the autoimmune antibodies responsible for the disease.
- Clinical improvement takes several days to occur and lasts up to 3 weeks.
- The factors predicting better clinical response are severe myasthenia gravis, absence of thymoma, early onset myasthenia gravis, and higher removal rate for IgG[534].
- Because of the delayed onset of beneficial effects, plasmapheresis has limited utility in the ED setting, but often is used in the ICU setting.

IMMUNOTHERAPY

- With **intravenous gamma globulin (IVIG)** appears to diminish the activity of the disease for unknown reasons.
- The benefit begins within 2 weeks and may last for several months. Approximately 65% of patients with myasthenia gravis respond to intravenous gamma globulin.

THYMECTOMY

- Thymectomy as a treatment of myasthenia gravis (in the absence of thymoma) has been the practice for several years. The young age and the absence of thymoma have been shown to predict a better response in some studies, though age did not have any effect on the response in a recent study[535].
- The need for anticholinesterase medication fluctuates significantly in the postoperative period but overall is less than it was prior to thymectomy.

TRANSFER, CONSULTATIONS, MONITORING

- Patients with severe exacerbations of myasthenia gravis or cholinergic crisis should be transferred **only after they have been stabilized** and the airway has been secured. Persistent hypoxemia, hypercarbia, dysrhythmias, or unstable vital signs make transfer unwise, unless appropriate care cannot be delivered at the original facility.
- Emergent consultation with a neurologist is indicated.
- Patients with severe exacerbations requiring intubation and mechanical ventilation are managed in an intensive care setting with appropriate consultation.
- With regard to patient monitoring, all patients with myasthenia gravis should be referred to a neurologist for ongoing care.

534 *Chiu HC*, Chen WH, Yeh JH. *The six-year experience of plasmapheresis in patients with myasthenia gravis. Therapeutic Apheresis 2000;**4**:291–5*

535 *Abt PL*, Patel HJ, Marsh A, et al. *Analysis of thymectomy for myasthenia gravis in older patients: a 20-year single institution experience. J Am Coll Surg 2001;**192**:459–64.*

VII. MULTIPLE SCLEROSIS IN THE ED

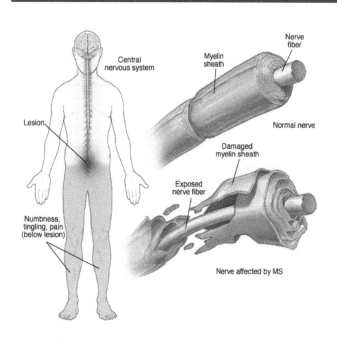

Multiple sclerosis (MS) is an immune-mediated inflammatory disease that attacks myelinated axons in the central nervous system, destroying the myelin and the axon in variable degrees and producing significant physical disability within 20-25 years in more than 30% of patients. The hallmark of MS is symptomatic episodes that occur months or years apart and affect different anatomic locations.

SIGNS AND SYMPTOMS

Classic MS signs and symptoms are as follows:

- Sensory loss (ie, paresthesias): Usually an early complaint
- Spinal cord symptoms (motor): Muscle cramping secondary to spasticity
- Spinal cord symptoms (autonomic): Bladder, bowel, and sexual dysfunction
- Cerebellar symptoms: Charcot triad of dysarthria (scanning speech), nystagmus, and intention tremor
- Optic neuritis
- Trigeminal neuralgia: Bilateral facial weakness or trigeminal neuralgia
- Facial myokymia (irregular twitching of the facial muscles): May also be a presenting symptom
- Eye symptoms: Including diplopia on lateral gaze (33% of patients)
- Heat intolerance
- Constitutional symptoms: Especially fatigue (70% of cases) and dizziness

- Pain: Occurs in 30-50% of patients at some point in their illness
- Subjective cognitive difficulties: With regard to attention span, concentration, memory, and judgment
- Depression: A common symptom
- Euphoria: Less common than depression
- Bipolar disorder or frank dementia: May be a late finding but is sometimes found at initial diagnosis
- Symptoms associated with partial acute transverse myelitis

DIAGNOSIS

MS is diagnosed on the basis of clinical findings and supporting evidence from ancillary tests.

Tests include the following:

- **MRI:** The imaging procedure of choice for confirming MS and monitoring disease progression in the CNS
- **Evoked potentials:** Used to identify subclinical lesions; results are not specific for MS
- **Lumbar puncture:** May be useful if MRI is unavailable or MRI findings are nondiagnostic; CSF is evaluated for **oligoclonal bands** and **intrathecal immunoglobulin G (IgG) production.**

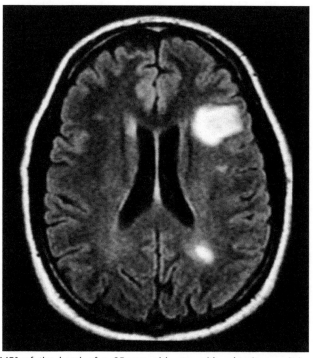

MRI of the head of a 35-year-old man with relapsing-remitting multiple sclerosis. MRI reveals multiple lesions with high T2 signal intensity and one large white matter lesion. These demyelinating lesions may sometimes mimic brain tumors because of the associated edema and inflammation.

CLASSIFICATION

MS is divided into the following categories, principally on the basis of clinical criteria, including the frequency of clinical relapses, time to disease progression, and lesion development on MRI[536]:

- Relapsing-Remitting MS (RRMS): Approximately 85% of cases
- Secondary progressive MS (SPMS)
- Primary progressive MS (PPMS)
- Progressive-relapsing MS (PRMS)

The following 2 subgroups are sometimes included in RRMS:

- **Clinically isolated syndrome (CIS):** A single episode of neurologic symptoms
- **Benign MS:** MS with almost complete remission between relapses and little if any accumulation of physical disability over time

EMERGENCY DEPARTMENT MANAGEMENT

Medical management goals that are sometimes achievable in the emergency department are to relieve symptoms and to ameliorate risk factors associated with an acute exacerbation. In patients with fulminant MS or disseminating acute encephalitis, management involves the following:

- Stabilize acute life-threatening conditions
- Initiate supportive care and seizure precautions
- Monitor for increasing intracranial pressure

Consider intravenous steroids, IV immunoglobulin (IVIG), or emergent plasmapheresis.
One study suggested that plasmapheresis may be superior to IV steroids in patients with acute fulminant MS[537].

Identification and control of known precipitants of MS exacerbation include the following:

- Aggressively treat infections with antibiotics
- In patients with a fever, normalize the body temperature with antipyretics, as even small increases in temperature can strongly affect conduction through partially demyelinated fibers
- Provide urinary drainage and skin care, as appropriate

Preoperative considerations for emergency surgery in patients with fulminant MS are as follows:

- Gastric emptying may be delayed secondary to autonomic GI dysfunction
- Lability of the autonomic nervous system may precipitate hypotension during anesthesia and surgery
- Spontaneous ventilation may be disrupted

Treatment of MS has 2 aspects: immunomodulatory therapy (IMT) for the underlying immune disorder and therapies to relieve or modify symptoms.

Treatment of acute relapses is as follows:

- **Methylprednisolone** can hasten recovery from an acute exacerbation of MS
- **Plasma exchange (plasmapheresis)** can be used short term for severe attacks if steroids are contraindicated or ineffective.
- **Dexamethasone** is commonly used for acute transverse myelitis and acute disseminated encephalitis

The following Most of the disease-modifying agents for MS (DMAMS) have been approved for use only in relapsing forms of MS:

- Interferon beta-1a (Avonex, Rebif)
- Interferon beta-1b (Betaseron, Extavia)
- Peginterferon beta-1a (Plegridy)
- Glatiramer acetate (Copaxone)
- Natalizumab (Tysabri)
- Mitoxantrone
- Fingolimod (Gilenya)
- Teriflunomide (Aubagio)
- Dimethyl fumarate (Tecfidera)
- Alemtuzumab (Lemtrada)
- Daclizumab (Zinbryta)

A single-use autoinjector is also available for self-injection of interferon beta-1a (Rebif) in patients with relapsing forms of MS. The following agents are used for treatment of aggressive MS:

- **High-dose cyclophosphamide** (Cytoxan) has been used for induction therapy
- **Mitoxantrone** is approved for reducing neurologic disability and/or the frequency of clinical relapses in patients with SPMS, PRMS, or worsening RRMS

Treatment of the symptoms of MS involves both pharmacologic and nonpharmacologic measures. The following symptoms may be amenable to pharmacologic therapy:

- **Fatigue:** Off-label treatments include amantadine, methylphenidate, and fluoxetine.
- **Depression:** Selective serotonin reuptake inhibitors are preferred.
- **Spasticity:** Baclofen is effective in most cases
- **Pain:** Tricyclic antidepressants are first-line drugs for primary pain.
- **Sexual dysfunction:** Oral phosphodiesterase type 5 inhibitors (eg, sildenafil, tadalafil, vardenafil)
- **Optic neuritis:** Intravenous methylprednisolone may speed recovery.

536 Poser CM, Paty DW, Scheinberg L, et al. New diagnostic criteria for multiple sclerosis: guidelines for research protocols. Ann Neurol. 1983 Mar. 13(3):227-31.

537 Rodriguez M, Karnes WE, Bartleson JD, Pineda AA. Plasmapheresis in acute episodes of fulminant CNS inflammatory demyelination. Neurology. 1993 Jun. 43(6):1100-4.

VIII. TETANUS IN THE ED

OVERVIEW

- Potentially lethal condition characterised by muscular rigidity and spasms, caused by the tetanospasmin toxin produced by **Clostridium tetani,** that may lead to life-threatening respiratory failure and autonomic dysregulation in severe cases.
- Rare in the developed world, but accounts 1 million deaths worldwide per year.

TYPES

Tetanus may be categorized into 4 clinical types:
- Generalized tetanus
- Localized tetanus
- Cephalic tetanus
- Neonatal tetanus

CAUSE

- **Clostridium tetani**
  - Caused by toxin from *Clostridium tetani* -> able to survive in the environment as highly resistant spores
  - Anaerobic spore forming gram positive bacillus
  - Once in a suitable environment -> spores germinate -> bacteria multiply -> toxins released (**tetanospasmin and tetanolysin**)
  - **Tetanolysin** – This substance is a hemolysin with no recognized pathologic activity
  - **Tetanospasmin** – This toxin is responsible for the clinical manifestations of tetanus[538]; by weight, it is one of the most potent toxins known, with an estimated minimum lethal dose of 2.5 ng/kg body weight.

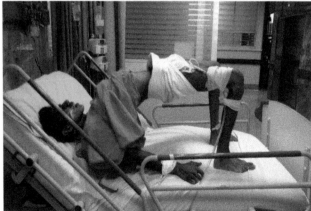
Opisthotonus | courtesy SciELO

CLINICAL FEATURES

- Clinical triad of **rigidity**, **muscle spasms** and, if severe, **autonomic dysfunction.**
  - Contaminated wound (may be trivial) or umbilical stump in neonates
  - **Incubation period:** 3-14d (1-60 at the extremes) = time to first symptom
  - **Onset time:** 1-7d = time from first symptom to first spasm
  - Rigidity (persists > 2 weeks)
    - Trismus, Dysphagia, Increased Tone In Trunk Muscles – Greater On Side Of Injury Initially
  - Spasms (reduce after 2 weeks)
    - Spontaneous or provoked by physical or emotional stimuli, laryngospasm, risus sardonicus, opisthotonos (severe spasm in which the back arches and the head bends back and heels flex toward the back)
  - **Autonomic disturbance** (onset after spasms, lasts 1-2 weeks)
    - Tachycardia and hypertension may alternate with bradycardia and hypotension, dysrhythmia, cardiac arrest.
    - Salivation, bronchial secretions
    - Gastric stasis, ileus, diarrhoea
  - **Respiratory compromise**
    - Chest wall rigidity
    - Laryngospasm
    - Aspiration
    - Retained secretions

DIFFERENTIAL DIAGNOSIS

- **Diagnosis of tetanus is made clinically**[539]:
  - Strychnine poisoning
  - Trismus due to orofacial infection
  - Stiff person syndrome
  - Acute dystonic reaction
  - Seizure disorder
  - Hypocalcemic tetany
  - Psychogenic
  - Meningism

- **Neonatal tetanus may resemble:**
  - Seizures
  - Meningitis
  - Sepsis

---

[538] *World Health Organization. WHO Technical Note: Current recommendations for treatment of tetanus during humanitarian emergencies. January 2010.*

[539] *Patrick B Hinfey, Tetanus Differential Diagnoses [Medscape Online]*

INVESTIGATIONS
- Urinary strychnine to exclude this as a cause
- CK, U&E, CMP for rhabdomyolysis and to rule out low Ca
- ABG (respiratory failure)

MANAGEMENT
- **RESUSCITATION**
  - **A** – intubate as requires large doses of sedatives to control muscle spasm and to overcome laryngospasm
  - **B** – at risk of aspiration and have copious bronchial secretions requiring frequent suctioning, often ventilated for **2-3 weeks** until spasms subside
  - **C** – autonomic dysfunction necessitate monitoring in a critical care environment, fluctuant haemodynamics so use **short acting agents; fluid loading.**
  - **D** – **benzodiazepines** in large doses (up to 100mg/h diazepam) -> non-depolarsing NMBD

- **SPECIFIC THERAPY**
  - **Metronidazole** (first choice); penicillin is used throughout most of the world but is a GABA antagonist
  - **Anti-tetanus immunoglobulin:** 100-300IU/kg of human Ig IM
  - **Benzodiazepines**; adjuncts include barbiturates, propofol, chlorpromazine
  - **Magnesium** to 2-4mmol/L as useful in spasm treatment and limits autonomic instability
  - Consider **dantrolene** (unproven)
  - Consider **intrathecal baclofen**

- **TREAT UNDERLYING CAUSE AND COMPLICATIONS**
  - **Clean and debride wounds** (source control)
  - **Immunize** (infection does not confer immunity) – Q10 yearly

- **Supportive care and monitoring – usual cares with emphasis on:**
  - Calm environment
  - Cardiac monitoring
  - Nutrition e.g. Enteral feeding
  - Often require tracheostomy
  - Prevention of pressure sores and GI stress ulcers

COMPLICATIONS
- **Respiratory**
  - Aspiration
  - Laryngospasm/obstruction
  - Sedative-associated obstruction
  - Respiratory apnoea
  - Type I (atelectasis, aspiration, pneumonia) and type II respiratory failure (laryngeal spasm, prolonged truncal spasm, excessive sedation)
  - ARDS
  - Complications of prolonged assisted ventilation (e.g. pneumonia)
  - Tracheostomy complications (e.g. tracheal stenosis)
- **Cardiovascular**
  - Tachycardia, hypertension, ischaemia
  - Hypotension, bradycardia, asystole
  - Dysrhythmias
  - Cardiac failure
- **Renal**
  - High output renal failure
  - Oliguric renal failure
  - Urinary stasis and infection
- **GI**
  - Gastric stasis
  - Ileus
  - Diarrhoea
  - Haemorrhage
- **Other**
  - Dehydration
  - Weight loss
  - Thromboembolus
  - Sepsis and multiple organ failure
- **Musculoskeletal**
  - Fractures of vertebrae during spasms
  - Tendon avulsions during spasms
  - Rhabdomyolysis

PROGNOSIS
- **Mortality**
  - Untreated: >50% (usually due to respiratory failure)
  - High level ICU care available: 10-25% (usually due to autonomic failure)
- **Survivors**
  - Severe cases usually require 3-5 weeks in ICU
  - Often make full recovery
- **INDICATORS OF POOR PROGNOSIS**
  1. Incubation of < 7 days
  2. Period of onset < 48 hours
  3. Portal of entry from umbilicus, uterus, burns, open fracture or IM injection
  4. Presence of spasms
  5. Temperature > 38.4
  6. HR > 120 (adults), > 150 (neonates)

IX. BOTULISM IN THE ED

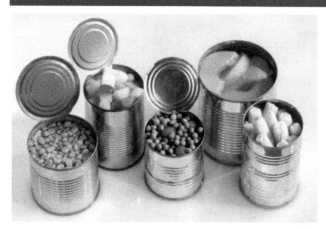

OVERVIEW

- Endotoxins from **Clostridium botulinum** (and other Clostridia) -> prevents the release of Ach -> neuroparalytic disorder
- Spore forming anaerobes with heat resistant spores
- Found in soil and marine sediment

TYPES

- Food-borne botulism
- Wound botulism
- Infant intestinal botulism
- Adult intestinal botulism
- Inhalational botulism
- Iatrogenic botulism

CLINICAL FEATURES

- Cranial neuropathies
- Descending paralysis
- Bilateral symptoms
- No fever
- Clear sensorium
- Lack of sensory findings

- **Food-borne**
  - Toxin absorbed from small intestine
  - Home-canned fruit and vegetable ingestion
  - Symptoms within 12-36 hrs
  - GI distress -> neuro symptoms
  - Parasympathetic dysfunction: dry mouth, blurred vision, dilated pupils, cardiovascular instability
  - Severity proportional to amount of endotoxin

- **Wound**
  - From *in vivo* toxin production in abscessed devitalised tissue
  - 7- day incubation period
  - No GI upset prodrome otherwise identical

- Physicians need to be alert to recognize botulism, especially in patients who use black-tar heroin or in those with a history of injection drug-associated botulism[540].

- **Infant intestinal**
  - Ingestion of spores -> colonise large intestine -> toxin production
  - 2-4 months of life
  - Constipation, poor feeding, lethargy -> acute tetraparesis and respiratory failure
  - Hypotonia
  - Head lag
  - Ptosis
  - Reduced facial expression
  - Reduced suck and swallow
  - Loss of reflexes
  - Slowly improves after weeks

- **Adult intestinal**
  - Adult intestinal toxemia results from enteric colonization with *C botulinum* that progresses to toxin production. The pathophysiology of the changes in the gastrointestinal flora that facilitate colonization is unclear[541].

- **Inhalational**
  - Bioweapon
  - Iatrogenic
  - Used to treat: dystonia, spasticity, cosmesis

INVESTIGATIONS

- Collect possible source + gastric, stool, serum samples
- Mouse toxicity and neutralisation assay
- **LP**: rule out GBS
- **Edrophonium test:** rule out MG
- **EMG:** normal nerve conduction, small motor response seen on repetitive nerve stimulation

MANAGEMENT

- Notify public health
- Antitoxin
- Supportive
- IV human botulism globulin
- Wound Botulism: Debride, Penicillin

---

540 Yuan J, Inami G, Mohle-Boetani J, Vugia DJ. Recurrent wound botulism among injection drug users in California. Clin Infect Dis. 2011 Apr 1. 52(7):862-6.

541 Centers for Disease Control and Prevention. Kinds of Botulism. CDC. Available at https://www.cdc.gov/botulism/definition.html. May 8, 2017;

INDEX

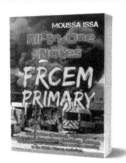 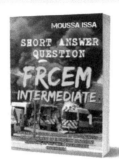 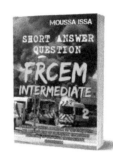
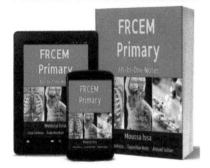 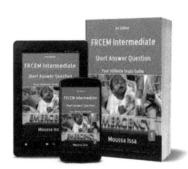 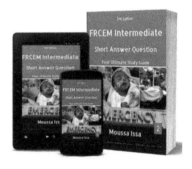
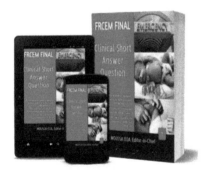 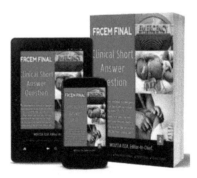 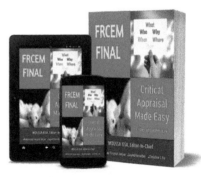
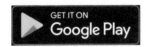
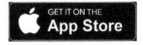

Lightning Source UK Ltd.
Milton Keynes UK
UKHW051557200221
378984UK00001B/2